SO-ALE-497

5A2950

Nursing Skills for Clinical Practice

THIRD EDITION

Edited by

BEVERLY J. RAMBO, R.N., M.A., M.N.

Assistant Professor of Nursing
Mount St. Mary's College
Los Angeles, California

and

LUCILE A. WOOD, R.N., M.S.

Director of Nursing
Bay Area Hospital
Coos Bay, Oregon;
formerly,
Associate Director of the Nursing Occupations
Allied Health Professions Project
University of California Extension, Los Angeles

Illustrations by Sharon Belkin
New revisions by Ruth Ann Barmettler

W. B. SAUNDERS COMPANY
Philadelphia □ London □ Toronto □ Mexico City □ Rio de Janeiro □ Sydney □ Tokyo

W. B. Saunders Company   West Washington Square
Philadelphia, PA 19105

1 St. Anne's Road
Eastbourne, East Sussex BN21 3UN, England

1 Goldthorne Avenue
Toronto, Ontario M8Z 5T9, Canada

Apartado 26370–Cedro 512
Mexico 4, D.F., Mexico

Rua Coronel Cabrita, 8
Sao Cristovao Caixa Postal 21176
Rio de Janeiro, Brazil

9 Waltham Street
Artarmon, N.S.W. 2064, Australia

Ichibancho, Central Bldg., 22-1 Ichibancho
Chiyodo-Ku, Tokyo 102, Japan

Library of Congress Cataloging in Publication Data

Nursing skills for clinical practice.

Third ed.: Nursing skills for allied health services/edited by
Beverly J. Rambo and Lucile A. Wood. 1977-1980.

Issued also in single volume.

Includes index.

1. Nursing. 2. Care of the sick. I. Rambo, Beverly J.
   II. Wood, Lucile A. III. Wood, Lucile A. Nursing
   skills for allied health services. Vols (1) & (2) 80-54857

RT41.N89 1982b   610.73   Single 81-5757

ISBN 0-7216-7458-5 – Single volume   AACR2

ISBN 0-7216-7456-9 – Volume 1

ISBN 0-7216-7457-7 – Volume 2

Nursing Skills for Clinical Practice   Volume 1 ISBN 0-7216-7456-9
                                              Volume 2 ISBN 0-7216-7457-7
                                         Single Volume ISBN 0-7216-7458-5

©1982 by the Regents of the University of California, Division of Vocational Education
Allied Health Profession Projects. Copyright 1972 and 1977 by the Regents of the Uni-
versity of California, Division of Vocational Education, Allied Health Profession Projects.
Copyright under the Uniform Copyright Convention. Simultaneously published in Canada.
All rights reserved. This book is protected by copyright. No part of it may be reproduced,
stored in a retrieval system, or transmitted in any form or by any means, electronic, mechanical photocopying, recording, or otherwise, without written permission from the publisher.
Made in the United States of America. Press of W. B. Saunders Company. Library of Congress catalog card number 80-54857.

Last digit is the print number: 9   8   7   6   5

FOREWORD

The Allied Health Professions Publications Program is part of University of California Extension, Education Extension, Los Angeles. It is an outgrowth of a research project, "Development and Validation of Instructional Programs for the Allied Health Occupations," supported by the U.S. Office of Education and conducted by the Division of Vocational Education, now also a part of University of California Extension. The research program generated curriculum materials such as occupational analyses and instructional manuals. These were sold to those who had use for them, and the Allied Health Professions Publications Program was set up to print and distribute some of the materials, and to work out publication agreements with private publishers for others, particularly the instructional manuals.

When the original research grant program ended, the Allied Health Professions Publications Program continued, supported entirely by earnings from sales of some publications and royalties on others. As earnings increased, new publications were undertaken, working with outside writers, illustrators, and editors on a contract basis. All of these publications are instructional manuals in various health-care fields, produced and distributed for the program by private publishers on a royalty basis.

This manual, *Nursing Skills for Clinical Practice*, is based on tasks validated by a nationwide study that produced the occupational analysis *A Study of the Nursing Occupations*. The analysis indicated what tasks workers in the nursing occupations did, and what they had to know to do them, the frequency with which they did them, and the criticality of both the tasks and their performance. The writers who prepared this manual described and illustrated how to perform each task, and explained the scientific and technical knowledge needed by the worker to perform the task. The educational philosophy exemplified in these materials is task-oriented instruction in which the emphasis is on helping the student learn to *perform* the tasks of the occupation and to *use* the basic scientific and technical knowledge related to them. This approach is designed to shorten the learning process so that the goal of "more learning in less time with greater retention" can be achieved. If these materials make a significant contribution toward accomplishing this goal, they will help solve the health manpower problems, and we will feel that the endless hours we have labored on the development of this manual were not in vain.

MILES H. ANDERSON, Ed.D., Director (Emeritus)
Allied Health Professions Publications
University Extension
University of California, Los Angeles

PREFACE

The Third Edition of *Nursing Skills for Clinical Practice* is a major revision that introduced a new look and title. From the time of their initial publication, Volumes 1 and 2 of *Nursing Skills* have been well received and used as basic texts to teach nursing skills in countless nursing programs, both in this country and abroad. They have been popular in programs teaching nursing assistants for entry into nursing, as well as students in programs leading to licensure as practical, vocational, or registered nurses. The books have been utilized in hospitals, nursing homes, and other health agencies as procedure manuals and have been translated into several foreign languages.

As before, the key concept of Volumes 1 and 2 involve the student's performance of the skill. In this revision, greater emphasis is placed on the recognition that these skills are not just motor but also psychomotor in nature. We all know that merely carrying out the steps of a procedure is not enough. Nursing activity requires communication with the patient; use of knowledge of normal and abnormal behavior, of attitudes, and of judgment; and other uses of the thought processes. This information has been extracted from the Key Points and is described in more detail in the content items preceding the skill. The depth of knowledge required varies according to the level of nursing, but even beginning students are expected to be able to (1) discern changes in patients that indicate problems in meeting their needs, (2) make use of the nursing process to solve these problems, (3) take appropriate action, and (4) use sound judgment when providing nursing care.

Each unit begins with behavioral objectives the student is expected to be able to perform and the introductory items that explain the conditions or reasons for performing the task or activity. The skill activity is divided into a logical and orderly sequence designated "Important Steps" and supported with practical information under the heading of "Key Points." Key Points include safety factors, related scientific principles, rationale, suggestions for communication or making this step easier to do, and pertinent ethical or legal concepts. A Performance Test follows the procedures in the Unit, and its satisfactory completion is crucial. The written Post-Test provides a test for understanding of the theoretical content underlying the purpose of the procedure, or the cognitive portion of the skill.

Another important change in this revision has been a focus on basic human needs as a unifying theme for the background information about patients and understanding the principles and rationale for carrying out the various procedures. This approach leads the student to focus not so much on the task as an end in itself, but on the patient's needs as a reason for carrying out the procedure. It provides a method of encouraging the beginning nurse to implement the nursing process. Content in the unit provides information about normal or expected values of measurement, how needs are met, and how to determine inadequacies leading to problems.

Many additional changes made in this revision of *Nursing Skills* were in response to comments made by those of you who have used the book. First, the books have been divided into sections of related skills. Each section includes a list of the units, an explanation of the section content, directions for the student, and selected references that provide a starting point for enrichment reading and study.

Section 1, on patient rights, has been expanded, and basic needs of individuals and the utilization of the Kardex nursing care plan have been added. The unit on charting and medical terminology has been rewritten with emphasis on what is charted and how. The subject of consents has become more complex, and guidelines are given for who may sign various types of consents or releases. Section 2 deals with skills related to movement and activities and includes directions for using the patient turning frames. Skills associated with the hygiene needs of the patient are in Section 3, while Section 4 deals with skills needed to help meet the other basic needs. The unit on cardiopulmonary resuscitation is included here, since it is a skill employed to provide for oxygen needs. Section 5 contains various units that contain procedures related to carrying out the medical therapy prescribed for the patient.

Duplication has been reduced by moving student directions to the Sections, setting off workbook questions to distinguish them from the rest of the content, listing the equipment and supplies under the heading of Items Needed for each procedure, and using the concept of Universal Steps. With few exceptions all of the procedures involving care of the patient contain a number of steps that are identical. These are described in Section 2 as the Universal Steps of washing the hands, collecting the items needed, approaching and identifying the patient, providing for privacy, and at the conclusion of the procedure providing for the patient's comfort, removing all used items, and recording the activity. These Universal Steps are listed in the first procedure of every unit, and in subsequent procedures the student is instructed to carry out these steps.

Most of the units contain a Post-Test and the questions are primarily matching or multiple choice. The questions relate to the theory presented in the Unit and test the student's ability to remember factual material, to understand relationships, analyze situations, and make nursing judgments.

The units permit students to move at their own pace through the background information on the subject and to familiarize themselves with the steps of the procedure. The instructor is released from the need to repeat instructions or information for each student and is therefore available to better help students polish their skills, expand their interest and understanding, and apply these skills in the clinical care of patients. With the emphasis on the performance of skills, we have found that students have less stress in the skill learning laboratory and develop positive attitudes about their nursing activities. They become involved "up to their elbows" in their own learning.

BEVERLY J. RAMBO

ACKNOWLEDGMENTS

I would like to thank all of the people who have been involved in the preparation of this revised edition and those who have made previous contributions to *Nursing Skills*. Foremost, I am grateful to Dr. Miles Anderson for his wholehearted support of the revisions. He allowed me freedom and time to proceed. He has served as a stabilizer in times of change and as a sounding board for new ideas. To Christine Ford, his able assistant, my thanks for her help with the manuscript and for handling many of the necessary details. I'm grateful to Katherine Pitcoff, Nursing Editor for W.B. Saunders Company, for her cooperation and support. She is a facilitator who has been open to suggestions and has an understanding of issues in the field of nursing. Special thanks go to Ruth Ann Barmettler, who prepared the new illustrations with so much sensitivity for the smallest detail.

Most of all, I am indebted to my colleagues who contributed so much of the original format and content of *Nursing Skills:* Lucile Wood, the former editor, who has been unable to continue owing to other professional demands; Inice Chirco, Chairman of Allied Health Department, Rio Hondo College; Adrienne Ardigo, Nursing Instructor, Los Angeles Trade Technical College; Jane Kahn, former Director of Nursing, Hollywood Presbyterian Medical Center; Bettie Rich, Chairman, Health Occupations, Mt. San Jacinto College; Frances Rogozen, Nursing Instructor, Los Angeles Trade Technical College.

Finally, I want to express my appreciation to the instructors and the students who have used the books and shared their comments and suggestions of ways in which the contents contributed to their nursing skills or could be improved to better meet their needs. It is my hope that these volumes continue to spark the interest and enthusiasm of students to gain more knowledge and skill to provide the highest quality of nursing care to their patients.

BEVERLY J. RAMBO

CONTENTS

pital Gown. Changing a Gown for Patient with an IV. Assisting the Patient with Robe and Slippers. Assisting with Pullover Garments. Assisting with Pants-Type Garments. Use of Diapers. Assisting with Elastic Stockings.

A.M. Care. P.M. Care, or H.S. Care. Mouth Care for the Conscious Patient. Mouth Care for the Unconscious Patient. Care of Dentures. The Back Rub. Types of Baths. Giving a Bed Bath. The Partial Bath. The Tub Bath. The Sitz Bath.

Skin Care for Incontinent Patients. Care of the Pressure Sore. Skin and Cast Care. Traction. Skin Care for the Patient with a Colostomy. Use of Permanent Stoma Bags. Care of Fingernails and Toenails.

Principles of Hair Care. Combing and Brushing Hair. Braiding Hair. Shampoo for the Bed Patient. Stretcher Shampoo.

Dealing with Patient Embarrassment. Perineal Care for the Female Patient. Patient Self-Care of the Perineum. Perineal Care for the Male Patient.

VOLUME 2

Section 4
SKILLS RELATED TO OTHER BASIC NEEDS   399

Body Temperature. Normal Body Temperature. Problems of Temperature Regulation. Types of Thermometers Used. Taking an Oral Temperature. Taking a Rectal Temperature. Taking an Axillary Temperature. The Arterial Pulse. Measuring the Radial Pulse. Taking the Apical Pulse. The Respirations. The Blood Pressure. Equipment Used for Measuring BP. Principles Related to Blood Pressure. Measuring the Blood Pressure. Charting Vital Signs.

Nutrition. Giving an Intermittent Tube Feeding. Wound Draining Tubes. Collection of the Sputum Specimen. Collection of a Gastric Specimen.

Unit 34

Principles Related to Heat and Cold. Important Considerations. Use of Disposable Hot and Cold Packs. The Aquathermia Pad (K-Pad). The Electric Heating Pad. The Hot Water Bottle. The Heat Cradle. The Ice Bag or Ice Collar. Full Body Hypothermia and Hyperthermia Treatment. Ultraviolet and Infrared Heat Treatments.

Unit 35

Purposes for Bandages and Binders. Types of Bandages. The Circular Bandage. The Figure-8 Bandage. The Spiral Bandage. The Spiral Reverse Bandage. The Recurrent Bandage. The Scultetus Binder. The Sling. The T-binder or a Double T-binder.

Unit 36

Spread of Infectious Diseases. Body Defenses Against Infections. Ways to Kill or Control Microorganisms. Comparison of Medical and Surgical Asepsis. Types of Medical Precautions. General Principles Regarding Isolation. Setting up an Isolation Unit. Putting on a Face Mask. Using an Isolation Gown. Putting on Gloves. Serving Diet Trays. Taking TPR and BP. Removal of Linens. Double-Bagging Technique. Collection of Specimens. Assisting a Patient to Sign a Document. Transporting a Patient Out of the Unit. Terminal Disinfection. Reverse Isolation Technique. Keeping Yourself Healthy.

Unit 37

Coping with Approaching Death. Caring for the Dying Patient. Religious Beliefs and Practices. Signs of Death. After Death Occurs. Postmortem Care.

Section 1

SKILLS NEEDED TO PREPARE
FOR DIRECT PATIENT CARE

INTRODUCTION

Nurses use a number of skills every day that do not involve direct care of the patient but are nevertheless important and necessary as a basis for such care. These skills require the nurse to use information about the physical setting of the hospital or nursing facility and the ways in which nursing services are provided to patients or work is managed.

The ethics that guide the behavior of the nurse and the laws and regulations that govern nursing practice are described in Units 1 and 2. Information is provided in Units 3 and 4 about the patient care units and factors that affect the comfort and safety of both the patients and other workers in the area. Unit 5 introduces the student to the principles of charting and to selected medical terms and abbreviations. Nurses are then required to make out a number of other records to document the care given to the patient, assign patients to a room, and record the movement of patients from one nursing unit to another. Units 6 and 7 discuss the procedures of admission, discharge, and transfer of patients, and the purposes and preparation of consents, releases, and incident reports. The handwashing procedure used by nurses is presented in Unit 8, and Unit 9 includes the skills involved in operating hospital beds and making the unoccupied, occupied, and anesthetic types of beds. Brief mention is made of orthopedic attachments that are often used on patients beds.

DIRECTIONS FOR THE STUDENT:

In the study of this section, you should read the objectives for each unit carefully, as these will tell you what you are expected to know or be able to perform. The vocabulary provides a list of words and medical terms that are pertinent to the material presented and will help you enlarge your knowledge of medical terminology. The nursing procedures are described in two sections: The important steps are listed in sequence, and the key points provide the rationale or scientific principles that are involved as well as information and helpful hints from actual practice. In the past, much of the practical information in the key points was passed on to the student verbally or "on the job"; sometimes such information, which contributes greatly to the "art" of nursing, was overlooked.

The essential part of each unit is the performance test. You are asked to demonstrate your ability to carry out the steps of the specified procedure correctly. This is the crucial element in learning nursing procedures and interventions — can you actually perform the task? In addition, nurses must know the principles and factual information about the nursing procedures in order to make decisions about the patient's care that are appropriate.

Post-tests at the end of most units are used to test your understanding of the rationale and principles underlying the steps of the procedure and the process involved, as well as your recall of factual material.

When you have completed your study of the unit, arrange with your instructor to take the performance test and to demonstrate your skill in carrying out the nursing procedures.

SELECTED REFERENCES

Unit 1: Ethics in the Healing Arts

Ethics. Special feature. Am J Nurs 77:845–876 (May) 1977.

Code for Nurses With Interpretive Statements. Kansas City, MO: American Nurses' Association, 1976.

Silva, Mary C.: Science, ethics, and nursing. Am J Nurs 74:2004–2007 (November) 1974.

Unit 2: The Nurse and the Law

American Hospital Association: Statement on a Patient's Bill of Rights. Chicago: American Hospital Association, 1972, pp 2–4.

Bandman, Elsie, and Bandman, Bertram: There is nothing automatic about rights. Am J Nurs 77:867–872 (May) 1977.

Creighton, Helen: Your legal risks in nursing coronary patients: How you can (and should) minimize them. Nursing 77 7:65–71) (January) 1977.

Helmet, Mary D., and Mackert, Mary E.: A nursing '79 handbook: Your legal guide to nursing practice. Part 1. Nursing 79 9:57–64 (October) 1979. Part 2. Nursing 79 9:57–64 (November) 1979. Part 3. Nursing 79 9:49–56 (December) 1979.

Lipman, Michael: Defamation: A rash comment could get you sued. RN 38:48–51 (February) 1975.

O'Sullivan, Ann L.: Privileged communication. Am J Nurs 80:947–950 (May) 1980.

Regan, William: How gossip backfires: The $12,000 tidbit. RN 42:65–66 (November) 1979.

Springer, Eric W. (ed.): Nursing and the Law. Pittsburgh: Aspen Systems Corp., 1970.

Symposium on current legal and professional problems. Nurs Clin North Am 9:391–586 (September) 1974.

Unit 5: Charting and Medical Terminology

Bloch, Doris: Some crucial terms in nursing: What do they really mean? Nurs Outlook 22:689–694 (November) 1974.

Blount, May, et al.: Documenting with the problem-oriented record system. Am J Nurs 78:1539–1542 (September) 1978.

Eggland, Ellen T.: Charting: Document your care daily and fully. Nursing 80 10:38–43 (February) 1980.

Frenay, Sister Agnes Clare: Understanding Medical Terminology. 5th ed. St. Louis, MO: Catholic Hospital Association, 1973.

Jones, Cathy: Glasgow Coma Scale. Am J Nurs 79:1551–1553 (September) 1979.

McCloskey, Joanne C.: The problem-oriented record vs the nursing care plan. Nurs Outlook 23:492–495 (August) 1975.

Rambo, Beverly: Ward Clerk Skills. New York: McGraw-Hill Book Co., 1978.

Weed, Lawrence L.: Medical Records, Medical Education, and Patient Care: The Problem-Oriented Record as a Basic Tool. Chicago: Year Book Medical Publishers Inc., 1971.

Wolff, LuVerne, Weitzel, Marlene, and Fuerst, Elinor: Fundamentals of Nursing. 6th ed. Philadelphia: J.B. Lippincott Co., 1979.

Unit 6: Admissions, Transfers, and Discharges

Anderson, Cynthia: Home or nursing home? Let the elderly patient decide. Am J Nurs 79:1448–1449 (August) 1979.

Connolly, Mary G., and Vlack, Jessie E.: When a nursing home is the best choice. Am J Nurs 79:1450–1451 (August) 1979.

Fanslow, Cathleen, and Masset, Evelyn: Building staff rapport between institutions. Am J Nurs 79:1441–1442 (August) 1979.

Rambo, Beverly: Ward Clerk Skills. New York: McGraw-Hill Book Co., 1978.

Smith, Jennifer, Buckalew, Judith, and Rosales, Suzanne: Coordinating a workable system. In Making the right moves in discharge planning. (Special feature.) Am J Nurs 79:1439–1440 (August) 1979.

Unit 7: Consents, Releases, and Incident Reports

Besch, Lina: Informed consent: A patient's right. Nurs Outlook 27:33 (January) 1979.

Brandman, Elsie, and Brandman, Bertram: There's nothing automatic about rights. Am J Nurs 77:867–872 (May) 1977.

California Hospital Association: Consent Manual. 19th ed. Sacramento, CA: California Hospital Association, 1978.

Carnegie, M. Elizabeth: The patient's bill of rights and the nurse. Nurs Clin North Am 9:557–562 (September) 1974.

Doll, Anne: What to do after an incident. Nursing 80 10:73–79 (January) 1980.

Etzioni, Amatai: The right to know, to decide, to consent and to donate. Nursing Dig October, 1974, pp 43–50.

Mancini, Marguerite: Nursing, minors, and the law. Am J Nurs 78:124–126 (January) 1978.

Murray, Malinda: Fundamentals of Nursing. 2nd ed. Englewood Cliffs, NJ: Prentice-Hall, Inc., 1980, pp 283–297.

Notter, Lucile: Protecting the rights of research subjects. Nurs Res 18:483 (November/December) 1969.

Quinn, Nancy, and Somers, Anne: The patient's bill of rights: A significant aspect of the consumer revolution. Nurs Outlook 22:242, 1974.

Unit 1

ETHICS IN
THE HEALING ARTS

GENERAL PERFORMANCE OBJECTIVE

You will demonstrate your understanding of the importance of ethics in the roles of the nurse and other health-related hospital workers. You will answer questions with 80 per cent accuracy or better to demonstrate understanding of ethical behavior in health service situations.

SPECIFIC PERFORMANCE OBJECTIVES

Upon completion of this unit you will be able to:

1. Define ethics.

2. State the differences between ethical behavior and legal requirements in nursing.

3. Discuss the statements contained in the Code of Ethics for Nurses and the Code of Ethics for the Licensed Practical Nurse.

4. Apply guidelines from codes of ethics in judging appropriate choices of action and behavior in six hypothetical health-related situations.

VOCABULARY

breach—breaking of a law or of any obligation, tie or contract.
conduct—one's actions in general; behavior.
custom—long-established practice; accepted behavior.
ethics—a code of conduct that represents ideal behavior for a particular group.
expire—to breathe one's last breath; to die.
hygiene—rules designed for the promotion of health; sanitary science.
hypothetical—involving a supposition for the purpose of reasoning; fictitious with a logical purpose.
overt—open; not hidden.
P.N. student—practical nursing student; when such students complete their course and become licensed, they are called LPN's, except in California and Texas where they are called LVN's (Licensed Vocational Nurse); all must be graduates of accredited practical nursing programs.
solvent—solution that dissolves a substance, converting it to a liquid.
unethical—not ethical; not representative of ideal behavior.
utilization—to make use of.
value systems—a pattern of conduct or set of behaviors or ideals that is accepted as worthwhile or meaningful.

INTRODUCTION

Nursing is a vital human service provided for and to people by another person, the nurse. It is a service based on trust that the nurse will do what is right, what is needed, and what will benefit the patients and their well-being. Because people behave in such diverse ways when interacting, guidelines have been formed to define how they should act, what is the proper behavior, and what their rights and responsibilities are. For example, there are implicit rules that govern the way people act in certain situations or roles; more explicit guidelines can be seen in national or local law, in religious tenets, and in the codes of ethics for the various professions.

Ethics represent judgments about actions and conduct that are deemed to be right, correct, or moral for a specific group. Many professions, including the law, medicine, and nursing, have devised statements of their beliefs about what constitutes ethical behavior by their members. Many ethical guidelines impose responsibilities or duties for the members that are more stringent than those legally required for other people. Members of professions have specialized knowledge or skills that they use to make decisions affecting other people, so the code of ethics is a method to prescribe the right and moral way to use this power.

ETHICS AND NURSING

ITEM 1. NURSING CODES OF ETHICS

Students in registered nursing programs generally study ethical issues in the senior year, just before graduation. They examine various issues that involve ethics and problems that nurses face in their clinical practice. Problems involving ethics seem to be more complex today, and the right or moral response to difficult questions seems less clear-cut. The questions that follow are examples:

Should any female be given an abortion upon demand or should there be limitations?

When does life begin — in the embryo, or in a fetus capable of living outside the womb?

Should medical research and experiments be carried out on humans?

When terminally-ill patients die, should efforts be made to revive them with CPR?

Should life-support systems be discontinued on terminally-ill patients, and if so, when?

Although these are serious issues of great interest to society and the professions, there are many other less complex issues you will encounter in your nursing practice that involve ethics and, more specifically, guidelines for behaving on the job. Examine the Code of Ethics for Licensed Practical Nurses. It is quite specific in some areas and can be used as a guide for behavior by students in various nonprofessional nursing programs as well. Registered nurses who supervise the activities of licensed nurses should be acquainted with this code of ethics and should note the ways in which it is similar to and different from the Code for Nurses.

CODE OF ETHICS FOR THE LICENSED PRACTICAL NURSE

The Licensed Practical Nurse shall:

1. Practice her profession with integrity.

2. Be loyal to the physician, to the patient, and to her employer.

3. Strive to know her limitations and to stay within the bounds of these limitations.

4. Be sincere in the performance of her duties and generous in rendering service.

5. Consider no duty too menial if it contributes to the welfare and comfort of her patient.

6. Accept only that monetary compensation which is provided for in the contract under which she is employed, and she does not solicit gifts.

7. Hold in confidence all information entrusted to her.

8. Be a good citizen.

9. Participate in and share responsibility of meeting health needs.

10. Faithfully carry out the orders of the physician or registered nurse under whom she serves.

11. Refrain from entering into conversation with the patient about personal experiences, personal problems, and personal ailments.

12. Abstain from administering self-medications, and in event of personal illness, take only those medications prescribed by a licensed physician.

13. Respect the dignity of the uniform by never wearing it in a public place.

14. Respect the religious beliefs of all patients.

15. Abide by the Golden Rule in her daily relationship with people in all walks of life.

16. Be a member of The National Federation of Licensed Practical Nurses, Inc., and the state and local membership associations.

17. Not identify herself with advertising, sales, or promotion of commercial products or service.

Adopted by The National Federation of
Licensed Practical Nurses

The Code for Nurses was adopted by the American Nurses' Association in 1950. It consists of 11 statements that are revised periodically. The statements are more general in nature and a number refer to the nurses' responsibility to remain competent in nursing, participate in bettering the conditions of employment, help inform the public, carry out further nursing research, and cooperate with others in handling health matters. Both codes mention handling personal information about the patient in a confidential manner.

CODE FOR NURSES*

1. The nurse provides services with respect for human dignity and the uniqueness of the client unrestricted by considerations of social or economic status, personal attributes, or the nature of health problems.

2. The nurse safeguards the client's right to privacy by judiciously protecting information of a confidential nature.

3. The nurse acts to safeguard the client and the public when health care and safety are affected by the incompetent, unethical, or illegal practice of any person.

4. The nurse assumes responsibility and accountability for individual nursing judgments and actions.

5. The nurse maintains competence in nursing.

---

*Code for Nurses With Interpretive Statements. Kansas City, MO: American Nurses' Association, 1976, p. 3. Reprinted with permission of ANA.

6. The nurse exercises informed judgment and uses individual competence and qualification as criteria in seeking consultation, accepting responsibilities, and delegating nursing activities to others.

7. The nurse participates in activities that contribute to the ongoing development of the profession's body of knowledge.

8. The nurse participates in the profession's efforts to implement and improve standards of nursing.

9. The nurse participates in the professional's efforts to establish and maintain conditions of employment conducive to high quality nursing care.

10. The nurse participates in the profession's effort to protect the public from misinformation and misrepresentation and to maintain the integrity of nursing.

11. The nurse collaborates with members of the health professions and other citizens in promoting community and national efforts to meet the health needs of the public.

ITEM 2. ETHICS IN EVERYDAY NURSING

Now let us take a look at ethics in the hospital setting as it relates to nurses and the various other health workers. The hospital employs many workers in a number of categories in order to provide smooth operation and uninterrupted service for the patients. All must observe some form of ethical behavior so that patients are not maltreated or taken advantage of because of their weakened conditions.

The following brief dramatic presentation illustrates the application of ethics in the hospital setting. You may find it more stimulating to have the parts read aloud by various members of your class.

The Setting: Orientation of new hospital employees.

List of Characters:

Miss Johnson	Instructor
Mrs. Sayre	New LPN
Miss Sands	Nursing Student
Miss McGuire	Nursing Student
Mrs. Deeds	Housekeeping Assistant
Mr. Thomas	Orderly
Mrs. Boyd	Nursing Assistant
Miss Boyne	Ward Clerk
Mrs. Acala	Diet Assistant
Mr. Troyle	Maintenance Man

MISS JOHNSON
Instructor

We're happy to have the nursing students from the Community College join our hospital orientation session for new employees. Technically, the students are not employees of our hospital, but they do have their clinical assignments here and are therefore part of the hospital team. Our topic for discussion today is Ethics in the Healing Arts.

MISS SANDS
Nursing Student

Miss Johnson, what does "ethics" mean?

MISS JOHNSON

It comes from a Greek word that means "custom." There are many definitions we could use, but let's try this one: "Ethics is a code of behavior that represents the ideal conduct for a particular group."

MISS McGUIRE
Nursing Student

Well, I expect to become a licensed practical nurse (LPN), so will my ethical conduct be different from yours as a registered nurse?

MISS JOHNSON	Each profession or vocation requiring a license in the health occupations has a written code of conduct that has been approved and adopted by its membership. These codes whether for the physician, registered nurse, licensed practical nurse, or other health group member, have many things in common. For example, (1) the rules are based on reason, good judgment, and an understanding of the difference between right and wrong behavior; (2) they strive to respect the dignity and rights of the individual patient.
MISS SANDS	I've noticed that I have a tendency to judge all nurses by the actions of the few I know.
MISS JOHNSON	That's a common reaction and one good reason for each member of a group to strive for ideal behavior. Ethical conduct by the individual members of the group presents the whole group in a favorable light to the public.
MRS. DEEDS *Housekeeper Assistant*	What do you mean by right and wrong? Maybe what is right for me is not right for you.
MISS JOHNSON	It is true that every person has his own "customs" and perhaps his own value system for what is right or wrong based upon his personal life experiences. However, by accepting employment in a hospital, the worker must accept the "ethics" or "customs" required by the employer.
MR. THOMAS *Orderly*	Why are ethics necessary? Couldn't the employer just give us a handbook of rules when we apply for a job?
MISS JOHNSON	Sometimes this is done, but through the ages societies and groups have established codes of conduct as a method of preventing friction between people, improving personal and group status, and encouraging growth and development in one's life. For example, Hippocrates, the Greek "Father of Medicine," proposed a code of conduct for physicians before the birth of Christ.
MRS. BOYD *Nursing Assistant*	I'd like to know how ethical conduct differs from my legal requirements as a hospital employee.
MISS JOHNSON	That is a point that needs careful explaining. Ethical conduct codes are written and adopted by the membership of the groups. Ideal behavior is encouraged through education, example, and discussion. It is to be hoped that enforcement is seldom needed. But sometimes a person whose conduct is highly unethical may be disciplined by the group or even lose his membership in the group. As one of you mentioned earlier, the group is judged by the behavior of its members, so an unethical member is expected to conform, or lose membership privileges. None of you is as yet a member of a professional group, but you are members of the hospital group and as such, unethical conduct that reflects upon the hospital could result in reprimand or expulsion from the hospital — that is, loss of employment.
MRS. SAYRE *New LPN*	Miss Johnson, could you explain this a little more and perhaps give us some examples of the difference between unethical and illegal conduct?

MISS JOHNSON   Ethics have to do with our moral responsibilities or behavior, as we said, and violation of an ethical concept means that we are not living up to ideal moral or ethical behavior. Legal requirements (laws) are set by the society as a whole, that is, by national, state, or local governments. Violation of these laws places the guilty person in trouble with the law enforcement agencies. For example, ethical conduct for a registered nurse or licensed practical nurse requires that the uniform and cap should not be worn in public places. A nurse who does so is unethical, but she has not violated any laws that will cause her to be arrested. However, if the nurse takes money from the wallet of an unconscious patient, she has violated the law, and the action could result in her arrest and punishment. She has, of course, also committed a serious breach of ethics by her lack of ideal conduct.

MR. THOMAS   I don't seem to fit in any group. I don't wear a cap, and I'm not an RN nor an LPN. Where do I get my ethical guidelines?

MISS JOHNSON   As an orderly giving direct patient care, you belong to the hospital group. And since you will be working under the direct supervision of the registered nurse and also with the licensed practical nurses, why don't you read the codes of ethics for these two groups?

Read the Code for Nurses and the Code of Ethics for the Licensed Practical Nurse again. When you have completed your study of these two codes, fill in the following blanks.

1. a. Ethics is a code of _____

    b. that represents _____ conduct

    c. for a particular _____ .

2. A violation of ethical behavior may result in discipline by _____ .

MISS JOHNSON   Now that you have read the codes of conduct for two groups of health workers, let's continue our conversation by writing a list of specific situations in which a hospital worker would have to make a choice in his or her behavior, based upon an ethical judgment. Mr. Thomas, can you name a principle or describe a situation that you have experienced along this line?

MR. THOMAS   Yes, I must give the best possible care to all patients regardless of financial status, religion, race, or creed.

MISS JOHNSON   Very good.

MR. THOMAS   And I must respect religious beliefs and try not to convert their/them to mine.

MRS. SAYRE   That certainly follows our basic guideline of respecting the dignity and basic rights of the individual.

MISS JOHNSON   Miss Boyne, how do you think that "ethics" affect your relationship with your employer?

MISS BOYNE
Ward Clerk

I guess I should report for work on time, and not leave early, and not take sick time off unless I'm really ill.

MRS. SAYRE

How about doing a day's work for a day's pay, and always doing your share of work so that your coworkers can rely on you?

MISS McGUIRE

Miss Johnson, I'd like to add to that list. You told us in class that we must stay with our patient if needed until relieved; isn't that part of ethical conduct, too?

MISS JOHNSON

Yes. If you were to leave before your relief came, and your patient suffered harm, it might also carry a legal penalty. So you see that the line between ethical (ideal) behavior and legal requirements is sometimes a little hazy. However, the worker who consistently holds to ideal behavior should not have to worry about meeting the requirements of the law.

MRS. BOYD

I read in the employee's handbook that I can't wear any jewelry on duty, or any nail polish except very pale or clear. Why is that in the handbook?

MISS JOHNSON

Organized nursing had its roots in both military and religious disciplines and adhered quite strictly to the dignity of the uniform as a "symbol" of the profession. However, a great deal more latitude is allowed now — the introduction of pantsuits and colored hose are examples. Although there is a gradual decrease in strict adherence to the symbolic uniform, you must still adhere to the basic principles of cleanliness to prevent disease and infections for your own protection as well as the protection of your patients. Soiled uniforms, jewelry, and other adornments may carry germs which can cause disease or infection. It is your ethical duty to prevent the transfer of germs from patient to patient. This can be easily done by keeping your uniform and hands clean.

In some agencies, particularly in caring for children or the emotionally ill, the nurses wear streetclothes or colored uniforms without the cap. Your employer has the right to establish the standards of apparel for his employees and, by accepting employment, you have agreed to accept such standards. Another point about uniforms — try to wear your uniform only to and from work, and not to the grocery store or on shopping errands. When hospital workers wear their identifying uniforms outside of the health setting, it is similar to a doctor wearing a stethoscope and carrying a "black bag" to do errands. Items used in our work often become contaminated with germs, and we may carry them to the unsuspecting public when we wear our duty clothes and equipment in public places.

Nail polish is affected by some of the solvents we use and is difficult to keep undamaged and attractive. Therefore, it is usually neater and less bothersome for you if you do not wear nail polish while you are on duty.

MISS BOYNE
Ward Clerk

Does personal grooming come under the topic of ethics?

MISS JOHNSON

I would think so. Good hygiene and careful attention to cleanliness and grooming make your patients' environment more pleasant. They surely are entitled to that. Incidentally, good grooming includes careful and minimal use of cosmetics. Avoid heavy eye makeup, obvious perfumes, extremes of any sort, which are not in good taste for wear in any situation. Frequently, cosmetics have a heavy, sweet odor which may be nauseating to an ill patient. Therefore, if you are concerned about your patient's welfare, you will refrain from excessive use of cosmetics.

MRS. BOYD

Miss Johnson, last week Mr. Goldrocks tried to give me two dollars when I finished his bathtime care. I told him I wasn't permitted to accept. it. How could I have handled this situation better?

MISS JOHNSON

Did you notice in the codes of ethics we read that you are supposed to accept only the money given by your employer? Tipping to ensure service could be disastrous in a hospital, couldn't it? It would violate the fundamental concepts of ethics — respect for the dignity and basic rights of the person. How do you think you would react in such a situation?

MISS SANDS

Maybe I could let my patient know that assisting him isn't just a job to me but that it is very satisfying for me to be able to help another person. I can let him know this by my attitude and by the way I respond to his needs.

MISS McGUIRE

I think I might suggest that if he feels like making a cash donation, perhaps he would like to give it to the hospital fund for furnishing the new patient lounge, or whatever current project the hospital has. I think there is a difference between a patient offering me a gift or money when he first comes into the hospital, and his giving me a handkerchief, card, or candy when he leaves. It is unethical to accept the latter?

MISS JOHNSON

I don't think so, Miss McGuire, because if the patient has gone home, he could hardly expect preferential service as a result of his gift. It would be nice, though, if you received a gift, to share it with the other team members who also cared for the patient. I guess that would be following the Golden Rule.

MRS. ACALA
Diet Assistant

Something I saw yesterday bothers me. One of the hospital workers took the dessert from the patient's tray and put it in the utility room and later I saw her eating it.

MISS JOHNSON

Of course, we don't know all the circumstances, but taking what is not ours is stealing, and that is a violation of the law. I wonder if the worker would have openly eaten the dessert if the head nurse or hospital administrator had been present? You are not responsible for the actions of others, but by being responsible for your own actions, you set a good example for others. In some agencies, eating food from a patient's tray is considered cause for immediate termination.

MR. THOMAS

What should be done when a person observes someone violating either the law or ethical concepts; doesn't it show consent if nothing is done?

MISS JOHNSON

You are full of hard questions today, Mr. Thomas. No list of rules could be given that would fit every circumstance. Who is involved, the nature of the infraction, and the circumstances must all be taken into consideration. Sometimes it is best to speak directly to the person involved and allow him a chance to alter his behavior, and sometimes a private discussion with your superior will give you appropriate help in deciding what to do.

One of your most important legal and ethical responsibilities in a health care situation is to guard the privacy of your patient. Privacy is one of the basic rights. When people are sick, they are dependent upon other people to do many things that they cannot do themselves. They are entitled to privacy in all respects — concerning their condition, personal data, illness, and everything that you might learn because they are patients. Sometimes it is tempting for a hospital worker who is "on the inside" to reveal information about patients. It is exciting to tell something nobody else knows. This is illegal in some instances and unethical in all instances.

MRS. DEEDS   Sometimes patients ask me questions when I'm cleaning their rooms. Last week one of them asked me if the patient across the hall had died. I didn't know what to say, although I had just finished cleaning the unit after the body was taken away.

MISS JOHNSON   Patients are often curious about other patients, particularly about one who is very ill or who may have expired. Your ingenuity will be challenged to evade the question without appearing rude or dishonest. How do you class members think Mrs. Deeds might have answered her patient?

MISS McGUIRE   Could she have evaded answering by saying something like, "I'm not involved with assigning patients their rooms or in moving them from one room to another"?

MISS SANDS   How about a simple, courteous "I don't know."

MISS JOHNSON   That could be a truthful reply, for perhaps the patient did not expire, but was moved to the intensive care unit or to some other room. However, another way to handle the situation is to ask the patient in return, "Why do you ask?" The patient may only want to talk about the worries or concerns he has for his own health.

MR. TROYLE   I'm a new employee, and my neighbor was hurt in an accident and
Maintenance Man   brought here. I was looking at his chart to see how he was and the head nurse jumped all over me.

MISS JOHNSON   Some of you will see information on a patient's chart. You may have reason to use the chart or see it by accident. Unless your work requires you to make notations on the chart or to use it in order to give care to the patient, do not read it or even take it from the chart rack. The chart is a legal document. It belongs to the hospital and the material in it is known as "privileged information" — that is, it is very private and is meant only for those people who need it to care for the patient. Privacy of everything surrounding the patient is his right.

Another point about privacy. It is highly unethical to discuss your patients in the cafeteria, hallways, or public places. Family and friends often overhear conversations and misunderstand what is said. Sometimes they think you are talking about their loved one or friend. Loose gossip can be very upsetting to others. Guard your conversation at all times! Discussion of your patient should be limited to those team members who assist or share in his care and then the discussion should occur in the appropriate place, so it is not overheard or misinterpreted by outsiders.

MISS BOYNE   I think the topic of ethics is quite complex, but I'm glad we had this class today, because I have some guidelines to help me in my work. I'm going to try to be an ideal employee because it should help to keep me out of trouble with my employer and the law.

MISS JOHNSON   No doubt that is true, but aren't there other good reasons?

MRS. BOYD   Yes, I feel good when I know I'm doing the right thing and when I have done a good job.

MRS. SAYRES   There has been a lot in the news lately about violations of ethics, if not by law, by prominent prople in many professions. Do you think that the standards for ethical conduct are changing with the times?

MISS JOHNSON   The basic principles upon which ethics are founded, that is, respecting the rights and dignity of the individual, are changeless. In fact, in some ways a greater emphasis is being placed upon the individual rights of *all* people in the fields of education and employment as well as their right to adequate health care. Although we hear about the spectacular breaches of conduct by prominent people, each of us needs to remember that we are primarily responsible for our own ethical conduct.

We have made quite a list of ethical guidelines today from our discussion. We can summarize by saying, whenever you are faced with a situation involving a moral or ethical decision, ask yourself these questions:

1. How will my action or choice affect the patient?
2. How will my action or choice affect my employer or coworker?
3. How will my action or choice affect me?

You have probably made a sound choice if your answer to all three questions is positive. Your behavior would uphold the dignity and basic rights of the patient and your employer and maintain your own self-respect.

ITEM 3.   APPLICATION OF PRINCIPLES OF ETHICS

Let's try out our new concepts of ethics by reading the following hypothetical situations and filling in the blanks or circling the appropriate *italicized* word or words.

Situation A

Mr. Brown in Room 201 is in critical condition, and although you have not cared for him, you have heard one of the other nurses mention that the doctor feels the patient will not live much longer. A relative of the patient asks you in the corridor if Mr. Brown has improved. Your answer might be, "You probably should speak to the doctor about that."

3. Ethically, who is being considered here?

   a. _____   b. _____

   c. _____

4. In any situation in which the answer is not clear to you, it is appropriate to refer the question to your *(supervisor) (coworker)*.

5. In doing the above, you recognize your *(legal) (ethical) (both legal and ethical)* limitations.

Situation B

A young girl has been brought by ambulance to the Emergency Room. You are the ward clerk there and note that she has swallowed an overdose of sedatives and is now having her stomach emptied of its contents. Since this was an attempted suicide, the police reporters were in the hallway. When you go to lunch, the other ward clerks want to know why the ambulance had its sirens sounding, how old the girl is, and why she was brought in. You were the person who recorded the emergency room notes and so you have some information.

6. When asked why the girl took the overdose, you might answer: (Circle the letter of the correct answer.)

   a. I assume because she is pregnant and unmarried.

   b. She must have had a desire to die.

   c. This information is confidential.

7. In this situation, to discuss the patient not only violates her right to privacy, but could result in a *(legal action) (loss of employment) (both of these)*.

Situation C

Carol Brown, nursing assistant, has always been conscientious and reliable in her work habits. She is scheduled to work on the weekend and receives an invitation from an old friend to spend the weekend at Yosemite National Park. Carol has never been to Yosemite and does not often have such opportunities. She ponders long and hard before arriving at a decision.

8. Persons considered in her decision-making would be:

   a. _____   b. _____

   c. _____   d. _____

Situation D

Mr. Grimm in Room 410 always orders his meals from the hospital's special gourmet menu. At noon on Sunday he didn't touch any of the food although the dinner was excellent. The filet and strawberry pie were indeed tempting. You are the dietary aide who is responsible for taking trays back to the kitchen.

9. In an effort not to waste such delectable food, you decide: (Circle correct letter.)

   a. To eat it yourself.

   b. To give it to a fellow employee who is quite needy and doesn't eat properly.

   c. To ask the dietitian to confer with the patient about ordering smaller portions.

Situation E

Your doctor has observed that you are very tense about your job as a ward clerk in the hospital unit, and has recommended a common tranquilizer for you to take three times a day. You know that often when patients go home, they leave their medications, which are then returned to the pharmacy. You ask the medication nurse if she could give you the tranquilizers that are left on a patient's discharge, saving you the expense of having your prescription filled.

10. This is a distinct breach of _____ on your part.

11. Your ethical behavior is lowered. However, if the nurse grants your request, she is

prescribing or dispensing medicine without a license and this is a _____ offense.

Situation F

You are a nurse's aide and have cared daily for Mrs. Johann. She has come to rely on you and, when she is ready to go home, wants to give you a sum of money in appreciation for the "lovely things you have done for her."

12. What would you do? (Circle the correct letter.)

   a. You must explain to her that the service is part of her care.

   b. You may accept the money because, although you are paid a salary by the hospital, patients should pay for the service you render them individually.

   c. Accept the gift of money and tell nobody so that no one else will feel hurt that she selected only you.

13. Mrs. Johann insists you must take the money or you will hurt her feelings. Therefore you (Circle the correct letter.)

   a. Tell her of some specific need the hospital has to which she could make a contribution.

   b. Suggest a fund in her name with suitable recognition.

   c. Accept the gift so that there are no hurt feelings in the situation.

WORKBOOK ANSWERS

1. (a) behavior, (b) ideal, (c) group

2. by the group, or lose membership in the group.

3. a. Patient — his privacy is respected.

   b. Employer or group — you are representing high ideals of confidence

   c. Yourself — self-respect is maintained

4. Supervisor

5. Both legal and ethical

6. c

7. Both of these

8. The following in any order: the patient, coworkers, employer, and herself (any of these)

9. c

10. Ethical standards

11. Legal standards

12. a

13. a

POST-TEST

Directions: Circle the letter indicating whether the statement is true (T) or false (F).

T   F   1. All professions follow the same code of ethics.

T   F   2. Ethics applies only to the doctors and nurses who are licensed professionals.

T   F   3. You enter into an agreement to follow institutional policy when you take a job with the hospital.

T   F   4. Since patients are in a dependent position, they must expect their privacy to be invaded during illness.

T   F   5. Information about patients can be discussed freely as long as it is not detrimental to their character.

T   F   6. Personal hygiene and good grooming are related to ethics.

T   F   7. Wearing the symbols of your job while shopping helps to enhance your image in the community and is therefore ethical.

T   F   8. A patient's chart is simply a convenient place for everyone caring for the patient to put notes and findings.

T   F   9. Food that has been taken into a patient's room is meant only for the patient and should not be eaten by others.

Directions: In the statements below, indicate the word "ethical," "unethical," "legal," or "illegal" to describe what guideline or principle is being considered or violated. If two are appropriate, write in both.

10. _____ Mary Brown constantly comes to work in a soiled uniform that smells strongly of cigarette smoke.

11. _____ A patient's chart is left lying open near your station and you as the maid read it, since the patient is your neighbor and friend.

12. _____ At a party you tell about a prominent socialite who had given birth to an illegitimate child.

13. _____ You delight your classmates in the lounge with an account of the antics of a patient who was coming out of anesthesia.

14. _____ You ask the medicine nurse to save any unused antibiotics of a certain kind for you to give your child.

15. _____ When the returned medications are ready for Pharmacy, you carry them over yourself and take out whatever medicines you need for your own use, since they will not be charged to any specific patient.

16. _____ An elderly lady gives you $25 when she leaves the hospital and thanks you for the extra-special way you took care of her plants and flowers during her hospital stay. You accept and keep the money.

17. _____ Because you failed to convince a wealthy gentleman not to give you a sizeable amount of money upon his discharge without causing a scene, you accept the money and give it to the supervisor who puts it in a fund for some special equipment.

18. _____ Although your contract clearly states that your hours are from 8:00 A.M. to 4:40 P.M., you find you can get to work at 8:30 and leave shortly before 4:00 because your supervisor is away at a conference.

19. _____ A discharged patient leaves a lovely dinner ring in the bedside table. You find that it fits you and slip it into your pocket while cleaning the room.

Directions: Fill in the blanks indicated.

20. Ethics is a code of _____ for a _____ group representing ideal _____ .

21. Having to rely on another person for help or support of any kind makes a person _____ .

22. Breaking an obligation or contract, or an infraction of behavior is often called a _____ of ethics or contract.

23. A common substitute for the word "die" in hospital usage is _____ .

24. Rules designed for the promotion of health and good grooming are collectively called _____ .

25. Behavior that is unethical may result in _____ from the group.

26. Ethics involve moral decision and a knowledge of the difference between _____ and _____ .

27. Ethical conduct always respects the basic _____ of the patient.

28. My hospital conduct involves myself, my employer, coworkers, and the _____ .

POST-TEST ANSWERS

1.	F	15.	unethical, illegal
2.	F	16.	ethical
3.	T	17.	ethical
4.	F	18.	unethical
5.	F	19.	unethical, illegal
6.	T	20.	conduct; specific behavior
7.	F	21.	dependent
8.	F	22.	breach
9.	T	23.	expire
10.	unethical	24.	hygiene
11.	unethical	25.	discipline; expulsion
12.	unethical	26.	right; wrong
13.	unethical	27.	rights
14.	unethical, illegal	28.	patient

THE NURSE AND THE LAW

GENERAL PERFORMANCE OBJECTIVE

You will answer questions based on definitions of legal terms and an understanding of legal problems that might occur during a patient-professional relationship with at least 80 per cent accuracy.

SPECIFIC PERFORMANCE OBJECTIVES

Upon completion of this unit you will be able to:

1. Define the term "law" as used in this study.

2. Distinguish civil from criminal law.

3. List the main sources for the law, specifically "medical" law.

4. Demonstrate your knowledge of the patient's rights under the law and the ways in which these rights might be violated.

5. Recognize in given situations when an act might be interpreted as malpractice or negligence.

6. Demonstrate your knowledge of responsibility in relation to legal records.

7. List several basic rules to follow for the prevention of legal suits.

VOCABULARY

assault—either a threat or an attempt to injure another in an illegal manner.

battery—unlawful touching of another person without his consent, with or without resultant injury. Assault and battery are often charged together because of successful attempt to injure.

civil law—pertains to legal relationships between private individuals.

common law—a term given to unwritten law, customs with authority of law, of precedents established by judges and juries in past cases.

consent—permission voluntarily granted by a person who is competent; written consent is preferred because it is easier to prove.

crime—an act that is forbidden or the omission of a duty that is commanded by a public law and that makes the offender liable to punishment by that law.

criminal law—defines legal obligations between the individual citizen and the state.

defamation of character—the wrongful injury of another's reputation or character without good reason or cause.

false imprisonment—holding or detaining a person against his will.

felony—a serious crime, for which the penalty is imprisonment in the state prison for more than one year.

invasion of privacy—a civil wrong that unlawfully makes public any private or personal information without the consent of the wronged person.

libel—a civil wrong; to communicate in writing to a third party defamatory matter about an individual or group.

licensure—authorization by the state to practice one's profession or vocation; involves control of educational standards, licensing examinations, and prohibitions for individuals who are not licensed.

litigation—another word for law suit.

malpractice—literally "bad practice," that is, improper or injurious practice by a professional person; unskilled and faulty medical or surgical treatment.

misdemeanor—a crime less serious than a felony, punishable by imprisonment in the county jail for a term of less than one year.

negligence—failure to perform in a reasonably prudent manner.

privileged communication—any personal or private information related to his care that a patient gives medical personnel.

slander—spoken statement of false charges or misrepresentations that defame or damage another's reputation, as distinguished from libel, which is written.

standard of care—the obligation under law for a nurse or other health worker to perform services for a patient that meet the common standards of practice expected in the community for a comparable worker.

statutory law—that law which has been enacted by a legislative branch of the government.

tort—a civil wrong occurring between two or more persons.

will—a written document, legally executed, by which a person disposes of his property; to take effect after his death.

INTRODUCTION

Why does the nurse need to be concerned with the law? Why is such emphasis placed on legal matters, and why must a unit on the subject be included in a book devoted to nursing skills? Nurses just take care of sick people, so why is it necessary to spend time on such things as rights, laws, legal terms, and so forth?

Nursing is primarily a service provided by people (nurses) for other people (patients) who are sick. Sick people are most often helpless, uncomfortable, anxious, and unable to look after all of their own needs. They depend on other people to help them, and they are powerless to control many of the events in their immediate vicinity that affect their lives. They are at great risk of having other, less scrupulous people take unfair advantage of them, subject them to cruel or debasing treatment, or force them to do things against their will. Rules and laws have been enacted to reduce the possibility of making victims out of patients.

In this unit we will examine the rights of patients and the types of laws that protect these rights. A number of legal terms are introduced, along with descriptions of the common kinds of illegal practices that occur in medical settings and some of the nurse's responsibilities for safeguarding the patient's rights.

LEGAL CONCEPTS IN NURSING

ITEM 1. TYPES OF LAWS

Laws (as the term is used in this unit) are regarded as the rules or standards that control the conduct of members of society, and set limits or guidelines for curbing natural impulses. The purpose of laws is essentially to safeguard both individuals and society as a whole. There are various types of laws, each with a specific frame of reference and application; the following types are among the best known:

Common Law. Based on customs and precedent, common laws refers to decisions of similar cases tried previously. It comprises a large body of English and American law.

Legislative Laws and Statutes. These include written laws passed by the legislative branch of federal, state, and local governments. Also included are the "enabling" bills that allow a created agency to develop its own regulations, which are then binding on the people and have the effect of law.

Moral Laws. Moral laws are based on a divinely appointed system or order; examples include the Mosaic law, the laws of the Old Testament, the Koran, and the laws of other religious bodies.

Physical Laws. These laws are based on certain conditions or sequence of actions that invariably take place, such as Newton's law of gravity.

Protective Laws

Many of the laws passed by federal and state governments involve health care or have some effect on the health and safety of people. One of the methods of protecting the public is through the licensing of hospitals and health care facilities to ensure that they meet minimum standards. The standards include details of construction such as the size of doors, with width of hallways, the size of floor space for each patient, fire safety measures, and sanitation requirements. Other laws regulate the purity of foods sold to the public, the methods of manufacturing and selling drugs, the control of harmful or toxic products, and many other public health matters.

Other important protective laws involve the registration or licensing of various professional groups as a means of indicating that certain educational requirements have been met or that the individual has the specified qualifications to practice a particular profession. Among the professionals who must be licensed or registered in order to practice in most states are doctors of medicine, dentists, podiatrists, registered nurses, practical or vocational nurses, medical technologists, pharmacists, and physical therapists. The first state to pass a nurse registration law was North Carolina in 1902, and other states soon followed. The nursing practice acts adopted by each of the states set standards for schools of nursing, policies for safe practice, and methods for handling violators. By 1934, 10 states had licensing laws for practical nurses, and today all states have similar laws to regulate practical nursing practice.

Civil and Criminal Cases

Laws are further classified as civil law and criminal law. Criminal law is concerned with the rules that govern the society as a whole. Under it certain acts are forbidden that would cause harm, injury, or death to another person or that might deprive others of their health or safety. The government prosecutes anyone discovered breaking these laws and punishes those found guilty of such crimes. The serious crimes are called felonies and carry with them severe punishment, while the less serious crimes are called misdemeanors. Depriving patients of civil rights is a crime, and these cases are tried in criminal courts along with cases for assault, robbery, or murder.

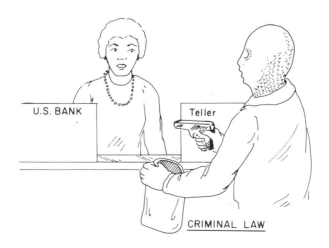

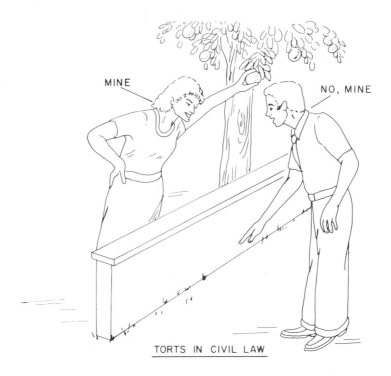

TORTS IN CIVIL LAW

Civil law cases are those in which one party claims that another party has caused some type of harm and therefore seeks compensation from the second party. The accusation of wrong-doing by one party is called a "tort," and the case is tried in civil courts. Medical malpractice suits generally fall into this category, as the patient seeks compensation from the doctor and others who may have been involved for some harm claimed to have resulted from the treatment rendered. Other civil cases involve libel, slander, breaking or not meeting the terms of a contract, and similar disputes between two parties.

ITEM 2.   THE RIGHTS OF PATIENTS

People have a basic right to protection and safety. When they become ill, they expect nurses to provide for their comfort, give the care that is needed, and protect their lives and their rights. The patient does not give up the civil rights previously held, but, may in fact, gain additional rights pertaining to the role of a patient. In the past, patients were reluctant to speak out or voice complaints about their care, but with the encouragement of consumer groups, more are speaking out now and demanding that their rights be observed.

Civil Rights

Each individual is guaranteed certain civil rights by the Bill of Rights in the Constitution of the United States. It specifies that no one is to be discriminated against on the basis of race, religion, or political beliefs. Even the most basic rights are often jeopardized when a person becomes ill or is hospitalized; among those most susceptible to infringement are the right to privacy; the right to freedom of movement; and the right to make decisions, to send or receive mail, to make telephone calls, or to vote. Under certain legally specified conditions, some individual rights may be temporarily suspended; for example,

1. When it is essential for medical treatment.

2. When it is necessary to protect the patient from harm.

3. When necessary to protect the public from harm.

A Patient's Bill of Rights

In 1972, the American Hospital Association adopted a group of statements called A Patient's Bill of Rights. The document specified what patients could expect from their doctors and the hospital staff who provided for their care. Accordingly, the patient has rights to the following:

1. Considerate and respectful care.

2. Information from the doctor about the diagnosis, treatment, and prognosis of the condition in terms that can be understood.

3. Information from the doctor that is adequate so that informed consent can be given for any treatment or procedure.

4. Refusal of treatment to the extent that is permitted by law.

5. Consideration for privacy concerning the patient's own medical care program.

6. Confidential treatment of all communications and records about the care.

7. A reasonable response by the hospital to requests for service.

8. Knowledge of the relationship of the hospital to other educational and health facilities and to the individuals involved in the treatment.

9. Awareness of human experimentation projects being considered and freedom to refuse to participate in such research.

10. Reasonable continuity of care during and following hospitalization.

11. Inspection and explanation of the hospital bill.

12. Knowledge about the hospital rules and regulations that apply to him or her as a patient.

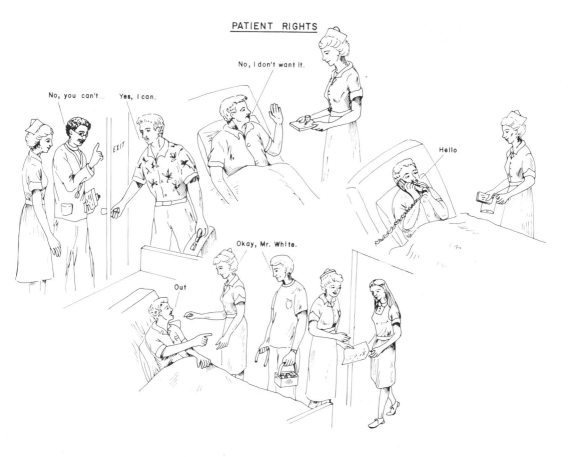

Although these rights are not enacted into law, the list does specify rights that patients should have and the kind of care they should receive. Their rights include the power to make decisions, such as refusing specific medications or treatments, and the freedom to refuse all treatment by leaving the hospital, except when such actions would result in danger to the patient or to others, or when the patient is not competent to make these decisions. The question of competence is discussed in more detail in Unit 7.

Psychiatric Patient's Rights

Not too many years ago, patients who were confined in psychiatric units were denied as many as 16 of their civil rights, while criminals confined to prison were deprived of only 6 of theirs. Since that time, many states have passed laws to ensure that patients with mental illnesses retain more of their rights even though hospitalized. The current principle is to protect the right of harmless individuals to be different, to act in odd or unusual ways, to disagree with the majority, to live their own lives, and to seek their own solutions to their private difficulties. In most states, mentally disturbed people cannot be held in hospitals against their will for more than two or three days. They may be detained for longer periods of time only under conditions such as these: (1) The person poses a distinct danger to himself, or to others; (2) The person is gravely disabled as a result of a mental disorder. "Gravely disabled" means unable to provide for one's own basic needs for food, shelter, or clothing.

ITEM 3. MEDICO LEGAL TERMS

There are a number of legal terms that you should know, since they often apply to torts and crimes that reach the courts. Customarily the person with the highest level of educational training and licensure is held responsible for the consequences of the medical treatment rendered to the patient. In the past, the doctor was the one most likely to be named in a lawsuit instituted by the patients or their families; however, decisions by the courts have held various health workers responsible for their actions and so the trend is to name all persons in suits who have been involved in the action being contested. Although nursing enjoys a good public image, nurses may still be summoned to testify in court cases.

Malpractice

Malpractice means bad or faulty practice, and it specifically refers to negligence by the professional person. When caring for patients, the professional is able to perceive risks and problems that are not apparent to the lay person by virtue of advanced training, knowledge, and skills. All medical malpractice must be based on negligence, but all cases of neligence are not necessarily malpractice, because nonprofessionals may also be negligent.

Negligence

Negligence is defined as failing to perform some act that a reasonably prudent person would carry out in similar circumstances or as acting in ways that the reasonably prudent person would not. Taking the wrong action and failing to act reasonably both constitute negligence. In order to show negligence, the following factors must be shown:

1. A standard of care existed to show what should have been done.

2. A failure to meet the standard of care took place.

3. There was knowledge that harm might result from failing to meet the standard.

4. Harm did occur.

Standard of Care.   Nurses are responsible for providing patients with safe and competent care. The law states that "safe and competent care" is the level of care that would be given by a comparable worker in similar circumstances. Nursing procedure books define a standard of care to be used by nurses; failure to perform these procedures correctly constitutes negligence when the nurse knows that harm might result to the patient and harm actually does occur.

Many examples could be given to illustrate negligent actions by nurses. In one case, an elderly man complained to the nurse making rounds that his feet were cold. The nurse obtained an order from the doctor for a hot water bottle and then directed the practical nurse to apply it. The man suffered first and second degree burns to the feet. The practical nurse was negligent because the prudent nurse knows that poor circulation in the elderly makes the skin more susceptible to burning and that the water temperature must be adjusted so it is not hot enough to cause burns. Other cases of negligence by nurses include carrying out doctor's orders incorrectly or overlooking them, changing an order without the doctor's authorization, or failing to notify a superior when the patient's condition indicates the need for a change in orders. Many cases involve the incorrect administration of medications, such as when the nurse has given the wrong dose, administered the wrong medication, used the wrong route, or given the drug to the wrong patient.

Assault and Battery

Assault refers to approaching or handling another person in such a way that it poses a threat to the person. The threat may be a verbal statement, such as the following example: "If you don't stay in bed, we'll have to tie you up in restraints." Bumping, shaking, or otherwise touching others without their consent may also lead to charges of assault. Battery is the extension of the threat through violent contact with or forcible restraint of the person. Examples of battery include acts such as hitting, pinching, roughness, as well as forcing the patient to take medications or to submit to a procedure or treatment.

Patients have the right to refuse medical treatment and care even when this care is clearly indicated for their benefit and welfare. Medical treatment is often disturbing or uncomfortable, and people ordinarily do not choose to submit to discomfort voluntarily unless it is necessary. For this reason, it is important that the patient's consent be obtained before any treatment is given. Ordinarily, patients sign a consent form on admission to the hospital agreeing to general medical care, nursing care, and laboratory and x-ray tests; however, additional consent must be obtained for each surgical operation or for other unusual or complex procedures. See Unit 7 for more information about consents.

False Imprisonment

As the name implies, false imprisonment is charged when a person is held without just cause. Using restraints to keep a patient in bed, locking a person in a room, or holding a patient in the hospital because the bill has not been paid may lead to charges of false imprisonment.

In one court case, the patient sued the doctor for admitting her to a psychiatric unit of a private hospital and forcibly keeping her there. Her husband had requested Dr. X to treat his wife, who repeatedly claimed she wasn't mentally ill but just upset by her husband's affair with another woman. She refused hospitalization but was restrained and forcibly given an injection of a sedative by Dr. X. The next thing she remembered was waking up in the hospital a week later and being forced to stay there for another week. The court found that the treatment by the doctor and others constituted assault and battery. In addition, hospitalization against her will was false imprisonment, since expert testimony supported her claim that she was not mentally ill.

Invasion of Privacy

Patients have a right to privacy concerning their body and its function and to information about their condition.

Physical Privacy. The right to privacy is often jeopardized in hospitals unless constant vigilance is kept to preserve it. Nurses provide physical privacy for patients by draping for procedures, drawing curtains around the bed, closing the door of the room, and protecting the patients from unwelcome visitors. The hospital releases limited information about patients, usually just the name, and accident victims or newsworthy patients are shielded from reporters or photographers. Groups of students who gather at the bedside to observe a procedure, study a medical condition, or make an examination should avoid invading the patient's privacy by obtaining his or her permission.

Confidential Information. Much of the information that patients provide to the doctors and nurses is of a highly personal nature. Since it is privileged communication and not common knowledge, it should not be shared with other people without the patient's knowledge or consent but should be treated as confidential. This includes the medical history, results of tests or examinations, and other material entered into the patient's hospital record. Confidential information is to be shared only with those who have a need to know it in their care of the patient. Nurses should not discuss this confidential information in places where it can be overheard by the public or by others not involved in the patient's care, nor should it be used in the form of gossip.

Defamation of Character

Any written or oral statement that blackens or damages the reputation of another person falsely and without good cause may be the basis of a defamation of character suit. The two kinds of defamation are slander and libel.

Slander. Spoken or oral statements that are untrue or injurious to another's reputation constitute slander. The statements generally subject the person to contempt or ridicule. An example is making a false statement to the effect that a doctor is a butcher and unfit to practice medicine.

Libel. Libel consists of defamation that is written or printed. Making false or malicious statements on the patient's hospital chart, such as "Patient is a complainer and uncooperative" or "Is addicted to narcotics and demands shots every hour," may constitute defamation of character. Cartoons and pictures that subject the person to ridicule are other forms of libel.

Define and give an example of each of the following terms:

1.	standard of care	5.	criminal law
2.	negligence	6.	invasion of privacy
3.	malpractice	7.	slander
4.	civil law	8.	assault and battery

ITEM 4. LEGAL DOCUMENTS

The basic purpose of medical records is to provide a written history of the patient during the course of treatment. The patient's hospital chart contains written reports of the medical history, the findings of examinations, the results of laboratory tests and x-rays, the progress of the illness, and the daily nursing care that was given. Doctors, nurses, therapists, and other involved staff members refer to the chart for information about the patient's condition, the response to treatment, and signs of progress. The chart contains the signed consent forms that indicate the patient gave permission for the action or procedure to be done.

There is always a possibility that the medical records of one of your patients may become a legal document in a court action. The chart is often used to verify facts in a lawsuit, in disputes over insurance claims, or in other matters of litigation. As a legal document, the chart records are in written form, given evidence of events and actions that took place in the past, and are subject to scrutiny by lawyers, judges, and even the public.

Accurate, factual, and legible charting of nursing care is essential and provides the best protection for the nurse. Other legal documents you may come in contact with are the personal legal papers of the patient, such as wills, agreements, contracts of various kinds, or other similar legal instruments.

The Chart. Let us examine a patient's chart in these respects. Is it complete? Is it signed? Is it in ink and in no way altered? These questions are asked when the acceptability of the chart as a legal document is being determined. In other words, if the nurse were to appear in court, the lawyer showing an entry in the patient's chart would be expected to ask, "Is this your signature? What did you mean by what you said here?" Later in this course you will learn how to chart your nursing care on the patient's chart. With the knowledge you have gained from this unit, you will be more aware of how important it is to chart legibly, accurately, and according to prescribed charting rules.

Consents. Another highly important legal record is the "signed consent." Without proper consents signed by the patient we can be accused of illegal acts. Specific information concerning consents is discussed in Unit 7, Consents, Releases, and Incident Reports. In court action, the lawyer can be expected to ask any or all of the following questions:

"Is there a consent form available for use in this instance?"

"Was the patient competent to sign?"

"If the patient was not competent to sign, is the signature on the consent that of the legally authorized person?"

"Was this an informed consent? Was the person told the risks, the extent of the procedure, and the expected results?"

"Was the consent signed before the treatment was given?"

Witnessing Wills and Personal Legal Papers. People often put off making wills to dispose of their personal property after death until they become sick or until the threat of dying is more apparent. Nurses may be asked then to witness the signature of the patient signing his or her will. When this is done, the patient must indicate that the paper is a will and sign it in your presence. Your signature as a witness indicates that the patient was of sound mind and signed the will voluntarily, not under duress.

Personal legal papers signed when the person is a patient in a hospital are more apt to be challenged and end up in court suits. Relatives or business partners may have brought undue pressure on the sick person, or their actions may be so interpreted by others. Because of this, many agencies specify that the patient's personal legal papers be witnessed by a specific individual other than a nurse. Whenever possible, the patient is encouraged to have these papers witnessed by friends or acquaintances rather than by the nurses.

Nursing Responsibilities

Perhaps you can think of ways in which you might prevent becoming involved in a lawsuit. If you responded with comments along the following lines, you are to be commended for your understanding of your legal responsibilities for your patient's care:

"I will be a conscientious worker because the patient is my responsibility, no matter how I feel or how distracted I am."

"I will be observant of the patient's rights and avoid any violation of them."

"I will be careful with the paperwork for which I will be responsible. I will do all in my power to see that all documents are legally correct."

"I understand what is meant by being responsible for one's own actions. At all times I will do only those things for which I have been trained and supervised to do."

ITEM 5. CONCLUSION

You have completed the lesson on The Nurse and the Law. You should have a good idea of the law as it relates to you while performing your job of caring for patients.

When you feel sure you understand this lesson, ask your instructor to allow you to take the post-test. You will be expected to pass the test with at least 80 per cent correct answers.

WORKBOOK ANSWERS

The terms are defined in the vocabulary, and any appropriate example could be given.

1. Worker performs services in the same way as a comparable worker in similar circumstances would do. Example: Follows correct procedure when giving colostomy care.

2. Failure to perform in a reasonably prudent manner. Example: A health worker fails to notify the nurse or doctor when a patient with a fresh cast complains of pain and swelling.

3. Faulty or improper practice by a professional person. Example: A registered nurse fails to heed signs of toxic overdose of medication and continues to administer the drug causing harm to the patient.

4. Laws that refer to claims of one party against another and for compensation. Example: A patient sues nurses for defamation of character and seeks thousands of dollars in damages.

5. Laws that refer to crimes against the state or the public. Examples include robbery, manslaughter, murder, and so on.

6. Violating the right to privacy concerning one's body and private information without the person's consent. Example: Two ward clerks discuss the number of abortions a patient may have had.

7. Oral statements that are false or that injure another's reputation. Example: A nurse makes a false statement that another nurse forged a registration card and is not entitled to be a nurse.

8. Assault is the threat of harm to an individual; battery is the forceful or violent action of carrying out the harm to another, i.e., the illegal contact. Example: A nurse threatens a patient with forcible detention when the patient expresses a desire to leave; when the patient attempts to get out of bed, the nurse pushes him down and straps his arms to the bed rails.

POST-TEST

Directions: Match statement on the right to the most appropriate term on the left.

_____ 1. standard of care

_____ 2. statutory law

_____ 3. invasion of privacy

_____ 4. slander

_____ 5. crime

_____ 6. negligence

_____ 7. privileged communication

_____ 8. battery

_____ 9. tort

_____ 10. misdemeanor

a. laws made by legislature

b. verbal defamation of character

c. unlawful handling of a person without his consent

d. information kept in trust by medical personnel

e. illegal act between persons

f. less serious crime

g. making personal information public without due consent

h. failure to give reasonable care

i. performing duties and services in an expected manner

j. threatening to injure another person

k. detaining unlawfully

l. an illegal act against society

Directions: Select the one best answer.

11. Marie a ward clerk never saw a certain patient in the hospital but was accused by the family of defamation of character. She was most likely guilty of:

    a. assault and battery

    b. felony

    c. slander

    d. negligence

12. A practical nurse inserted a rectal thermometer in an unconscious patient and left the room to finish another task. The patient moved, broke the thermometer, and sustained injury. Which of the following might the nurse be sued for?

    a. reasonable care

    b. felony

    c. assault

    d. negligence

13. The nurse knows that Mrs. Green needs her heart medications, so when the patient refuses to take them, the nurse forces them down her throat. This is an example of which of the following?

    a. assault and battery

    b. invasion of privacy

    c. standard of care

    d. misdemeanor

14. The doctor orders a treatment procedure for the patient that the registered nurse does not know how to perform; however, the nurse proceeds anyway and the patient is injured. The person(s) most likely to be held for negligence is(are):

    a. the doctor

    b. the registered nurse

    c. the supervisor

    d. the hospital

15. A will is not valid if when signing it the patient can be proved to have been

   (1) under the influence of pain medication

   (2) not mentally competent

   (3) coerced by the family

   (4) displeased with the witnesses

   a. all of the above   c. 1, 2, and 3

   b. none of the above   d. 2 and 3

16. A patient may not be detained at the hospital until the bill is paid because this may be considered an illegal act of

   a. invasion of privacy   c. defamation of character

   b. false imprisonment   d. libel

17. A malpractice suit can be brought against a hospital or health worker for the following:

   a. a stroke patient falling from a wheelchair when being transferred

   b. a diabetic not receiving insulin as ordered owing to fasting lab tests

   c. a sponge left in the abdomen when the patient was operated on

   d. a patient losing a valuable ring

18. A nurse may be said to have acted with reasonable care if he or she:

   a. is a specialist in emergencies

   b. has been a supervisor

   c. has nursed for 20 years

   d. did what other nurses of similar background would have done in similar circumstances

19. A nurse's aide was instructed by a licensed practical nurse to place a hot water bottle for comfort at the feet of a patient who is paralyzed from the waist down. It resulted in severe tissue damage. Who will probably be held responsible for an act of negligence?

   a. the aide   c. the hospital

   b. the doctor   d. the licensed practical nurse

20. Which of the following will help the health worker avoid litigation?

   a. consistent practicing of conscientious care

   b. obtaining written consents

   c. always considering human rights

   d. staying within the limits of her training

   e. all of these

POST-TEST ANSWERS

1.	i	11.	c
2.	a	12.	d
3.	g	13.	a
4.	b	14.	b
5.	l	15.	d
6.	h	16.	b
7.	d	17.	c
8.	c	18.	d
9.	e	19.	a
10.	f	20.	e

Unit 3

GENERAL PERFORMANCE OBJECTIVE

In a written test you will demonstrate your knowledge of ten hospital environmental factors that affect patients' comfort, recovery, and safety.

SPECIFIC PERFORMANCE OBJECTIVES

Upon completion of this unit you will be able to:

1. Definition of the terms presented in the vocabulary.

2. The responsibilities of the nurse in environmental management.

3. The desirable ranges for room temperature and humidity and acceptable methods of modifying these conditions.

4. Correct methods of providing ventilation.

5. Ways to control offensive odors.

6. Common noises in the hospital and ways to minimize their effects on patients.

7. Methods of light adjustment.

8. Methods used to maintain patients' privacy.

9. Safety precautions used in the patient's environment.

VOCABULARY

anesthesia— partial or complete loss of sensation, with or without loss of consciousness, such as may result from disease, injury, or administered drug or gas.

anesthetic—an agent or drug that produces insensibility to pain or touch.

ecology—the relationship between living things and the environment.

environment—the surroundings; any condition that affects life or development.

emotional environment—conditions that influence our emotional life.

external environment—those conditions outside the body that affect it, such as temperature and noise.

internal environment—the fluid surrounding the body cells.

humidity—the amount of moisture in the air.

photophobia—fear of light; a condition in which light is painful to the eyes.

sedated—state of being calmed, usually effected by means of a drug.

ventilation—the movement of air.

INTRODUCTION

"Environment" is a word frequently used by today's news media. Any condition that affects the life or development of a person is part of that person's environment or surroundings.

"Ecology" refers to relationships between living things and their environment. Environmental and ecological conditions worldwide as well as local can affect our health and that of our patients. The explosion of an atom bomb thousands of miles away can result in radiation fallout that can contaminate local food and water supplies. Most of us are all too familiar with an unpleasant environmental factor called "pollution." Eye and respiratory irritants in the air affect all of us.

The Internal Environment. The physician is greatly concerned with our "internal environment," or the composition and volume of the fluids that surround the body cells. You will be responsible for helping the patient to maintain good internal environment through such measures as (a) keeping accurate records of fluid intake and output or (b) restricting salt intake.

Another factor rising from within us is the emotional mood or condition that affects our lives. In nursing, the terms "therapeutic environment" and "emotional environment" are increasingly discussed. We can be surrounded by emotional factors that are helpful or detrimental. The hospital worker is responsible for using communication skills and good interpersonal relationships to reduce tensions, anxiety, and fear in order to provide a good emotional environment for the patient.

The External Environment. The rest of this lesson will be confined to those factors concerning the immediate external environment of patients for which the hospital team is responsible. Many things are involved to provide the patient with shelter that is safe, comfortable, and healthy. Many departments and workers are required to provide services of heat, light, water, furnishings, food, cleanliness, linens, and other services that contribute to and influence the patient's care.

Circle the letter or letters of the appropriate answer.

1. The *interrelationship* between people and their surroundings is called:

    a. external environment

    b. therapeutic environment

    c. ecology

    d. internal environment

2. Nurses help to make a therapeutic environment for the patient when they:

    a. get along well with coworkers

    b. explain to the patient what they are going to do

    c. lessen a tense situation with communication skills

    d. tell the patient their honest opinion about the patient's physician

3. What is meant by the "internal environment"?

4. How does the nurse help maintain the patient's internal environment?

MANAGING THE PATIENT ENVIRONMENT

ITEM 1. MAINTAINING THE EXTERNAL ENVIRONMENT

In the modern hospital many people share the responsibility of maintaining the patient's external environment, from the engineers, who maintain temperature through control of heating, cooling, and ventilation, to the housekeeping personnel, who provide cleanliness and order throughout the building. In promoting cleanliness, housekeeping carries out the dual function of maintaining a pleasant appearance and preventing the spread of disease-causing germs. Their activities such as mopping up spills also prevent accidents.

In some hospitals the housekeepers clean and restock the patient units after each patient has been discharged. Thorough, careful technique is most important, because the patient's unit is his immediate external environment.

The nursing team has an important and continuing role in patient environment. Providing safety, privacy, neatness, and order, as well as controlling of odor and noise, is a continuous process.

The maintenance crew keeps up the painting and repair of the building and equipment; these factors are also important to the patient's well-being and safety.

The entire hospital team works together to see that the patient's surroundings are safe, clean, and comfortable.

---

5. In the following blanks, indicate a specific duty of each person which contributes to the hospital environment.

     a. Engineer: _____

     b. Housekeeper: _____

     c. Nursing assistant: _____

     d. Maintenance person: _____

ITEM 2. TEN ENVIRONMENTAL FACTORS

Let's examine in detail ten specific external environmental factors of concern to the nurse when providing care to patients. These ten are temperature regulation, humidity control, ventilation, light, use of color, control of noise, neatness and order, elimination of noxious odors, safety, and privacy. Each is now examined in more detail.

Regulation of Temperature. Temperature affects our comfort and even our disposition. A range between $68°$ and $72°$ Fahrenheit ($20°$ to $22°$ Centigrade) is maintained in most air-conditioned hospitals. For patients in the nursery or for the elderly, or at bath time, a slightly higher temperature, perhaps $80°F$ ($26.7°C$), might be required.

When the environmental temperature is high, perspiration cools the body by evaporation. It is essential then to offer additional fluids to patients (unless contraindicated) to replace the fluids lost. Remember also to replace fluids that *you* lose when *you* are perspiring heavily.

Some air-conditioned hospitals have individual controls in the patient rooms to allow for flexibility in temperature control. When this is not available, fans, coolers, and heaters may sometimes be used. Adding an extra blanket, shawl, or bed socks can provide warmth for the patient who feels cold. Remember that the sick person may feel cold or hot even though the temperature of the room is in the so-called ideal range. Hot water bottles are rarely used today because of the danger of burns, especially when caring for the aged, infants, diabetics, and those with decreased feeling such as patients who are sedated, anesthetized, or paralyzed. There are effective and safe heating and cooling devices such as the K-pad and the hypothermia machine with the hypothermia blanket, which use warmed or cooled fluids circulating through tubes in the pad. The temperature is automatically maintained by thermostats. A refreshing bath or alcohol rub may temporarily cool and refresh the patient even though the room temperature cannot be lowered.

||||||||||||||||||||||||||||||||||||||||||||||||||||||||||||||||||||||||||||||||||||||||||||||||||||||||||||||||||||||||||||||||||

6. A desirable temperature range for most hospital rooms is between _____ and

   _____ .

7. Two occasions on which it may be desirable to raise the room temperature slightly are:

   a. _____

   b. _____

8. List three methods of providing a patient with additional warmth (a doctor's order is required for some):

   a. _____

   b. _____

   c. _____

9. List the three types of patients who require *very special care* if external heat is applied because they could be burned easily:

   a. _____ ,   b. _____ ,

   c. _____

||||||||||||||||||||||||||||||||||||||||||||||||||||||||||||||||||||||||||||||||||||||||||||||||||||||||||||||||||||||||||||||||||

Humidity Control. "It's not the heat — it's the humidity" is a common expression. Humidity is the amount of moisture in the air, and a range of 30 to 50 per cent is normally comfortable. Very *low* humidity dries the respiratory passages. As the temperature increases, air can hold more water. At $50°F$, $(10°C)$ saturated air holds 4.2 grains of water per cubic foot of air. (A grain is a measurement of weight.) At $90°F$ $(32.2°C)$, nearly three times as much water is retained. With the air already saturated by moisture, perspiration does not evaporate, and the patient loses a major cooling device.

Unfortunately, there is no simple method of decreasing humidity; it has become a technical problem for air-conditioning experts and is accomplished by modern engineering methods. However, a vaporizer or humidifier is sometimes ordered for patients to *increase* humidity in some respiratory conditions.

Ventilation Control. Ventilation refers to the movement of air. Stale air can be oppressive. The use of fans increases comfort because the air is in motion even though the temperature and humidity remain unchanged. In home care, opening windows — top and bottom — increases circulation when the warmer air rises to be replaced by cooler air. In most hospitals, air-conditioning is used for ventilation and temperature control. Windows are not used for these purposes and should not be opened.

Use *caution* to avoid a chilling draft on the patient. The use of screens between the source of cool air and the patient will prevent drafts.

Circle the "T" if the statement is more true than false, and circle the "F" if the statement is more false than true.

10.   T   F   The higher the air temperature, the more water it can hold.

11.   T   F   Evaporation of perspiration is increased in high humidity.

12.   T   F   The use of a vaporizer increases humidity.

13.   T   F   A humidity of 30 to 50 per cent is considered most comfortable.

14.   T   F   Humidity refers to movement of air.

15.   T   F   Cold air rises.

Regulation of Lights. Lighting contributes to our well-being. However, some illnesses cause "photophobia," a condition in which light is painful to the eyes. Bright light must be avoided during the acute phase of measles. Also, patients who have had certain types of eye surgery must avoid glaring lights.

A sunny room is cheerful and can improve your patient's spirits. Adequate light should be provided for reading and all other close work. This means a light that is bright enough to see without *glare* and to avoid eye strain. Good light is *soft* and *diffused*. It does not make sharp shadows. Overhead fluorescent lighting is generally effective. You can check for glare by holding a pencil or similar object 4 to 6 inches above a piece of light-colored paper. If the outline is sharp, there is enough glare to be troublesome; if the outline is fuzzy and soft, glare should be no problem.

Most people prefer lights dimmed when going to sleep. Adjust the shades, blinds, and drapes to help regulate light. The use of a night-light provides safety for the person who gets up to go to the bathroom at night. This also permits nursing personnel to observe the patient throughout the sleeping hours.

Use of Color. In the patient environment, some bright colors stimulate; other colors are soothing. The location of the source of light influences color. Decorators are aware of this, and colors in patient rooms are usually subdued pastels. In solaria and workrooms, however, bright colors may be used. It is rare now to find the cold, all-white hospital room; most have colorful bedspreads, pictures, and draperies. Many convalescent hospitals are using attractive wallpapers and color combinations to provide a cheerful, homelike atmosphere.

Complete the following statements:

16. A good light is bright enough to avoid straining the eyes in order to see, but it should

     be diffused or without _____ .

17. Why is a night-light desirable in a hospital room? _____

_____ .

Circle the best response:

18. The colors in a room *(can) (cannot)* affect a person who is not colorblind.

19. Most patient rooms in hospitals have *(subdued pastel colors) (bright stimulating colors)*.

Noise Control. Noise is a negative environmental factor (one that patients frequently note and that they complain about) and can affect one's health. People who are careless or thoughtless about talking and laughing cause unnecessary noise. Voices carry loudly in corridors, which seldom have drapes or other sound-absorbing materials. Equipment and machinery, such as floor polishers and carts being rolled down hallways, are often noisy. Dropping equipment causes startling noises. Many hospitals use carpeting, resilient floor materials, sound-absorbing ceilings, and plastic equipment in an effort to decrease noise. This still does not reduce the major source of noise — people.

The hospital should be a place for rest and quiet, and you can help to reduce "people noise." Tact is required when one patient's radio or television is disturbing another. Skill in human relations, which involves both tolerance and courtesy in dealing with people, is very important for nurses. This is a skill that you should continue to develop throughout your lifetime.

Provision of Neatness and Order. Some people seem to thrive in clutter; others are offended by a picture that hangs even slightly crooked. The unit should be kept in sufficient order to be safe, but you must avoid imposing rigid standards on patients who enjoy being surrounded by their possessions.

Remove soiled dishes and unused equipment promptly. Check the unit several times during your tour of duty to maintain neatness and order.

20. List three common sources of hospital noise.

    a. _____

    b. _____

    c. _____

21. How do you think *you* can best reduce undesirable noise in your hospital?

    a. _____

    b. _____

Prevention or Control of Odors. Odors can be pleasant or unpleasant. Unfortunately, unpleasant smells seem to predominate in a hospital. Illness alters our sensory perceptions; for example, the scent of cooking food might produce nausea rather than hunger. Some ways to reduce and control unpleasant odors follow:

a. Dispose of refuse properly. Dressings and refuse should be wrapped in paper or placed in a paper bag provided for the purpose. Place refuse in the proper container with a tight cover to prevent odors for escaping. *Do not* put such items in the patient's waste basket.

b. Remove old, disintegrated flowers and stagnant water, which may be a source of unpleasant odors.

c. Reduce offensive odors from body discharges of the sick person's feces, flatus, and emesis by covering the bedpan, urinal, and emesis basin.

d. Avoid being a source of odors yourself. Odors that may be offensive to others, and particularly those who are ill, include the lingering smell of cigarette smoke; strong foods like garlic on the breath; perspiration or body odors that can be eliminated by bathing and wearing clean clothes; and heavy scents, perfumes, or highly fragrant lotions. All of these are important. The nurse with a spotless uniform and impeccable grooming inspires confidence in patients concerning their own care.

Good ventilation and cleanliness are far more effective in controlling odors than scented air sprays and other masking devices. "Hospital Clean" should be a reality as well as an expression. Prompt and proper disposal and scrupulous cleanliness can decrease odors.

Provision of Privacy. Privacy is essential for the patient's well-being. Always knock gently when the door to a patient's room is closed, and identify yourself before entering. Closing the curtain around the patient's cubicle can spare embarrassment to the patient, worker, and visitors.

Hospital workers become accustomed to situations and functions that would be embarrassing to the nonmedical person. A discreet withdrawal from the room provides privacy for the shy patient to perform necessary functions such as defecating, urinating, or even washing dentures.

Visitors come to see the patient. A polite greeting and withdrawal by the worker allows privacy for patients and their guests. Lack of privacy, like noise, is a frequent source of patient irritation. The thoughtful nurse can do much to decrease these irritations.

22. List two ways in which the patient may be a source of unpleasant odors.

   a. _____

   b. _____

23. List two ways in which the worker may be a source of unpleasant odors.

   a. _____

   b. _____

24. List two ways in which the room or hospital might be a source of odors.

   a. _____

   b. _____

25. List three ways in which you can provide privacy for your patient.

   a. _____

   b. _____

   c. _____

ITEM 3. PROVISION OF A SAFE ENVIRONMENT

We shall talk about *Safety* more than once — it is a fundamental guideline in the unit "Guidelines for Nursing Skills." Remember that safety is necessary in preventing accidents and in reducing the possibility of lawsuits. Various types of accidents occur among patients; the most common are falls, burns, cuts or bruises, altercations with others, loss of a personal possession such as false teeth or money, choking, or electrical shock. The alert nurse is on the lookout for safety hazards and corrects them so that accidents can be prevented.

Patients at Risk of Having Accidents

Some patients are more likely to have accidents than others. One group at risk are those patients who are confused. They may be elderly, on medication, or emotionally disturbed. Their safety is *your* concern. Elderly patients often need special attention. They may be forgetful or have decreased sensory perceptions such as dimmed vision or decreased hearing that deprives them of some of their "danger warning" capabilities.

Another group of patients at risk are children. They climb, touch, taste, and eagerly explore their environments. They need special protection to prevent their curiosity from causing injury.

Patients who are sedated with drugs or anesthesia also need special safety measures such as siderails, straps, and close observation to ensure their well-being.

Falls and Their Prevention

Falls are particular hazards in hospitals. Falls can be prevented by removing foreign objects from the floor that might cause a patient to trip. Handrails and grab bars should be installed in the bathroom and in the corridors to assist the weak or debilitated patient. Siderails are a common safety device. Usually the bed is left in *low* position when the patient is not receiving care that requires the high position. This decreases the danger of falls. You will learn more about siderails in future units.

Mop up spills immediately. Post "Slippery" caution signs when the floor is being mopped. Usually only one side of the floor is mopped at a time, allowing half to remain dry for use.

Soft ties and other restraints may be ordered to prevent falls. These, too, will be discussed in a later unit.

Patients who have poor vision should be given assistance in order to prevent accidents. It is especially important that scatter rugs and clutter be removed and that furniture remain in customary locations.

Burns and Their Prevention

The alert nurse looks out for safety hazards and corrects them so that burns can be prevented. Testing the temperature of solutions used for soaks, baths, irrigations, and heating devices is necessary to prevent burns. Remember that persons with diabetes, those with impaired circulation, those who receive drugs to reduce pain, the paralyzed, and those not mentally alert can be burned much more easily than can a person in good health.

Inspection of all electrical plugs, cords, and equipment before use can prevent accidents. Most agencies require that any electrical appliance brought in by the patient (e.g., radio or heating pad) must be thoroughly checked by the electrician to ensure their safety.

Oily rags and other combustible materials usually are stored in mental containers that have tight lids. Oxygen tanks and other gas containers under pressure should be secured with straps or by other means to prevent falling.

The danger of burns to the patient is decreased by prohibiting smoking while in bed, or careful supervision if it is permitted. Patients who are sedated, confused, or irrational may set the bed and mattress on fire or drop hot ashes in a waste basket, which can start a fire in the room. Smoking is not allowed when oxygen is used in the treatment of the patient. "No Smoking" signs must be posted, and electrical equipment that might cause a spark is removed from the area.

Fire in a hospital is always a possibility; therefore, know the rules for fire safety. Generally, the agency's fire regulations will be taught in the first few days of employment. Many local fire departments hold regular fire safety classes for employees in health agencies in their area. These are required in most states if a health agency is to receive its fire safety clearance from the fire department. Know the location of extinguishers, fire doors, and so forth. Many institutions have occasional fire drills; make sure you know what to do in case of a fire or other disaster.

26. Falls cause many accidents in and out of hospitals. List five ways in which you might prevent falls.

a. _____

b. _____

c. _____

d. _____

e. _____

In summary, the ten external environmental factors with which you as a health worker will need to be concerned in your care of the patient are: temperature, humidity, ventilation, light, color, noise, odor, neatness and order, privacy, and safety. It is your ethical responsibility to your patient, your coworkers, your employer, and yourself to maintain a pleasant and safe environment.

WORKBOOK ANSWERS

1. c

2. a, b, and c

3. composition and volume of fluid around cells, and emotional environment

4. accurate measurement of fluid intake and output, restricting salt intake if ordered by the physician, communication, and good interpersonal relationships.

5. a. oversees air-conditioning, heating and cooling, ventilation

  b. provides cleanliness, order, safety

  c. maintains,safety, cleanliness, order, light, privacy, odor and noise control

  d. carries out painting, repairs, safety

6. $68°$ to $72°$F

7. a. a bathtime in the nursery

  b. when bathing the elderly

8. a. add blankets, shawls, bed socks, K-pad

  b. hot water bottle

  c. hypothermia machine with blanket

9. any three of the following: diabetics, infants, aged, or patients with decreased feeling or sensory abilities

10. T

11. F

12. T

13. T

14. F

15. F

16. giare

17. so the patient can get up safely if permitted; so nurses can observe him at night

18. can

19. subdued pastel colors

20. any three of the following: people talking, equipment, dropping equipment, radio, TV

21. any two of the following: avoid loud talking, care in handling equipment, encourage others to be quiet, keep radios and TV at reasonable levels, avoid noisy activities during patient's rest periods (could be many other similar answers)

22. any two of the following: discharges (feces, urine, pus, emesis), breath, perspiration, flatus, dressings, medications, and others

23. any two of the following: bad breath, strong perfumes, body odor, or the odor of tobacco on clothes, hands, or hair

24. any two of the following: cooking odors, improper waste disposal, lack of general cleanliness, incontinent patients who have not been kept dry and clean, use of heavy masking spray to cover odors

25. any three of the following: close door, pull screen, knock before entering, leave patient alone to use bedpan (could be many others)

26. any five of the following: remove clutter, avoid scatter rugs, mop up spills immediately, post "Slippery" signs when appropriate, encourage use of siderails and grab bars, use restraints when indicated, keep bed in low position, assist patients who have poor vision to walk, avoid moving furniture

POST-TEST

Directions: Circle the letter in front of the correct response or responses. More than one may be right.

1. Management of the hospital environment is the responsibility of:

    a. the nurse

    b. housekeeping

    c. maintenance

    d. all of these

2. The most comfortable range of temperature and humidity in a hospital room is usually:

    a. 70 to 76°F, 50 to 60 per cent humidity

    b. 65 to 70°F, 20 to 30 per cent humidity

    c. 68 to 72°F, 30 to 50 per cent humidity

    d. 72 to 80°F, 40 to 70 per cent humidity

3. Effective and desirable methods of decreasing offensive hospital odors are:

    a. prompt and proper disposal of refuse

    b. use of fragrant perfume by employees

    c. good personal hygiene by employees

    d. good ventilation

4. Bright (non-glaring) light in the room is undesirable in or during the following circumstances:

    a. when the patient is reading

    b. period of rest or sleep

    c. some types of illness (measles, eye surgery)

    d. when the patient is depressed

5. Noise can have the following effects on patients:

    a. cause irritation

    b. disturb sleep or rest

    c. increase fatigue

    d. none of these

6. Ways to provide patient privacy include:

    a. the closed door

    b. cubicle curtain

    c. visitors

    d. withdrawal from unit by nurse

7. Ventilation means:

    a. surroundings

    b. moisture in the air

    c. environment

    d. movement of air

8. A vaporizer in the room increases:

    a. temperature

    b. ventilation

    c. humidity

    d. external environment

9. The *one* major source of noise in hospitals is:

    a. equipment

    b. street noise

    c. people

    d. elevators

10. Fill in the blanks:

    Safety is a fundamental responsibility for all hospital personnel. A safe environment is especially needed by certain categories of patients who cannot regulate their own environment. List four of these:

    a.

    b.

    c.

    d.

POST-TEST ANSWERS

1. d

2. c

3. a, c, d

4. b, c

5. a, b, c

6. a, b, d

7. d

8. c

9. c

10. any four of the following: infants and children, aged, mentally confused, sedated or anesthetized, unconscious, blind, deaf, or paralyzed (could be others)

Unit 4

GUIDELINES FOR NURSING SKILLS

GENERAL PERFORMANCE OBJECTIVE

In a written test using questions representing patient situations, you will demonstrate your knowledge of the guidelines for performing a nursing skill and use the nursing process to plan nursing care to meet the needs of the patient.

SPECIFIC PERFORMANCE OBJECTIVES

Upon completion of this unit you will be able to:

1. As a nurse with beginning skills, carry out the Kardex nursing care plan developed by other nurses for the care of the patient.

2. Use the nursing process of assessing the patient's needs, then plan, implement, and evaluate the nursing tasks used to meet these needs.

3. Prepare to perform the task safely and effectively by assessing the condition of the patient, the abilities and limitations of the student, and the environmental factors that could help or hinder performance.

4. Implement the nursing task using the following guidelines:

   a. Preparing the patient physically and mentally.

   b. Preparing the required equipment.

   c. Performing the task utilizing applicable principles from biological and physical sciences.

   d. Performing follow-up care of the patient.

   e. Performing follow-up care of the equipment.

   f. Reporting the recording accurately and appropriately.

5. Evaluate the outcome of the task by answering the following questions:

   a. Did the task accomplish the intended purpose?

   b. Was it performed safely for the patient? For the worker?

   c. Was it performed in a manner economical of time, effort, and supplies?

VOCABULARY

assessment—the gathering of information from a variety of sources and through any means.
evaluation—judging or comparing the results of those that were expected, or measuring the amount of change and the direction of the change.
implement—put into action; carry out the actions.

nursing process—a problem-solving approach used by nurses to determine the patient's problems or needs by assessing, planning to meet the needs, carrying out the plan, and evaluating its effectiveness.

self-actualization—using more of one's potential abilities; expanding the areas of one's interests and skills.

INTRODUCTION

Healthy people are able to carry out all of the usual activities of their daily life without any problem or assistance from others. They get up each day, dress, brush their teeth, eat breakfast, and go about their work, school, or play. When illness strikes, however, it interferes with their ability to meet their basic needs and carry out their usual activities. They need the help of others, such as family members, doctors, and nurses, to provide for them until they recover. As one entering the field of nursing, you need to understand about the basic needs of people, how to identify problems that arise when needs are not satisfied, the procedures or skills used to solve such problems, and how to carry these out.

Everyone has certain basic needs that must be met in order first, to survive, and then, to grow and function. The physiological needs related to survival must be met first of all, and these take priority over other needs. The most crucial need is for a continuing supply of oxygen, which is required by every tissue in the body in order to keep functioning. Without respiration — the intake of oxygen and removal of carbon dioxide — a person would die within a few minutes. As an illustration of the need for oxygen, consider how long you could hold your breath. The adequate intake of fluids and certain substances called electrolytes are also essential to keep the internal environment of the body constant. Food is needed to provide energy for all of the body functions and activities, and waste products in the form of urine, feces, and perspiration must be eliminated or excreted from the body. Activity or movement to stimulate the body growth and well-being also are necessary, as is the need for adequate rest. Sensory input through the five senses — vision, hearing, taste, smell, and touch — provide information about the world and reality. It is through the senses that we meet our needs for comfort, safety, and stimulation. These needs, along with the psychological needs for love and belonging, for self-esteem, and for self-actualizing, or developing one's potential, have been described by Maslow as the hierarchy of needs. The basic physiological needs have a greater priority over those higher on the pyramid.

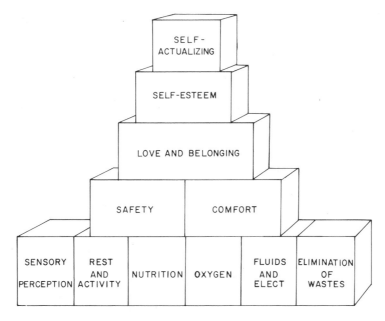

HIERARCHY OF BASIC NEEDS

During sickness or injury, some of the body's energy is used to deal with the damage to the tissues and begin the healing process. This leaves less energy for the sick person to use to carry out routine activities of life and to meet personal needs. During hospitalization, the doctors, nurses, and therapists carry out various procedures and tasks to insure that the essential needs are met. As patients enter the convalescent stage of their illness, they are able to meet more of their own needs. They are able to move about unaided, bathe and feed themselves, perform their toilet functions without help, and begin to make plans to go home in the near future.

In this unit, the nursing process is introduced as a method for determining the patient's difficulties in meeting his or her basic needs and as a basis for planning the nursing care help the patient overcome these difficulties. Guidelines are presented for carrying out these procedures. The practice of nursing involves the nurse's ability both to solve the patient's problem and to carry out nursing procedures competently.

PLANNING NURSING CARE

ITEM 1. A CASE PRESENTATION

The call light is flashing at Room 212. You are about to answer it. This is your fourth week as a student in a nursing class at the local community college. The four hours a day you spend at Hills Memorial Hospital as a student fly by as you perform your duties.

Who is the patient in Room 212 and how can I help her? It may be Mrs. Mary Jones in bed "C" who is the reason for the flashing red light. You observe that the top bedding is pushed back, revealing a very damp drawsheet. This is your chance to be a "good nurse." Of course, you can change a drawsheet in no time at all;

but wait —

Mrs. Jones is a 76-year-old lady who is confused. She is partially paralyzed from a stroke, and she weighs 198 pounds! Are you still confident?

Try this —

Just suppose she is another Mrs. Jones, not the 198-pound lady at all. Instead, she is a 32-year-old housewife with a ruptured stomach ulcer who is getting a blood transfusion and oxygen and has a tube in her nose leading to her stomach and connected to a suction device. Her anxious family clusters about the bed. Remember, all she needs is a dry drawsheet and, of course, you can provide that!

— Or can you?

Don't give up. Room 212 "C" might be yet another Mrs. Jones, who is a 22-year-old new mother and who speaks only Spanish. She will be going home within the hour, taking that adorable baby boy from the nursery. Of course, you can handle this one — just whisk off the wet sheet and pop on a clean, dry one.

You get the idea: It's not simply a matter of changing a drawsheet; these people have needs that require you to plan what to do and how to do it.

Circle the letter of the *best* answer.

1. In order to perform even the simplest nursing skill you need to:

   a. Plan what to do.

   b. Plan how to do it.

   c. Consider the individual needs of the patient.

   d. All of these.

ITEM 2. THE NURSING PROCESS

As you can see, nursing consists of more than following the steps of a procedure or carrying out a task. Nurses at every level use the nursing process to some degree as a method of problem solving. It focuses on identifying the patient's problems in order to meet a basic need, developing the nursing actions required to solve the problem, and then judging the effectiveness of the actions. The nursing process consists of these steps: the assessment phase, the planning phase, the implementing phase, and the evaluation of the results.

The Assessment Phase

Assessment means gathering information about your patients and their needs through a variety of ways. Communication is one of the most important skills, and it is used throughout the nursing process, in assessing, planning, implementing, and evaluating. The communication between the nurse and patient or others may be verbal — talking and listening — or nonverbal, which involves facial expressions, body posture and movement, and gestures. Information is gathered from observing, using the five senses, reading the chart or other sources of information, and consulting with others. The best source of information, however, is the patient, and the assessment begins on admission, when the nurse interviews the patient to find out the major complaints, takes the vital signs, and obtains other pertinent information.

Assessment is important whenever you are faced with a nursing situation. Consider the case of Mrs. Jones as described in the example. Her problem is simple: She has a wet drawsheet that causes some discomfort because it should be dry. But is that really the problem? What happened? Why was the drawsheet wet? Was Mrs. Jones unable to move about? Did she then spill the glass of water while trying to get a drink? Was she confused and unable to call for a bedpan in time to avoid wetting the bed? Might she be running a fever, and the wetness is due to profuse perspiration? Or is the dampness due to bloody drainage? More information is needed in order to identify her basic problem, beyond the discomfort of the wet drawsheet.

The Planning Phase

Once the information has been gathered, the nurse has to sort it out to find what it means and what the problem is. In order to solve the patient's problem, it is necessary to correctly identify it. Mrs. Jones may continue to have one wet drawsheet after another until attention is focused on the underlying problem. Once the problem is defined, then the nurse plans what to do to resolve it. As you plan the appropriate nursing actions and procedures, you will need to consider these factors: the condition of the patient, the size of the patient, the patient's ability to assist, the patient's ability to hear, and the patient's ability to understand our language. (Remember the three different Mrs. Joneses.)

After assessing the patient, assess yourself: Is this task within the personal capacities of my training, policy, physical skills? Should I get assistance? Do I need some special equipment? (You would need help in changing the drawsheet on two of our Mrs. Joneses.)

Last, assess the environment. Will I have to move some equipment? Should I modify the temperature of the room? What are the provisions for privacy?

In addition, these guidelines should be considered when planning your nursing actions.

Safety. Think safety. Plan for safety. Safety means following routines or the procedures so that the expected result occurs. Laws, rules, regulations, and steps of a procedure exist in order to insure that the outcome can be predicted. Accidents occur when shortcuts are taken or changes are made, so the outcome is different from the one that was expected. Whenever steps are omitted, or precautions not taken, the risk of accidents increases. Tossing the wet drawsheet onto the floor could pose a safety hazard to anyone walking by. If it is placed on furniture, the germs from the sheet contaminate the surfaces and could be spread to other patients, causing an infection.

Legal and Ethical Limitations. Of course, it is legal for you to change the drawsheet for Mrs. Jones, and ethical, too. But how about giving Mrs. Jones a medication for headache, starting an intravenous infusion, changing a sterile dressing on the surgical incision, or even giving her a shampoo? In your role as a beginning nurse practitioner, you can legally perform only those tasks that you have been taught to do and which are defined in your job description. Even if you know how to draw blood from some previous work experience, you would not be allowed to do this unless your nursing job description included this as one of your tasks. In addition, when patients are under medical care in the hospital, you are limited in what can be done without the doctor's permission or a written order.

Economy of Time, Effort and Expense. Medical costs are very high, and nurses help curb costs by planning in the economical use of time and effort. Careless handling of equipment causes unnecessary expense. Discarding urine that should be added to a 24-hour specimen may mean an additional day in the hospital for the patient so that the test can be repeated. Making a second trip to the linen room to pick up a clean gown in addition to the drawsheet is wasteful of both your time and effort. Using supplies for a purpose not intended can also be wasteful, such as wiping up a spill on the floor with a washcloth, rather than using a paper towel or a rag.

Circle the best answer, or fill in the blanks.

2. The worker who is careful to work within legal limitations protects:

     a. self

     b. the employer

     c. the patient

     d. all of these

3. Remember the Mrs. Jones with the stroke? After changing her drawsheet, you make sure that the siderails were in place because nurses must provide _____ for their patients.

4. List at least four different methods you can use in assessing the patient.

     a. _____ .

     b. _____ .

     c. _____ .

     d. _____ .

5. When planning to carry out some nursing activity, what factors about the patient do you need to take into consideration?

Implementation

After planning comes implementation, or putting your plan into action. Our guidelines for this are as follows:

Step 1. Prepare the patient. Let them know what to expect. This helps prevent fear. Provide for safety. Pulling the curtain or closing the door provides privacy.

Step 2. Prepare the equipment. Inspect equipment for breaks, wear and safety. Collect as much as is practical at one time (economy of time). Remember, the patients comes first — it is poor planning to bring the bath water in at the same time as the linens because it would get cold before the bedding was removed and before you are ready to bathe the patient.

Step 3. Perform the task. Some of your tasks will have been taught in great detail. Every accredited hospital has a procedure manual that can help you review if necessary. Your team leader is available for help and guidance. Strive for the minimum amount of time, effort, and expense that provides safe care.

Step 4. Give follow-up care to the patient. Provide cleanliness, give explanations, and take safety measures as indicated. Siderails up? Call bell handy? Necessary personal items within reach? It is best to provide for your patient *before* caring for the equipment — remember, people are more important than things.

Step 5. Give follow-up care to the equipment. Proper care of equipment can prevent the spread of infection. Many items commonly used in the hospital are disposable. It is more economical to replace them than to clean and sterilize them. Nondisposable items should be stored in the proper place and marked with the patient's name as needed.

Step 6. Report and record. Reporting and recording are most important. They help provide continuity of care when you are off duty. They fulfill legal requirements and provide a word picture of the patient's progress from the nursing viewpoint. The chart is a legal record. Your recording should be accurate, concise, and appropriate.

Summary. Let's list the steps required to perform a given task:

1. *Prepare the patient.* This means communicating with the patient before beginning.

2. *Prepare the equipment* to save time and effort.

3. *Perform the task* using the techniques acceptable to your institution.

4. *Follow-up care of the patient* for comfort and safety.

5. *Follow-up care of equipment:* proper labeling, cleaning, or disposal.

6. *Report and record.*

━━

6. Place the numbers 1 through 6 in the blanks in the usual order of the steps for performing a nursing task.

_____ Give follow-up care to the equipment.

_____ Report and record.

_____ Prepare the patient.

_____ Explain the procedure to the patient.

_____ Give follow-up care to the patient.

_____ Perform the procedure.

━━

Evaluation

Now that the planning and implementation are complete, let us consider evaluating the outcome. In doing this, we might ask ourselves three questions:

1. Did I accomplish the purpose of the procedure?
   Has the problem been improved or resolved?

2. Was the procedure carried out with:

   a. *Safety for the patient?*
      For Mrs. Jones with the ruptured stomach ulcer, it would mean not disturbing the drainage tubes, managing oxygen tubing, and moving her in such a manner as to avoid an increase in bleeding. These are reasons why you would work under the close supervision of your team leader in this situation.

   b. *Safety for the worker?*
      In moving the paralyzed, 198-pound Mrs. Jones, you would need to apply techniques of proper body alignment and movement. You might need assistance to reduce the risk of injuring yourself.

    c. *Safety for others?*
        Proper disposal of the soiled drawsheet and careful handwashing prevent spread
        of germs that might cause infection in others. (See Unit 8 for handwashing.)

   3. Did you practice economy of time, effort, and money?

       Taking all needed supplies at one trip means economy of time and effort. Also, you
       took only what was needed and did not waste supplies — this showed economy of
       expenses.

ITEM 3. THE KARDEX NURSING CARE PLAN

As nurses assess their patients and develop a plan of care to meet their needs, the information is recorded on a special form that is placed in a visible file holder called the Kardex. The nursing care cards contain a current summary of the medications, treatments, and tests ordered for the patient, as well as the nursing care that is needed. The style and kind of information contained on the card vary greatly from hospital to hospital. Most nursing care cards provide space for a list of the medications the patient is receiving, special treatments, laboratory tests that have been ordered, the diet, the degree of activity the patient is allowed, and so forth.

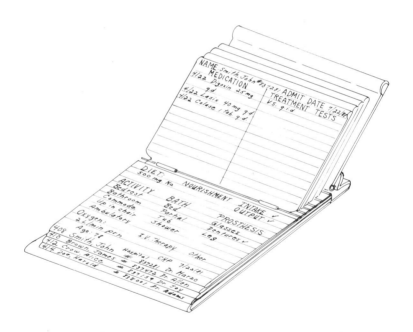

Who makes out the Kardex card and keeps it up to date? Under the nurse's supervision, the unit secretary or ward clerk generally transcribes the doctor's orders to the Kardex as they are written and erases the discontinued orders. The orders are written in pencil so they can be easily changed and kept up to date. All nurses contribute to the nursing care plan by identifying the individual patient's needs, and the nursing actions or approaches to meet these needs. Check with your nurse or instructor before you make changes in the patient's nursing care plan.

As a beginning nurse, you will consult the Kardex card for current information about your patients, their problems or needs, the medical treatments and restrictions, and the nursing care to be given. Your team leader or charge nurse will give you a brief report of the patient's condition, interpret the Kardex nursing care plan, and give you any special instructions that may be necessary. You should work closely with the nurses on your unit and report to them the care you have given, changes in the condition of your assigned patients, and other pertinent information.

ITEM 4. SUMMARY

As a nursing student, you will constantly be faced with changing situations. This is what makes nursing interesting. Skills can be learned and improved. This lesson has provided some principles and guidelines that can help you whenever the call light flashes and you go to help many Mrs. Joneses.

In summary, we have discussed the nursing process that will help to make your work easier as well as more efficient:

1. Assess the patient, yourself, and the environment to determine your course of action.

2. Plan your work.

   a. Consider the legal and ethical implications.

   b. Practice economy of time, effort, and expense.

3. Implement your plan:

   a. Prepare the patient.

   b. Prepare the equipment.

   c. Perform the task.

   d. Give follow-up care to the patient.

   e. Give follow-up care to the equipment.

   f. Report and record.

4. Evaluate the outcome of the action:

   a. Safety for the patient, worker, and others.

   b. Was the purpose accomplished?

   c. Were you economical (time, effort, and expense)?

If you believe you understand the guidelines that have been discussed, ask your instructor to allow you to take the post-test.

WORKBOOK ANSWERS

1. d

2. d

3. safety

4. Any four of the following:
   a. verbal communication
   b. nonverbal communication
   c. observation
   d. reading the chart
   e. books
   f. consultation with others

5. Any or all of the following:
   a. the condition of the patient
   b. patient's size
   c. ability to assist or help
   d. ability to hear
   e. ability to understand the language

6. 5 — Give follow-up care to the equipment

   6 — Report and record

   2 — Prepare patient

   1 — Explain procedure to the patient

   4 — Give follow-up care to the patient

   3 — Performing the procedure

POST-TEST

Matching. Match the activity in Column 1 with the need area most closely associated with it in Column 2.

Column 1	*Column 2*
1. Going out on a date with a close friend.	a. Physiological need
2. Preparing food for dinner.	b. Safety and comfort need
3. Playing a game of tennis.	c. Love and belonging need
4. Thinking well of oneself.	d. Self-esteem need
5. Having a bowel movement regularly.	e. Self-actualizing need
6. Teaching oneself to play the guitar.	
7. Dressing attractively in stylish clothes.	
8. Having pain in a surgical incision.	
9. Begging the nurse not to leave one alone.	
10. Feeling nauseated and vomiting after chemotherapy.	

Multiple Choice. Select the one best answer.

11. Everyone has basic needs that must be satisfied in order to grow and develop. Which one of the following needs has the highest priority and must be met first?

    a. the need for happiness.

    b. the need for oxygen.

    c. the need to move about.

    d. the need for freedom from pain.

12. One of the major effects that illness has on the body is

    a. the person has to be hospitalized for nursing care.

    b. it interferes with the person's plans for the future.

    c. the increase in the amount of sleep needed per day.

    d. it reduces the energy available for other activities.

13. Nurses use the nursing process as a method of

    a. solving problems.

    b. communicating with the patient.

    c. meeting the legal requirements in nursing.

    d. gathering information from the patient.

14. A summary of the current medical orders, treatments, and nursing care for the patient is provided by

    a. the charge nurse in report.

    b. the patient's chart.

    c. the Kardex card.

    d. the unit secretary.

Situation: The following questions pertain to this nursing care situation.

Mrs. Anders, a 72-year-old blind woman in Centerville Convalescent Hospital, has recently undergone surgery for a fractured hip and has a dressing on the operative area. She has been admitted from the acute hospital for convalescent and rehabilitation care. She is one of the patients assigned to your care during your clinical training.

15. It is time for Mrs. Anders' bath. Rank each of the following activities by placing the number "1" in front of the activity that you would perform first, the number "2" in front of the activity you would do second, and so on, to the last activity.

   a. _____ Take out the soiled linen.

   b. _____ Get help to turn Mrs. Anders.

   c. _____ Remove the top bedding.

   d. _____ Put on the bath blanket.

   e. _____ Bring in the necessary clean linen.

   f. _____ Get the bath water.

   g. _____ Pull the curtain about the unit.

   h. _____ Explain what you are going to do.

   i. _____ Go to the patient's unit and check it for supplies, i.e., soap, towels, bath blanket, and so forth.

   j. _____ Turn off the cooler in the room.

   k. _____ Report that Mrs. Anders has a reddened area on her unoperated hip.

16. By reporting the reddened area to the team leader and charting accurately about it, you are: (Place an X in the appropriate blank[s].)

   a. _____ Communicating.

   b. _____ Carrying out a legal obligation.

   c. _____ Providing safety for the patient.

   d. _____ Making use of your theoretical nursing knowledge.

17. You took all of the supplies needed for the bath and linen change. In addition, you took two extra sheets to hide in the closet because the linen supply is often low and you are going to be sure your patient has what she needs. This is being economical of: (Circle letter of best answer.)

   a. Time

   b. Effort

   c. Supplies

   d. All of these

   e. None of these

   f. "a" and "b" only

18. You requested assistance from a classmate to turn Mrs. Anders when you make the bottom of her bed. In getting assistance, you recognize your:

   a. Legal responsibilities

   b. Ethical responsibilities

   c. Personal limitations

   d. All of these

19. After completing the bath, you performed the following services. Place an "X" in front of each one that contributed to Mrs. Anders' *safety*.

    a. _____ Attached the call bell near her right hand and had her locate it.

    b. _____ Placed the bed in low position.

    c. _____ Left the siderail down so she could get up to the bathroom by herself.

    d. _____ Cleaned and filed her fingernails.

POST-TEST ANSWERS

1.	c	15.	a.	10
2.	a		b.	9
3.	a		c.	6
4.	d		d.	7
5.	a		e.	4
6.	e		f.	8
7.	d		g.	5
8.	b		h.	3
9.	c		i.	1
10.	a		j.	2
11.	b		k.	11
12.	d	16.	a, b, c, d	
13.	a	17.	f	
14.	c	18.	d	
		19.	a, b	

CHARTING AND MEDICAL TERMINOLOGY

GENERAL PERFORMANCE OBJECTIVE

You will be able to enter a written account on a patient's chart of the patient's health problems, the therapy given, the patient's reaction to therapy, and your observations of a patient situation.

SPECIFIC PERFORMANCE OBJECTIVES

Upon completion of this unit you will be able to:

1. State the purpose of charting.

2. Describe the two types of charting: the traditional narrative method and the problem-oriented record (POR) system.

3. Record your nursing observations of the patient's behavior, both objective and subjective information; describe the patient's health problems and ability to carry out activities of daily living; and record the nursing care provided and the patient's response to that care.

4. Follow the ABC's of charting by recording accurately and with specific meaning, making the entries brief, concise, and complete.

5. Develop a system of charting to ensure that pertinent information has not been omitted.

6. Correct errors made in your own charting in the approved manner.

7. Use and understand medical terminology with increasing skill.

8. Define and use standard abbreviations correctly.

INTRODUCTION

Charting is one of the most important activities performed by the nurse after giving care to patients. It is the method used to document the observations the nurses make about the patient's condition, the care and treatment that was given, and the patient's response to the therapy. The hospital chart or medical records provide a written history of the patient's illness and can be used as evidence of what occurred or what was done. When the nurse makes certain observations about the patient or administers nursing care but does not chart these, the legal implication is that they were not done or did not exist. Accurate and complete charting gives evidence of the quality of care rendered to the patient and is often the nurse's best defense when something goes wrong.

When you are working in hospitals and health facilities, you will be expected to use and understand medical terms, or the technical language used in the healing arts. Medical terminology conveys precise information to others regarding the biological structures of the body and medical activities. It is used extensively for diagnosis, in operative reports, in the physician's progress reports, and in reports of various examinations and procedures. Although medical terminology is generally not used by the nurse when charting on the nurse's notes, a number of standard abbreviations may be. In this unit, you will be introduced to the hospital chart and the principles related to charting. You will be given a brief introduction to medical terminology and provided with groups of abbreviations that are commonly used in hospitals and other medical settings.

REPORTING AND RECORDING PATIENT CARE

ITEM 1.   THE HOSPITAL CHART

The medical record of the patient's care while in the hospital is called the hospital chart or record. The chart consists of a collection of sheets or forms used to document and record information about the patient. Since it contains much information of a private nature, the chart is handled in the same way as other confidential information. Only those people who are involved in the care of the patient are authorized to read the chart or have access to it. Although the patient, family members, relatives, friends, lawyers, insurance agents, and others may have an interest in reading or gaining copies of records in the chart, they must go through the legal steps of obtaining administrative approval of the hospital before they can see chart information. The chart is the property of the hospital, not of the patient or the doctor.

Following the discharge of the patient, the hospital record or chart is sent to the Medical Record department for safekeeping. Even charts of patients who die must be kept and not destroyed. The old chart from a previous admission is often requested by the doctor when treating the patient again. Old charts are also often used by the hospital to provide needed information regarding insurance claims, and in court cases it is used as legal evidence of events in the patient's hospitalization, and the care that was provided.

Basically, there are now two approaches to charting by those giving care to patients: (1) the traditional narrative style, which focuses on the patient's disease, and (2) the problem-oriented record system, commonly referred to as POR, which focuses on the problems experienced by the patient as a result of being ill. Each health facility uses chart forms designed to meet the needs of that institution, and you must use your own institution's chart forms. Although the chart forms differ in some specific details, most have a similar format and use either the traditional approach or the POR form of charting.

ITEM 2.   TRADITIONAL NARRATIVE CHARTING

The hospital care of patients has traditionally been divided into medical care and nursing care, with each recorded in separate parts of the chart. Doctors complete the history and physical examination forms, write orders for medical treatment on the order sheet, and record notes concerning the patient's progress on a special form. The nurses record vital signs on the graphic sheet and document their nursing care on the nurse's notes and the medication record. Intake and output forms, the diabetic record sheet, the neurological check list, and other special forms are used as required.

On most nursing units, the forms of the chart are placed in a specific order in the chart cover, usually with the most frequently used forms in the front and those used less often in the back. Some forms are made out for every patient; other, special forms, such as the report of an operation or a diabetic record, are used only for those patients who have had surgery or who are being treated for diabetes.

Every form in the patient's chart should bear the patient's name, hospital number, room number, and other required information. In most hospitals this information is entered on a patient identification card and is stamped onto the form by means of the card and an imprinter; if this is not available, it must be written in by hand. The date and time should be included whenever narrative entries are made in the chart, such as when the vital signs or nursing care is recorded on the nurse's notes or when the doctor writes new orders. Entries in the chart are made in black or blue ink, which reproduces better on microfilm. Many larger hospitals microfilm their old patient records for storage in a smaller space. Some hospitals may use red ink for night charting, but it doesn't show up if records are microfilmed.

Forms for Traditional Charting

Although there are some variations in the forms used, the traditional hospital chart contains the following general forms, in addition to whatever special forms that may be required in the treatment of the patient.

General Forms and the Information They Contain

1. *Physician orders:* the physician's directives for patient care

2. *Graphic sheet:* temperature, pulse, respiration, blood pressure, and sometimes weight

3. *Medication administration record (MAR):* medications and intravenous fluids

4. *Nurse's notes:* patient complaints (subjective symptoms); nurses' observations (objective symptoms); notes on patient morale and reactions to therapy; and nursing care administered

5. *History and physical:* physician's record of examination

6. *Progress sheet:* physician's continuing account of patient's progress

7. *Laboratory sheet:* results of laboratory tests

8. *Admission forms:* information on patient identification; conditions for admission; consent for general medical and nursing care

Special Forms and the Information They Contain

1. *Social history:* patient's name, address, religion, nearest of kin, and other similar information

2. *Respiratory therapy sheet:* information regarding the administration of oxygen and respiratory care

3. *Physical therapy sheet:* records of physical therapy treatments

4. *Consultation sheet:* records of physicians called in for referral by attending physician

5. *Surgical or treatment consent:* patient authorization for surgery or treatment

6. *Other:* may contain records concerning blood pressure, fluid intake/output, diabetic information, and so forth.

ITEM 3. PROBLEM-ORIENTED RECORDS (POR)

Since the late 1960's, a new system of recording has gained acceptance as a method of focusing on patient care, not medical or nursing care. This is the problem-oriented record, or POR, first introduced by Dr. Lawrence Weed. POR provides a method of communicating *what, when,* and *how* things are to be done in order to meet the needs of the patient. The problem-oriented record contains four basic parts: the data base, the problem list, the plan, and the progress notes. The precise form these records take will vary greatly between agencies.

The Data Base

The data base contains information of a routine nature about the patient, including a general health history, the findings of the physical examination, and the results of physiological and laboratory tests. It also contains information about the patient's lifestyle, family, and social relations, as well as response to illness as determined in the nurse's assessment. The data base is a collection of information that can follow the patient from the hospital to an outpatient facility and back again. It isn't necessary to make out a new data base every time someone else takes care of the patient, but new information is added to the record to provide and up-to-date description of the patient.

The Problem List

In the POR, a problem is some situation or aspect of the patient's health that interferes with physical or psychological comfort, or the ability to function, or that threatens survival. From the information provided by the data base, the patient's problems are identified and listed on a form that is usually the first document in the patient's chart. The list of problems is dynamic; new problems are added as they develop and others become inactive as they are resolved. If POR is used in your agency, the problem list provides you with immediate information about the patient's needs for care.

Progress Notes: The SOAP Format

The POR progress notes are a section of the chart that contains the findings, assessment, plans, and orders of the doctors, nurses, and other therapists involved in the care of the patient. All chart on the same form, and the progress notes are charted using the SOAP format.

S = Subjective information obtained from the patient or the patient's parent.

O = Objective information based on the health team's observations of the patient, the physical examination, or diagnostic or labroatory tests.

A = Assessment, which refers to the analysis of the patient's problem.

P = Plan of action to be taken to resolve the problem.

Progress notes contain the date and the title of the problem, with the information recorded in the SOAP format. It is not necessary to chart all problems each day, nor will it be possible to include each SOAP element in each note. After the initial plan, additional plans are the changes and revisions made as a result of the evaluation of the previous action.

Example 1. SOAP format (initial admission)

Date	Time	Problem	Progress Notes
6/11	7 P.M.	1	Admitted at 6:30 P.M.

		S	Complains of feeling warm and restless.
		O	Face appears flushed, skin warm to touch. T 103°F. P 120. R 24. B/P 160/90.
		A	Fever of unknown origin.
		P	Call physician for treatment orders; provide tepid water sponge bath.
			Retake temperature 10–15 minutes after sponge bath. Take vital signs q 15 minutes.

U
N
I
T
5

Example 2.

1/5	8 A.M.	2	Abdominal Pain

S   Complains of pain in upper right quadrant. States pain radiates to right shoulder and is precipitated by meals. States he feels nauseated but has not vomited.

O   Patient is pale and appears acutely ill. Diaphoretic and splints abdomen. Patient is taking $FeSO_4$ at present. T 100°F.   P 112.   R 22.

A   Recurring abdominal pain.

P   Put on NPO and notify physician.

PORS Flow Sheets

An essential element of the POR system of charting is the flow sheet. Flow sheets are used to record routine information, recurring observations, and data that are repeatedly entered. Flow sheets are designed by the agency to include the information needed to show routine nursing care and specific treatments. Vital signs, baths, bowel movements, diet, pain, medications, and other activities are included on these forms. Flow sheets may be used for specific assessment data, such as in the CCU for cardiac function and blood gases, for diabetes, for head injuries, and so forth.

In summary, POR charting accomplishes the following:

1. Focuses on the patients and their problems.

2. Reduces the cost of health care by deleting needless duplication of information and recording.

3. Provides for confidentiality by allowing release of information on specific problems, and separation of sensitive data without the need to release the whole chart.

4. Provides control of the quality of care by making the patient data, assessments, and plans available to those giving care so there is less chance that some problem will be overlooked.

5. Provides a method for evaluating the importance and meaning of the patient's concerns.

ITEM 4. WHAT IS CHARTED?

Charting is a skill that takes time to master. As a student, you may feel overwhelmed by instructions to chart your observations of the patient and the care that you performed. You may find it difficult to think of something significant to write down if the patient is recovering without incident, or you may be overwhelmed by so much information that you are afraid of omitting some action or skin blemish that might be important. Guidelines are presented in this unit, and examples of charting are included as part of the procedures described in subsequent units.

Patient Behaviors and Nursing Activities

Your charting should provide a record of the patient's condition and activities or events that occurred; it is not a diary of the nurse's activities. The focus is on the patient, and your nurse's notes should describe the patient's needs, problems, and activities in terms of the patient's behavior. By describing the actual behavior of the patient, the nurse focuses on what exists and is factual and avoids making assumptions and errors in judgment or drawing other conclusions; the chart is kept in the "here and now" of the present, rather than dwelling on past events or speculating about the future. Do not chart, "Patient will ambulate down the hall and back three times today"; rather, chart the ambulation after the patient actually has walked.

Behavior of the patient consists of two types of information: (1) subjective information in the form of statements made by the patient, complaints of pain, or other verbal reports of emotions or thoughts, and (2) objective information in the form of the actual things that can be measured or observed by the nurse. Examples of objective information include the drainage of urine through the Foley catheter, the vital signs, the amount of food or fluids ingested by the patient, and the inability to feed oneself. The POR form of charting emphasizes the behavioral approach in charting by including subjective and objective information in the SOAP format.

The ABC's of Charting

Your charting should be characterized by the ABC's: Be accurate, be brief, and be complete. When these guidelines are followed and when coupled with recording objective behavior observed by the nurse and the subjective information supplied by the patient, the charting gives a meaningful description of the patient's condition.

Be Accurate. Accuracy in charting requires that you be specific and definite in using words or phrases that convey the meaning you want to express. Avoid using the words "appears" or "seems" in phrases such as "appears to be resting." In charting behavior, the patient either is or is not resting. Some words used by other nurses in charting have little common meaning. For example, how much is a little, small, moderate, or large amount? What do phrases like "ate well," "taking fluids poorly," or "decubitus on sacrum" mean? Although they give a general idea of what is meant, they are not specific. We do not know if the patient who "ate well" consumed one half slice of toast and a cup of coffee, or ate a breakfast consisting of a bowl of cereal, scrambled eggs, bacon, a Danish roll, orange juice, milk and coffee. Rather than chart a conclusion such as "taking fluids poorly" it would be preferable to list the behaviors of the patient and the amounts of liquids the patient had taken in a specified amount of time, such as "Given fluids at frequent intervals, but takes only a few small swallows. Intake from 0700–1000: 30 ml coffee, 60 ml orange juice, and 50 ml water." Pressure areas develop quite rapidly in debilitated bed patients, so while an entry on the chart of "decubitus on sacrum" points to a nursing problem, a better description is "Skin of back clear, except for reddened area 1½ inch in diameter over the sacrum" Specific information about size, amounts, and other measurements provides a means for determining whether the condition is getting better, getting worse, or staying the same.

Be Brief. Not every behavior of the patient or observation made by the nurse is charted. To do so would result in such lengthy nurse's notes that no one would have time to read them to find out what was going on. Important information would be difficult to find in the mass of material. Charting must be concise, and that means that you must select the pertinent and more significant behavior and observations to record. Avoid repetition of chart entries such as "Up to the bathroom and voided," before breakfast, again after breakfast, and later in the morning. It is not necessary to make three separate notes; these could be condensed into one by stating, "Up to the bathroom and voided × 3 from 0700–1100." Many nurse's notes have a checklist for patient hygienic and physiological needs, such as type of bath, linen change, type of activity, voiding, bowel movement, and so on. No other notation is made on the nurse's notes about these activities unless there was a problem or some significance in that area.

You can determine whether a certain behavior or observation about the patient is significant or pertinent and should be charted or not. For example, your patient just coughed several times but did not spit out any mucus. Should you chart it? What about a red streak going up the inside of the patient's arm? Should it be charted? In both instances you need more information: How long has it been there? How often does it happen? What causes it? What effect does it have? Does it cause pain or discomfort? Is it part of the disease condition or is it a possible complication?

	Date		H. Day		P. O. Day	

	Chart Time and Initials			MEAL	Type of Diet	% taken
Shift	11 P–7A	7 A–3P	3 P–11P	Breakfast		
AM / PM / HS Care				Lunch		
Complete Bed Bath				Dinner		
Partial Bed Bath				Trips off Unit		
Shower – Tub				To:	To:	
Linen Change				Via:	Via:	
Ambulate				Left: Ret:	Left: Ret.	
Amb. with help				Time B/P P R	Assigned Nurse	
In Chair					11–7	
BRP only					7–3	
Dangle					3–11	
Side rails up						
Safety belt on						
Urine					* All nursing observation entries must be signed by nurse making them. First initial, last name, job classification. Continue Nursing observations on back of sheet.	
Stool						
Specimen to Lab						
MD Visits Dr. Dr. Dr.						

HOURS		* NURSING OBSERVATIONS
A.M.	P.M.	

Hourly check 11-7 shift-nurse initial in box at completion of rounds:

12 MN [ ] 1 AM [ ] 2 AM [ ] 3 AM [ ] 4 AM [ ] 5 AM [ ] 6 AM [ ]

FORM 1026 NRS (REV. 12-74)   24o NURSE'S CLINICAL RECORD

Legend: Sample nurse's note with check-off list for routine activities.

Be Complete. The completeness of your charting should never be sacrificed to the principle of keeping it brief. Not only do you record information about your patient's needs and problems, but the nursing care given for those needs or problems must be included. It is not enough to chart, "Skin of back clear except for reddened area 1½ inch in diameter over the sacrum"; your charting should include what you did about this. The complete entry would then read like this: "Skin . . . sacrum, back rub given and reddened area massaged gently. Reston foam pad applied around reddened area. Eggcrate pad placed over mattress.

Positioned at left side and instructed to stay off back as much as possible to promote healing." This charting is specific and accurate in describing the patient's behavior and the nursing care given; it also includes instructions that are a form of health teaching for the patient.

What constitutes complete charting may vary between hospitals, extended care facilities, or other health agencies. Long-term facilities may require only a monthly summary for patients in stable condition, while hospitals caring for acutely ill patients require continual documentation of the patient's condition, with entries made every hour or two to show that the patient was at least observed during this time.

Systems of Charting. When daily or continual documentation is required, it is helpful for the nurse to develop a system of charting that reduces the chances of omitting or forgetting something that should have been included. Any system that you use should meet the charting requirements set down by your hospital.

Many of the treatments and activities involving the patient occur at specified times during the day, and they should be recorded as having been done at these times, even if the charting is done later. These should remain in chronological order, but other observations may be added as another topic included in the entry, when appropriate. Most systems of charting feature a combination of time-related events and other observations.

In the head-to-toe system of charting, all of the pertinent categories are covered and recorded in sequence. Vital information from the nursing care plan, statements of the patient's problems, the patient's ability to carry out the activities of daily living (ADL's), visits by doctors and family, and other diversional activities are included. Avoid covering too many topics at any one time; otherwise, an entry for 0900 might look like this: "NPO since 2400. Urine specimen obtained, green in color, sent to lab. Dr. Jones visited. Patient complaining of headache."

A system based on charting behaviors that show how well patients can meet their own needs and their needs for nursing care has been found to be very effective in reducing the number of topics to remember to a more manageable number. Times are included to show relationship to activities on the day shift. Needs related to pain or discomfort are charted whenever they occur.

Between 0700 and 0900, chart on how well the patient meets these needs or problems that exist:

1. Oxygenation needs: Describe the level of consciousness, orientation, degree of response, vital signs. This provides a basis for comparison if there is a change later in the day. Notes concerning special equipment related to oxygen therapy, tracheostomy, respiratory or inhalation therapy, and so on, would be recorded when such means are employed.

2. Fluid and electrolyte needs: Describe the patient's fluid intake, as most will have had breakfast by this time; also record the use of IV fluids and abnormal loss of fluids by any route, such as by suction, wound drainage, or diarrhea.

3. Nutritional needs: Record how much the patient actually eats for those who have nutrition-related problems, such as patients on a special diet, and those who have had surgery, extensive burns, or debilitating diseases.

Between 0900 and the end of the shift several entries are made to show the nursing care related to these need areas:

1. General hygiene and condition of skin: Record or check the bath, AM care, back rub, and other hygienic measures. Inspect and record pressure areas, bruises, the presence of surgical incisions, draining wounds, rashes, and the condition of the skin on the back, especially in aged patients who are confined to bed.

2. Rest and activity needs: Chart what the patient can't do or needs assistance doing and include some of the things that he or she can do when progress is made. Most acutely ill patients spend from 20 to 24 hours a day in bed when in the hospital, so state the degree of activity and how it is tolerated.

3. Elimination needs: Record the number of times of bowel movements; flatulence; use of bathroom, bedside commode, Foley catheter; excessive perspiration; colostomy care.

4. Special treatments and equipment: If these have not been mentioned in the other need area reports, describe the use of suction, dressing changes, wound irrigation, use of traction, casts, braces, patient instruction, and so on.

ITEM 5. SPECIFIC CHARTING SUGGESTIONS

Whether a system of charting is used or not, the following subjects are included. Record the information on the proper form and in the space provided for it. In POR records, much of the daily care and routine treatment is checked off on the flow sheets. Many of the charting examples provided for the procedures in this book show how to describe the information needed.

1. Admission: Record the patient's full name, hospital number, room number, age, blood pressure, temperature, pulse, respirations, height, weight, and allergies; also record whether patient wears dentures or contact lenses. Note any prostheses and valuables, identification band number, the chief complaint, known diagnostic tests, and mode of admission (ambulating, wheelchair, gurney).

2. Body care: Chart the hour, area cared for (back, mouth, and so forth), type of bath, and positioning. Indicate special procedures or appliances used. State the patient's body position and describe any required supports.

3. Diet and fluids: Chart the type and amount of food taken, as well as the amount of fluids consumed.

4. Pain: Chart the onset, type, and location of pain and what was done for it.

5. Degree of activity: State whether patient is allowed bathroom privileges, up in chair, or ambulation. If ambulating, chart the distance and how patient tolerated walking.

6. Dressing: Chart the appearance of the wound, any drainage, and the type of dressing applied.

7. Output: Chart the character and amount of vomitus, BM (bowel movement), wound drainage, urine, and perspiration, and the amount obtained by suction.

8. Oxygen: Chart the time oxygen was begun, when discontinued, and the method of administration (mask, catheter, tent).

9. Mental state: Chart any mental symptoms, state of consciousness, convulsions, or untoward behavior. State the patient's general attitude and the time, place, and outcome of such symptoms.

10. Diagnostic tests: Note the time and type of such studies, any unusual occurrences, the patient's reaction, and the outcome.

11. Medications: Note the time, amount, and method of medication given.

12. IV infusions: Chart the time that IV was begun, the type, where given, and the number of drops per minute. Also record the time that the IV was completed, the amount, the condition of the tissue, and the patient's reaction. (Usually the entry-level nurse would not chart items mentioned in the first statement.)

13. Sleep: Chart the time the patient slept during the day as well as during the night.

14. Postoperative care: Chart the patient's pulse, respiration, blood pressure, general condition, time of reaction from anesthesia, condition of wound dressing, and other pertinent factors about the patient.

15. Doctor's visits: Note the time of the physician's visit, examination, and treatments.

16. Specimens: Identify and label each one. Chart the time and kind sent to the laboratory.

17. Procedures performed: Chart the type, time, outcome, and patient's reaction.

18. Death: Chart the time of death, the name of the doctor certifying the expiration, the date when the deceased patient was transferred to the mortuary, the disposition of the patient's belongings, and the name of the mortuary.

ITEM 6. CORRECTION OF CHARTING ERRORS

At times, an error is made in charting. Since the chart is a legal document, the error should not be removed by erasing or painting it out with liquid correcting fluid. Instead, a line is drawn through the incorrect word or phrase with the word "error" written above it; it is then initialed by the person who wrote it. Only errors in charting, such as a misspelled word, use of the wrong word, or an entry made on the wrong chart are handled in this way by the person doing the charting. It is not to be used to delete a charting entry or phrase made by someone else that may differ from what you observed.

A.M.	P.M.	
0930		T W E given. Expelled mod. amount of
		~~dark brown~~ *error* P.W. clay colored stool. P. Walls LN

You may want to write your charting on scrap paper before writing it on the chart until you know how you want to describe the patient's problems and your nursing care. You may need to look up words in a dictionary to be sure of the proper spelling and usage.

If you chart an entry on the wrong chart, you may need to recopy an entire page of nurse's notes, some of which had been charted by other nurses. When possible, have the nurse who charted the original note sign the one would have recopied. If this is not possible, sign your name following the copied signature of the original charter in this manner: Jane Doe, RN/Mary White, NA. The incorrect page is never destroyed but is placed at the back of the patient's chart.

ITEM 7. GENERAL RULES FOR CHARTING

1. Charting should be done by the person who made the observations or performed the nursing service and who thus is legally responsible for the accuracy and quality of the care. Do not chart or sign for someone else unless you are prepared to be responsible or vouch for the accuracy of the information.

2. Check with the hospital or health facility to learn the color of ink used there for charting. Usually blue or black ink is specified because it can be microfilmed. Red ink does not microfilm.

3. Print the proper headings on all new pages added to the chart. Addressograph each page.

4. Entries on the patient's chart should be printed or handwritten. After completing the account, sign the chart with one initial and your last name, and your title, e.g., J. Jones, RN; S. Smith, LVN; M. White, NA.

5. Ditto marks may *not* be used.

6. Record *after* completing each task for the patient and sign your name correctly after each entry.

7. Use the present tense. Never use the future tense, as in "patient to be ambulated."

8. It is not necessary to use the term "patient" on the chart; the chart concerns the patient, and all notations are about him or her.

9. Leave no blank lines in the charting. Draw a line through the center of an empty line or part of a line. This prevents charting by someone else in an area signed by you.

10. Be exact in noting the *time*, *effect*, and *results* of all treatments and procedures.

11. Chart the time that the patient leaves the unit for treatment, surgery, or diagnostic procedure, and the time of return.

12. Use standard abbreviations.

13. Spell correctly. If you are not sure about the spelling of a word, use the dictionary at the desk to look it up.

14. Do not erase. Erasures provide reason for question if the chart is used later in a court of law.

ITEM 8. MEDICAL TERMINOLOGY

Medical terms form a large part of the technical language used by members of the health team. The main purpose of medical terms is to communicate ideas in such a way so that everyone will understand exactly what is meant. Generally, words in our language have a number of different meanings, and their use can lead to their misunderstanding. The word "face" is easy to understand and you know what the speaker is referring to. Or do you? Is the speaker talking about someone's face or appearance, or the face of a clock, or the act of turning in some direction? Medical terms have a specific meaning that is accepted by everyone in the field. Bronchitis means an inflammation of the bronchi, and the bronchi are the air passages of the lungs. In addition, it is more convenient to write "bronchitis" than "inflammation of the bronchi." The use of medical terminology also allows us to convey confidential information about the patient to other health workers and still protect the patient's privacy.

Many of the medical terms we use today are from Latin and Greek sources. Often they are composed by two or more simple words or word elements. The word elements are the prefix, the stem word, and the suffix, and when added to the word they change the meaning. Not all medical terms contain all three elements, as shown by these examples:

Word	Prefix	Stem	Suffix	Meaning
appendicitis		appendix	–itis	inflammation of the appendix
diarrhea	dia–		–rrhea	flow through
gastroenteritis		gastro– entero–	–itis	inflammation of the stomach and small bowel
hydronephrosis	hydro–	nephro–	–osis	Condition of the kidney distended with water (urine)

To assist you in your study of medical terminology, a vocabulary list is provided for each unit that contains the terms used or described in that section. In addition, a short list of stem words and suffixes is included here so that you can try combining them to form different words. Included among the suffixes are those used to name various types of surgical operative procedures.

Common Stem Words

Term	Meaning
append–	appendix; blind pouch
arterio–	artery (carrying blood away from the heart)
arthro–	joint
cardio–	heart
cholecysto–	gallbladder
colo–	large intestine
cranio–	skull
encephalo–	brain
gastro–	stomach
laparo–	abdominal wall
leuko–	white
myelo–	spinal cord; bone marrow
thoraco–	chest or rib cage
tracheo–	windpipe

Common Medical Suffixes

Term	Meaning
–ectomy	to remove a part
–emia	blood
–esthesia	without feeling
–gram	the record made
–graph	the machine
–graphy	the process
–itis	inflammation
–ology	the study of
–oma	tumor
–orrhaphy	surgical repair
–ostomy	to make an opening
–otomy	to cut into
–pexy	to anchor or fixate
–plasty	revision; surgical molding of tissue

ITEM 9. STANDARD ABBREVIATIONS

Many of the medical terms derived from Greek and Latin have been abbreviated for convenience. The specific meanings of such terms have been accepted universally, and the abbreviations are used throughout the United States by those in the health professions. In addition, many doctors, nurses, and hospitals use abbreviations that are specific to their location or nursing unit, but these are not included in this section as standard abbreviations.

You should begin to learn and use the standard abbreviations that are listed here. Other groups of abbreviations have been included, but it may not be necessary for you to learn all of these at this time. They include abbreviations related to time, to body position or direction, to anatomical regions, to measurements, and to the general administration of medications.

Abbreviation	Meaning
abd	abdomen
ADL	activities of daily living
ad lib	as desired

Abbreviation	Meaning
amb	ambulatory
BM	bowel movement
BP, B/P	blood pressure
BRP	bathroom privilege
C	Celsius
$\bar{c}$	with
Ca	cancer, calcium
cal	calories
C/O	complains of
DC, dc	discontinue
D_x	diagnosis
ECG, EKG	electrocardiogram
EEG	electroencephalogram
ER	emergency room
F	Fahrenheit
F_x	fracture
GI	gastrointestinal
GU	genitourinary
Hgb, Hb	hemoglobin
H_2O	water
I & O	intake and output
ICU	intensive care unit
inv	involuntary
irrig	irrigation
K	potassium
lab	laboratory
Na	sodium
noc	night
NPO	nothing by mouth
(O)	orally
O_2	oxygen
OB	obstetrics
OOB	out of bed
OR	operating room
P	pulse
per	through, by
po	orally (per os)
postop	after surgery
preop	before surgery
PRN	when necessary
pt	patient
PT	Physical Therapy
R	respirations
R_x	prescriptions
RBC	red blood cells
RR	Recovery Room
s	without
sol	solution
spec	specimen
ss	one-half
SSE	soapsuds enema
stat	immediately
T	temperature
TWE	tap water enema
UA	urinalysis

Abbreviation	Meaning
URI	upper respiratory infection
wt	weight
WBC	white blood cells

ABBREVIATIONS RELATED TO TIME

Abbreviation	Meaning
AM	before noon
BID	twice a day
H, h	hour
HS, hs	hour of sleep
MN	midnight
PM	after noon
QD, qd	every day
QOD	every other day
QH, q1h	every hour
Q2H, q2h	every two hours
Q3H, q3h	every three hours
Q4H, q4h	every four hours
Q6H, q6h	every six hours
Q8H, q8h	every eight hours
QID, qid	four times a day
TID	three times a day

In many hospitals, time is recorded according to the 24-hour clock, a method commonly used in the military services. The hours are counted from one to 24 and the minutes from one to 59. Four digits are used: the first two numbers indicate the hour, and the third and fourth numbers indicate the minutes. For example 9:30 AM is written 0930, 7:25 PM is 1925. With the 24-hour clock, the 12 AM hours are added to any time after 12 noon.

Twenty-four-hour clock charting compared to regular time charting.

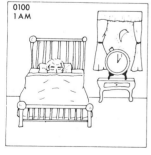
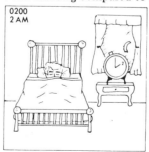
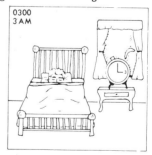
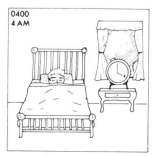
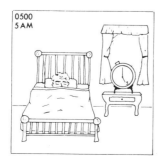
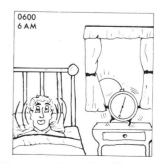

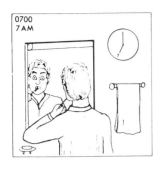
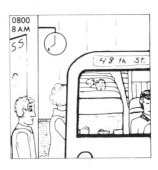
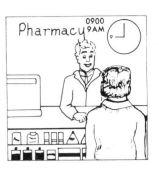
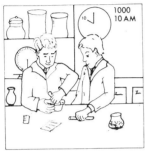
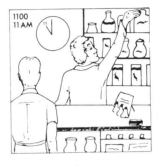
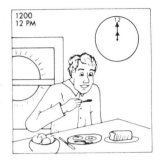
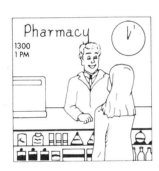
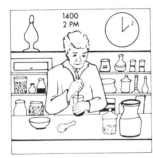
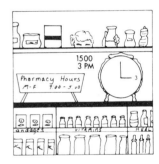
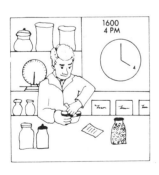
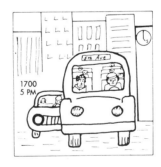
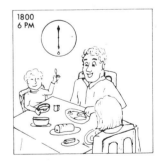
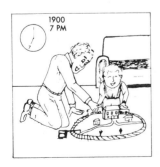
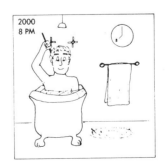
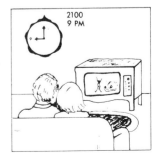

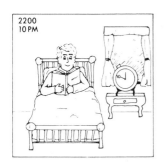
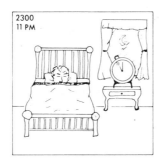
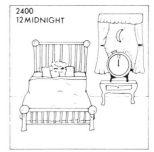

TERMS INDICATING POSITION OR DIRECTION

Term	Meaning
anterior	front of body or structure
posterior	back of body
superior	toward head or source
inferior	lower part, away from head or source
proximal	nearest head or source
distal	away from head or source
inguinal	lower abdomen near groin
lumbar	the loin, the middle of the back
ventral	front of body
dorsal	back of body or structure
lateral	toward the side
decubitus	lying down; bedsore
medial	toward the midline
peripheral	away from the head or source
sagittal	dividing into right and left halves
transverse	dividing into upper and lower halves

QUADRANTS OF THE ABDOMEN

1. Right upper quadrant: RUQ
2. Right lower quadrant: RLQ
3. Left upper quadrant: LUQ
4. Left lower quadrant: LLQ

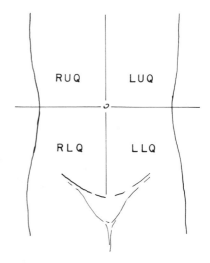

QUADRANTS OF THE ABDOMEN

UNIT 5

ANATOMICAL REGIONS OF THE ABDOMEN

1. Right hypochondriac area
2. Epigastric area
3. Left hypochondriac area
4. Right lumbar region (in back and side)
5. Umbilical (navel) area
6. Left lumbar area (side and back)
7. Right iliac
8. Hypogastric area
9. Left iliac
10. Genitourinary area

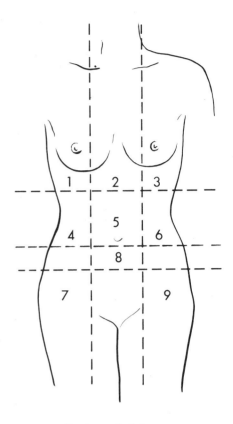

Regions of abdomen.

ABBREVIATIONS RELATED TO MEASUREMENTS

Abbreviation	Meaning
cc	cubic centimeter
cm	centimeter (0.39 inch)
ʒ	dram (about 4 ml or 1 teaspoon)
gm, g	gram
gr	grain (15 gr = 1 Gm)
gtt	drops
kg	kilogram (about 2.2 pounds)
L	liter (1000 ml, or about one quart)
meq, mEq	milliequivalents
mg	milligram
ml	milliliter
m	minim
ʒ	ounce (about 30 ml or 30 gr)
tsp	teaspoon (about 4 ml or 4 cc)
tbsp, T	tablespoon (about 15 ml or ½ ounce)
U	unit (amount as stated or defined)

ABBREVIATIONS RELATED TO MEDICATIONS

Abbreviation	Meaning
aa	of each
a.c.	before meals
amp	ampule, sealed glass flask
bucc	buccal, between cheek and gums
cap	capsule
comp	compound, two or more substances
dil	dilute
elix	elixir, solution containing alcohol
ext	extract; concentrated drug from plant or animal sources
H (H)	hypodermic, under the skin
ID	intradermal, between layers of the skin
IM	intramuscular, between layers of muscles
IV	intravenous, within veins
OD	right eye
OS	left eye
OU	both eyes
p.c.	after meals
pp	postprandial, after eating
tab	tablet

ITEM 10. COMMON DESCRIPTIVE TERMS

Word	Idea to be Charted	Terms Suggested
abdomen	appearance	bruised; ecchymotic; tympanitic; distended; sensitive to touch; tender; boardlike; rigid; protruding; soft; flaccid; flat
bleeding	in large amounts or spurts	spurting blood; profuse oozing;
	very little	minimum amount
	location	blood in vomitus/urine/sputum nosebleed or epistaxis
breath	taking in air	inspiration
	breathing air out	expiration
	difficult breathing	dyspnea
	short time without breathing	apnea
	rapid breathing	hyperpnea
	cannot breathe lying down	orthopnea
	snoring sounds of breathing	stertorous respiration
	unpleasant odor	halitosis
	increasing dyspnea with periods of nonbreathing	Cheyne-Stokes respiration
convulsion	muscles contract and relax	clonic tremor or convulsion
	muscle contraction maintained for a time	tonic tremor or convulsion
	localized muscle contraction	spasm
	began without warning	sudden onset
	abrupt start and end of spasm or convulsive seizure	paroxysm

Word	Idea to be Charted	Terms Suggested
cough	coughs all the time	continuous
	coughs up material	productive
	coughs over long period of time	persistent
	coughs without producing material	nonproductive
	coughs with a "whoop"	a whooping cough
	sudden attacks of coughing	paroxysmal
	various types of cough	loose; deep; dry; painful; exhaustive; tight; hacking; hollow
consciousness	aware of surroundings	alert — conversant; fully awake and conscious
	partly conscious	lethargic; semiconscious
	not conscious, but can be aroused; reponds to some stimuli	stuporous, semicomatose
	unconscious, cannot be aroused; does not respond to stimuli	comatose
drainage	water, from the nose	coryza
	sticky	viscous
	contains pus	purulent
	watery; bloody	sanguineous or serosanguineous
	fecal (contains bowel material)	fecal
	contains mucus and pus	mucopurulent
	from vagina after delivery	lochia
odor	not pleasant; pungent; spicy	aromatic
	like fruit	fruity
	unpleasant	offensive; foul
	belonging to a particular thing	characteristic
pain	amount of pain	use statement of patient; slight to severe
	comes in seizures	spasmodic
	spreads to certain areas	radiating
	begins suddenly	sudden onset
	hurts when moving	increased by movement
	other terms to describe type of pain	dull, aching, faint, burning, throbbing, gnawing, acute, chronic, generalized, superficial, excruciating, unyielding, cramping, shooting, darting, colicky, continuous, shifting, agonizing, piercing, intense, cutting, transient, localized, remittent, persistent
skin	terms to describe condition	pale, red, moist, dry, clear, coarse, tanned, scaly, thick, loose, rough,

Word	Idea to be Charted	Terms Suggested
		tight, infected, discolored, jaundiced, mottled, calloused, edematous, excoriated, abraded, bruised, oily, painful, scarred, black, brown, white, pink, clammy, rash, wrinkled, smooth
speech	unable to be understood	incoherent
	meaningless	rambling, irrelevant
	runs words together	slurs
	difficulty in speaking	dysphasia
	unable to speak	aphasia
	other terms to describe	stammering, stuttering, hoarse, feeble, fluent

U
N
I
T
5

POST-TEST

Multiple Choice.   Select the one best answer for each of the following items.

1. The record of the patient's medical and nursing care while in the hospital is the property of

     a. the patient.

     b. the doctor.

     c. the nurse.

     d. the hospital.

     e. the insurance company.

2. The primary purpose of charting the care of a hospitalized person is to

     a. provide a written history or record.

     b. provide a legal record for the courts.

     c. provide a defense for the nurse.

     d. to prove the high quality of nursing care.

3. The traditional narrative chart contains all of the following forms EXCEPT

     a. the doctor's progress sheet.

     b. the data base form.

     c. the history and physical form.

     d. the laboratory sheet.

4. The traditional narrative type of charting is characterized by

     a. a specific order of forms in the chart.

     b. the focus on the patient's problems.

     c. separation of medical care and nursing care.

     d. patient identification stamped on each form.

5. In problem-oriented charting, the data base contains all of the following types of information EXCEPT

     a. the results of laboratory tests.

     b. the SOAP progress notes.

     c. the report of the physical examination.

     d. data about the patient's family and life.

6. The purpose of the SOAP format in POR charting is to

     a. record the progress of the patient.

     b. list the medical problems of the patient.

     c. reduce the number of forms in the chart.

     d. provide for the confidentiality of the chart.

7. In the POR chart, routine information and recurring observations such as baths and the clinitest of sugar in the urine of diabetic patients is recorded on forms called

    a. the nurse's notes.

    b. graphic sheets.

    c. flow sheets.

    d. treatment sheets.

8. When charting the patient's condition and nursing care, the nurse records

    a. treatment planned for a later time in the future.

    b. goals for the medical treatment and evaluation.

    c. the activities and responses of the nurse.

    d. behaviors that are measured, observed, or stated.

9. The nurse charts accurately by observing the following principle:

    a. qualifies statements by using "seems" or "appears."

    b. uses specific and definite words or phrases.

    c. reports only assumptions and conclusions.

    d. uses general statements and measurements.

10. When an error is made in charting, the nurse remedies it by

    a. lining out the error and initializing it.

    b. recopying the sheet and destroying it.

    c. using an eraser to remove the error.

    d. painting over the error with liquid correction fluid.

    Matching. You are to form the medical term for the meaning given in Column 1 using the stem word that is given and select the proper suffix from Column 2.

Column 1	Column 2
11. to cut into the bladder; cyst–	a. –plasty
12. to remove the tonsils; tonsil–	b. –ectomy
13. to make an opening between the stomach and the small intestine; gastrojejun–	c. –ostomy
14. to repair a rupture; herni–	d. –orrhaphy
15. to make an incision into the abdomen; lapar–	e. –otomy
16. to remove a kidney; nephr–	
17. to revise tissue at the pyloric end of the stomach; pylor–	
18. to remove the uterus; hyster–	
19. to make a new opening in the large intestine; col–	
20. to repair a tendon; teno–	

Column 1	Column 2
21. a record of heart action; cardio–	a. –emia
22. an inflammation of the throat; laryng–	b. –oma
23. lacking white blood cells; leuk–	c. –gram
24. a malignant tumor; carcin–	d. –itis
25. an infection of the brain; encephal–	

Define. Give the correct meaning for each of the abbreviations in questions 26 to 35.

26. qd

27. c̄

28. (O)

29. PRN

30. ad lib

31. stat

32. BP

33. SSE

34. I & O

35. BR

POST-TEST ANSWERS

1. d		19. c	
2. a		20. a	
3. b		21. c	
4. c		22. d	
5. b		23. a	
6. a		24. b	
7. c		25. d	
8. d		26. every day	
9. b		27. with	
10. a		28. orally	
11. e		29. whenever necessary	
12. b		30. as desired	
13. c		32. immediately	
14. d		32. blood pressure	
15. e		33. soapsuds enema	
16. b		34. intake and output	
17. a		35. bathroom	
18. b			

ADMISSIONS, TRANSFERS, AND DISCHARGES

GENERAL PERFORMANCE OBJECTIVE

You will be able to admit, transfer, or discharge patients correctly while demonstrating concern for their physical and emotional well-being as well as for personal belongings.

SPECIFIC PERFORMANCE OBJECTIVES

After finishing this lesson, you will be able to:

1. Identify the types of admissions to the nursing unit as routine admissions, nonroutine and emergency admissions, and transfers from other nursing units.

2. Describe the admission procedure and the responsibilities of the admission office, escort service, medical staff, and the nursing staff.

3. Explain the types of information that are included in the orientation of the patient to the nursing unit.

4. Distinguish between the types of discharges from the nursing units: transfers to another unit, the planned discharge, discharge against medical advice (AMA), and deaths.

5. Carry out the procedure for discharging the patient from the hospital or through a transfer to another nursing unit.

VOCABULARY

assess—gather information or data through observation, the use of knowledge and resources, and communication.
autopsy—the examination of the body to determine the exact cause of death.
comatose—a prolonged state of unconsciousness following an illness or accident.
consciousness—the state of awareness and alertness to one's surroundings.
convalescence—the period of healing and recovery from an illness.
coroner—a public official charged with investigating all deaths not due to natural causes.
gurney—a stretcher or rolling cart used to transport patients.
imprinter—a machine used to stamp data from an identification card onto forms.

INTRODUCTION

The admission to a hospital or health care facility is an anxious time for patients and their families. Patients are usually worried about their health problem and often are having pain or discomfort. The first contact they have with nurses and other health workers is important in helping to allay anxiety and fears. You should greet the patient warmly by name and introduce yourself. Be helpful in any way you can by answering questions and providing information they may need to know about the hospital, the nursing unit, and the care that will be provided. This should be done by every health worker, not just the one assigned to care for the patient.

Patients are admitted to nursing units for care during their hospitalization. In most hospitals, patients with similar types of diseases or conditions are assigned beds on the same nursing units whenever possible. For example, patients admitted for treatment of heart conditions are admitted to coronary care units; those with fractures are treated on nursing units with other patients with orthopedic problems. In smaller hospitals with fewer patients, it may not be possible to segregate patients according to disease, but surgical patients may be grouped on one unit, and those with medical diseases on another.

PATIENT ADMISSIONS AND DISCHARGES

ITEM 1. TYPES OF ADMISSIONS

In the United States, the present health care system does not provide for a person to gain admission to a hospital without the authorization of a doctor, dentist, or other medical authority. Even though the person arrives at the emergency department of a hospital, the final decision to treat the individual in the hospital or a health care facility rests with the physician. While the individual has the right to refuse hospitalization, most people do follow their doctor's recommendations for hospital care.

Patients arrive on the nursing unit of the hospital in one of two ways: as an admission directly from outside the hospital or as a transfer from a different nursing unit within the hospital. Those who are admitted from the community are classified as routine admissions or as nonroutine, or emergency, admissions. The highest priority is given to those patients in the nonroutine category, and the available beds are provided for their care before patients are admitted for nonacute conditions.

Routine Admissions

Admissions are classified as routine when the illness or health problem of the patient does not pose an immediate or serious threat to the individual's life, functioning, or comfort. It is frequently employed for patients undergoing elective surgery, physical examinations, or diagnostic tests and procedures. The patient's admission is authorized by the doctor and may be scheduled days or weeks in advance in order to reserve a bed or a room. On the scheduled date, the patient arrives at the hospital during designed hours and is admitted for treatment. These patients often have X-rays, laboratory tests, and other procedures done before reporting to the nursing unit, since they are not acutely ill.

Emergency and Non-routine Admissions

Those who are acutely ill or injured are admitted immediately, and beds are made available for their care even when it involves cancelling other, routine admissions and prematurely discharging patients who are able to convalesce at home. The patients must be seen by a doctor, who authorizes admission and initiates the medical treatment. This may occur in the doctor's office, in a clinic, or in the emergency room of the hospital. Many emergency cases are transported to the hospital by paramedic units or ambulances, and in some hospitals, people who have suffered heart attacks are taken directly to the coronary care unit rather than to the emergency room.

The admission office is notified of every emergency and nonroutine admission, and the admission forms are completed in the office when the patient's condition allows, or at the patient's bedside if necessary. Required information may be obtained from a member of the family or from a friend, and the consent forms are signed by the appropriate person as soon as possible.

ITEM 2. THE ADMISSION PROCESS

A number of people are involved in admitting patients to the hospital or facility, including those in the admission office and the escort service, the staff assigned to the nursing unit, and the physician.

Admission Office Responsibilities

Clerks in the admission office interview the patient or a member of the family to obtain information needed to complete the required forms for the business records and the patient's hospital chart. The patient is assigned a hospital number, and this is used on all records pertaining to the current stay in the hospital. An admission sheet is completed that contains identifying information such as the patient's name, age, address, marital status, occupation, physician, and admitting diagnosis, and an identification band is fastened on the patient's wrist. A plastic or metal card for stamping identifying data on the chart forms and various records is made up. Consent forms such as the Conditions of Admission are completed, and the appropriate signatures obtained.

The Escort Service

From the admission office, routine admissions who are not acutely ill are accompanied by a volunteer or an escort to the nursing unit. The escort delivers the admission sheet, identification card, and other forms to the nurse or the unit secretary. Wheelchairs or stretchers are used to transport the acutely ill, disabled, or elderly patients to the unit.

Medical Staff Responsibilities

The doctor attending the patient and authorizing the admission to the hospital is responsible for directing the medical treatment, and this should begin as soon as possible. The doctor or, in some hospitals, residents and interns obtain a medical history, carry out the physical examination, and write the orders for medications, treatments, tests, and procedures. Often the doctor authorizing the admission sends or phones orders to the nurse on the unit so that the medical treatment begins from the moment the patient is admitted on the nursing unit. The medical treatment for each patient should include an order specifying the type of diet and the level of activity allowed, as well as other medications and treatments.

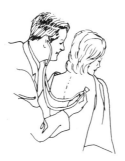

Nursing Staff Responsibilities

When the patient arrives on the nursing unit, the nursing staff assumes the responsibility for his or her care. In many hospitals, the nurse is assisted by the unit secretaries or ward clerks who take care of many of the clerical duties related to admissions. Those clerical duties include preparing the patient's hospital chart, recording the initial vital signs on the graphic sheet, making out nursing care cards and name tags, entering the patient's name on the various nursing unit records, ordering the diet, and transcribing the medical orders.

A member of the nursing staff is assigned to the tasks related to the admission of the patient. These include (1) orienting the patient to the unit, (2) taking care of the patient's property, and (3) planning and carrying out the nursing care.

Orienting the Patient. The degree to which the nurse orients the patient to the nursing unit and the hospital depends on the condition of the patient. For the acutely ill patient, it may be limited to only the essential things that the person needs to know; for those not as ill it is more detailed. Most patients need to know the location of their room, the operation of the call light or intercom system for calling the nurse, the location of the bathroom and the emergency call light, the way to operate the controls of the bed, and instructions about making and receiving telephone calls. The nurse should also explain the daily routine of the nursing unit, such as the times that meals are served, the usual bedtime, and other regulations affecting the patients.

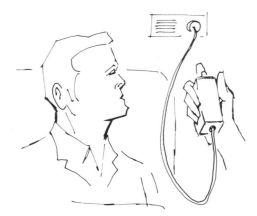

Visiting hours vary greatly from hospital to hospital, as well as for different nursing units within the same hospital. You will need to find out what they are for your agency and nursing unit. Some nursing units allow visitors from 10 A.M. until 8:30 or 9 P.M., while others limit visiting from 2 to 4 P.M. and from 7 to 8 P.M. Coronary care and intensive care units generally restrict visitors to no more than five minutes out of the hour to avoid overtiring the critically ill patient. In many hospitals, visitors are limited to two persons at a time owing to the limited space and number of chairs in the patient's room and to the need to keep the noise level down. Children under the age of 14 or 16 may be barred from visiting in order to minimize the possible exposure of the sick person to various infectious diseases. Furthermore, young children are often frightened and disturbed by tubes and equipment used in treating patients, especially when a loved one is involved.

Hospitals frequently provide a booklet for patients that gives general information about the hospital, the services available, regulations affecting patients, and so forth. It describes such things as the hospital gift shop and library and the hospital safe (for storage of valuables); the location of the chapel, lounges, and cafeteria or dining facilities for the public; the availability of chaplains, social service workers, or barber services; and the policy about smoking.

Care of the Patient's Property. Patients come to the hospital with various kinds of possessions; however, there is limited space in the room or patient unit for the storage of personal clothing, cosmetics, hygiene articles, and other belongings. In some hospitals, all of the items brought in by the patient are inventoried and a record of them is placed on the chart. If this is the policy at your hospital, you will need to fill out the patient clothing and property inventory form.

Although reasonable care is provided for the patient's possessions, the hospital is not held liable for loss of or damage to the items kept at the bedside, including those things of value. Valuables such as jewels, rings, watches, furs, and so forth as well as large amounts of cash, should be sent home or placed in the hospital safe. The nurse follows the hospital procedure to inventory valuables for safekeeping. Ordinarily, items that have a sentimental value such as pictures, letters, trinkets, keys, and pocket knives are not locked up as valuables. Patients are encouraged to keep only a few dollars or some change at the bedside for newspapers or incidental purchases.

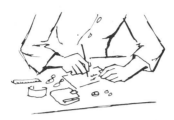

Medications brought to the hospital should be sent home or taken to the pharmacy for safekeeping during the patient's hospital stay. These are returned at the time of discharge. Only medications dispensed by the hospital pharmacy are used during the hospital stay. The reason for this policy is to ensure the accuracy of the contents of the medication; patient-owned medications might prove to be a legal liability if an error has been made or contents switched.

Providing the Nursing Care. In addition to carrying out the doctor's orders for the treatment of the patient, the nurse must gather information in order to plan and carry out the nursing care. It is important to know the condition of the patient upon admission, so the following information is obtained:

— the level of consciousness: whether the patient is alert, lethargic or drowsy, semicomatose, or comatose;

— the vital signs, including blood pressure;

— any difficulty in breathing, such as wheezing, dyspnea, and coughing;

— the weight and the general body build (heavy or obese, thin, or emaciated);

— the ability to communicate thoughts and needs; the language used (e.g., English, Spanish, French);

— nature of the complaints, such as pain, discomfort, or inability to do something;

— any restriction in movement;

— condition of the skin, for example, bruises, pressure areas, dryness, birthmarks;

— any difficulty in seeing or hearing;

— the use of prosthetic devices, including dentures, glasses, hearing aids, wigs, or artificial limbs.

Your nursing unit may also use a nursing history form that focuses on the patient as an individual who happens to be sick and provides useful information for making a nursing plan of care. Although such forms vary, they often include information about food likes and dislikes, the usual pattern of daily activities, types of interests, special needs of the patient, and feelings about the illness of hospitalization.

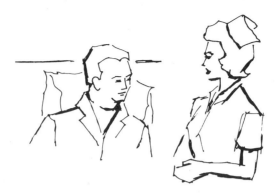

ITEM 3. PREPARATION OF ROOM FOR NEW PATIENT

Upon notification that a patient will be admitted, prepare the patient's room for the new arrival.

EQUIPMENT NEEDED:

Sphygmomanometer and stethoscope	Admission checklist, if used
Thermometer	Urine specimen container

Important Steps	Key Points
1. Open the bed.	Turn back the covers, fluff the pillow, and adjust lights, temperature, and ventilation.
2. Lower the bed.	This makes it easier and safer for the patient to get in. (Place the bed in high position if the patient comes to the room by stretcher.)
3. Place a gown on the bed.	Patients usually change into hospital gowns in preparation for the examination by the doctor and the beginning of their treatment. If not too ill, some patients may prefer to wear their own sleeping garments.

ITEM 4. PATIENT'S ARRIVAL ON THE UNIT

Upon arrival of the patient to the unit:

Important Steps	Key Points
1. Greet the patient and introduce yourself.	Call patient by name and check the identification band. Give the chart to the ward clerk or nurse. Tell the patient and the family, "I'm Miss Olsen, the nurse assigned to take care of you." Be warm, friendly, and courteous. First impressions should make the patient feel that he has been expected.
2. Take the patient to the room.	Introduce the patient to his or her roommates if admitted to a multiple bed unit.

Important Steps	Key Points

3. Provide privacy for the patient to undress.

Pull the curtains to give patient privacy for changing into either the hospital gown or own sleeping garments. Provide assistance if needed and prepare for tests or treatment to begin. Be sure the room is warm and free of drafts. When a screen or curtain is not available close the door to the corridor.

4. Obtain a urine specimen, if required.

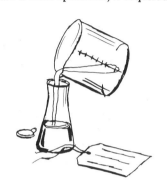

Ask the ambulatory patient to go to the bathroom and void into the container. Have the patient on bedrest use the bedpan or urinal. (Refer to Unit 24, Urine Elimination.)

Excitement or apprehension often acts as a stimulating force in elimination, making this a good time to obtain the urine specimen. If the patient is unable to void, however, leave the container at the bedside for later use.

U
N
I
T
6

5. Help the patient put belongings in the appropriate storage place.

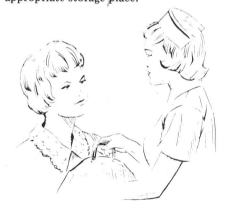

Hang clothes neatly in the closet. Place personal hygiene articles in the bedside stand (toothbrush, comb, brush, and deodorant). Put the empty suitcase in the closet or ask the family to take it with them.

Make out a clothing list and inventory the patient's belongings. Follow your hospital's procedure for placing valuables in safekeeping.

Many hospitals issue patients an admission pack containing disposable plastic utensils such as bath basin, bedpan, emesis basin, and water pitcher. The cost is added to their bills, so the items are part of their belongings.

6. Assess the patient's physical and emotional well-being.

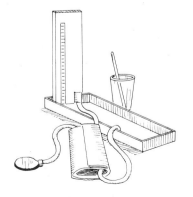

Record the information on the admitting record as you proceed. Later, transfer it to the patient's chart.

   a. Take the T, P, R, and BP.

   b. Weigh the patient (use either the portable scales or the health scales in the treatment room).

   c. Observe the patient carefully during the entire procedure for level of consciousness; difficulty breathing; limited movement; complaints of pain or discomfort; ability to communicate, hear, and see; the condition of skin; and the use of any prosthetic devices.

Important Steps	Key Points
7. Explain the use of hospital equipment.	Demonstrate how to use the *call button* and intercom (communication system) for calling the nurse. Attach the call light conveniently within the patient's reach; demonstrate the use of the bathroom emergency call button. Explain how to operate the bed controls for the bed; demonstrate the operation of the TV controls; and explain how to use the telephone for outside calls. Be sure that the telephone is easy to reach.

8. Explain the hospital routine.

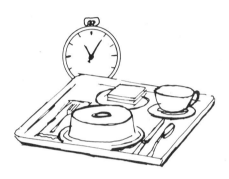

Tell the patient when meals will be served and explain the visiting hour regulations.

Explain what the patient is expected to do for laboratory tests, X-ray examinations, or special treatments that have been ordered. If the patient is scheduled for surgery, explain that surgical preps (shaves) are usually done in the evening by someone from the operating room. Mention the volunteer service for obtaining newspapers, toilet articles, reading materials, and so forth.

Describe the various personnel the patient will have contact with, such as nursing assistants, orderlies, LPNs, RNs, student nurses, and personnel from other departments (housekeeping, dietary, and maintenance).

9. Provide for the patient's safety.

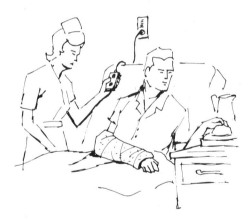

Place the bed in the low position. Raise the siderails if indicated. Place the call light and TV and bed controls within easy reach. Put the bedside table near the bed and within easy reach. Make sure the patient is in good body alignment.

10. Report and record.

Transfer information from your admission form to the nurses' notes. Report any unusual findings to your team leader. Take the urine specimen (properly labeled) immediately to the laboratory. Charting example:

1445. Admitted per stretcher to Room 604. Put to bed. Dr. Healer notified. Alert and oriented. Stated that he injured his back in a fall. Skin is clear with no redness or rash noted, except for a bluish brused area 4 inches in diam. in the left lumbar area. Tender to touch. B/P—156/88, T—98, P—80, R—18. No dyspnea. Voided 250 ml of dark straw-colored urine, spec. sent to the lab.   B. Olsen, SN

ITEM 5. TYPES OF DISCHARGES

Millions of people are admitted to hospitals in this country each year for an average stay of five to seven days. The length of the hospital stay depends on the seriousness of the disease, the patient's rate of progress toward recovery, and the age of the patient. Older patients tend to be sicker, have more chronic conditions affecting their health, and require longer periods of hospitalization. As patients enter the convalescent stage of their illness, they begin to look forward to leaving the hospital. When they are able to care for themselves, or have someone to take care of them, they are discharged to their own homes. Others are discharged to convalescent hospitals or extended care facilities when they need more care and help than is available in the home.

While the vast majority of patients admitted to a nursing unit in the hospital receive treatment, recover, and are discharged back into the community, other patients are transferred from one nursing unit to another owing to changes in their need for specific types of care. Many aspects of the transfer procedure are similar to the procedure for the discharge of a patient, since both involve the patient's release from the unit and removal from the census count. Finally, about 80 per cent of the people who die annually expire in hospitals and other health care facilities. After death occurs, the body is released to the mortuary and the hospital chart and other records are closed according to the discharge procedure.

In summary, patients are discharged from the nursing unit, or from the hospital, in one of the following ways: planned discharge home or to another facility in the community, transfer to another nursing unit within the hospital, discharge against medical advice, or discharge by reason of death. For each type of discharge, the nurse assists the patient as needed, takes care of the personal possessions, and completes the patient's chart and other records. Nursing care of patients continues until they leave and are safely out of the hospital. Most hospitals require that patients be discharged by wheelchair, even though they are able to walk. As an added safety precaution, patients are escorted to the exit by one of the staff. If at all possible, discharged patients are encouraged to have a family member or friend accompany them.

ITEM 6. PLANNED DISCHARGE OF THE PATIENT

A number of people may be involved in planning the discharge and continued care of the patient after release from the hospital. The planned discharge is initiated by the doctor, who advises the patient that he or she is well enough to leave the hospital and writes an order to this effect on the patient's chart. The services of social workers are often needed when planning the discharge of elderly or poor patients who need continuing care, a housekeeper, visiting nurses, or other special arrangements. Utilization review committees make recommendations about the hospitalization and continuing care of patients who receive medical benefits from governmental programs such as Medicare and Medicaid. Law enforcement officers must be consulted when discharge is planned for patients who are on a "police hold" and are being detained on criminal charges by the authorities.

Many of the clerical tasks related to the discharge of patients are carried out by unit secretaries or ward clerks. They complete and rearrange the hospital charts for the medical records department, record the discharge on census records, arrange for the return of the valuables envelope from the hospital safe, and notify other departments such as dietary, housekeeping, and the business office. Before the patient can be released from the nursing unit, financial arrangements for paying the bill must be made in the business office by the patient or a member of the family.

Patients may be discharged by ambulance service, and a time is usually scheduled for the departure. Make sure that the patient is completely ready for discharge when the ambulance personnel arrive. Again, be courteous and helpful as you assist the patient in packing personal belongings and leaving the hospital.

U
N
I
T
6

Important Steps	Key Points
1. Wash your hands, identify the patient, and explain the procedure.	Determine the expected time of discharge and the time when family, friends, or ambulance will arrive.
2. Obtain the patient's valuables from the safe.	The patient must sign the release tab on the valuables envelope; this indicates that the items have been returned. The signed receipt will either be attached to the patient's chart or returned to the business office for filing.
3. Provide instructions for home care as indicated.	Make certain that the patient or family has received prescriptions or medications and instructions concerning a. special diet (from the dietitian) b. future appointments with the doctor c. activities that are permitted and those that are restricted.
4. Assist the patient to dress and pack. 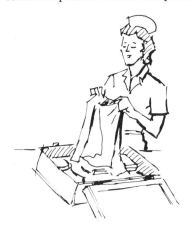	Help patient to pack belongings; check the bedside stand and clothes closets. Assist patient to dress as needed.
5. Verify that the business office procedure has been completed.	Most agencies require a special release form that must be completed by the business office before the patient can leave. The patient or a member of the family goes to the business office to take care of the financial arrangements.
6. Obtain a wheelchair.	Assist the patient into the wheelchair, and secure the safety belts. The excitement of "going home" often causes patients to overestimate their physical strength, and feel the wheelchair is not necessary. However, most institutions require the use of wheelchairs for patients being discharged.
7. Transport the patient and belongings to the exit.	Most agencies have a discharge area where the patient is protected from the weather when getting into the car. Assist the patient to the car.
8. Return the wheelchair to the storage area.	Some agencies have a special area for returning supplies so they can be cleaned before reuse. In any event, when you return the equipment, be sure it is clean and in good working order.

Important Steps	Key Points
9. Prepare for terminal cleaning of the patient's unit by stripping the bed.	In most agencies, nursing personnel are responsible for this activity, but the actual cleaning is done by the housekeeping department.
10. Report and record.	Report to your team leader and ward clerk that the patient is gone. Chart the discharge on the nurses' notes. Information should include the time, the means of transport (stretcher or wheelchair), a statement about the patient's general condition, the destination (home or another health facility), and any other appropriate comments. Remove the chart from the chart holder and put it in the area designated for discharge charts. Charting example: 1430. Discharged via wheelchair to home with dietary instructions and prescriptions. <div align="right">B. Olsen, SN</div>

U
N
I
T
6

In addition, the nurse or unit secretary carries out these additional steps when patients are discharged:

Important Steps	Key Points
1. Return unused drugs and items for credit.	Make out the correct forms, and return items such as suction machines and trapezes to Central Supply.
2. Discharge patient from unit records.	The name is listed on census forms as a discharge; the diet is cancelled; and Kardex cards, identification card, and nursing care plans are disposed of according to agency policy.
3. Complete the patient's hospital record.	All charting on graphic sheet, nurses' notes, and medication record should be complete. The chart is removed from the chart cover and arranged in the order required by medical record department.

ITEM 7.   TRANSFER TO ANOTHER NURSING UNIT

Patients are often transferred from one nursing unit of the hospital to another as their need for care changes. In addition to the general nursing units, many hospitals have set up special care units that provide complex and highly technical care. Patients are transferred to these units when acutely ill and requiring that type of care, and then transferred back to general nursing unit when the special care is not longer required. These special care centers include intensive care units, coronary care unit, burn units, hemodialysis units, and rehabilitation units.

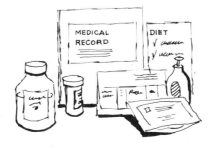

The procedure for transferring the patient to another unit is similar to the discharge procedure, except that the patient remains in the hospital. The patient's chart, the Kardex card, the nursing care plan, the identification plate, and related records are sent to the new unit with the patient and the personal belongings. In most cases, the transfer is made using a wheelchair or stretcher, although acutely ill patients may be taken to the new unit in their beds.

Important Steps	Key Points
1. Wash your hands, identify the patient, and collect his personal items. 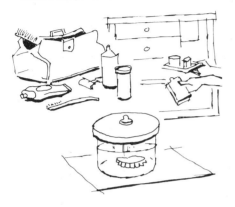	Explain the reason for the transfer to the patient. Check the bedside stand, clothes closets, dressers, and bathroom. Be sure to take all of the clothes, luggage, personal items, and dentures. If these items are lost during the transfer, you may be held responsible. Collect all equipment, such as the bedpan, washbasin, and emesis basin, and take them with the patient.
2. Transfer the patient.	Take the patient's chart and medications with you and move the patient by wheelchair or stretcher, to the new unit. Remember to use good body movement both for yourself and your patient during this procedure.
3. Check in with the nurse on the receiving unit.	Give the chart, medications, and related records to the nurse. Take the patient to the room or bed number as directed. Report to the nurse and give information about the patient's condition and needs as appropriate. The nursing staff on the receiving unit then carries out the admission procedure. Your assistance may be needed to help get the patient into bed before you return to your assignment unit.
4. Return the wheelchair or stretcher to the storage area.	Remove soiled linen from the stretcher and replace it with clean linen, ready for the next usage.
5. Prepare the patient's former unit for terminal cleaning.	Strip the room of used linens and supplies. Make it ready for terminal cleaning by housekeeping personnel or nursing personnel, according to your agency procedure.
6. Report and record.	Note the transfer on the patient's chart, including the time and means of transfer (wheelchair or stretcher). Chart any unusual occurrences. Charting example: 1030. Continues to complain of chest pain. O_2 per nasal cannula at 3 L/min. 1045. Transferred to coronary care unit per stretcher. K. Overhill, SN

ITEM 8. DISCHARGE AGAINST MEDICAL ADVICE (AMA)

From time to time, a patient may exercise his or her right to refuse further treatment and leave the hospital, even though the doctor does not agree to discharge. Often the patient is angry or upset with the doctor, the hospital routine or regulations, or the kind of care that was given. When the patient insists on leaving, the nurse notifies the doctor. The doctor advises the patient of the need for continued hospitalization and the possible consequences or results of leaving at that time and asks the patient to sign a form indicating that he or she understands that the action of leaving the hospital is against medical advice. Threats to refuse patients medical or hospital care in the future should not be used to force them either to sign the form or to remain in the hospital against their will. If the patient refuses to sign the form, this should be indicated on the form, and this is placed in the chart.

ITEM 9. DISCHARGE BY DEATH

In comparison to the number of patients who recover and are discharged from the hospital, the number who die in health care settings is very small. Since the majority of deaths occur in hospitals, however, nurses and other health care workers are more apt to be involved in the care of the critically ill or dying person than are the general public. When the nurse finds a patient who has stopped breathing or has no detectable pulse, cardiopulmonary resuscitation (CPR) is started immediately, unless there are orders on the patient's chart stating "No CPR." Many patients have been revived through CPR and saved from a premature death. The CPR team is summoned to the bedside by an announcement of "Code Blue in Room _____ ."* Members of the team bring the crash cart with emergency supplies and provide supportive treatment. If CPR is not done or is unsuccessful, the patient is pronounced dead and medical care is terminated.

Pronouncement of Death

Recent advances in organ transplantation have led to the belief that the doctor is the best qualified person to determine when death occurs and that it is preferable if the person is pronounced dead by a doctor rather than by a nurse, police officer, military corpman, or others. After death has been determined, the nursing staff prepares the body for release to the mortuary (see unit 37). The doctor also signs the death certificate, which is required by every state. The death certificate contains information identifying the person, the cause of death, and the date and time of death.

Autopsies

An autopsy is an examination conducted after death to determine the cause of death. It may be requested by the doctor, who must obtain the signature of the next-of-kin on a special consent form. Autopsies may be requested by the coroner, who is a public official, when persons die under specific conditions, including deaths by murder, by suicide, in accidents, under suspicious circumstances, and when the person had not been under a doctor's care.

---

*Your hospital may use a different code.

Discharge by Death

The following procedure is followed:

Important Steps	Key Points
1. Pronouncement of death by a doctor.	Record the time and the name of the doctor. A death certificate is prepared for the doctor to sign and the cause of death is stated.
2. Postmortem care of the body.	Refer to Unit 37 for steps of the procedure.
3. Removal of the body by authorized agent.	The body is sent to the hospital morgue or released to the mortuary or the coroner.
4. Collect the personal belongings and valuables.	Follow the appropriate hospital policies to inventory the items and release them to the next-of-kin or other designated agent. Be careful not to give the personal possessions to just any family member, because it is now part of the deceased person's estate.
5. Return unused drugs and items for credit.	
6. Discharge the deceased from the unit records.	List on census form as a death or expiration; cancel diet and other therapy; dispose of Kardex cards, nursing care plan, identification plate, and so forth, according to agency policy.
7. Complete the patient's hospital chart.	Describe the incidents leading up to the pronouncement of death, the time of death, and the name of the doctor. Prepare the chart for the medical record department.

PERFORMANCE TEST

1. Read through the following situation. Record the appropriate information on the nurses' notes.

   On December 22, 1970 at 2:15 P.M., a Caucasian male, age 63, was admitted via wheelchair to room 466. He undressed and was assisted to bed. Vital signs 98.2—82—22, BP 122/82, Wt. 152 lbs., Ht. 6 ft. He was alert but appeared to have difficulty moving his right arm and leg. He complained of nausea and vomiting, and stated his stomach hurt. While assisting him to bed, you noticed a small bruise on his right ankle and a large reddened area on his sacrum. A urine specimen was obtained and sent to the lab. His doctor was notified.

2. Given a partner in the skill laboratory, you will prepare the "patient" and carry out the procedure for admission, transfer, or discharge. You will assemble the necessary equipment, supplies, and records, explain to the patient what you are going to do, follow the procedure established in the lesson, and practice the charting of your activity on the nurses' notes. Explain *what* you are doing and *why* so that both the "patient" and your instructor will be able to follow your line of reasoning.

U
N
I
T
6

PERFORMANCE CHECKLIST

ADMISSION

1. Adjust the height of the bed: low if the patient is ambulatory, high if on a stretcher.

2. Prepare the environment: open a bed, adjust the lights, temperature, and ventilation.

3. Provide a hospital gown and towels.

4. Assemble the admitting equipment: urine specimen container, sphygmomanometer, stethoscope, thermometer, and admission checklist.

5. Await the patient's arrival.

6. Greet the patient and check the identification band.

7. Give the chart to the nurse.

8. Introduce yourself.

9. Take the patient to the room.

10. Wash your hands.

11. Pull the screen.

12. Assist the patient into a hospital gown.

13. Obtain a urine specimen.

14. Hang patient's clothes neatly in the closet.

15. Inquire about valuables and medications, take the necessary steps.

16. Assess the patient's temperature, blood pressure, and weight; observe objective symptoms and elicit subjective symptoms from the patient.

17. Explain hospital procedures: the call signal and emergency call system, and the television and bed controls.

18. Explain the agency schedules and procedures: meals, visiting, laboratory and X-ray exams, prep, volunteer service, and types of personnel.

19. Provide for safety: lower the bed, position the siderails, check the controls, and make sure there is a bedside stand nearby.

20. Leave the patient comfortable and in good body alignment.

TRANSFER

1. Wash your hands, identify the patient, and explain the procedure.

2. Collect the patient's personal items.

3. Obtain a stretcher or wheelchair to transport patient.

4. Transfer the patient to the new unit.

5. Take the chart and medications and deliver to charge nurse.

6. If needed, assist the nursing staff on the receiving unit to transfer the patient into bed.

7. Return the stretcher or wheelchair to the storage area.

8. Return to the patient's former unit and strip the bed for a terminal cleaning.

9. Chart the procedure on nurses' notes.

DISCHARGE

1. Obtain the discharge order.

2. Wash your hands, identify the patient, and explain the procedure to the patient.

3. Obtain the valuables.

4. Check to see if special instructions have been carried out, e.g., take-home medications provided, special diet instructions given.

5. Assist the patient to pack and dress (make sure all personal items are packed).

6. Verify the final business office clearance.

7. Obtain a wheelchair for transportation.

8. Transport the patient and belongings to the discharge area.

9. Assist patient to car.

10. Return the wheelchair to the storage area.

11. Return to the patient's room, strip it, and make it ready for a terminal cleaning.

12. Record the activity on nurses' notes.

POST-TEST

Directions: Choose the one best answer for each item.

1. The admission of patients to hospitals for care is authorized by

    a. the nurse

    b. the doctor.

    c. the admission clerk.

    d. the hospital administrator.

2. The patient scheduled to report to the hospital one week from today in order to have an operation a few days later is classified as what type of admission?

    a. Nonroutine admission.

    b. Emergency admission.

    c. Short-stay admission.

    d. Routine admission.

3. Highest priority for hospital beds and care is given to which group of patients?

    a. Those with an acute illness or injury.

    b. Those with a chronic disease.

    c. Those scheduled to have elective surgery.

    d. Those undergoing diagnostic tests and examinations.

4. Who is responsible for obtaining information about the patient's address, birth place, and employer; name of party who will pay the bill; and the consent for hospital treatment?

    a. The patient's doctor.

    b. The nurse on the unit.

    c. The admission office.

    d. The business office clerk.

5. When does the medical treatment of the patient begin?

    a. As soon as the patient arrives at the hospital.

    b. After the nurse takes the vital signs.

    c. When the patient is put to bed on the unit.

    d. As soon as the doctor's orders are received.

6. The responsibilities of the nurse admitting the patient include all of the following, except for

    a. prescribing the diet.

    b. orienting to the unit.

    c. caring for patient's belongings.

    d. carrying out the nursing care.

7. Most hospitals prohibit children under the age of 14 or 16 from visiting patients. The main reason for barring them is

 a. to provide more rest and quiet for the patient.

 b. to reduce the exposure of patients to infectious diseases.

 c. that they don't understand about illness.

 d. there is no place for them to play.

8. Medications brought to the hospital by patients are routinely sent home with the family or placed in storage until time of discharge. The reason for not allowing their use during the hospital stay is

 a. that the hospital sells medications through the pharmacy.

 b. to save the drugs so the patient can take them at home.

 c. that no one can be sure the drug is what the label says it is.

 d. that the hospital and nurses prefer to use unit-dose type of medications.

9. Which of the following types of valuables would be placed in the hospital's safe?

 a. The house and car keys.

 b. A photo with a bronze frame.

 c. A gold and diamond watch.

 d. All of these.

10. When discharging the patient from the hospital, your nursing duties include all of the following, except

 a. providing instructions regarding home care as needed.

 b. recording the time and mode of discharge.

 c. writing the discharge order.

 d. taking care of the patient's personal belongings.

11. Patients recovering from an illness or operation are generally discharged from the hospital by wheelchair. The reason for this is

 a. to ensure their safety.

 b. it is required by hospital regulations.

 c. it is ordered by the doctor.

 d. the family expects it.

12. The patient asks, "When can I go home?" The doctor replies, "Tomorrow," and writes on the chart that the patient can go home tomorrow. What is this type of discharge called?

 a. a transfer to home.

 b. a planned discharge.

 c. a delayed discharge.

 d. an informed discharge.

13. When transferring a patient from your nursing unit to an intensive care unit, which one of the following is NOT one of your responsibilities?

   a. Collecting and packing the patient's belongings.

   b. Delivering the chart and other records to the receiving nurse.

   c. Recording the transfer on the nurses' notes.

   d. Orienting the patient to the new unit.

   e. Reporting the patient's condition to the receiving nurse.

14. A patient, Mr. Doe, states that he is sick of the hospital, can't stand the treatment he has gotten, has called a cab, and is leaving immediately. Which of the following actions does the nurse take?

   1. Tell him he can't go because there is no order for discharge.

   2. Call for help to detain the patient and put him back to bed.

   3. Ask him to wait until his doctor can talk to him.

   4. Call the doctor and explain the situation.

   5. Insist that Mr. Doe sign the form "Discharge Against Medical Advice."

      a. all   b. 1 and 2   c. 3 and 4   d. 1, 3, and 5

15. When a patient is found not breathing and no pulse can be detected, the pronouncement of death is made by

   a. the CPR team.

   b. the doctor.

   c. the nurse.

   d. the coroner.

POST-TEST ANSWERS

1. b	9. c
2. d	10. c
3. a	11. a
4. c	12. b
5. d	13. d
6. a	14. c
7. b	15. b
8. c	

Unit 7

CONSENTS, RELEASES
AND INCIDENT REPORTS

GENERAL PERFORMANCE OBJECTIVE

You will know how to obtain consents and releases and complete incident reports according to legal requirements.

SPECIFIC PERFORMANCE OBJECTIVES

Upon the completion of this unit you will be able to:

1. Describe at least five rights of the hospitalized patient and the factors that constitute an informed consent.

2. Explain the different consents and releases commonly used in hospitals and other similar agencies, including the admission agreement and the operative permit.

3. Explain the release from use of siderails form to the patient or the family, and obtain a valid signature.

4. State at least five types of events that are reported as patient incidents.

5. Prepare a patient incident form for submission to the hospital administration.

VOCABULARY

biopsy—the excision of a small piece of tissue for the purpose of examination and diagnosis.
bone marrow—the soft (spongy) tissue in the hollow of long bones; the center bone marrow is yellow and is chiefly fat; the surrounding tissue is called the red bone marrow because it manufactures red blood cells.
emancipated minor—a person age 16 or over who lives apart from parents or guardian and is responsible for handling own finances.
guardian—a person who is legally entrusted with the care of the person and/or the property of a minor or one who is legally incapable of managing his own affairs.
informed consent—agreement given by a patient to undergo treatment or therapy after having been supplied sufficient information regarding its advantages and disadvantages.
lumbar puncture—the procedure of inserting a needle into the lumbar spine in order to withdraw spinal fluid or inject a drug.
radiology—a branch of medicine that deals with X-rays and other radiations for diagnosis or treatment.

INTRODUCTION

Consents and releases are legal records of agreements between two parties, such as those between the patient and the hospital. The hospital provides printed documents that state the services that will be provided and the general treatment that the patient can expect. By signing the consent, the patient indicates agreement to what has been specified and to the limits set. Both parties are protected legally. The patient who signs an operative permit for the repair of a hernia authorizes a specific operation to be performed. The doctor and the hospital staff in the operating room agree to repair the hernia, and do only the procedures necessary to achieve this.

PATIENT RIGHTS AND CONSENTS

ITEM 1. RIGHTS OF HOSPITALIZED PATIENTS

When people become ill, the need for medical treatment often affects some of their personal and property rights. At times, unfortunately, it seems that patients who are powerless and dependent on others for care are called on to give up their rights for the convenience of the doctor or the hospital routine. The patient's ability and freedom to move about is often severely restricted by pain, traction, or bed rest. The number of personal possessions that can be brought to the hospital is limited, and little security, if any, is provided for those articles kept at the bedside. Patients may be required to share a room with others, and this impinges on their rights to privacy. Privacy is further reduced by the stream of nurses, technicians, and therapists who approach the bedside in order to provide care.

Only in recent years has much attention been given to the rights of patients. In 1973, the American Hospital Association approved a document called "A Patient's Bill of Rights," which describes what patients might reasonably expect of their care in the hospital. The document states that patients are entitled to considerate and respectful care without regard to sex, race, social background, or the ability to pay for health care. They are entitled to know the name of the doctor coordinating the medical care and the names and professional relationships of others who are involved in the treatment. An additional right is to be informed of the type of treatment planned, the risks involved, the alternatives, and the names of people providing the treatment in order to make a reasonable decision consenting to or refusing it. Patients also must be informed of plans for continued care following discharge from the hospital, and they must be given information about hospital rules and policies that affect them.

Further, patients have the right to actively participate in decisions regarding their care; this includes their right to refuse any treatment, medication, or procedure. They have the right to leave the hospital without the doctor's permission, except when this is prohibited by law. The laws are specific regarding the circumstances under which people can be detained against their will. Patients have the right to privacy in matters related to the illness and the course of medical care. All records concerning the care and stay in the hospital are confidential. Information about the illness and treatment is handled discreetly and restricted to those who are directly involved in the care. In this regard, patients may request that no observers be allowed during a procedure or examination. The patient's permission must be obtained, usually in writing, before medical information is released to anyone else, including insurance companies. The effect of the Federal Privacy Act of 1974 and various state laws further limits the release of information about patients. Finally, the patient has the right to examine the bill for services and to have it explained regardless of who pays it.

In order to safeguard the rights of patients, consent forms are obtained for the procedures that are part of the medical treatment. The general rule is that a consent is obtained from the patient before any treatment is rendered, since any treatment given before a consent carries a risk of liability with it. The exception is a medical emergency, when treatment is required immediately to prevent deterioration or aggravation of the patient's condition that poses a danger to life.

ITEM 2. WHO MAY SIGN CONSENTS OR RELEASES?

The patient's signature is obtained on a consent form by the agency in order to have written verification of the agreement. Can anyone sign a consent for his or her own treatment? For someone else's treatment? What about a child? At what age can a teenager give consent for medical treatment? What if the person is unable to sign a signature? Although the laws in your state may be different, the following will provide some guidelines when you are considering who should sign the consent or release form.

Adult Patients

Competent adult patients must consent to their own medical treatment. An adult is anyone who has reached the age of 18 or has entered into a valid marriage, even if the marriage was later dissolved by divorce, annulment, or separation. The competent person is one who has the ability to understand the nature and the consequences of the matter under consideration. Unless there is reason to think otherwise, any person seeking nonemergency medical treatment is assumed to be competent. Adults who are considered mentally incompetent are those who have been legally declared incompetent, as well as those who are permanently or temporarily incapable of giving consent, such as in cases of mental deficiency, head injury, drug abuse, or alcohol abuse.

Although the adult may be married, the spouse does not have the legal right to sign for the patient. Even adult patients who are in the custody of law enforcement officers must give permission for nonemergency treatment, examination, and operations, except in states where the law permits such procedures as blood alcohol tests. In cases in which an adult is incompetent, no treatment of a nonemergency nature is given until consent is obtained from the guardian or conservator.

Patients Who Are Minors

Children under the age of 18 are regarded as minors and lack the legal right to consent to treatment, except as allowed by law in some states. Consent is given by the parent(s) or by a legal guardian, if one has been appointed. If the parents of the child are divorced, it is customary to gain the consent from the parent who has custody. A stepparent cannot consent ordinarily, unless the child has been legally adopted. (See table for legal consent requirements.)

Under certain circumstances, minors may give consent for medical purposes. The emancipated minor of 16 years of age or older who lives away from the home of the parent or guardian and who manages his or her own financial affairs can give consent for care without the parent or guardian's knowledge or consent. Other minors who can give consent are those on active duty with the armed forces and, in some states, those receiving treatment for pregnancy or its prevention, those who have been raped, other victims of sexual assault, those suffering from communicable diseases that must be reported, those over age 12 with a drug or alcohol problem, and married minors.

ITEM 3.   GENERAL PRINCIPLES FOR OBTAINING SIGNED CONSENTS

The consent for treatment may be oral, written, or implied, but it is recommended that the consent be in written form in case a dispute arises at some time in the future.

Consent Freely Given

The consent must be given free of duress in order to be valid — *the person must not be pressured into signing the form.* Even though the consent has been signed, the patient may change his or her mind and revoke it anytime before the procedure or treatment is carried out.

Form of the Signature

Patients may sign their name in any way, and it is customary to accept the name as written. In most instances, a nickname is not used as part of the signature. When the person is unable to write, an "X" is made on the form, and must be witnessed by two people. For

LEGAL CONSENT REQUIREMENTS FOR MEDICAL TREATMENT OF MINORS IN VARIOUS CIRCUMSTANCES*

If patient is:	Is Parental Consent Required?	Are Parents Responsible for Cost?	Is Minor's Consent Sufficient?	May M.D. Inform Parents of Treatment?
Under 18, unmarried, no special circumstances	Yes	Yes	No	Yes
Under 18, married or previously married	No	No	Yes	No
Under 18, emergency and parents not available	No	Yes	Yes (If capable)	Yes
Emancipated (over 16, not living at home, manages own financial affairs)	No	No	Yes	Yes
Not married, pregnant, under 18 (care related to pregnancy) (including consent to an abortion)	No	No	Yes	Yes
Not married, pregnant, under 18 (care not related to pregnancy and no other special circumstances)	No	No	Yes	No
Not married, under 18, determination if pregnant, no other special circumstances	Yes	Yes	No	Yes
Under 18, on active duty with Armed Services	Probably not	Probably not	Probably yes	Probably not
Under 18, over 12, care for contagious reportable disease	No	No	Yes	No
Birth control, under 18	No	No	Yes	No
Under 18, over 12, care for rape	No	No	Yes	Yes
Under 18, care for sexual assault	No	No	Yes	Yes Usually
Under 18, over 12, care for alcohol or drug abuse	No	No	Yes	Yes Usually

*From California Hospital Association: Consent Manual. 10th ed. Sacramento, CA, 1978. Reprinted with permission of CHA.

UNIT 7

this procedure, the nurse writes the patient's name and "his" or "her mark," the patient then makes an "X," and the two witnesses also sign.

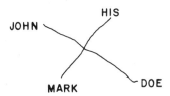

Witnesses

It is recommended that the actual signing of a consent form by the patient be witnessed by another person, and for some types of consent, two witnesses are required by law. Persons signing the form as witnesses should be 18 years of age or older. In most agencies, the admitting clerks, registered nurses, licensed practical or vocational nurses, ward clerks, and those with similar responsibilities serve as witnesses.

Nurses and other members of the nursing staff are increasingly being discouraged from witnessing the patient's signature on documents that are of a personal nature, such as wills, business agreements, contracts, and other similar types of papers. When these documents require the signature of the hospitalized patient, they tend to be important and more apt to have their validity challenged at a later time. Rather than witness these documents, suggest that the patient arrange to have a friend do this. If that is not possible, you might call a notary public, if there is one in the hospital's business offices, or refer the request to the Nursing Service Office for handling.

"Informed Consents"

The law requires that any person who signs a consent for any procedure of a complex nature must know enough about the matter to make a reasonable decision. This means that patients asked to sign an operative consent must know the need for the surgery or procedure, who will do it, basically what is involved, the expected results, the disadvantages, and the risks. It is the physician's responsibility to provide this information. Usually, the patient who is admitted to the hospital for elective surgery, or that of a nonemergency nature, has been informed of the need for surgery by the physician; what it will do; the consequences if it is not done; and, if a serious or complicated operation, what the risks are. If the patient verbally agrees to have the operation, the doctor schedules the operation and instructs the patient to be admitted to the hospital on a certain date. If the patient later indicates that he or she doesn't know anything about the operation, it may be that patient wasn't asked the right question or that he or she is extremely anxious.

When you are requested to obtain the patient's signature on the consent form, be sure that the patient understands what is being signed. The patient should read the consent form; responses to a question such as "What has the doctor told you about your surgery (or this procedure)?" will give you an idea what the patient does understand about the operation. If the patient does not understand, postpone getting the signature on the consent form and notify the doctor. Avoid rushing patients to sign a consent form or appearing to force them to complete the form. Some patients may ask to wait until they can discuss the matter with others in their family. Decisions are not always easy to make when the procedure may be painful, pose a high risk, or result in alterations or changes in the body.

In an emergency situation, when surgery is indicated to save the patient's life, the surgeon may operate without a consent form signed by the patient. In the case of a minor, however, every effort must be made to obtain permission from a parent or guardian, even if by telegram or telephone or by an order from the court.

ITEM 4.   COMMON TYPES OF CONSENTS

Patients are required to sign a number of consents and forms when entering a hospital or nursing care facility. In some agencies, you may be expected to help secure the patient's

CONDITIONS OF ADMISSION

PATIENT NO.	NAME

1. **MEDICAL AND SURGICAL CONSENT:** The undersigned is under the control of his/her attending physician and the hospital is not liable for any act or omission in following the instructions of said physician, and the undersigned consents to any x-ray examination, laboratory procedures, anesthesia, medical or surgical treatment or hospital services rendered the patient under the general and special instructions of the physician. The undersigned recognizes that all doctors of medicine furnishing services to the patient, including the radiologist, pathologist, and the like are independent contractors and are not employees or agents of the hospital. I also agree to remain in the hospital until the physician recommends my discharge. Should I leave before the physician or physicians in charge of my case have discharged me I agree to assume all responsibility for any untoward results which may follow. I do hereby authorize and direct the pathologist of the Brotman Medical Center to use his discretion in the disposal of any member or organ, that may be amputated from or removed from my body at the time of any surgery performed on my body by my physician or physicians.

2. **PERSONAL VALUABLES:** It is understood and agreed that the hospital maintains a safe for the safekeeping of money and valuables. If I do not desire to avail myself of the safekeeping facilities, I do hereby agree that the hospital shall not be liable for the loss or damage to any money, jewelry, glasses, hearing aids, dentures, documents, furs, fur coats and fur garments or any articles of unusual value and small compass, or any personal effects and other valuables of any kind or nature retained by me or kept in my accommodations while I am at the hospital. ·

3. **RELEASE OF INFORMATION:** The hospital may disclose all or any part of the patient's record to any person or corporation which is or may be liable under a contract to the hospital or to the patient or to a family member or employer of the patient for all or part of the hospital's charge, including, but not limited to, hospital or medical service companies, insurance companies, workmen's compensation carriers, welfare funds or the patient's employer. All such information would be available after a written request and the approval of the physician who was the doctor in the case. I hereby authorize any insurance company, administrator, prepayment organization, employer, hospital or physician to release all information with respect to myself or any of my dependents which may have a bearing on the benefits payable under any plan providing benefits or services.

4. **RELEASE OF LIABILITY:** I agree to hold the hospital and its agents, servants and employees harmless and free from all responsibility for injuries or losses received by me as a result of falling from bed, or falls on the floor, or from other cause while out of bed contrary to the instructions of doctors or nurses.

5. **GUARANTEE OF PAYMENT:** The undersigned agrees, whether he/she signs as agent or as patient, that in consideration of the services to be rendered to the patient, he/she hereby individually obligates himself/herself to pay the account of the hospital in accordance with the regular rates and terms of the hospital. Such account to be paid at the time of discharge, or to make such additional deposits, or contracts, from time to time as the hospital may request. Should the account be referred to an attorney for collection, the undersigned shall pay reasonable attorney's fees and collection expenses. All unpaid balances at time of discharge to bear interest at the highest legal rate.

6. **GENERAL DUTY NURSING:** The hospital provides only general duty nursing care. Under this system nurses are called to the bedside of the patient by a signal system. If the patient is in such condition as to need continuous or special duty nursing care, it is agreed that such must be arranged by the patient, or his legal representative or his physicians, by private contract with the nurse, and payment for services shall be made direct to the special duty nurse. The hospital shall in no way be responsible for failure to provide special duty nursing and is hereby released from any and all liability arising from the fact that said patient is not provided with such additional care.

7. **SIDE RAILS:** The undersigned has been informed that the hospital has placed protective side rails on the bed for the personal protection of the patient, and I agree that, should the patient remove them or have them removed, the hospital and its employees shall be held harmless in the event of any injury or damage by failure of the side rails to be in place.

8. **MEDICARE: PATIENT'S CERTIFICATION, AUTHORIZATION TO RELEASE INFORMATION AND PAYMENT REQUEST:** I certify that the information given by me in applying for payment under Title XVIII of the Social Security Act is correct. I authorize any holder of medical or other information about me to release to the Social Security Administration or its intermediaries or carriers any information needed for this or a related medicare claim. I request that payment of authorized benefits be made on my behalf.

9. **INSURANCE ASSIGNMENT:** I hereby authorize payment directly to Brotman Medical Center the UCD benefits plus any other benefits payable to me, including disability insurance and payment under Title XVIII of the Social Security Act which is applicable to my account, but not to exceed the hospital's regular charges for this period of hospitalization. I understand that I am financially responsible to the hospital for charges not covered by my hospitalization plan.

10. **PATIENT'S RIGHTS:** I have read the "Patients Rights" posted in the admitting area and/or have been given a copy at my bedside and acknowledge its contents and am fully informed in this regard.

The undersigned certifies that he has read the foregoing, receiving a copy thereof, and is the patient, or is duly authorized by the patient as patient's general agent to execute the above and accept its terms.

PLEASE NOTE: CHECKOUT TIME IS 11.00 A.M. IF DUE TO THE FAULT OF THE PATIENT, CHECK OCCURS AFTER 11.00 A.M. THE PATIENT SHALL PAY AN ADDITIONAL CHARGE.

SIGNATURE OF PATIENT _____

WITNESS _____

SPOUSE, GUARDIAN, NEAREST RELATIVE OR GUARANTOR _____

DATE _____ TIME _____

ADDRESS _____

State law provides that upon an inquiry as to the presence or general condition of the patient, the hospital may, unless otherwise requested by the patient, next of kin, or provider of health care release at its discretion none, part or all of the following information: the patient's name, address, age and sex, reason for admission, general nature of injuries, or the general condition of the patient

WITNESS _____

SIGNATURE OF PATIENT _____

DATE _____

SPOUSE, GUARDIAN, NEAREST RELATIVE OR GUARANTOR _____

TIME _____

ADDRESS _____

FORM 3502 (11) (REV. 2-80)   **DISTRIBUTION:** WHITE - CHART COPY · YELLOW - PATIENT COPY – PINK - INSURANCE COPY

California Hospital Association: Consent Manual. 10th ed. Sacramento, CA, 1978. Reprinted by permission of CHA.

UNIT 7

signature on these forms. Usually, this will be done by the admission clerk or the nurse. However, you will need to know about the types of consents and be able to explain them to the patients and their families.

The Admission Agreement. Hospitals routinely require that patients or their legal representatives sign the admission agreement. This document describes the type of care and services the patient can expect the hospital to provide; in return, the patient assumes responsibility for the costs. The admission agreement states that the hospital will provide general staff nursing care and the usual medical treatment prescribed by the physician. It also states the limits of responsibility for the patient's personal property kept at the bedside and for valuables kept in the hospital safe. The agreement outlines the patient's financial obligation for the care rendered and provides for the release of certain information to insurance companies, worker's compensation, or other similar agencies for payment purposes.

The medical care that is covered in the admission agreement includes obtaining specimens for examinations in the clinical laboratory, X-rays that may have been ordered, and other medications and treatments commonly used in the treatment of disease.

Often the admission agreement form consists of several copies, one of which is given to the patient; another copy is placed in the patient's chart.

The Operative Consent. The operative consent is called by a variety of names, including the *Surgical Permit* and the *Consent to Operation and Administration of Anesthesia*; it is obtained when the physician operates on the patient's body with hands or instruments. Most people know about the operations that are done in surgery and involve some sort of incision and cutting into body tissue. All surgical procedures and biopsies require that an operative consent be signed preoperatively to authorize the surgery, the giving of the anesthesia, and the services of pathology or other departments when needed. It is the doctor's responsibility to explain the operation or procedure so that the patient can give "informed consent." If the patient seems confused or to have doubts, do not pressure him or her to sign the consent; rather, notify the physician. An operative consent form is shown.

The operative consent, or a similar form specified by your agency's policies, is used for procedures and examinations of an "invasive" nature when the physician uses an instrument or introduces a substance into one of the patient's body spaces or cavities. The procedures that need an operative consent vary, so you should consult your agency's policies. Generally the list would include, but should not be limited to, the following:

1. Arteriogram
2. Bone marrow puncture
3. Bronchoscopy
4. Cardiac catheterization
5. Cystoscopy
6. Encephalogram
7. Lumbar puncture
8. Myelogram
9. Paracentesis
10. Pneumoencephalogram
11. Thoracentesis

Other Types of Consents. You may be asked to prepare other types of consents and obtain the signatures on them. Others may be more appropriately obtained by the nurse or the physician.

1. **Autopsy Permit.** The nurse or physician fills out the form and obtains the signature of the next of kin for a postmortem examination of the body to determine the cause of death.

2. **Authorization for Treatment of a Minor.** The nurse prepares the agency form and obtains the signature of the parent or legal guardian to authorize care for the minor.

3. **Consent for Photographs.** The agency form is used and the patient's signature is obtained. The consent also states the purpose of the photographs.

4. **Consent for Use of Experimental Drugs or Treatment.** The agency form is used and is initiated by the physician or the nurse. The physician prescribing the

CONSENT TO OPERATION, ADMINISTRATION OF
ANESTHETICS, AND THE RENDERING OF OTHER
MEDICAL SERVICES

....
Name of Patient

Date ....

Hour ....M.

1. I authorize and direct ....M.D.

my surgeon and/or associates or assistants of his choice to perform the following operation upon me

....

and/or to do any other therapeutic procedure that (his) (their) judgment may dictate to be advisable for the patient's well-being. I have been informed by my Doctor, of the nature and intended result of this operation, as well as its foreseeable risks and possible alternatives. I further understand that no warranty or guarantee has been made as to the result or cure.

2. I hereby authorize and direct the above named surgeon and/or his associates or assistants to provide such additional services for me as he or they may deem reasonable and necessary, including, but not limited to, the administration and maintenance of the anesthesia, and the performance of services involving pathology and radiology, and I hereby consent thereto.

3. I understand that the above named surgeon and his associates or assistants will be occupied solely with performing such operation, and the persons in attendance at such operation for the purpose of administering anesthesia, and the person or persons performing services involving pathology and radiology, are not the agents, servants or employees of the above named hospital nor of any surgeon, but are independent contractors and as such are the agents, servants, or employees of myself.

4. I hereby authorize the hospital pathologist to use his discretion in the disposal of any severed tissue or member, except ....

Patient's Signature ....

Witness ....

Witness ....

(If patient is a minor or unable to sign, complete the following:)

Patient is a minor, or is unable to sign, because ....

....
Father

....
Mother

....
Guardian

....
Other Person and Relationship

FORM 1054-A (REV. 2-74)   ARTISTIC PRESS, P.O. BOX 20540
LOS ANGELES, CALIF. 90006   CONSENT TO OPERATION

U
N
I
T
7

experimental drugs must follow guidelines set by federal agencies. The patients must give an "informed consent" for experimental drugs or treatments.

5. **Permit to Use Personal Electrical Appliances.** Some agencies require that patients sign a request to use their own electrical appliances, such as a radio, shaver, or television set. The agency form is initiated by the nurse.

ITEM 5. COMMON TYPES OF RELEASES

A release is another type of legal record that is used to excuse one party from responsibility or liability. The release is an administrative form and is usually made out in duplicate, with one copy going to the administration and one copy on the patient's chart. You should follow instructions provided by your agency, however. The release forms are simple to prepare: Stamp the form with the Addressograph card and fill in the date and any other information requested.

Common releases you may encounter include the following:

1. **Release from Use of Siderails.** Hospitals frequently require that siderails on the beds be used for patients whenever they are in bed as a safety measure. Some patients oppose the use of siderails, refuse to cooperate or follow the agency policy, or believe that there is no need to use siderails; therefore, they sign a release. The form indicates that they are aware of the possible hazard of not using the siderails and will not hold the hospital responsible for any harm that might occur as a result of not using them.

2. **Discharge Against Medical Advice.** This form is prepared whenever a patient demands to leave the hospital without an order from the doctor authorizing the discharge. The doctor or the nurse should talk with the patient and explain the reasons that continued hospital care is needed. If the patient insists on leaving, however, make out the discharge against medical advice (also abbreviated to AMA) in duplicate and offer it to the patient to sign. The form states that the hospital is released from responsibility for the patient's conditions because he or she left the hospital AMA. If the patient refuses to sign the form, this should be noted and witnessed. Discharge of a patient AMA is reported immediately to the attending physician, the nursing supervisor, and the administration. One copy of the form remains on the patient's chart.

3. **Other releases** may be used for a number of conditions, including the release of information, the release of responsibility for personal property, and so forth.

ITEM 6. PROCEDURE FOR GETTING SIGNATURES

Given a patient scheduled to have surgery, you are to prepare the operative consent and obtain the patient's signature.

Important Steps	Key Points
1. Obtain the form and equipment: consent, pen, and surface (e.g., clipboard) to write on.	If you are responsible for securing consents, make sure that the patient's name, age, sex, room number, physician, and type of surgery or procedure are correct before you take it to the patient. Forms are usually stored in a designated place in the nurse's station.
2. Wash your hands, identify the patient, and explain the procedure.	

Important Steps	Key Points
3. Give the consent form to the patient to read.	Allow the patient time to read over the form. Through discussion or questions, make sure that the patient understands the nature of the treatment or operation.
4. Obtain the patient's signature.	Indicate the appropriate space for the signature to be written in ink. Write the date and time in the space provided. If the patient refuses to sign the consent, refer to your charge nurse, who will notify the physician. The consent is the physician's responsibility. If you obtain the patient's signature, you *must* witness the signature. Sign your full name and title with a pen. This form becomes a part of the patient's chart or record.
5. Place the completed consent or release on the patient's chart.	

U
N
I
T
7

ITEM 7. PATIENT INCIDENT REPORTS

Patient incident reports are made out if there is an error in treatment or if a patient accident occurs. They are not part of the patient's chart, as are consents and releases, but are intended for the use of the hospital administration and attorneys. They alert the hospital administration to the possibility of litigation (law suits).

What Constitutes a "Patient Incident"?

The following generally constitute incidents that are reportable:

1. Falls or injuries to the patient.

2. Burns resulting from treatment, or careless smoking.

3. Lost or damaged personal articles.

4. Medication errors.

5. Errors in patient identification, e.g., giving the treatment to the wrong patient.

6. Injection injuries, e.g., needle injury to a nerve during medication injection.

7. Treatment injuries.

8. Thermometers broken in the patient's mouth, rectum, bed, and so forth.

9. Fights and assaults.

10. Damage to property belonging to the hospital or others.

Who Completes Incident Reports?

The nursing personnel who are most familiar with the incident or who observed its happening should complete the account of the incident according to the agency policy.

If an incident occurs, provide emergency and safety measures for the patient; call for help, either verbally or by using the patient call light. Your team leader will notify a house physician or the patient's own physician.

NOTIFICATION FORM

THIS REPORT IS CONFIDENTIAL --
     NOT A PART OF THE MEDICAL RECORD

Addressograph Plate

SECTION I
If no addressograph plate, complete following two
(2) items:

_____
          Name of Person Involved

_____
          Identification Number

Cost Center/Location_____

Print Name of Person Filling out Form

WITNESS: Name_____

          Address_____

          Phone #_____

Name_____

Address_____

Phone #_____

For administrative use only:
     1) _____   2) _____   3) _____

SECTION II

AGE | If under 1 year, circle one:
       YRS. 0-14 DAYS ___ 15-364 DAYS ___

SEX: M   F   (Circle One)

Check One: If patient, check one:
[ ] Inpatient   [ ] MED   [ ] PSYCH
[ ] Outpatient/ER   [ ] SURG   [ ] REHAB
[ ] Visitor/Volunteer   [ ] OB

DATE OF OCCURRENCE   ___/___/___
                      MM DD YY

TIME   _____   AM   PM   (Circle One)

DATE OF FORM COMPLETION   ___/___/___
                           MM   DD   YY

DESCRIPTION OF OCCURRENCE-Briefly describe what
happened. Name the equipment, drug, treatment or
procedure involved, and parts of the body affected.
Do not mention names of individuals in this section: _____

_____

_____

_____

_____

_____

Copyright © 1980 by the
California Hospital Association

SECTION III

A. 1.0 [ ] LOST/DAMAGED PROPERTY ONLY
            (If checked, skip all other information.)

Check One Box in Each of the Following Groups:

B. EVENT HAPPENING DURING THIS ADMISSION

    2.00 [ ] Not Applicable or Unknown
    2.10 [ ] Consent for Procedure
    2.20 [ ] Diet
    2.30 [ ] Elopement
    2.35 [ ] Equipment
    2.40 [ ] I.V. Infusion
    2.50 [ ] Fall
    2.60 [ ] Fire
    2.70 [ ] Medication
    2.80 [ ] Transfusion
    2.90 [ ] Treatment/Procedure
    2.95 [ ] Other_____

C. EFFECT HAPPENING DURING THIS ADMISSION

    3.00 [ ] No Apparent Effect
    3.10 [ ] Aspiration - Foreign Matter
    3.15 [ ] Burn
    3.20 [ ] Cardiac Arrest
    3.25 [ ] Decubitus Ulcer
    3.30 [ ] Drug Reaction or Toxic Effect
    3.35 [ ] Fracture
    3.40 [ ] Infection
    3.45 [ ] Laceration
    3.50 [ ] Neurological Impairment
    3.55 [ ] Postoperative Hemorrhage
    3.60 [ ] Pulmonary Embolism
    3.65 [ ] Retained Foreign Body
    3.70 [ ] Vascular Impairment of an Extremity
    3.75 [ ] Wound Disruption
    3.95 [ ] Any Other Effect_____

D. SEVERITY OF EFFECT

    4.10 [ ] Effect Nonexistent / Unknown
    4.20 [ ] Effect Inconsequential
    4.30 [ ] Effect Consequential
    4.40 [ ] Death

E. SPECIAL CIRCUMSTANCES DURING THIS ADMISSION

    5.10 [ ] None of the following circumstances were present
    5.20 [ ] Return of a patient to the Operating
               Room.
    5.30 [ ] Occurrence of acute myocardial infarction.
    5.40 [ ] Newborn infant with evidence of cerebral
               dysfunction.
    5.50 [ ] Unplanned removal of an organ or structure.
    5.60 [ ] Prior care - 30 days.

Incident Report form California Hospital Association, Sacramento, CA. Reprinted by permission of CHA.

After the patient's comfort and safety are provided, try to obtain an account of the incident. You will need this to complete the report. Carry out the doctor's order for care if the incident necessitates follow-through; for example, the patient falls and breaks an arm — the doctor orders an X-ray.

ITEM 8. PREPARING AN INCIDENT REPORT

Given a patient who has fallen in his room, provide assistance and prepare the patient incident report for the hospital administration.

Important Steps	Key Points
1. Provide for the patient's safety and comfort.	Call for help verbally or by signaling with the patient's call light. Do not try to move the patient until an examination has been performed by the doctor or nurse for signs of injury. Remove any safety hazards such as broken glass. Provide warmth for the patient.
2. Notify physician to examine for injury.	Follow the doctor's orders, if given; for example, call for an X-ray or discontinue a blood transfusion.
3. Return the patient to bed.	Do this as soon as possible. Get assistance as needed.
4. Get the patient's account of the incident.	Ask the patient to relate what happened to cause the incident. Write this information in the space provided in the report. It is desirable (when appropriate) to quote the patient's own words. You will start the comment on the form: "The patient states that . . ."
5. Complete an incident report form.	Ask your team leader for assistance in completing your history of the incident and other patient information. Charting should be clear, concise, and accurate.
6. Distribute copies of the completed form according to instructions.	The physician will sign in the appropriate place; one copy is forwarded to the nursing office, and one to the administration. It is an administrative form and does not become part of the patient's chart.

UNIT 7

PERFORMANCE TEST

1. Complete a patient incident report form from the following information:

   At 3:45 A.M. Mrs. Mary Volk, room 223, bed 2, fractured hip, 87 years old, patient of Dr. G. Marshall, fell out of bed while trying to get up to the bathroom. Siderails were down, and the bed was in the low position. Patient had received Nembutal gr 1ss h.s.

2. Complete a Surgical Consent form for Mr. Victor Welk, room 257, bed 1, patient of Dr. S. First, for a right inguinal herniotomy. He is scheduled for surgery at 9:00 A.M. on Thursday, December 1.

3. Complete a Release of Siderails Form for Mr. V. Welk in Question #2.

PERFORMANCE CHECKLIST

COMPLETION OF A PATIENT INCIDENT FORM

1. Obtain the proper form.

2. Fill in the preliminary information.

3. Wash your hands.

4. Identify the patient.

5. Explain the procedure to the patient.

6. Verify the patient's understanding of the form.

7. Complete the history of the incident as related by the patient; for example: "The patient states that _____."

8. Document the report if possible; i.e., list all individuals familiar with the incident.

9. Transmit the form to the appropriate departments.

COMPLETION OF A SURGICAL CONSENT FORM

1. Obtain the proper form and the necessary equipment.

2. Fill in all preliminary information.

3. Wash your hands.

4. Identify the patient and explain the procedure.

5. Permit the patient to read the form, and clarify his understanding of the form.

6. Ask the patient to sign the form.

7. Write in the date and time that the form is signed.

8. Witness the form as required.

9. Place the completed form with the patient's chart.

10. In the event that the patient will not sign, notify the nurse.

11. In the event that the patient cannot write his name and makes an X, obtain the signature of two witnesses.

12. In the event that the patient is a minor, obtain the parent's or guardian's signature.

COMPLETION OF RELEASE FORM

1. Obtain the proper form and necessary equipment.

2. Fill in all preliminary information.

3. Wash your hands.

4. Identify the patient and explain the procedure.

5. Permit the patient to read the form, and clarify his understanding of the form.

6. Ask the patient to sign the form.

7. Write in the date and time that the form is signed.

8. Witness the form as required.

9. Place the completed form with the patient's chart.

10. In the event that the patient cannot write his name but can make an "X" or mark, obtain the signatures of two witnesses.

11. In the event that the patient is a minor, obtain the parent's or guardian's signature.

POST-TEST

Matching. For each of the patients listed in Column 1, select the category of person from Column 2 who must sign the consent form or legally give consent for the medical treatment.

Column 1

1. A woman, age 38, married, who is unconscious from an overdose of a tranquilizer.

2. A girl, age 17, married, with an upper respiratory infection.

3. A woman, age 22, single, mentally retarded, for breast biopsy.

4. A male, age 16, living in nearby city with friends, for abdominal pain.

5. A male, age 45, severe injuries from car accident following an evening of drinking.

6. A boy, age 14, adopted, for a broken wrist.

7. A girl, age 14, for treatment of pregnancy.

8. A baby, 6 months old, with pneumonia.

9. A woman, age 50, for diagnostic tests and treatment of headaches.

10. A man, age 63, collapsed on the street with chest pain, and shock.

Column 2

a. by the parent

b. by the patient for own self

c. by a guardian

d. by spouse

e. by implied consent

Multiple Choice. For each of the following questions, select the one best answer.

11. Which consent form is used to show the patient has consented to have blood drawn for laboratory tests, treatments by the nurses such as dressing a wound or catheterization, and treatment by the physical or respiratory therapist?

    a. consent for surgery

    b. "informed consent"

    c. conditions of admission

    d. consent for special procedures

12. Mr. Rarely was admitted for a cystoscopy that is scheduled for tomorrow. When asked to sign the consent form, he states that he doesn't know anything about an operation. What should the nurse do now?

    a. Explain what a cystoscopy is in terms he can understand.

    b. Tell him to sign the form, since this is the treatment his doctor ordered.

    c. Call the patient's wife and get her signature on the form.

    d. Leave and notify the physician of the patient's doubt and lack of knowledge.

13. The term "informed consent" includes which of these factors or components?

    1. Name of each complication that might occur.

    2. State what the procedure is expected to do or correct.

3. Describe the nature of the operation or procedures.

4. Give the names of the persons performing the procedure.

    a. all   b. all but 1   c. all but 2   d. all but 4

14. Most hospitals require the patient to sign a consent for special procedures or examinations that are considered as "invasive" of the body. Which of the following are invasive and require a special consent?

1. lumbar puncture

2. angiogram

3. chest X-ray

4. cystoscopy

5. blood transfusion

    a. all   b. all but 3   c. 1, 2, and 4   d. 2, 4, and 5

15. The responsibility of ultimately ensuring that the patient is informed about the procedure or treatment requiring consent rests with

a. the nurse

b. the person securing the signature

c. the patient's physician

d. the person performing the procedure

16. Hospitalized patients have a number of rights outlined in the Patient's Bill of Rights. Which one of the following is not included as one of those rights?

a. the right to refuse medications.

b. the right to watch TV as late as he or she wishes.

c. the right to know the names of doctors and others giving care.

d. the right to be examined by their physician in private.

17. In cases of an emergency such as when the patient is unconscious or unable to give verbal or written consent, what is the justification for providing medical care without the consent?

a. It is implied that the person would give it if able to.

b. There isn't any, and medical care must be delayed until a consent is obtained.

c. Consent is obtained from a parent, spouse, or other close relative.

d. The doctor has a professional responsibility to do whatever is necessary.

18. A patient becomes very upset and insists on going home against medical advice. What should the nurse do when the patient refuses to wait for the doctor and refuses to sign the "Discharge Against Medical Advice" form?

a. Force the patient to stay in the room until the doctor arrives.

b. State on the form that the patient refuses to sign.

c. Notify the hospital security officer to keep the patient on the unit.

d. Give a tranquilizing drug by injection to calm the patient.

19. All of the following occurrences are considered a patient incident and should be reported on an Incident Report, except for

     a. a fall to the floor while getting out of bed.

     b. a hole burned into the mattress from a smoldering cigarette butt.

     c. giving the patient the wrong medication.

     d. the patient's having developed a pressure area on the sacrum.

20. What happens to the incident report after it is made out?

     a. It is put on the patient's chart.

     b. It is sent to Medical Records.

     c. It is sent to Administration office.

     d. A copy is given to the patient.

POST-TEST ANSWERS

1. e		11. c
2. b		12. d
3. c		13. b
4. b		14. c
5. e		15. c
6. a		16. b
7. b		17. a
8. a		18. b
9. b		19. d
10. e		20. c

HANDWASHING TECHNIQUE

GENERAL PERFORMANCE OBJECTIVE

Employ the correct technique for washing the hands at all appropriate times in order to maintain standards of cleanliness that will minimize the risk of contracting or transmitting infections.

SPECIFIC PERFORMANCE OBJECTIVES

Upon completion of this lesson you will be able to:

1. Name the routes by which bacteria can be transmitted, recognize the conditions that are favorable and unfavorable to their growth, and take appropriate handwashing precautions against bacterial contamination.

2. State at least five circumstances that necessitate washing your hands as a result of direct or indirect contact with contaminated materials.

3. Wash your hands without any contamination of hands, body, or clothing.

4. Explain and demonstrate correct handwashing technique to others.

VOCABULARY

abrasion—an injury resulting when a portion of skin or mucous membrane is scraped away.
anaerobic—anything that lives or grows in the absence of oxygen.
antiseptic—preventing or arresting the growth or action of microorganisms.
asepsis—the absence of germs, freedom from infectious material.
bacteria—one-celled microorganisms, some of which cause disease.
contaminate—to soil or pollute; to render unclean or unsterile.
debris—rubbish or ruin.
friction—the rubbing of one thing against another.
genitourinary—pertaining to the organs of reproduction and excretion.
germ—a common term for disease-causing microorganisms.
medical asepsis—the absence of germs or infectious material in medical settings.
microorganisms—exceedingly small living bodies not visible to the naked eye.
palm—concave area of the hand between the base of the fingers and the wrist.
pathogenic—related to or causing disease.
virulence—the ability of an organism to cause severe disease or symptoms in the host.

INTRODUCTION

One of the most important tasks you have in the health field is providing a healthy environment for both your patient and yourself. A clean, dry, light, and airy atmosphere goes a long way toward preventing the growth of germs or killing those that already exist.

One of the simplest methods we have to prevent the spread of disease and germs is the handwashing technique. It is a safety skill not only for you personally but also for your patient, coworkers, visitors, and your family. It assists in protecting you and others from the spread of infections and disease. You will wash your hands before and after doing any procedures that involve direct or indirect contact with a patient, after contact with any wastes or contaminated materials, before handling any food or food receptacles, and at any other time when your hands are soiled.

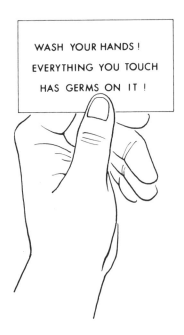

HANDWASHING FOR ASEPSIS

ITEM 1. UNDERSTANDING THE GERM THEORY

As you enter your career in caring for sick people, you need to develop an understanding of how germs cause disease and how nurses use principles of medical asepsis to carry out one of the most important nursing goals: that of protecting the patient from infection. Medical asepsis includes the techniques and skills used to render any medical setting free of disease-causing microorganisms, although nonharmful microorganisms may still be present. The most crucial of these skills, and one of the most effective actions in preventing the spread of infection, is handwashing.

Our world is teeming with microorganisms — extremely small bits of plant or animal life, too small to be seen with the naked eye. They can be seen and studied with the use of a microscope. Only a small number of microorganisms are harmful and capable of causing diseases; these are referred to as germs, or pathogenic organisms. Bacteria are one-celled microorganisms. Some are pathogenic and cause infections, whereas others are nonpathogenic.

People come in contact with microorganisms and germs constantly, but the body's defenses are strong enough to protect us from diseases most of the time. Microorganisms consist of protein, have a certain amount of weight (although it is very minute), and are unable to move about on their own. Because they are exceedingly small, they are picked up and carried by the slightest air current, and they settle on any convenient surface. Because they have weight, they drift lower and lower until they settle on a surface, so the heaviest concentration of microorganisms is usually found on floors. No matter what you touch, microorganisms will be present; even on sterile items that have been exposed to the air for a short period of time.

Microorganisms are found on all of our skin surfaces. Large numbers are found within the body, especially in the air passages of the respiratory tract, in the mouth, and along the entire length of the digestive tract. Normal, harmless residents of the intestinal tract include *Escherichia coli (E. coli)* and *Proteus vulgaris.* Such organisms, however, may cause an infection if introduced into a different part of the body, such as the urinary bladder, or into an open wound. The skin is an effective barrier against pathogenic organisms and protects the delicate organs within the body. Vigorous washing removes most of the microorganisms on the surface of the skin that are picked up when we come in contact with objects, but it cannot remove all of those that reside in the grooves and crevices that are present in the outer layers of skin. Additional protection against microorganisms is provided by the immune system of the body.

Infections are caused by germs that invade the tissues of the body and set up a chemical reaction that causes the tissues to react in the symptoms associated with the disease: fever, swelling, redness, pain, and some loss of function of the part. Generally, people develop infections when one or more of these conditions exist: (1) The body is exposed to a large number of pathogenic organisms; (2) the body is attacked by germs that are very strong and virulent or capable of causing a more serious illness or severe symptoms; or (3) the individual has low resistance.

Through the use of medical asepsis, nurses provide a safe environment for sick patients who are particularly susceptible to infections. They have low resistance owing to the disease and to the anxiety it produces. Medical asepsis includes various actions and skills that reduce the number of pathogenic organisms present in the immediate vicinity. It is necessary to reduce the number of all microorganisms in order to lower the number of pathogens, and this is done by frequent handwashing, cleaning dirty or soiled surfaces, disposing of highly contaminated dressings or items, using clean or sterile equipment and supplies, and so on.

From this brief look at how germs cause disease, we can form several general principles:

1. Microorganisms are everywhere in our environment.

2. Microorganisms are unable to move by themselves and must be carried or transported from one location to another.

3. Germs, or pathogenic organisms, are opportunists just waiting to attack when conditions favor their growth and survival.

4. The severity of the infection caused by germs depends on the number of pathogenic organisms present, the virulence of the organisms, and the resistance of the infected individual.

ITEM 2. CONDITIONS FOR THE GROWTH OF MICROORGANISMS

Because microorganisms are living organisms, they need certain environmental conditions to help them live and grow — just as you do:

Moisture: Needed in the process of nutrition to break down solid food particles to permit their utilization as nutrients for the body cells. Moisture also enables waste materials to be expelled from the body.

Food: Needed to assist in the growth process of the organism.

Oxygen: Most living organisms need an oxygen supply to live, but there are some organisms that do not; they are called anaerobic (without oxygen). Some common anaerobic pathogens you may have heard about are tetanus and gas gangrene organisms.

Temperature: The normal body temperature (98.6°F) is the best temperature for most bacteria to grow and multiply. High temperatures (over 170°F) kill most bacteria. Therefore, heat in various forms is often used to disinfect objects — to kill the germs, in other words. Below-freezing temperatures (under 32°F) inhibit the growth of bacteria, although many bacteria cannot be killed in this manner.

Darkness: Most microorganisms die when exposed to light; they multiply rapidly in darkness. This is why airing and sunning of articles from a patient's home or room are highly effective ways of killing germs.

When pathogenic organisms enter the body through a break in the skin or one of the body openings, the internal conditions favor their growth. It is warm, dark, moist, with tissues of the body supplying nutrients and oxygen as needed. Germs multiply in as little as 20 minutes and grow in any place that provides these conditions. In hospitals, they can grow profusely in air-conditioning systems, in mopping water, in wet soap dishes, on bed linens and pillows used by patients, and in similar places. Cleanliness of all areas of the hospital is essential because germs multiply so rapidly and pose such a serious threat to people who are already ill. Since nurses and other care-givers come in direct contact with patients, it is important that the number of organisms harbored on the skin be reduced by handwashing and attending to personal cleanliness.

ITEM 3. HOW MICROORGANISMS ARE SPREAD

Microorganisms are incapable of moving by themselves, so they must rely on other vehicles for transportation from one site to another. For an infection to occur, the pathogens have to escape from the reservoir or host where they have multiplied, and be transmitted to another host. They are carried in the following ways:

1. by human, animal, or insect carriers;

2. on objects such as furniture, clothing, dressings, medical equipment;

3. by air currents produced by winds, drafts, sneezing, or coughing; and

4. in foods, water, milk, and other ingestible materials.

Probably the most common method of transporting microorganisms is by direct contact with an infected person, contaminated materials, or supplies; thus they are carried on the hands or skin to another susceptible person. In the hospital setting, microorganisms are spread in the various ways shown in the illustrations: from worker to worker, from contaminated equipment to the patient or a worker, from patient to patient, or from worker to patient.

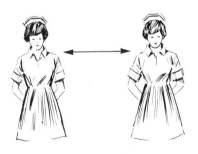

Worker to worker.

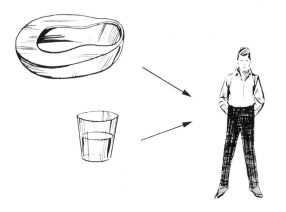

Hospital equipment to patient or worker.

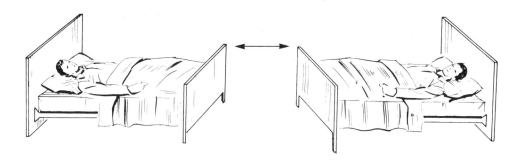

Patient to patient.

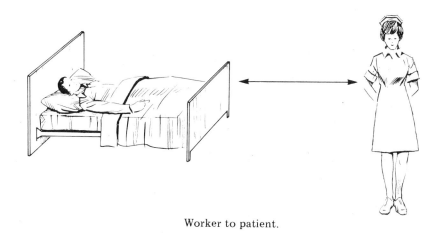

Worker to patient.

How Microorganisms Are Transferred.

ITEM 4. SPECIAL INSTRUCTIONS FOR HANDWASHING

In order to provide a safe environment for the patient and to reduce the number of microorganisms as well as the total number of pathogens, the nurse washes hands frequently when providing nursing care. Hands should be washed before and after giving care to patients; after touching contaminated materials or objects such as soiled dressings, blowing your nose, or going to the bathroom; and before handling food.

In addition to washing your hands frequently, you should follow these guidelines regarding temperature of the water, types of soap to use, length of time to scrub, and use of towels.

Care of Your Hands. Jewelry should not be worn when giving patient care because microorganisms become lodged in the settings or stones of rings. The only exception is a plain wedding band. Fingernails should be kept clean and short. By following these two requirements, you minimize the accumulation of bacteria on the hands or nails, which in turn can be spread to other persons. Proper hand care includes prevention of hangnails and skin abrasions, which might provide entry of bacteria into your body and cause you to become ill.

Types of Soaps. Soap combines with foreign matter on the skin and lowers the surface tension (clinging effect) of grease and dirt, thus permitting them to be easily removed from the skin surfaces. Most health agencies prefer to use liquid soaps. When an investigation was made of soap bars and soap dishes in use, many bacteria were found to be growing on them. The bar of soap can be a germ-carrier itself when it is contaminated by dirty water. Care must be taken to rinse the soap well before returning it to the soap dish. This reduces the chance that the next person will use contaminated soap.

Bacteria-inhibiting (bacteriostatic) liquid soaps may be used for special handwashing and disinfecting of skin surfaces. The active ingredient in these types of soaps is hexachlorophene, which has a cumulative effect in reducing bacteria on the skin; the more often it is used, and the longer it remains on the skin, the fewer the bacteria that grow. However, you should use preparations such as pHisoHex and others with care and as directed, since hexachlorophene may produce other effects as well.

Water and Temperature. Running water carries away dirt and debris. If a water faucet is not available, secure a pitcher of clean water and ask someone to pour the water over your hands and forearms.

Warm water makes better suds than does cold water and is preferred to hot water because it removes less protective oil from the skin. Extremely hot or cold water tends to dry the skin. With repeated washing, your skin may become chapped or cracked, thus providing the prime site for germs to enter the body.

Towels. Paper towels are best because they are disposable. If only cloth towels are available, wipe hands on clean, unused areas and discard when soiled.

Container for Soiled Towels. Wastebaskets should be placed beside each lavatory for paper towel disposal. Linen hampers should be available in each wash area where linen towels are used.

Recommended Handwashing Schedule

1. Beginning tour of duty: 2 minute (120 strokes). Since the hands are the most grossly soiled, they are washed first. After the wrists and forearms have been washed and rinsed, the hands are washed again to remove any bacteria that may have been picked up by washing the arms and wrists.

2. Between patients: 30 seconds (30 strokes) for patients not grossly contaminated; 60 seconds (60 strokes) for grossly contaminated patients.

ITEM 5. 2-MINUTE HANDWASH FOR MEDICAL SEPSIS

Important Steps   Key Points

1. Remove all jewelry.

Important Steps   **Key Points**

2. Approach the sink.

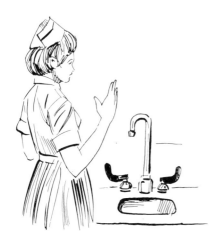

Stand in a comfortable position, leaning slightly toward the sink. Maintain good body alignment. Avoid contaminating your uniform by touching the sink or getting it wet. Usually there are many microorganisms around the sink area, because they grow and multiply rapidly in moist surroundings.

3. Turn on the water.

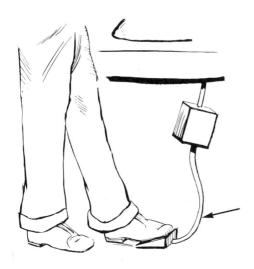

Keep the water running continuously throughout the handwashing procedure. You may find one of three main types of faucet at your agency:

    a. Hand-operated faucets. Because of the bacteria usually present in the sink areas, the faucet handles and the inside of the sink are considered contaminated. You can turn on the water with your hands, but you should protect your clean hands from contamination by using a paper towel to turn off the water.

    b. A sink with a foot pedal enables you to turn on and regulate the flow of the water without contaminating your hands.

    c. A sink with elbow levers is used frequently in hospitals, particularly in the operating room area.

4. Adjust the temperature of the water.

Important Steps   **Key Points**

5. Wet your hands with water.

Hold your hands down toward the sink, lower than your elbows. Water will then drain from the wrists to the fingertips and carry the bacteria away.

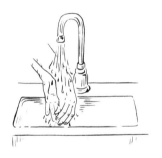

6. Apply soap (or detergent).

Use approximately 2 to 4 cc (one teaspoon) of a liquid soap.

If bar soap is used, rinse it well before returning it to the soap dish at the end of the handwashing procedure. The soap dish should be the kind that permits the bar of soap to dry on all sides before reuse. (Remember that dry surfaces help to stop the growth of bacteria.)

If you accidentally drop the bar of soap on the floor while washing, pick it up, rinse it thoroughly, and then begin again at Step 1 of the handwashing procedure!

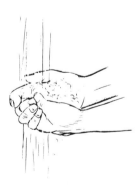

7. Wash your hands.

This step will take about 30 seconds: 10 seconds for the palms; 10 seconds for the backs of the hands; and 10 seconds for the fingers.

Important Steps	**Key Points**

Wash the palms of the hands using ten rotary (circular) motions and friction (strong rubbing movements).

Wash the back of each hand with ten rotary motions.

Wash your fingers with ten rotary motions. The fingers and thumbs should be interlaced to clean the spaces between the fingers quickly and efficiently.

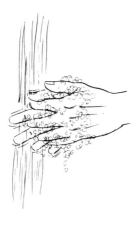

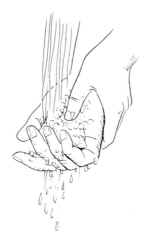

8. Rinse well.

Hold your hands with the fingers pointing downward. Avoid touching any portion of the sink with your hands.

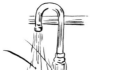

9. Wash your wrists and forearms with soap.

Use soap and wash one wrist and forearm for 10 to 15 seconds, using firm rotary and friction action. Then wash the other wrist and forearm in the same manner, moving from the wrist up toward the elbow. Total strokes for both arms = 30.

10. Rinse your arms and hands.

Again, remember to drain the water from the forearm to your fingertips.

U
N
I
T
8

Important Steps	Key Points
11. Repeat Steps 5 through 9.	60 strokes. All remaining bacteria and soil should now be gone.
12. Inspect your knuckles.	The knuckles frequently harbor excessive bacteria and germs in the folds of the skin and need additional attention. If so, cleanse with soap, using firm friction and rotary action.
13. Clean your fingernails.	Fingernails should be cleaned at the beginning of your tour of duty and as needed during the shift. An orange stick or a curved end of a flat toothpick will remove the dirt and help prevent breaks in the skin; discard it after use.
14. Dry your hands well.	Because you wash your hands many times throughout your tour of duty, it is necessary to dry them very gently and carefully to avoid chapping. Chapped skin frequently breaks open, thus permitting bacteria to enter your system.

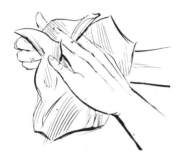

Dry hands well.

15. Turn off the running water.	Use a paper towel to turn off the hand faucet. Discard the towel into the wastebasket.
16. Apply lotion.	Use lotion as desired to keep your skin soft.

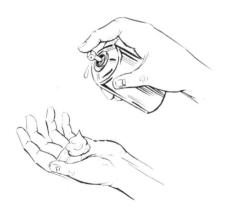

Apply lotion.

17. Leave sink area neat and clean.	Wipe the surfaces surrounding the skin with a paper towel. Remember that germs thrive on moist surfaces! Discard the towel. A clean, dry environment promotes health.

ITEM 6. ENRICHMENT

The Nature of Bacteria and Microorganisms

There are many kinds of microorganisms; bacteria represent only one type.

You have learned that handwashing is a way of preventing the spread of bacteria and other microorganisms in order to protect the patient, others, and yourself.

You now know that bacteria enter the body through the mouth, the nose, and the genitourinary tract. Each of these tracks has secretions that serve as barriers to bacteria. Threadlike cilia (hairs) and the mucous membrane of the nose are so effective in removing dust and bacteria that the lungs are kept relatively free of these microorganisms. There is an acid reaction to urine and vaginal secretions that prevents growth of most bacteria in the genitourinary tract. Digestive juices kill some of the bacteria that enter through the mouth, and the mucous membranes of the intestines are effective in keeping bacteria from invading the tissues.

One kind of bacteria that is generally found on the skin is the staphylococcus (plural, staphylococci), commonly called "staph." All health facilities are plagued by this disease-causing organism. When staph enters the body, usually through a break in the skin, it causes local infection or soreness with pus. Staph is also one of the agents responsible for boils, styes on eyelids, infections in surgical wounds, infections around fingernails, and food poisoning.

Drugs called antibiotics are used to fight this type of infection, but staphylococcus and certain other microorganisms are highly resistant to most antibiotics.

Staphylococci are present on your skin most of the time, even when you are in good health. This is one reason why handwashing is so important. Like all bacteria, "staph" thrives in moist, dark places. Direct sunlight is its enemy because it dries and kills "staph" when it is exposed for a given time.

Escherichia coli are common inhabitants of the alimentary tract and are present in feces. This bacteria may cause an inflammatory condition of the urinary bladder, gallbladder, or peritoneal cavity. Washing your hands is very important after handling a bedpan or coming in contact with feces at any time.

Pseudomonas aeruginosa is a pathogenic microorganism found in draining wounds, infant diarrhea, otitis media (ear infections), and some other conditions that cause one who is infected to become very ill.

Harmful microorganisms are spread more by hands than by any other method. Proper handwashing can prevent the spread of such germs.

U
N
I
T
8

PERFORMANCE TEST

In the skill laboratory, correctly demonstrate the handwashing procedure for medical asepsis, carefully observing the proper sequence of steps listed in the unit.

PERFORMANCE CHECKLIST

Demonstrate the correct handwashing technique:

1. Stand away from the sink in order to keep your clothing from touching the sink.

2. Turn the water on; adjust it to warm temperature. Keep the water running during the entire procedure.

3. Wet your hands.

4. Apply soap thoroughly — under the nails and between the fingers.

5. Wash the palms and the backs of your hands with strong frictional motion (ten rotary movements for at least 20 seconds).

6. Wash the fingers and spaces between them, interlacing the fingers, rubbing them up and down for 10 seconds (ten strokes).

7. Wash the wrists and three or four inches above the wrists, using rotary action (10–15 times).

8. Repeat steps 4 through 7 (completion of two-minute scrub, 120 strokes).

9. Pay special attention to problem areas.

10. Rinse well; run the water from wrists to fingers (final rinse).

11. Dry hands thoroughly with a paper towel from wrists to fingertips.

12. Turn off the water faucet with a paper towel and discard the towel into a receptacle.

13. Use hand lotion if desired.

POST-TEST

Multiple Choice: Select the one best answer for each of the questions.

1. One of the goals of nursing care is to keep the patient free of infection. The foremost method the nurse uses to achieve this goal is to

    a. give antibiotic drugs to kill the organisms.

    b. use only sterile items or supplies for the patient.

    c. follow principles of surgical asepsis.

    d. wash hands between patients and when contaminated.

2. Which of the following terms most clearly defines the word "germ"?

    a. nonpathogenic organism

    b. pathogenic organism

    c. a bacterium

    d. microorganism

3. The reason that people are free of infection most of the time is that

    a. there are few disease-causing organisms around.

    b. microorganisms gain entrance to the body only through a break in the skin.

    c. microorganisms do not adhere to the skin of the body.

    d. the body's defense mechanisms protect it from invading germs.

4. The body is protected from infections caused by microorganisms by means of

    a. the skin and mucous membranes.

    b. the muscular-skeletal system.

    c. the gastrointestinal tract.

    d. the urinary system.

5. Microorganisms are normally found within all of the following portions of the body except

    a. the urinary bladder.

    b. the nose and mouth.

    c. the air passages to the lungs.

    d. the digestive tract.

    e. none of these.

6. Microorganisms have which of the following characteristics?

    a. They are exceedingly small.

    b. They have weight.

    c. They move by sliding.

    d. All of the above.

    e. a and b

U
N
I
T
8

7. The effect of vigorous handwashing is that it

    a. renders the skin free of microorganisms.

    b. makes the skin chapped and reddened.

    c. removes the microorganisms from the surface.

    d. removes organisms from grooves and creases of the skin.

8. Any of the following conditions must exist in order for a person to develop an infection, except which one?

    a. The presence of a large number of pathogenic organisms.

    b. Exposure of the organisms to direct sunshine.

    c. The organism invading the body is more virulent than others.

    d. The individual has lowered resistance to fight off an infection.

9. Sick people are much more susceptible to developing infections because

    a. they are in hospitals or extended care facilities.

    b. they have lowered resistance.

    c. there are more microorganisms in the air.

    d. health workers handle more contaminated materials.

10. Germs grow and multiply when the conditions include all of the following except

    a. open basins of disinfectant solution.

    b. any dark, moist location.

    c. temperatures within the normal body range.

    d. available supply of oxygen.

11. The most common method of transmitting pathogenic organisms to another person in the hospital setting is by

    a. wounds draining pus.

    b. a contaminated instrument.

    c. air currents.

    d. another infected person.

12. When conditions favor their growth, how long does it take germs to multiply?

    a. 2 to 3 days.

    b. 24 hours.

    c. 20 minutes.

    d. 2 to 3 minutes.

13. The main reason the nurse should not wear jewelry or rings, other than a plain wedding band, is

    a. the setting or item might be lost.

    b. they harbor pathogenic organisms.

    c. the brilliance is dulled by using hand lotions.

    d. patients may be scratched by the stone or setting.

    e. it is a traditional custom in nursing.

14. The biggest disadvantage in using bars of soap for handwashing in hospital settings is

    a. the bars wear down so quickly.

    b. the cost of bars is higher.

    c. they slip so easily fron one's grasp.

    d. organisms grow in damp soap dishes.

15. When washing at the sink, the nurse's hands should have the fingers pointed downward with the fingers below the level of the elbows because

    a. it will be easier to inspect the nails and knuckles.

    b. they are contaminated and should be below the waist level.

    c. sudsy water containing debris is not rinsed back over clean hands.

    d. it aids circulation and prevents chapping of the skin.

16. The length of time the nurse should wash hands after giving the patient AM care and a bed bath is

    a. 2 minutes.

    b. 90 seconds.

    c. 30 seconds.

    d. 1 minute.

POST-TEST ANSWERS

1. d		9. b	
2. b		10. a	
3. d		11. d	
4. a		12. c	
5. a		13. b	
6. e		14. d	
7. c		15. c	
8. b		16. c	

UNIT 8

Unit 9

GENERAL PERFORMANCE OBJECTIVE

Upon completion of this unit, you will be able to prepare the unoccupied (closed), occupied, and anesthetic hospital bed in a way that presents a neat appearance, remains intact with use, and provides a safe and comfortable environment for the patient. You will also be able to operate the controls of the bed in order to adjust the position of the bed as may be required.

SPECIFIC PERFORMANCE OBJECTIVES

When you have completed this lesson you will be able to:

1. Adjust the hospital bed in the following positions, either manually or using the electrical control panel: high bed, low bed, Fowler's, semi-Fowler's, Trendelenburg, reverse Trendelenburg, and contour positions.

2. Remove blanket and spread from bed and fold for reuse, using longitudinal or horizontal center fold method.

3. Make an unoccupied bed starting from the bare mattress by selecting the required bed linens, placing them correctly and securely on the bed, and adjusting the bed to the appropriate position. This must be accomplished in *6 minutes or less.*

4. Make an occupied bed, which has a patient in it who is able to move without assistance, by selecting the required bed linens. Change all but the top linen by giving the patient the correct directions for moving and by adjusting the bed to the proper position for your work. This should take from 10 to 12 minutes to accomplish.

5. In *6 minutes or less*, make an anesthetic or surgical bed by selecting and using the appropriate items of bed linen, with the top bedding pie-folded or fan-folded on one side of the bed to permit easier transfer of a helpless patient into the bed; then adjust the position of the bed appropriately.

6. Identify special equipment attached to the hospital bed, including bedboards, IV rods, overbed frame, trapeze, and Balkan frame.

VOCABULARY

anesthetic bed (postoperative, recovery, or surgical)—a bed made with top linens folded in such a way as to permit easy, rapid transfer of a patient from stretcher to the bed.

closed bed—a clean bed with linens on it that is ready for a newly admitted patient; the top spread covers the entire bed and protects the bottom linens from dust until the bed is occupied by patient.

contour bed—the head, knee, and foot sections of the bed are elevated.

drawsheet—a special sheet (rubber, plastic, or cotton) that is about one-half the size of a regular sheet and is placed across the middle third of the bed to protect the bottom sheet from soiling; may be used to assist in moving heavy patients.

foundation sheet—the bottom (lower) sheet placed directly over the mattress pad or the mattress.

Gatch—the notch that fits into a ratchet on the underframe of the bed to maintain it in a sitting position; the Gatch bed was named after Dr. William Gatch, an American surgeon, who invented it in the late 1800's.

miter—a method of making equal angles so that sheets, blankets, and bedspreads fit corners properly and hold firmly.

occupied bed—the complete linen change with a patient lying in the bed.

pleat (tuck)—folded or double layer of material; a method of providing additional room in the top linens on a bed to prevent pressure on the patient's feet and toes.

reverse Trendelenburg—the head elevated and the foot section of the bed lowered.

taut—tense, or pulled tightly.

Trendelenburg—the head of the bed lowered and the foot of the bed elevated.

INTRODUCTION

Patients in a hospital spend a great part of their time in bed. Wrinkles and bumps or improperly placed top covers may cause them to feel uncomfortable and to become irritable. Hospital beds can be made skillfully so that wrinkles are reduced and the bed is comfortable.

A hospital bed must be made so that it is easy for the patient to get into it despite physical disabilities. It must also be convenient for hospital workers to put a helpless patient into bed. This may require adjusting the position of the bed and making the bed in special ways. The patient's condition and the usual procedure of the hospital are considered when determining the method for making the bed.

In this unit, you will learn how to operate manually or electrically controlled beds and to put the bed into various positions. There are routine ways of making beds in hospitals efficiently, uniformly, and neatly so that they meet the needs of most patients. You will learn how to make an unoccupied and a closed bed, an occupied bed, and an anesthetic or surgical bed.

MAKING HOSPITAL BEDS

ITEM 1. PRINCIPLES RELATED TO BEDMAKING

Although bed rest is an important part of the medical treatment of patients in hospitals and extended care facilities, the goal of nursing care is to get patients out of bed as soon as possible and increasingly active as they recover. You will find that most of your patients can get up to sit in a chair and that you can make the unoccupied bed during this time. When the physical debility and weakness of other patients prevent them from getting out of bed, you will be required to change the linens while the patient is in bed. Procedures for making both the unoccupied and the occupied bed are given in later items of this unit.

Supplies of linen are delivered to the nursing units for distribution. A common practice is to supply a linen pack or set that contains the routine amount of linen for the patient's daily use, and this is delivered to the patient's bedside or picked up by the nurse. The pack includes one or two large sheets, a drawsheet (if used), pillowcase, patient gown or pajamas, wash cloth, hand towel, and bath towel. The general hospital patient has linens changed daily following the bath and as needed when it becomes wet or soiled during the day. Although adequate supplies of linen are provided, clean linens should be used as needed and not wasted.

As you handle linens, make beds, and operate beds, there are a number of principles to observe:

1. Avoid contaminating clean linen. Linen taken into the patient's room is considered to be exposed to that patient's microorganisms, a possible source of contamination. While it can be used for that patient, it should not be returned to the clean linen

U
N
I
T
9

supply if unused, nor should it be used for another patient. Take only the amount of linen you will need into the patient's room and do not store extra linen in room closets, dressers, or bedside stands.

2. Linens should be unfolded and placed on the bed, not flipped or fanned. Fanning bed linens stirs up air currents that carry microorganisms far beyond the bed.

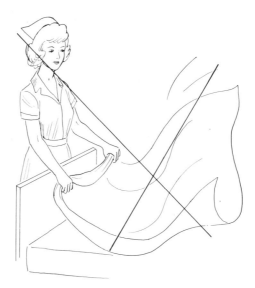

3. Bed linens, pillows, and blankets used by patients are contaminated with their microorganisms, some of them also disease-causing bacteria, and these items should be handled carefully to prevent the spread of infection. Avoid placing used or soiled linen from one patient's unit on the bed, table, or other furniture belonging to another patient's unit.

4. Use good body alignment and a wide base of support when making beds. Avoid reaching across the bed to the extent that you have to raise one foot off the floor in order to maintain your balance.

5. Work on one side of the bed and finish changing the linen there before going to the other side. Do not stand at the foot of the bed to unfold linen or tuck it under the mattress. It is very difficult to work at the foot of the bed and use good body alignment. Back muscles are more easily strained by these kinds of movement than are the stronger muscles of your thighs, hips, and arms.

6. Discard soiled linen in closed linen hampers. Carry it in your hands and avoid letting it touch your uniform, since it is contaminated with the patient's microorganisms. Wash your hands after disposing of the soiled linen.

7. When making an occupied or unoccupied bed, keep the patient in your field of vision as much as possible in order to continue your observations of his or her condition.

ITEM 2. OPERATING HOSPITAL BEDS

Manually Operated Bed. The hand-cranked bed requires effort and muscle power. When you operate this bed, it is essential that you use good body alignment and movements.

The manually operated bed has hand-cranks at its foot that are used to adjust the position of the bed.

To raise and lower the entire bed, pull out the hand-crank at the center of the bed and turn it clockwise to *raise* the bed. Turn it counterclockwise to *lower* the bed.

To place the bed in Fowler's and semi-Fowler's positions, pull out the hand-crank at the foot of the left side of the bed and turn it clockwise to *raise* the head of the bed. Turn it counterclockwise to *lower* the head of the bed. Fowler's position is that in which the head of the bed is elevated, usually between 30 and 60 degrees. The foot of the bed is not elevated but remains flat. Semi-Fowler's position is that in which the head of the bed is in Fowler's position and the knee or foot of the bed is elevated about 15 degrees. *To raise and lower the knees*, pull out the handcrank at the foot of the right side of the bed and turn it clockwise to *raise* the knee portion of the bed. Turn it counterclockwise to *lower* the knee portion of the bed.

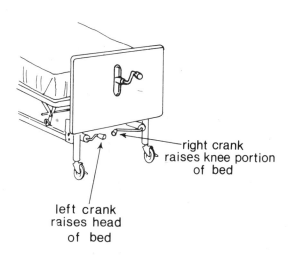

right crank raises knee portion of bed

left crank raises head of bed

Electrically Operated Bed. First introduced in 1956, the electric bed is operated by a motor that adjusts the bed to the desired position for treatment or for comfort. The patient may operate the bed controls by touch, unless the controls have been purposely locked to ensure a prescribed position.

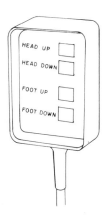

Hand controls.

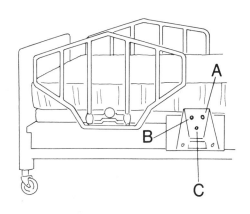

Electric controls located at side of bed.

Electric beds are made by a number of manufacturers who produce different types of adjustment controls used to operate the bed. Generally, the controls are sliding levers attached to a panel on the side of the bed, or push-buttons located on a moveable device connected to the bed by a cable. The controls enable the patient or the nurse to change the position of the bed with little effort.

To raise the backrest, push the "Head Up" button, or move control lever "A" toward the foot of the bed. *To lower the backrest,* push the "Head Down" button, or move control lever "A" toward the head of the bed.

To raise the knee rest, push the "Foot Up" button, or move control lever "B" toward the foot of the bed. *To lower the knee rest,* push the "Foot Down" button, or move control lever "B" toward the head of the bed.

To raise the bed to the high position, push the "Bed Up" button, or move control lever "C" vertically to its highest setting. *To lower the bed to the low position,* push the "Bed Down" button, or move control lever "C" downward to its lowest setting.

ITEM 3. SIDERAILS

Siderails are used to provide for the safety of the patient and are in no way to be considered a restraint. Siderails range in size from half the length of the bed side to the full length. Each type of siderail has special levers for raising or lowering; check with your agency for proper instructions.

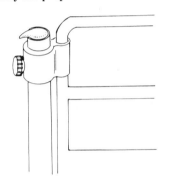

Pull knob to move siderail up or down.

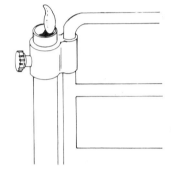

Flip cover up to remove one end of siderail from the bed.

Siderails are used to:

1. Prevent patients from falling out of bed.

2. Protect the restless patient.

3. Remind the patient when he or she is near the side of the bed and may be in danger of falling off the edge.

4. Provide security to the patient.

5. Assist ambulatory patients to get into and out of bed safely.

6. Give the patient support to grasp and hold when moving about.

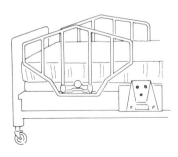

A half-length safety siderail in high position.

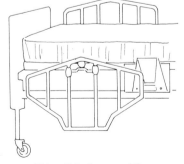

Siderail in low position.

ITEM 4.   BED POSITIONS

Most hospital beds can be adjusted to meet various needs of the patient for treatment or comfort. Some of the common positions are:

Fowler's. The backrest is raised 30 to 60 degrees above the bed level. This is used for any patient who is permitted to have the head of the bed elevated and assume a sitting position rather than remain flat in bed.

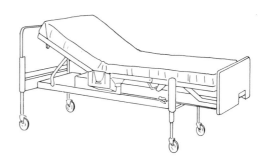

Fowler's Position (head of bed 30 to 60 degrees above bed level).

Semi-Fowler's. The backrest is raised 45 degrees. Knees may be raised 15 degrees. This is used for the general comfort of the patient; it may prevent sliding down in bed. Raising the knee rest, however, may impair circulation in the lower extremities, so check with the charge nurse before elevating the knee rest.

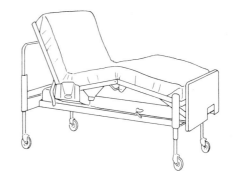

Semi-Fowler's Position (with knee position raised 15 degrees).

Trendelenburg. The head section of the bed is lowered; foot section is elevated. (Sometimes the foot of the bed is placed on "shock blocks," raised by a mechanical jack or lifter, or placed on a chair if the foot section cannot be elevated by mechanical means.) This position may be used for patients in shock from severe blood loss or other causes.

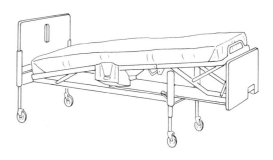

Trendelenburg's (shock).

Reverse Trendelenburg. The head section of the bed is elevated; foot section is lowered. (The head of the bed can be raised on "shock blocks" or by a mechanical jack or lifter, or placed on a chair if the head section cannot be mechanically placed in this position.) This position is used for patients with certain circulatory diseases.

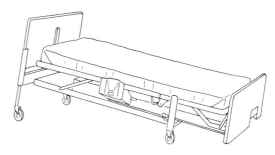

Reverse Trendelenburg's.

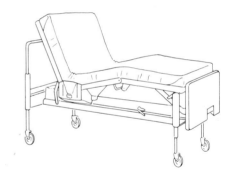

Contour. The head section is elevated; the knee and foot sections are elevated. The contour position is used for certain injuries or diseases of the lower extremities.

Contour (head section elevated and knee and foot section elevated).

ITEM 5. HANDLING LINENS

The method of handling linen is not crucial in making the hospital bed; the goal is to have a neat and clean bed that is comfortable and free of wrinkles. However, the nurse who folds and unfolds linens skillfully has more control of the articles and works in an organized way. The folded articles that are to be reused are placed neatly over the back of a chair for easier handling when used again. Stripping linen from the bed by gathering it up in a bunch and putting it on a chair until it is reused is not time- or energy-saving when you consider that each article has to be separated from the others, spread on the bed, and then rearranged until it is in place.

Linens used in the care of your patient are folded with the initial fold along the length of the article — that is, longitudinally — or with the fold across the width of it, or horizontally. When using folded linen such as sheets, spreads, and blankets in a controlled and organized manner, you need to find the first centerfold that resulted in folding the article in half. The centerfold edge is the only one with just two layers of material and determines whether the article was folded along the length of the material or across the width.

To unfold clean linen on the bed, follow these steps:

1. Identify the centerfold and determine whether the article was folded longitudinally or horizontally.

2. Place the centerfold on the proper half of the bed. If folded longitudinally, place the centerfold along the midline of the length of the bed. If folded horizontally, place the centerfold at the midline of the width and the quarterfold at the midline of the length of the bed.

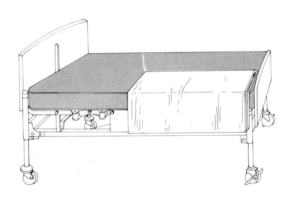

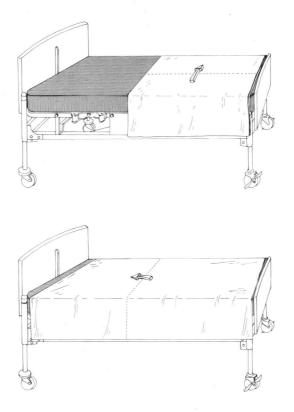

Placing horizontally folded linen on the bed.

To fold linen for reuse,

1. With one hand, select two adjacent corners of the article and line them up together.

2. Run the other hand along the two side edges for half the distance to be folded. For a large sheet this is about one yard or meter, which is equal to the distance of the width of the body and one outstretched arm.

3. Drop the corners, and pick up the centerfold directly opposite the half way point.

4. With the centerfold now in both hands, bring the corners together to fold the article in fourths and repeat once more if needed.

5. Place over the back of a chair until ready for use.

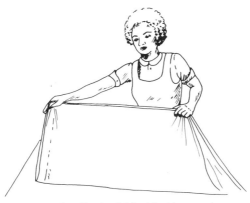

A. Centerfold at bottom

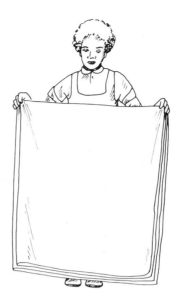

B. Centerfold in right hand

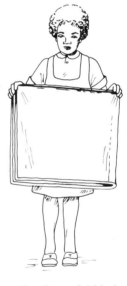

C. Centerfold in both hands

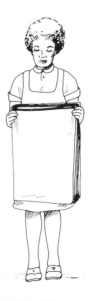

D. Final fold of linen

ITEM 6. MAKING AN UNOCCUPIED BED

In your classroom or skill laboratory, practice the following procedure for making an unoccupied bed. There should be a bed frame with mattress available for your practice use, and linen to make the bed.

▬▬

Supplies Needed

Large sheet (2)	Drawsheet (1)
Pillows (1 or 2)	Pillowcase (1 or 2)
Blanket	Spread

Optional Supplies (used in some agencies)

Mattress cover or pad	Plastic or rubber drawsheet

▬▬

U
N
I
T
9

Important Steps	Key Points
A. Prepare for Bedmaking	
1. Wash your hands.	
2. Assemble the linen supplies needed.	
3. Place the bed in a high position.	Having the bed in a high position puts your work at a comfortable level and helps to reduce or prevent back strain.
4. Move the mattress to the head of the bed.	Mattresses slip down when the head of the bed is raised. Stand at one side of the bed facing the head and grasp the mattress about the center and at the bottom edge. Move it toward the head of the bed, using good body alignment and movements.

B. Make the Bed on One Side	
Important Steps	**Key Points**
1. Place the large sheet at foot of bed and unfold toward the head.	Place the *centerfold* at the *center of the bed*, working from the foot of the bed to the head. The lower hem of the sheet should be even with the edge of the mattress at the foot. Then unfold the top layer onto the distal half of the bed.
2. Tuck in excess sheet at the head of the bed.	
3. Miter the corner at the head of the bed.	Pick up the side edge of the sheet so that the sheet forms a triangle with the head of the bed and the side edge is perpendicular to the bed.
	Use the palm of your hand to hold the sheet against the side of the mattress and tuck the excess sheet under the mattress.

Important Steps   **Key Points**

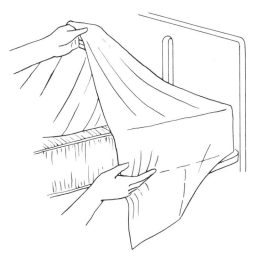

Stand facing head of bed.

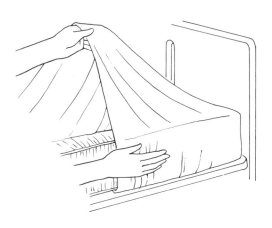

Tuck sheet under mattress.

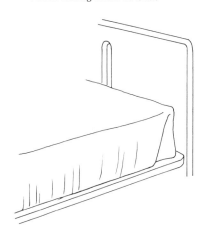

Drop the sheet over your hand, then withdraw
your hand and tuck the rest of the sheet under
the mattress.

Completed square corner.

4. Tuck the sheet under the mattress from
    head to foot of bed on one side.

5. Place a drawsheet over middle section of
    the bed and unfold, then tuck in.

Place the centerfold of the drawsheet at the
center of the bed and unfold the top layer
toward the distal side of the bed. Tuck the
proximal edge nearly under the mattress. This
step is optional in many agencies: Patients who
are up during the day may not need a drawsheet, and some agencies do not use them;
other agencies, however, may use a plastic
drawsheet covered with a cloth drawsheet to
protect the bottom linen from being soiled.

6. Place large top sheet at head of bed and
    unfold toward the foot.

Start at the head of the bed with the edge of
the sheet even with the mattress, seam side up.
Place the centerfold of the top sheet along the
center of the bed and unfold the upper layer
over on the distal half of the bed.

Important Steps	Key Points
7. Place blanket at head of bed and unfold toward the foot.	Start at the head of the bed, about 4 inches from the top of the mattress, and place the centerfold of the blanket along the center of the bed. Unfold the remaining half toward the distal side of the bed.
8. Place spread at head of bed and unfold toward the foot.	Start at the head of the bed, about 4 inches from the top of the mattress, and proceed in the same manner as with the blanket in step 7.
9. Tuck in the excess sheet, blanket, and spread at the foot of the bed.	

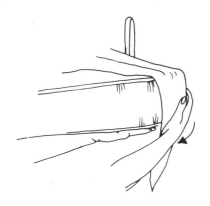

10. Miter the corner of the top linen at the foot of the bed.	Pick up the edges of the sheet, the blanket, and the spread, and smooth around the corner so that the side edge is perpendicular to the bed. Use the palm of your hand to hold the sheet, blanket, and spread against the mattress. Tuck the hanging portion under the mattress.
	Bring down the upper portion, which had been picked up, and smooth it into a neat line.
11. Make a toe pleat.	The toe pleat provides room for the feet to move in bed, and prevents pressure and strain on the toes or ankles. In some agencies, the top linens over the toes are simply elevated slightly to provide additional toe space.

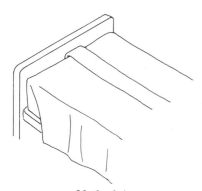

Method A
Longitudinal toe pleat.

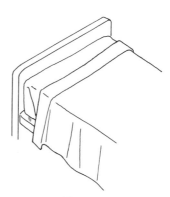

Method B
Horizontal toe pleat.

Important Steps	Key Points

Method A—At the center of the foot of the mattress, make a 6-inch lengthwise pleat in the sheet. Tuck the end of the sheet under the mattress.

Method B—About 6 to 8 inches from foot of bed, fold a 2-inch pleat across the sheet. Tuck the end of the sheet under the mattress.

C. Go to Other Side and Complete Making the Bed

1. Fan-fold top linen back toward the center of the bed while you complete the foundation.

2. Tuck in excess bottom sheet at the head of the bed.

   See steps listed in Section B.

3. Make a mitered corner.

4. Tightly tuck in bottom sheet from head to foot of bed.

   Grasp the edges of the sheet tightly in both hands with your knuckles on top, pull them tightly and smoothly down over the side of the mattress and tuck them under the mattress. Repeat the pulling and tucking all along the side, working toward the foot of the bed. Finally, pull sheet diagonally to remove wrinkles.

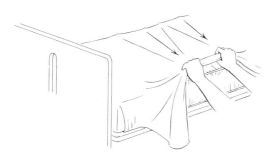

Grasp sheet; pull tight.

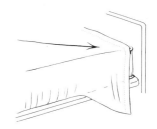

5. Tightly tuck in drawsheet.

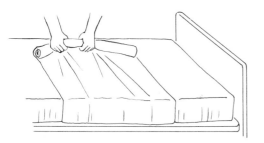

Grasp drawsheet and pull tight over mattress.

Important Steps	Key Points

6. Straighten top linen in place from head to foot of bed.

7. Fold excess sheet, blanket, and spread under the mattress at foot of bed.

8. Miter the corner of the top linens as one unit.

At the foot of the bed, miter the corner of the top linens, using the top sheet, blanket, and spread as one unit.

9. Move to the head of the bed and fold back the top sheet over the top edge of the blanket and spread.

This makes a cuff over the spread and blanket and protects them from becoming soiled when drawn up under the patient's chin. It also prevents irritation to the patient's chin by covering the rough blanket with the smooth sheet.

D. Dress the Pillows

1. Open the pillowcase.

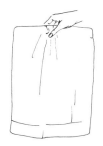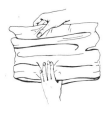

With one hand, grasp the center of the closed end of the case. With your other hand, gather the open pillowcase (as you would a stocking before putting it on) up over the hand at the closed end.

(1) Grasp center.   (2) Gather open pillowcase.

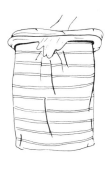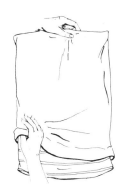

Grasp the pillow with your covered hand while holding it away from your body. With the other hand on an open edge, pull the open edges down over the pillow. Do this until the pillow is completely covered. Adjust the pillow inside the case, keeping it from contaminating your uniform.

(3) Grasp pillow.   (4) Pull pillowcase over pillow.

2. Place the dressed pillows on the bed.

Put them at the center of the head of the bed one on top of the other. Position them so that the open ends of the cases are away from the door of the room. This gives the bed a neater appearance.

E. Prepare the Bed and Unit for the Patient

1. Open the bed by folding the top covers back for easy entering.

Fan-fold the top covers toward the foot of the bed, *or* pie-fold the covers.

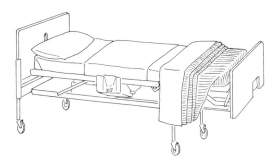

Fan-fold covers.

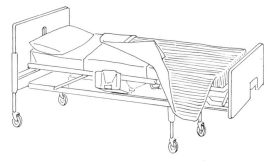

The pie-fold.

Fold accordion-type pleats 6 to 8 inches wide from the head of the bed to the foot, *or* fold half of the top cover toward the foot of the bed, and accordion pleat once or twice so that all covers are at the foot of the bed.

Place one finger at the center of the top covers facing the head of the bed. Lift the edge of the top covers and fold it back toward the center of the bed, making a triangle.

2. Place the bed in its lowest position.

This is most convenient for newly admitted, ambulatory, and semiambulatory patients to get into bed. Apply the brakes at the foot of the bed. The brakes should be in the locked position to prevent the bed from moving when the patient attempts to get into bed.

3. Attach the signal cord to the bed in a place where the patient can reach it easily.

Many cords have a special clip that clamps onto the pillowcase or foundation sheet.

4. Put the linens for the patient in the proper places.

Put towels and washcloth in the bathroom or in the bedside stand; put the hospital gown on the bed or in the bedside stand. (Use your agency procedure.)

5. Tidy the unit.

Neatly arrange the furnishings in the room; remove linen and other items not needed for the patient's use.

ITEM 7. THE CLOSED BED

The designation "closed bed" indicates that no patient occupies the bed. It is made so that the top covers and spread cover the bed completely to protect the linen beneath from soil or dust.

The procedure for making the closed bed is identical to that followed in making the unoccupied bed except for the spread. In the closed bed, the bedspread is put on as follows:

1. Place the centerfold of the spread on the bed, seam side toward the mattress. Begin at the head of the bed, and place the top edge of the spread even with the edge of the mattress.

2. Unfold the spread over the other half of the bed.

3. Tuck the spread under the bottom edge of the mattress.

4. Miter the corner on each side of the foot of the bed, making a smooth, neat corner.

5. Place the dressed pillows in the correct position with the open end of the case away from the door. Carry out the procedure in Section E to prepare the unoccupied bed and unit for the arrival of a new patient.

ITEM 8. THE ANESTHETIC OR SURGICAL BED

The anesthetic bed is also called the postoperative bed (post-op), the recovery bed, or the surgical bed. The object is to make the bed with all top bedding folded out of the way so the patient can be transferred from a stretcher to the bed with a minimum of time and movement, and then covered with the top bedding. This type of bed can be made for use when the patient undergoes medical treatments or has severe physical limitations of movement due to his condition or his disease. It is not restricted to patients who undergo surgery.

Basically, the bed is made in the same manner as the "unoccupied bed." There are some minor changes, which you should practice in the classroom or skill laboratory.

Supplies Needed

Large sheets (2)	Pillows (1 or 2)
Drawsheet (1)	Pillowcases (1 or 2)
Blanket	Towel
Spread	

Important Steps	Key Points
1. Make the bed according to Item 6, except that the top sheet, blanket, and spread *are not tucked* under the mattress at the foot of the bed, nor are the corners mitered.	Instead of tucking the top linens under the mattress, fold the covers back toward the head of the bed to make a 6- to 8-inch cuff that is even with the edge of the mattress at the foot of the bed.
2. Fold the top covers to the side or to the foot of the bed.	a. Fan-fold the top covers lengthwise to the side of the bed. Fold the overhang of the covers up onto the bed, even with the side of the bed. Lift the covers with both hands and make a 6- to 8-inch fold; repeat once more so that all covers are folded lengthwise on the far side of the bed.
	b. Or fan-fold them widthwise to the bottom of the bed.

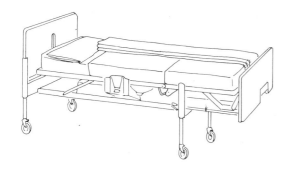

Fan-fold lengthwise.

3. Place a towel or disposable pad at the head of the foundation bed.	This is intended to protect the sheet if the patient should vomit (have an emesis).

Important Steps	Key Points
4. Place the pillows.	Put pillow either on a chair near the bed or in an upright position at the head of the bed.
5. Prepare the unit for the arrival of the patient.	
a. Check to see that siderails are attached to the bed, are in working order, and are in the lowered position.	
b. Attach the signal cord to the bed.	
c. Leave the bed in a high position.	The high level of the bed is approximately the same level as a stretcher in order to make it easier to transfer the patient from one to another.
d. Lock the brakes of the bed.	This prevents it from moving when the patient is being transferred into it.
e. Move furniture away from the bed.	Clear a space to allow room for the easy passage of the stretcher and for workers to transfer the patient from the stretcher to the bed.
f. Tidy the unit and remove linen and other items not needed for the postoperative care of the patient.	Other items that are required for the care of a patient returning from surgery will be discussed in the unit on postoperative care.

ITEM 9. MAKING AN OCCUPIED BED

In the day-by-day care of patients, it is often necessary to change some of the linen while the patient is still lying in bed. Not all patients are able to get out of bed while it is being made up with fresh linen.

The amount of linen that is changed each day varies from agency to agency. When patients are ambulatory or out of bed most of the day, bed linens are changed once or twice a week and when soiled. When patients spend most or all of the day in bed, linen is changed more frequently. Some hospitals change all of the linen each day; others change part of the linen daily. For example, a large sheet, drawsheet, pillowcase, towels, and patient gown may be provided daily for the patient's use. The usual method is to reuse the top sheet as the bottom sheet, replace the used drawsheet, change the pillowcase, and use the clean sheet as the top sheet. Spreads are reused and replaced when soiled.

Practice the procedure of making a bed with a patient in it by having one of your classmates play the part of the patient while you make the bed in the classroom or skill laboratory. This must be accomplished in 10 to 12 minutes. Remember to use good body alignment and movements as you work.

***

Supplies Needed:

Large sheet (1 or 2)	Pillowcase (1 or 2)
Drawsheet	Bath blanket

Reusable Items:

Spread	Pillows
Blanket	Linen hamper

Important Steps	Key Points
1. Wash your hands, identify the patient, explain what you plan to do, and enlist patient's cooperation.	While doing so, you can check the condition of the linens on the bed and estimate what you will need to change it.
2. Provide for the patient's privacy.	Close the door of the room, pull the bedside curtains, or use screens to provide privacy.
3. Obtain the articles of linen you will need.	Place the clean linen on the seat of a chair or on a dresser near your work area. You should plan to change the bottom sheet by reusing the current top sheet as the bottom sheet. However, some agencies may use entirely clean linen each day. You may have to share a linen hamper with other workers who are also making beds. In other hospitals, all soiled linen is carried to a central area and put in hampers that are kept there.
4. Place the bath blanket over the patient and the top covers.	Lower the siderail on one side and complete your work on that side of the bed before going to the other side. Unfold the bath blanket and ask the patient to hold the top edge, or tuck it under the shoulders to secure it. Reach under the bath blanket, grasp the top bedding (sheet, blanket, and spread) and fold to the bottom of the bed.
5. Loosen the top bedding from foot of bed and remove.	Remove the spread, fold it in half — top edge to bottom edge — or longitudinally, with side edge to side edge. Grasp the center and fold it in half, then in half one more time. Place it over the back of a chair for reuse. Remove the blanket and fold for reuse, then do the same for the top sheet.
6. Move the mattress to the head of the bed.	Have the patient help, if able, by grasping the head of the bed and pulling upward while you grasp the side edges of the mattress and move it toward the head of the bed. See Item 6, Making an Unoccupied Bed. You may need to obtain help to move the mattress with the patient on it. When moving a mattress with a helper, one person should stand at each side of the bed, grasp the mattress with both hands, and on your cue, slide it toward the head of the bed.
7. Move the patient to the distal side of the bed.	Turn patient away from you and on his side according to the instructions in the unit on positioning the patient. Patient may hold onto the siderail on the far side of the bed for support. If he is unable to hold on, you may place a pillow at the patient's back for support.
8. Make the bed on one side.	a. Loosen the foundation linens (sheet, drawsheet, and plastic drawsheet) from the top and side of the bed.
	b. Fold or roll the drawsheet toward the patient, then the plastic drawsheet, then the bottom sheet; tuck the soiled linen rolls as close to the patient's back as possible.

UNIT 9

Important Steps

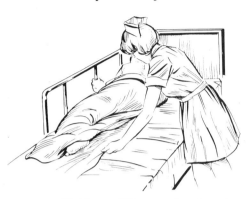

Fold or roll linen as close to
patient as possible.

9. Move the patient to the clean side of the bed.

10. Move to the other side of the bed and complete making the other side.

Key Points

c. Straighten the mattress pad to remove wrinkles.

d. Take the used large top sheet from the back of the chair and put it on the bed as a bottom sheet.

e. Unfold or unroll the plastic drawsheet, bringing it over both rolled bottom sheets; smooth it free of wrinkles and tuck it firmly under the mattress.

f. Place a clean cloth drawsheet on the bed.

g. Place the clean sheet, blanket, and clean spread on the bed according to Item 6, Making an Unoccupied Bed.

a. Reach under the top covers and hold them as you help the patient to roll over the folded linen and onto the the clean side of the bed.

b. Position the clean top covers over the patient and remove the bath blanket. Hold onto the top covers with one hand, and remove the bath blanket with the other. Avoid exposing the patient. Fold the bath blanket for reuse and put it away.

c. Raise the nearest siderail and ask patient to hold on to it for support.

d. Dress the pillow, and place it under the patient's head. (See Item 6, Making an Unoccupied Bed.)

a. Lower the siderail so that you can reach your work without straining.

b. Loosen the foundation linen on this side of the bed and remove the soiled drawsheet and large bottom sheet.

c. Straighten the mattress cover and remove wrinkles.

d. Pull and straighten the bottom sheet, tuck it under the head of the bed, miter the corner, and pull the sheet tightly along the side of the bed to remove wrinkles as you tuck it under the mattress.

e. Bring the plastic drawsheet toward you over the bottom sheet, pull it tightly to remove wrinkles, and tuck it under the mattress.

f. Bring the cloth drawsheet over the plastic drawsheet, pull it tightly to remove wrinkles, and tuck it under the mattress. When the foundation of the bed is completed, the patient can return

Important Steps	Key Points
	to the center of the bed in a dorsal recumbent position (flat on his back).
	g. Straighten the top sheet, blanket, and spread on the proximal side of the bed. Tuck top linens under the mattress at the foot of the bed. Miter the corner and complete the cuff at the top of the bed (see Item 6, Making an Unoccupied Bed).
11. Attach the patient's signal cord within his reach.	Never leave your patient without some means of summoning help.
12. Provide for the patient's safety and comfort.	Adjust the siderails according to the agency regulations. Place the bed in the low position, and the patient in a Fowler's or semi-Fowler's position if this is allowed. Position the pillows under the patient's head for good alignment and place the bedside stand and table nearby or within the patient's reach.
13. Tidy the room.	Put clean towels, a washcloth, and the patient's gown in the proper place (bathroom, bedside stand), then neatly arrange the top of the bedside stand. Remove from the room other equipment that is no longer being used, and return it to its proper place. Remove the soiled linen and the linen hamper if used.

UNIT 9

ITEM 10. SPECIAL ATTACHMENTS FOR BEDS

During the acute phase and convalescence from an illness, bed rest is one of the most essential parts of the treatment, and it is essential that hospital beds be versatile and adaptable to the many different needs of patients. In addition to adjusting the height of the bed and raising or lowering the head and foot sections, the nurse can modify the modern hospital bed through the attachment of various poles, frames, and equipment used for traction. Several of these are shown in the figures and described briefly.

Bed Boards

Bed boards, usually made of plyboard and often with a canvas cover to prevent splinters, are placed under the mattress to make the bed firmer and to prevent the mattress from sagging. Bed boards are available in two sections: one for the head of the bed and one for the foot section, so the head of the bed can be elevated for the patient's comfort. They are used for patients who have low back pain or spinal or other orthopedic problems.

IV Poles

Some hospital beds have a storage space for the IV rod and as many as six convenient receptacles for the placement of the rod. In a typical model, two receptacles are located on the head panel, two on the foot panel, and two in the center frame of the bed. A locking type notch secures the rod in place when it is inserted into the receptacle. It turns clockwise to lock in place and is turned counterclockwise to unlock and remove it.

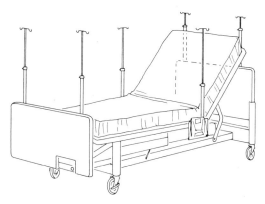

The six locations where
IV rod may be used.

Overbed Frame and Trapeze

The overbed frame is a single overhead bar that is attached to upright supports at the head and foot of the bed. It forms the frame for the attachment of trapezes, poles, pulleys, bars, and other orthopedic equipment. The trapeze is a swinging bar that is suspended from an overhead frame. By grasping it, patients can help lift themselves up in bed, move about, or turn more easily by themselves. In many agencies, there is a fee for the use of this equipment, so the physician's approval may be required. Overbed frames, trapezes, and other orthopedic attachments are applied or set up by a designated person, usually an orthopedic technician, and not the nurse. The use of the frame does not interfere with changing the linen on the bed.

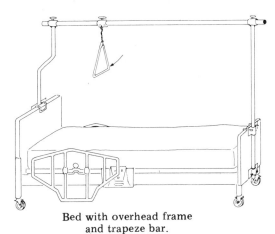

Bed with overhead frame
and trapeze bar.

Overbed frame and trapeze bar used to provide
balanced traction.

Balkan Frame

A larger type of overbed frame is the Balkan frame. It consists of a rectangular frame of pipes about the same size of the bed and supported by upright poles attached to the head and foot of the bed. The frame provides the basis for other bars, pulleys, trapezes, splints, and equipment used in various types of balanced suspension or skeletal traction. As with the overbed frame, it is set up by a designated person, usually not the nurse. The linen is changed on the bed in the same way as in the foregoing procedure, except that the top bedding is folded over the patient's body, not tucked under the mattress, if one or both extremities are in traction.

ITEM 11. CONCLUSION OF THE LESSON

You have completed the unit on making the hospital bed. After you have practiced operating the hospital bed, placing it in the various positions, and making the unoccupied bed, the anesthetic bed, and the occupied bed, you should arrange with your instructor to take the performance test. You will be expected to demonstrate your skill in performing these activities.

UNIT 9

PERFORMANCE TEST

In the classroom or skill laboratory, your instructor will ask you to demonstrate the following activities and procedures. You are to perform these without reference to the instruction book, notes, or other source materials.

1. Check the siderails of the bed. Locate the button or lever to release the siderail so that you can raise and lower the siderail several times. Notice how the siderail is attached to the bed.

2. · Given a hospital bed set in a low horizontal position, you are to adjust the bed to a number of different positions. Your instructor will tell you what position to adjust the bed to. When you have completed the adjustment, step back from the bed; the instructor will tell you the next position from among the following:

   a. Adjust the bed to Fowler's position.

   b. Adjust the bed to semi-Fowler's position.

   c. Adjust the bed to the contour position.

   d. Adjust the bed to the Trendelenburg position.

   e. Adjust the bed to the reverse Trendelenburg position.

   f. Adjust the bed to the position in which you would leave a completed *unoccupied* bed.

   g. Adjust the bed to the position in which you would leave a completed anesthetic bed.

3. Given a hospital bed adjusted to a low position with the brakes off and the siderails down, make an unoccupied bed in 6 minutes or less. Obtain the following supplies before beginning:

Large sheets	Pillowcase
Cloth drawsheet	Blanket
Pillow	Bedspread

   Notify your instructor when you are ready to begin.

4. Given a hospital bed without any linen on it, and with siderails down, brakes off, and signal cord unattached, obtain the linens listed above, and make an anesthetic bed. Inform your instructor when you have collected your supplies and are ready to begin.

5. Given a hospital bed occupied by a patient, make the bed and change all linen except for the spread, blanket, and top sheet, which you will use again. The bed is adjusted to a low position, siderails up, brakes off, and signal cord unattached. Collect the linen you will need to change the bed: a large sheet, a drawsheet, and a pillowcase. Inform your instructor when you are ready to begin.

PERFORMANCE CHECKLIST

ADJUSTMENT OF BEDS

The student will show the proper procedures for adjusting the hospital bed.

Adjust the bed correctly in the following positions without errors in selection and movement of controls:

1. Fowler's position.
2. Semi-Fowler's position.
3. Contour position.
4. Trendelenburg position.
5. Reverse Trendelenburg position.
6. Unoccupied bed position.

MAKING AN UNOCCUPIED BED

1. Select and assemble all materials required before beginning to make the bed.

2. Adjust the bed to the highest position without errors in your selection and use of controls.

3. Place the sheets, drawsheets, and blankets, and spread them in the proper sequence; position each item correctly, making one side of the bed first, then going to the other side and completing the bed.

4. Tuck each piece of bedding under the mattress neatly and make sure that each is smooth and taut.

5. Form all required mitered corners smoothly and neatly.

6. Form a toe pleat correctly at the foot of the top linens.

7. Fold back the top sheet and adjust the spread correctly in relation to the top sheet. Fan-fold or pie-fold the covers correctly to open the bed.

8. Handle and dress the pillow correctly, keeping it from contact with your body and clothing.

9. Position the pillow correctly with the open end away from the door.

10. Attach the signal cord within the patient's reach.

11. Lower the bed to its lowest position and set the brakes.

12. Adjust the siderails to the "up" position.

13. Observe good body alignment principles at all times.

14. Complete a neat and correctly made bed within 6 minutes.

MAKING AN ANESTHETIC BED

1. Select and assemble all materials needed before beginning to make the bed.

2. Wash your hands.

3. Raise the bed to working height.

4. Make one side of the bed first, then go to the other side and complete making it.

5. Place the sheets, drawsheets, blankets, and other materials in the proper sequence, positioning each piece correctly.

UNIT 9

6. Tuck each piece under the mattress correctly, making sure that each is smooth and taut.

7. Form all required mitered corners smoothly and neatly.

8. Fan-fold the top bedding to the side of the bed or to the foot of the bed, or pie-fold the top bedding to one side of the bed.

9. Place the pillows correctly, either on a chair or at the head of the bed, in a horizontal position.

10. Handle and place the pillow slip on the pillow while keeping the pillow from contacting your uniform.

11. Attach the signal cord within the patient's reach.

12. Place the bed in the correct position with the siderails down and set the brake.

13. Move furniture to make room for the stretcher.

14. Observe the principles of body alignment and proper movement at all times.

15. Reduce or eliminate contact and contamination as far as possible.

16. Proceed smoothly from one step to another in the procedure, working on one side before going to the other.

MAKING AN OCCUPIED BED

1. Wash your hands.

2. Assemble all materials before beginning to make the bed and stack the materials on a chair in order of use.

3. Identify the patient.

4. Raise the bed to its highest position.

5. Place the bath blanket correctly to cover the patient.

6. Remove the top covers and fold them correctly.

7. Move the mattress toward the head of the bed.

8. Make one side of the bed first, then go to the other side, and complete making it.

9. Remove the bottom sheet and drawsheets on each side of bed, and unfold and tuck in the new linen, performing all operations in the correct sequence.

10. Move the patient to the correct position for each step of the procedure.

11. Give appropriate explanations, directions, and assistance to the patient each time he is moved. Observe techniques of good body alignment when moving patients.

12. Remove the bath blanket from under the top sheet without exposing the patient.

13. Place sheets, drawsheets, blanket, and spread in the proper sequence, positioning each piece correctly.

14. Tuck each piece under the mattress neatly and make sure that each is smooth, free of wrinkles, and taut.

15. Form all required mitered corners smoothly and neatly.

16. Form a toe pleat correctly at the foot of the top linens.

17. Fold back the top sheet and adjust the spread correctly in relation to the top sheet.

18. Remove the soiled pillowcase and dress the pillow with a new case, handling the pillow correctly.

19. Position the pillow correctly with the open end away from the door.

20. Place the soiled linen in a laundry bag.

21. Attach the signal cord within reach of the patient.

22. Lower the bed to the lowest position and set the brake.

23. Adjust the siderails to the "up" position.

24. Adjust the bed to a comfortable position as requested by the patient.

25. Complete a neat and correctly made bed within 10 to 12 minutes.

Section 2

SKILLS RELATED TO ACTIVITY AND MOVEMENT

INTRODUCTION

One of the individual's basic needs is for activity, or the ability to move about and to change position. Any position becomes uncomfortable in a short period of time if unrelieved by movement, a fact well known to any student who has tried to sit still in a classroom for an hour. Movement of parts of the body is essential for health, and limited movement affects all systems of the body. Immobility, or the lack of movement, produces adverse effects on the body within hours; some of these prolong illness, and others may cause permanent damage.

Illness interrupts the individual's ability to move about. Physical immobility may be induced by injury, disease, pain, weakness, or fatigue; it can also be caused by medically prescribed treatment in the form of bedrest, the use of traction or casts, and the use of catheters, tubes, or equipment that interferes with movement. An important part of your nursing care involves helping patients meet their needs for movement and activity, since the majority of patients in general hospitals and long-term care facilities have impaired ability to move about freely or without assistance.

This section deals with movement and activity for the nurse as well as the patient. Units 10 and 11 explain the function of muscles, the types of actions involved in the various joint movements, and the principles of proper body alignment. The principles are included that relate to movements the nurse uses in performing nursing activities. Methods for changing the position of bed patients, preventing the adverse effects of pressure on the body, assisting to dangle and ambulate, and putting affected joints through the range-of-motion exercises are presented in Units 12 and 13. Then Units 14 and 15 discuss the principles and procedures for using various mechanical aids such as wheelchairs, crutches, braces, and patient-turning frames.

DIRECTIONS FOR STUDENTS

Read the objectives for the unit carefully to learn what you are expected to know or do, and review the words and medical terms included in the vocabulary. Although you have used these movements throughout your life, practicing in the skills laboratory will enable you to give your patients step-by-step instructions, turn and position patients correctly, and use the various mechanical devices that enable the patient to move or provide support for the body. For some of the procedures, such as range-of-motion exercises, the only thing you will need will be your own hands and body. Other procedures require certain items or equipment, and a list is provided of the things you will need.

In each procedure that involves the patient, the nurse performs certain steps such as washing hands, approaching the patient to explain what is to be done at the start of the procedure, providing for the patient's comfort, removing the used items, and making a record of the procedure and its completion. These universal steps are explained in detail in the Appendix. Hereafter, the steps are listed for the first procedure in each unit, but not explained in detail. Subsequent procedures in the unit instruct you to carry out the universal steps and then to proceed to perform the specific steps of that procedure.

The Universal Steps A, B, C, and D are carried out as necessary before the main steps of the procedure, and steps X, Y, and Z at its conclusion.

A. Collect the equipment needed.
B. Wash your hands.
C. Approach and identify the patient, explain the procedure, and gain patient's cooperation.
D. Provide for privacy and drape the patient as needed.

Following the procedure, these steps are carried out:

X. Collect the used items and equipment and dispose of these correctly.
Y. Provide for the patient's comfort.
Z. Record and report the procedure.

After you have practiced the procedures and feel that you can perform them correctly without referring to sources such as your book, arrange with your instructor to take the performance test. You should be able to perform the procedures in the skills laboratory before employing them in the actual case of patients. In addition, most units include a written post-test covering much of the factual material and principles underlying the procedures. Continue studying the unit until you are able to answer these and similar questions about the content.

NEED FOR ACCURACY IN PERFORMING NURSING SKILLS

All nurses are legally required to perform nursing care of patients in a safe and competent manner, as they have been taught. Safe practice requires that the nurse use good judgment and make decisions that promote the welfare of the patient. While many of the nursing procedures demand the utmost accuracy in their performance, others allow the nurse considerable leeway in the way they are carried out as long as the task is completed. It is essential that procedures such as measuring the blood pressure, or preparing and giving medications be carried out accurately and without errors; on the other hand, nurses may use a variety of ways to give a back rub and make an unoccupied bed and still achieve the desired result of stimulating the circulation in the back and making a neat, smooth, and wrinkle-free bed.

Based on this approach, many of the tasks in nursing that are described in these volumes can be rated on how critical it is for the procedure to be performed accurately, without errors or omissions. Those tasks with a "high" critical factor rating must be performed consistently and accurately by the nurse to be considered as safe and competent practice. The definitions of the levels of criticality (the degree to which a task must be performed with accuracy) follow:

"High" critical factor:

• The task must be performed in strict accordance with procedure or regulations.
• Little or no deviation is allowed, because deviation or inaccuracy results in a risk to health or life, discomfort or pain, or increased cost of time or resources.

"Moderate" critical factor:

- Inaccuracies can be corrected or remedied easily.
- Errors or deviations result in minor delay or inconvenience.
- Modifications are allowed by following principles and using alternative actions.

"Low" critical factor:

- Some deviation is normally allowed if principles are followed.
- A wide range of individual actions are tolerated.
- Method is not as important as the outcome.

Although a list of tasks and their critical ratings cannot be used as an absolute scale, such a list provides a measure or guideline for the performance of nursing skills. Table 1 gives the criticality rating for a number of nursing skills. Many of the tasks that involve moving or carrying out treatments for the patient tend to have a "high" critical rating, but charting nursing care is also rated as "high" because the chart is a legal record. Most of the personal hygiene measures have a "low" or "moderate" rating because a wide range of individual methods are acceptable.

The errors or inaccuracies referred to in the criticality ratings lead to changes in the patient that are not intended or desired. Although the nurse may have forgotten an article, (necessitating another trip) or neglected to raise the bed to a better working level, these are not critical errors unless the patient suffers an adverse effect. Evaluation of the nurse's performance includes attention to accuracy in carrying out all of the steps of the procedure, but more importance and weight is given to critical errors that are committed. Examples of critical errors affecting patients are (1) inaccurate measurements of the vital signs, thus delaying treatment of a patient going into a state of shock; (2) not measuring the temperature of the water in a hot water bottle and consequently burning the patient's skin; (3) turning the patient by body segments rather than log-rolling him or her and thereby causing the patient pain; or (4) allowing a patient who is NPO and scheduled for an x-ray examination to eat breakfast, thus requiring the examination to be rescheduled and causing a delay in treatment or discharge.

Table 1

Actions, Skills and Procedures	Critical Rating	Actions, Skills and Procedures	Critical Rating
Bed making		Protect patient from pressure	High
unoccupied	Low	Support or immobilize body	
occupied	Mod	parts	High
anesthetic	Low		
		Personal Hygiene of Patient	
Movement & Activity			
		Provide for patient privacy	Low
Body alignment and movement		Explain procedure to patient	Mod
self	High	Use bath blanket for bath	Low
patient	High	Strip top bedding for bath	Low
Positioning patient in bed	Mod	Drape for treatments	Mod
Positioning of bed		Bed bath, partial or total	Mod
high level for working	Mod	Shower	Low
low level when occupied	High	Tub bath	Low
Range of motion exercises		Back rub	Low
active	Mod	Oral hygiene	Low
passive	High	Cleanse dentures	Low
Dangle patient	Mod	Clean, clip nails	Low
Assist to walk	Mod	Brush, comb hair	Low
Transfer from bed to chair	High	Shave	Low
Transfer from bed to stretcher	High	Perineal care	Mod

Table 1 *(Continued)*

Actions, Skills and Procedures	Critical Rating	Actions, Skills and Procedures	Critical Rating
Safety		Include significant or relevant behaviors	High
Use of side rails	Mod–High	Avoid repetition in day's entries	Mod
Wrist, jacket, or belt for safety or restraint	High	Use correct words, terms, or abbreviations	Mod
Stable support for objects	High	Include each problem or need area	High
Foreign objects off floor	High		
Fire and accident prevention measures	High		
		Medical Asepsis & Isolation	
Oxygenation		Handwashing pre and post care	High
O_2 by nasal cannula	High	Equipment and linen not put on floor or other unit	High
Monitor level of consciousness, mental function	High	Soiled linen and equipment carried away from body	High
Measure vital signs	High	Work from "clean" to "dirty"	High
Report changes promptly	High	Follow isolation instructions re-gown, gloves, and so forth	High
Recognize emotional states, responses	Mod	Double-bagging and proper technique to take items out of isolation	High
Fluids & Electrolytes			
Record intake of fluid	Mod	*Surgical Asepsis*	
Monitor fluid by output of urine or limiting intake	High	Avoid contaminating sterile field, gloves, or items	High
Monitor abnormal fluid losses	High	Sterile catheter care	High
Observe IV infusion rate	Mod		
		Health Team Relationships	
Nutrition		Listen to report	High
Serve tray to patient	Mod	Give report to team member	High
Assist or feed patient	Mod	Notify nurse when leaving floor	Mod
Act on patient food preferences	Mod	Participate in team approach to care	Low
Monitor patient's weight	Low		
Diet teaching	Mod		
Provide between-meal nourishments	Low	*Nurse-Patient Relationship*	
		Initiate relationship with ease	Mod
Elimination		Facilitate trust relationship	High
Place bedpan, urinal	Low	Provide accurate information	High
Collect urine and stool specimen	Mod	Keep promises made	High
Measure output	High	Accept patient and his feelings in the "here and now"	High
Maintain closed drainage system and Foley catheter	High	Use touch appropriately	Mod
Perform simple urine tests of sugar, and so forth	High	Involve patient in planning of care as appropriate	Mod
Check for impaction	Mod	Make decisions on patient's behalf when needed	Mod
Give enema, Harris flush	Mod	Go beyond own anxieties and needs to deal effectively with patient's needs	High
Insert rectal tube	Mod	Consider patient's rights	High
Insert catheter	High		
Charting			
Describe behaviors	High		

Representative nursing procedures and skills rated according to the degree of accuracy that is required for safe and competent care. Ratings range from the high critical factor, which allows little or no deviations from the regulations or routine, to the low critical factor, which permits considerable deviation, as long as the objective of the procedure is achieved. Note that this is a list of representative tasks; it is not all inclusive. The critical rating may change for a specific individual or situation, depending on other influencing factors. (From Rambo, Beverly: Nursing Practicum Syllabus. Unpublished material. Los Angeles: Mount St. Mary's College, 1978.)

SELECTED REFERENCES

Unit 10. Body Alignment Balance and Movement

Bilger, Annetta, and Greene, Ellen (eds.): Winter's Protective Body Mechanics. New York: Springer-Verlag, 1973.
Campbell, Emily B.: Nursing problems associated with prolonged recovery following trauma. Nurs Clin North Am 5:551–562 (December) 1970.
Foss, Georgia: Body mechanics. Nursing 73 3:30–31 (March) 1973.
Jensen, J. Trygve: Introduction to Medical Physics. Philadelphia: J.B. Lippincott Company, 1960, pp. 24–43.
Wolff, LuVerne, Weitzel, Marlene, and Fuerst, Elinor: Fundamentals of Nursing. 6th ed. Philadelphia: J.B. Lippincott Company, 1979, pp. 371–376.

Unit 11. Using Body Movement

Owens, Bernice D.: How to avoid that aching back. Am J Nurs 80:394–397 (May) 1980.
Works, Roberta: Hints on lifting and pulling. Am J Nurs 72:260–261 (February) 1972.

Unit 12. Positioning the Bed Patient

Berecek, Kathleen: Etiology of decubitus ulcers. Nurs Clin North Am 10:157–159 (March) 1975. (Describes the causes of skin breakdown, including the "shearing effect.")
Berecek, Kathleen: Treatment of decubitus ulcers. Nurs Clin North Am 10:171-210 (March) 1975.
Carnevali, Doris, and Bruechner, Susan: Immobilization — reassessment of a concept. Am J Nurs 70:1502–1507 (July) 1970. (Discusses the effects of various types of mobility.)
Foss, Georgia: The "how-to's" of bed positioning. Nursing 72 2:14–16 (August) 1972.
DuGas, Beverly W.: Introduction to Patient Care: A Comprehensive Approach to Nursing. 2nd ed. Philadelphia: W.B. Saunders Company, 1977.
Gruis, Marcia, and Innes, Barbara: Assessment: Essential to prevent pressure sores. Am J Nurs 76:1762–1764 (November) 1976.
Harvin, J. Shand, and Hargest, Thomas J.: The air fluidized bed: A new concept in the treatment of decubitus ulcers. Nurs Clin North Am 5:181–187 (March) 1970.
Meyers, Marvin, McNelly, Dorothy, and Nelson, Karen: Total hip replacement. Am J Nurs 78:1485–1488 (September) 1978.
Wolff, LuVerne, Weitzel, Marlene, and Fuerst, Elinor: Fundamentals of Nursing. 6th ed. Philadelphia, J.B. Lippincott Company, 1979, pp. 383–395.

Unit 13. Patient Movement and Ambulation

Brown-Skeers, Vicki: How the nurse practitioner manages the rheumatoid arthritis patient. Nursing 79 9:26–35 (June) 1979. (Describes exercises designed to maintain joint mobility and illustrates range-of-motion exercises.)
Brunner, Lillian, and Suddarth, Doris: Textbook of Medical-Surgical Nursing. 4th ed. Philadelphia. J.B. Lippincott Company, 1980, pp. 182–190. (Illustrations of various types of movements and of range-of-motion exercises.)
Carnevali, Doris, and Bruechner, Susan: Immobilization — reassessment of a concept. Am J Nurs 70:1502–1507 (July) 1970. (Classifies types of immobility as physical, emotional, intellectual, and social, and their causes are illustrated in a case study of a patient with a stroke.)
Ellis, Rosemary: After stroke: Sitting problems. Am J Nurs 73:1898–1899 (November) 1973.
Ford, J.R., and Duckworth, B.: Moving a dependent patient safely, comfortably. Part 1. Nursing 76 6:27–36 (January) 1976.
Frankel, Lawrence, and Richard, Betty: Exercises help the elderly live longer, stay healthier, and be happier. Nursing 77 7:64–70 (December) 1977. (Illustrates exercises for ambulatory and chair-ridden elderly people.)

Gordon, Marjory: Assessing activity tolerance. Am J Nurs 76:606–608 (April) 1976.

Greenberg, Barbara: Reaction time in the elderly. Am J Nurs 73:2056–2058 (December) 1973.

Hirschberg, G. G., Lewis, L., and Vaughan, P.: Promoting patient mobility. Nursing 77 7:42-47 (May) 1977.

Long, Barbara, and Buergin, Patricia: The pivot transfer. Am J Nurs 77:980-982 (June) 1977.

Lynn, Frances. Incidents — need they be accidents? Am J Nurs 80:1098-1011 (June) 1980.

Meyers, Marvin, McNelly, Dorothy, and Nelson, Karen: Total hip replacement. Am J Nurs 78:1485–1488 (September) 1978.

Pfaudler, Marjorie: After stroke: Motor skill rehabilitation for hemiplegic patients. Am J Nurs 73:1892–1896 (November) 1973.

Snyder, Mariah, and Baum, Rebecca: Assessing station and gait. Am J Nurs 74:1256 (July) 1974.

Wille, Natalie: Why the elderly fall. Am J Nurs 79:1950–1962 (November) 1979.

Wolff, LuVerne, Weitzel, Marlene, and Fuerst, Elinor: Fundamentals of Nursing. 6th ed. Philadelphia: J.B. Lippincott Company, 1979, pp. 377–380.

Unit 14. Mechanical Aids for Ambulation

Anderson, Beverly: Carole, a girl treated with bracing. Am J Nurs 79:1592–1597 (September) 1979.

Foss, Georgia: Breaking the architectural barrier with crutches, wheelchairs, and walkers. Nursing 73 3:16–31 (October) 1973.

Programmed Instruction. Teaching a patient how to use crutches. Am J Nurs 79:1111–1126 (June) 1979.

Wolff, LuVerne, Weitzel, Marlene, and Fuerst, Elinor: Fundamentals of Nursing. 6th ed. Philadelphia: J.B. Lippincott Company, 1979, pp. 377–383.

BODY ALIGNMENT, BALANCE, AND MOVEMENT

GENERAL PERFORMANCE OBJECTIVE

You will demonstrate your knowledge of good body alignment, balance, and movement by a performance test and a written test.

SPECIFIC PERFORMANCE OBJECTIVES

After you have completed this lesson, in the skill laboratory without reference to any source material, you will be able to:

1. Position your body in alignment and balance, and state the reasons for the position of your feet, knees, buttocks, abdomen, thorax, and head, according to the standards outlined in this lesson.

2. Demonstrate accurately the body movements of flexion, extension, hyperextension, adduction, and abduction, and describe the movements using terms given in the vocabulary and in the lesson.

3. Answer in writing and with at least 85 per cent accuracy the post-test questions about the following:

   a. The vocabulary presented in this lesson.

   b. Principles of good body alignment as presented in this lesson.

   c. Principles of good body balance as presented in this lesson.

   d. Effects of physical forces of gravity.

VOCABULARY

This may seem like a lengthy vocabulary to you, but you probably already know some of the words and understand their meaning. It may help to list some of the words that go together.

1. Systems of the body.
   cardiopulmonary system—the body system that includes the heart, lungs, blood, and blood vessels.
   digestive system—the body system that includes the mouth, stomach, and intestines.
   endocrine system—the body system composed of the ductless glands such as the thyroid, pancreas, and adrenals.
   urinary system—the body system that includes the kidneys, ureters, bladder, and urethra.

163

2. Movements of the body or joints.

abduct—to move a body part away from the midline of the body.

adduct—to move a body part toward the midline of the body.

extension—straightening of two segments of the body; movement that widens the angle between two adjoining parts.

flexion—the movement of bending; the narrowing of the angle between two adjoining parts.

hyperextension—the movement that goes beyond 180 degrees or a straight line, increasing the angle beyond its normal range.

3. Names of muscle groups.

"corset muscles"—the layers of muscles that support the abdominal and pelvic organs.

gluteal muscles—the thick extensor muscles that form the buttocks.

hamstring muscles—strong flexor muscles located on the posterior part of the thigh.

quadriceps femoris—strong extensor muscles located on the anterior side of the thigh.

4. Others.

abdomen—part of the trunk between the chest and the pelvis.

antagonist—one of a pair of muscles having an action *opposite* that of the other muscle of the pair.

anterior—front side.

balance—the action of becoming stable, fixed.

body alignment—the relationship of each movable body segment to the other segments so that no undue strain is placed on the skeleton or muscles.

buttocks—the rounded prominences formed by the gluteal muscles; the seat, or rump.

distal—the furthest from any point, such as the midline or origin.

extremities—the limbs of the body.

glucose—a simple sugar used by body cells for energy.

gravity—a force that pulls toward the earth.

hormones—powerful chemicals formed by endocrine glands that regulate many body processes.

intervertebral disc—a cartilage found between most vertebral bones that acts as a cushion.

joint—the juncture or meeting of two or more bones.

lateral—pertaining to a side.

ligament—a tough band of tissue that attaches bone to bone at a joint.

oxygen—a colorless, odorless gas forming approximately one-fifth of the content of air.

pelvis—a basin-shaped structure of bones at the lower end of the trunk of the body that contains in its cavity the organs of the lower portion of the abdomen.

posterior—the dorsal or back portion of the human anatomy.

proximal—the part nearest to the point of references, such as the midline or origin.

stability—quality of balance, firmness; not having a tendency to tip or fall.

thorax—the chest portion of the body.

trunk (torso)—the body, not including the head and extremities.

vertebral column—the spinal column of vertebrae; the backbone.

BODY MOVEMENT

ITEM 1. INTRODUCTION

Hospital workers are very active people. In performing their work, they use a variety of movements as they reach, lift, carry, push, pull, stoop, sit, stand, and walk. Your activities will require that you, too, use these movements as you reach for linen from a shelf, lift and carry objects, push wheelchairs or stretchers, stoop to pick up objects from the floor, walk, or stand at a bedside.

All of us have been performing these movements most of our lives, so why do we single them out for consideration now? What is the point? The answer is that with knowledge of proper body alignment and movement (a) your work may be easier, (b) you may prevent injury to yourself and your patient, and (c) you will present a more attractive appearance as you work. We want you to be conscious that you are using proper body alignment for yourself and the patient at all times, to know how to balance yourself correctly, and to avoid strain or injury to yourself.

One of the common injuries to hospital workers is severe muscle strain, usually of the lower back, although it may occur in the shoulders or the abdomen. Low back strain is painful; it takes time to heal. It may require hospitalization, bed rest, or traction, it is costly in lost salary and medical fees, and it is preventable. Low back strain and other muscle strains are caused by improper body alignment, loss of balance, or poor body movements.

Your employer and your coworkers prefer you to be a healthy worker rather than a patient with a preventable injury. The knowledge and use of proper body alignment, balance, and movement will help you to prevent injury to yourself.

Please complete the following:

1. List five movements that you might perform in your daily hospital work.

a. _____ b. _____ c. _____

d. _____ e. _____ .

2. Give three reasons for using good body alignment, balance, and movement.

a. _____

b. _____

c. _____

3. Circle the best answer:

a. Low back strain is a *(fairly common) (uncommon)* injury among hospital workers.

b. Severe muscle strain is the result of *(lifting a heavy object) (someone else's carelessness) (poor body alignment or movement)*.

4. If you suddenly sustained this type of injury (low back strain) and were hospitalized, how do you think this might affect the workload of your coworkers? _____

_____

ITEM 2. SYSTEMS INVOLVED IN BODY MOVEMENT

Let's take a brief look at this wonderful and complex body of ours. This will help you understand how to align and balance your body in order to perform body movements safely.

The Musculoskeletal System. The bony framework of the body is formed by the skeletal system. The bones and joints are the important parts of the skeletal system. The point where bones come together is called a joint, and it is the joint that allows the movement of the body.

Bones cannot move by themselves. Muscles attach to bones and are usually found in pairs whose members work opposite each other. If one muscle flexes or bends a joint, the other muscle can extend or straighten that joint. When the muscle contracts or shortens, it pulls one bone toward the bone on the other side of the joint, and decreases the angle between the two bones.

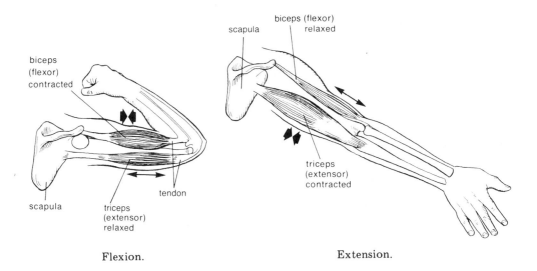

Flexion.   Extension.

These two body systems (the skeletal bones and the muscles) are often considered together and are referred to as the musculoskeletal system. In Item 3 you will learn more about this system.

The Nervous System. The brain, spinal cord, and nerves produce and conduct electrical energy impulses that allow the muscles to work in a smooth, coordinated manner. Muscles cannot function without the stimulation, or innervation, from the nervous system.

The Cardiopulmonary System. The heart pumps the blood through a vast system of tubes called blood vessels, and the blood carries oxygen, glucose, and other vital substances to the muscles and other body tissues where they are absorbed by the cells. The respiratory system supplies the oxygen needed by the cells to convert, or change, the glucose to energy. Air that we breathe contains about 20 per cent oxygen. The air is inhaled into the lungs where the oxygen passes through very thin air sac walls and is absorbed into the blood stream. The blood is then pumped throughout the body to deliver the oxygen to the cells.

The Digestive and Urinary Systems. The energy (or the fuel) used by the muscles is a simple sugar called glucose. The digestive system breaks down the food that we eat into simpler substances such as proteins, fats, and sugars, including glucose. In the digestive system, these substances are prepared to be absorbed into the blood stream.

When glucose is converted into energy by the body cells, not all of the substance becomes energy; some remains as waste material. When muscles have been used strenuously, waste material collects around the muscles, and this can slow down the functioning of the muscle. The waste material is absorbed into the many tiny blood vessels located throughout the muscle. These small vessels merge into larger vessels that take the blood to the kidneys, where the waste products are filtered out and eliminated from the body as urine: this is the function of the urinary system.

The Endocrine System. There is one more body system that is important in providing movement — the endocrine glands. There are seven main endocrine glands. You may already know some of them. They are the thyroid, parathyroid, pituitary, adrenals, thymus, pineal, and finally, gonads (ovaries or testicles). Each gland makes one or more powerful hormones that enter the blood stream directly from the gland. These hormones regulate many of the body's activities, including that of muscle action.

Do you see why we said that your body is very complex? Even the simple movements of reaching, standing, walking, pushing, and pulling require that many systems of your body work together in harmony.

Circle the appropriate number or numbers of your answer(s) to the following questions.

5. We could not align and balance and move our body without using the:

   a. muscular system
   b. skeletal system
   c. nervous system
   d. respiratory system
   e. all of these

6. Muscles need fuel to provide energy for contraction. Which statements correctly describe the nature of the "fuel" used by the body?

   a. Energy is provided by the simple sugar called glucose.
   b. The fuel is delivered to muscles by the circulatory system.
   c. The fuel comes from waste products carried in the blood.
   d. Oxygen is needed in order to release the fuel's energy.

7. The glands that produce powerful chemicals that help to regulate body functions form the:

   a. digestive system
   b. endocrine system
   c. nervous system
   d. none of these

ITEM 3. PARTS OF THE MUSCULOSKELETAL SYSTEM

If the framework of a building should sag, the whole building is weakened, is less sturdy and strong, and appears less attractive. Just so with the body. Since the skeletal system — i.e., the bones and joints — makes the body framework, it needs to be in good alignment to prevent sagging.

The major movable body parts are called segments and refer to the head, the trunk, and the extremities. Each of these segments has subparts. The movable parts of the head are the jaw and the neck. The upper extremity includes the shoulder, the upper arm, the forearm, the wrist, and the hand. The trunk of the body is composed of the chest, the abdomen, the pelvis, the back, and the buttocks. The parts of the lower extremity include the hip, the thigh, the leg, the ankle, and the foot. These are shown in the picture of the skeleton on page 168.

When we describe body surface or locations, we use terms that were included in your vocabulary: anterior, posterior, lateral, midline, proximal, and distal. You will need to learn these words and what they mean because they will be used frequently in many of your assignments and in your clinical experiences. *Proximal* refers to the body part that is nearest the midline or point of reference, and *distal* describes a part that is furthest away. *Anterior* refers to the front surface of the body or its parts. *Posterior* refers to the back surface of the body or its parts. *Lateral* refers to either side of the body or its parts. *Midline* refers to an imaginary line that divides the body or its parts into right and left halves.

Bones are held together by tough bands of tissues that are called ligaments. Muscles are attached to bones by other strong bands of tissues called tendons. When the body parts are in proper relationship to each other, each movable segment is aligned so that the least amount of strain is placed on these tendons, ligaments, muscles, and joints. Each part should be able to perform its intended function efficiently.

The backbone, which is also called the vertebral column or spine, is not really just a "bone." The vertebral column is a series of bones, or vertebrae, that supports the head on the upper end, provides the attachment for the back of the ribs, and joins with the pelvic bones near its lower end. The vertebrae also encase the spinal cord, which is composed of nerves going to and coming from the brain.

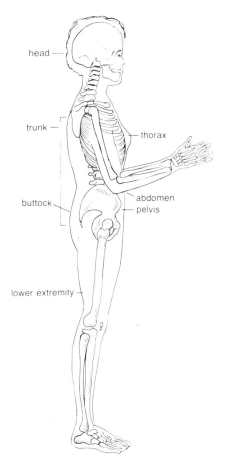

Side view of major body segments.

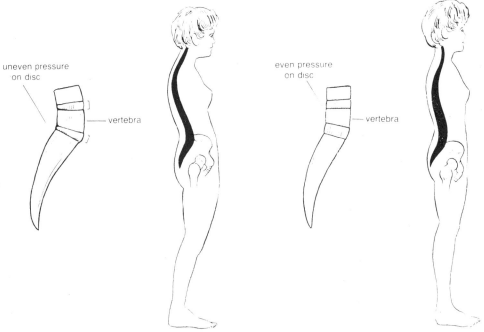

Poor alignment.   Good alignment.

Between each vertebra there is a cushion of cartilage called an intervertebral disc. These discs serve as shock-absorbers and decrease the jolting effect of the body movements. When the vertebrae are in good alignment, the pressure of the bones is more evenly distributed on the discs. Prolonged or severe and uneven distribution of pressure may cause the discs to become damaged.

This long, bony spinal column is most important in attaining proper body alignment and safe movement. The muscles that move the vertebral column are small and not very strong. They provide great flexibility of movement but are not designed for the heaviest work. The longer, thicker, and stronger muscles used for more strenuous work are found in the shoulder, upper arm, hip, and thigh. A rule in body function is this: *Structure determines function.* As an example, to raise an object you should stoop with your back straight. Use your strong thigh muscles to rise to a standing position, instead of bending with knees straight and back bowed.

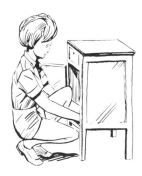

The worker will use strong thigh muscles to stand erect.

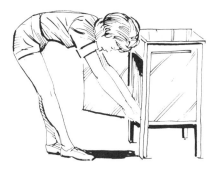

The worker is placing strain on the muscles of the back and legs. Poor alignment for body movement.

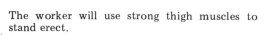

8. For each definition on the left, select the term or word that it best defines from those listed.

Definitions	Terms
1. back surface	a. intervertebral disc
2. spinal bones	b. ligaments
3. arms and legs	c. anterior
4. bind bones together	d. lateral
5. body without extremities	e. midline
6. imaginary line dividing body into equal halves	f. posterior
	g. trunk
7. cushions between spinal bones	h. extremities
8. refers to side	i. tendons
9. attaches muscles to bone	j. buttocks
10. refers to front surface	k. skeletal
	l. vertebral column

ITEM 4. BODY ALIGNMENT AND BALANCE

Alignment has been defined as the proper relationship of the body segments to one another. When the segments are properly aligned, it is easier to maintain body balance. Balanced means stable, steady, and not likely to tip or fall.

The main portions of the body (pelvis, thorax, head) are supported by structures below them that are often very small (e.g., small bones in feet, vertebrae). To maintain the proper relationship and balance of these anatomical parts, the ligaments and muscles must be used effectively. In the following figures, your common sense and past experience tell you that B is much more likely to tip or fall than A. That is, Figure A is more *stable* than Figure B.

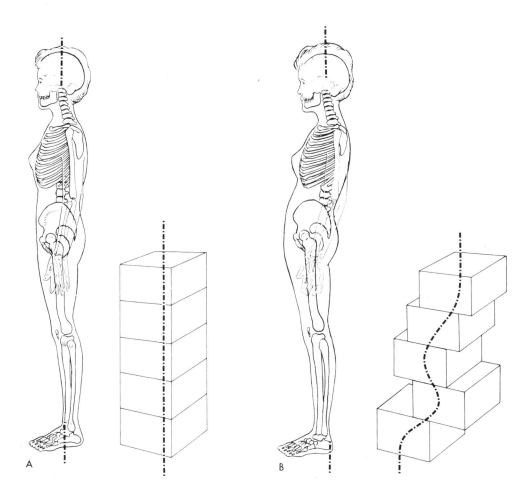

Good relationship of segments.   Poor relationship of segments.

Let us see why Figure A is more stable. The force of gravity affects balance because it is constantly pulling the body toward the earth. Three principles of gravity that affect our balance are:

1. *Center of gravity* — an area located in the pelvis about the level of the second sacral vertebrae. The exact location may vary slightly, depending on body structure.

2. *Base of support* — provides a stable stance for keeping the body from toppling over, as well as stability in movements such as lifting, pushing, or pulling.

3. *Line of gravity* — as documented by some well-known orthopedists (Lovett, Reynolds, Steindler), an imaginary line that falls in the frontal plane; i.e., it passes behind the ear downward just behind the center of the hip joint and then downward slightly in front of the knee and ankle joint. Individual variations may occur according to skeletal build and the curvatures in the spine.

When a person stands in an erect posture so that the line of gravity falls as stated above, body balance is preserved and there is minimal resistance needed to overcome the force of gravity. If the posture is out of alignment as seen on p. 172 the body weight distribution is shifted, the balance is upset, the muscles no longer work together, and the gravitational pull is increased.

To illustrate these three principles, the body may be compared to a plank of wood of the same length, or about 5 feet, 6 inches long. The body (or any object) has a point at which its "mass" or weight is centered. At this point, the weight of the upper body balances the weight of the lower body, and thus the weight of the entire body is balanced. This is called the center of gravity and it influences the stability of an object or a person.

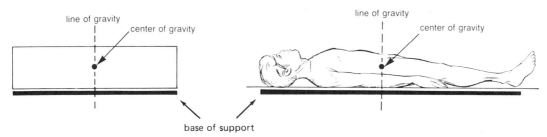

U
N
I
T
10

Stable objects have a broad base of support and a low center of gravity; the line of gravity passes through the base of support.

In the sketches shown above, note the center of gravity in the board and the body. It is quite low. The base of support is the part of an object in contact with the ground or other level surface. The base in the illustration is the length of the board, or the body, and is very

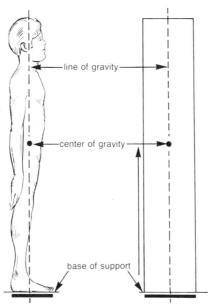

Unstable position.

broad. The line of gravity is an imaginary vertical line that passes through the center of gravity. Body balance is maintained when the line of gravity passes through the base.

Now let's see what happens to the center of gravity, the line of gravity, and the base when we stand up. Again, compare the body to a board of the same height. The body is most unstable when the

1. center of gravity is high,

2. base of support is narrow, and

3. line of gravity does not pass through
    the base of support.

In the following illustration, the figure is shown leaning over. See what happens to its stability.

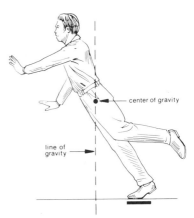

This figure would fall unless a force opposing gravity held it up. An opposing force could be the use of the arms pushing against an object to keep the body from tipping over.

Fill in the blanks with the most appropriate answer.

9. A force that pulls any object toward the ground is called _____ .

10. The point in the body where the mass is centered is called the _____ .

11. An imaginary vertical line that passes through this point is called the _____

_____ .

12. An object is said to be _____ if it is steady, not likely to fall.

13. We are least likely to fall if we follow these three principles:

    a. _____ .

    b. _____ .

    c. _____ .

ITEM 5. BODY MOVEMENT

You have studied some of the principles of good body alignment and balance and are now ready to learn more about body movement. The joints allow the movement when the muscles contract and pull on bones. Various terms describe these joint movements. We will now take up the movements of flexion, extension, hyperextension, abduction, and adduction.

First, notice that a full circle contains 360 degrees, while a straight line has half of that, or 180 degrees. The right angle has only 90 degrees.

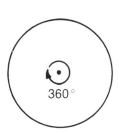

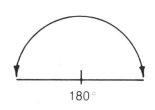

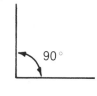

If you hold your arm out straight, the elbow joint forms a straight line — or a 180-degree angle. By bending the elbow joint, you decrease the angle, i.e., decrease the number of degrees from 180. This is called flexion. Extension is the joint movement opposite to flexion. When you straighten the arm that is bent at the elbow, or the leg that is bent at the knee, you are increasing the angle at the joint and extending the arm or leg.

Some joints allow for increasing the angle more than 180 degrees or beyond a straight line. This is called hyperextension. You hyperextend your neck each time you raise your chin and tilt your head backward. The knee joint also allows the movement of hyperextension. You can feel this movement if you stand normally with the knee joint nearly straight; then force the knee joint even straighter until the joint is locked or rigid.

Abduct is another term used to describe certain joint movements. Abduct means to move away from the midline of the body. (One way to remember this word and its meaning: if a child is kidnapped, he is abducted or taken away from his family.) The opposite movement of abduct is adduct — the movement to bring the part back toward the midline of the body. (A memory clue for this: "adds to" the body.)

The major body movements are flexion, extension, adduction, and abduction. The muscles that produce the movements are called flexors, extensors, adductors, and abductors.

U
N
I
T
10

----

14. Circle the appropriate answer.

   a. The *(skeletal system) (muscular system)* forms the framework of our body.

   b. The *(skeletal system) (muscular system)* produces movement.

   c. Muscles with opposite actions in pairs are called *(extensors) (antagonists)*.

15. Please carry out the following movements.

   a. Flex your lower leg (knee joint).

   b. Extend your lower leg (knee joint).

   c. Flex your head (neck).

   d. Hyperextend your head (neck).

   e. Hyperextend your lower leg (knee joint).

   f. Flex your hip joint.

   g. Abduct your arm.

   h. Adduct your arm.

ITEM 6. MUSCLE GROUPS

Muscles work in pairs and are called antagonists. Each muscle of the pair has an action opposite to that of the other. If one muscle flexes a joint, its antagonist will extend the joint. Abductors are antagonists of adductors. The following muscles represent some of the more important antagonist groups:

1. Muscles that bend the elbow and move the arm:
   Flexors: biceps and brachial muscles
   Extensors: triceps muscles

2. Muscles that bend the body at the hips and move the thigh:
   Flexors and adductors: the great, long, and short adductor muscles
   Extensors: the gluteus maximus muscle

3. Muscles that bend the knee and move the lower leg:
   Flexors: the hamstring muscles
   Extensors: the quadriceps muscles

4. Muscles that move the hand:
   Pronators: turn palm down or toward the back
   Supinators: turn palm up or toward the front

In the movements of lifting, carrying, and stooping, we will be referring to several specific muscle groups. Since standing erect and walking are essential to these movements, we will consider the two most powerful groups in the body. The quadriceps are extensor muscles and the hamstrings are strong flexors of the leg. The quadriceps are composed of four parts — hence the prefix "quadri." They are found on the anterior, or front, of the thigh and pass over the knee joint in order to extend the leg. Six muscles make up the hamstring group, which is on the posterior of the thigh. The hamstrings oppose the action of the quadriceps, so that they work to flex the leg at the knee joint.

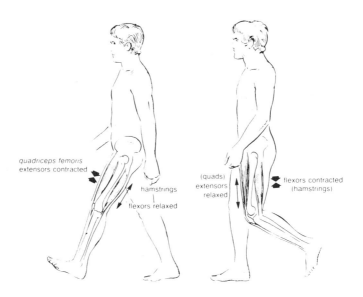

Extension of knee joint.   Flexion of knee joint.

The gluteal muscles form the seat or the rump. They are the thick muscles on which you sit. They function to extend and to hyperextend the hip joint. The adductor muscles, a group of strong, broad muscles that are attached anteriorly to the pelvis and the thigh bone, produce the flexion and adduction of the hip. The gluteals, hamstrings, and quadriceps are used in walking and other movements. When you are standing, they help to keep the femur, or thighbone, positioned on the tibia, which is the large bone of the lower leg.

There are other muscles around the hip joint and knee that act to stabilize the joint rather than to move it. (Stabilize means to set or prevent unnecessary or secondary movement.) These muscles are important in walking or lifting. They allow a joint to support the shifting weight of the moving body as the center of gravity changes.

We will consider another important muscle group at this time — the "corset muscles," or the "living girdle." The corset muscles are the muscles of your abdomen that are arranged in layers to form the wall of the abdomen and support the abdominal and pelvic organs. The abdominal muscles usually work in opposition to the diaphragm, so that when one is contracted, the other is relaxed. In lifting or carrying heavy objects, considerable strain is placed on the corset muscles. Before such exertion, these muscles should be contracted or "set" to provide good support and prevent possible injury.

‖‖

Circle the appropriate answer to the following questions.

16. The quadriceps muscles are found on the *(anterior) (posterior) (lateral)* part of the thigh.

17. The action of the quadriceps muscles is to *(flex) (extend)* the lower leg.

18. The hamstring muscles are located on the *(anterior) (posterior) (lateral)* part of the thigh.

19. The hamstring muscles *(flex) (extend) (hyperextend)* the lower leg at the knee joint.

20. The gluteal muscles form the *(thigh) (abdomen) (buttocks)*.

‖‖‖

ITEM 7.   CHECKPOINTS FOR GOOD BODY ALIGNMENT

Before beginning body movements, you should align and balance your body properly in order to prevent strain and injury. There are some checkpoints for you to remember and practice when aligning and balancing your body. In the skill laboratory, practice according to these checkpoints, then consciously check your alignment and balance every time you stand.

Important Steps	Key Points
1. Start from a good base of support.	Place your feet parallel and about 6 to 8 inches apart. You can widen your base if necessary, or if more comfortable. Then, for anterior-posterior stability, put one foot ahead of the other. This stable base of support will save your energy by minimizing the work the muscles must do to keep the body balanced. With your feet parallel, the joints are in good alignment. You will probably notice that the heels of your shoes will wear more evenly.
2. Distribute your weight evenly on both feet.	This permits the weight-bearing joints and their supporting structures to divide the weight and share the load.
3. Keep your knees slightly flexed.	Slight flexion produces a "shock-absorber" effect and prevents jolting movements of the entire body. It also prevents the strain caused by hyperextension of the knees, or "locked knees."

Important Steps	**Key Points**
4. Tuck in your buttocks.	By tucking in the buttocks, you tilt the pelvis forward and help straighten the lumbar curve of the spine. This prevents "swayback," and allows for even distribution of pressure of the intervertebral disc cushions. If you look at yourself in a mirror with the buttocks first protruding, then tucked in, you will see that the tucked-in position presents a better appearance.
5. Keep the abdomen up and in.	This will support the abdominal organs and decrease muscle strain on the back. Good abdominal muscle control permits your clothes to fit better and gives a more attractive appearance. Put your living girdle to work.
6. Raise your rib cage.	By holding your chest up, you allow for more complete expansion of the lungs. Keep the shoulders relaxed; you need not stand at military attention for good body alignment and balance. By raising the rib cage, you decrease the hump-shoulder appearance.
7. Keep your head erect.	Let your head "balance" on top of your spine. Holding the chin in and up prevents exaggerated curvature of the neck and the thoracic portion of the spinal column.

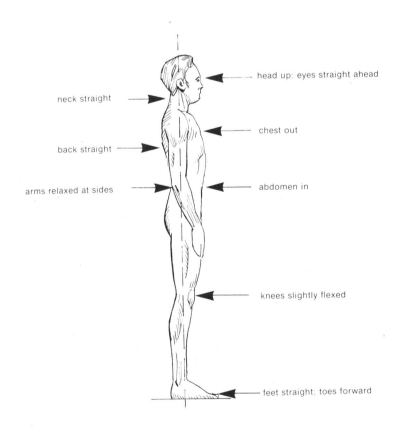

In summary, these checkpoints are listed again for you:

1. Start from a stable base of support with feet separated and one slightly ahead of the other.

2. Distribute body weight evenly.

3. Flex knees slightly to act as shock-absorbers.

4. Tuck buttocks under and tilt pelvis forward to prevent swayback.

5. Keep abdominal muscles up and in to support abdominal organs.

6. Keep rib cage up to allow full expansion of the chest.

7. Hold head erect to avoid curvature of neck and thorax.

‖‖‖

21. To demonstrate body balance, you should stand and check the alignment of your body:
Are your feet parallel?
Are your feet separated for good lateral stability?
Is your weight evenly distributed on both feet?
Are your knees slightly flexed, not locked or hyperextended?
Is your thorax up and in good alignment?
Are your shoulders relaxed?
Is your head in alignment and balanced?

22. Now, maintaining the alignment of your upper body, lean forward from your hips and to the side. Next, place both of your feet close together. Again lean forward from your hips and to the side.

    a. Were you able to lean as far without beginning to lose your balance?
    b. Did you feel unstable when you were leaning with your feet together?
    c. Why do you think this was so?

U
N
I
T
10

‖‖‖

ITEM 8. CONCLUSION OF THE LESSON

You have now completed the unit on body alignment, balance, and movement. The habit of good body alignment and balance will help you present an attractive appearance and may prevent strain or injury as you perform your duties. Obtain the written and performance post-tests. After you have completed the written test, make an appointment with your instructor to demonstrate your ability to understand and to practice good body alignment and balance.

WORKBOOK ANSWERS

1. a.–e. reach, lift, carry, push, pull, stoop, stand, sit, walk, turn (any five of these)

2. a. attractive appearance

   b. may prevent injury

   c. may make work easier
       (reduce fatigue; prevent added work for fellow employees; or other similar answer)

3. a. fairly common

   b. poor body alignment or movements

4. It would increase their workload because they would have to perform my work as well (any similar answer).

5. e. all of these

6. a., b., d.

7. b.

8. 1–f; 2–l; 3–h; 4–b; 5–g; 6–e; 7–a; 8–d; 9–i; 10–c

9. gravity

10. center of gravity

11. line of gravity

12. stable

13. a. The center of gravity is low.

    b. We have a broad base of support.

    c. The line of gravity passes through the base.

14. a. skeletal system

    b. muscular system

    c. antagonists

15. Confirm these movements by checking with the definitions in the text.

16. anterior

17. extend

18. posterior

19. flex

20. buttocks

21. The answer to each question should be *yes*.

22. a. No

    b. Yes

    c. The base of support was narrow and the line of gravity did not pass through the base.

PERFORMANCE TEST

In the skill laboratory, your instructor will ask you to demonstrate your ability to carry out the following instructions without reference to source material:

1. In a standing position, you are to position your body in proper alignment and describe the seven checkpoints that you are to use as a guide.

2. In a standing position using good body alignment, bend your right knee and take one step forward as you straighten your leg. Describe the body movements of the leg, and name and locate the muscles that were most involved.

3. In a standing position with good body alignment, take one step of 12 inches or more to your left, then bring the other foot parallel to your left foot. Describe the body action in the movement of the left foot and the action of the right foot.

4. You are to use your neck joints to perform these movements:

   a. flexion of the neck.

   b. hyperextension of the neck.

   c. abduction of the head.

   d. adduction of the head.

U
N
I
T
10

PERFORMANCE CHECKLIST

BODY ALIGNMENT, BALANCE, AND MOVEMENT

1. Student will demonstrate proper body alignment.

   - Feet in stride position, parallel or one slightly in front of the other.

   - Weight evenly distributed on both feet.

   - Knees slightly flexed.

   - Buttocks tucked in and pelvis tilted forward, spine straight, and lumbar curve reduced.

   - Abdominal muscles pulled up, held in.

   - Thorax raised, shoulders relaxed.

   - Head kept erect and balanced.

2. Student will demonstrate good posture while walking and be able to identify major muscles involved in producing the movement.

   - Body in good alignment.

   - Right knee flexed:
     Movement is flexion.
     Prime movers are the hamstring muscles.
     Location of muscles is on posterior thigh.

   - Extend right knee and step forward:
     Movement is extension.
     Prime movers are the quadriceps femoris.
     Location of muscles is on the anterior thigh.

- Shift weight to lead foot:
  Movement is extension of the hip.
  Prime movers are the gluteal muscles.
  Location of the prime muscles is the buttocks.

3. Student will perform sideward step.

  - Body in good alignment

  - With left foot, step 12 or more inches to left side:
    Movement is abduction.
    Prime movers are abductor muscles.
    Location of abductors is on outer lateral thigh.

  - Move right foot 12 or more inches to left to parallel other foot:
    Movement is adduction.
    Prime movers are adductor muscles.
    Location of adductors is medial aspect of thigh.

4. Student will demonstrate the following movements:

   a. Flexion of the neck.

   b. Hyperextension of the neck.

   c. Abduction of the head.

   d. Adduction of the head.

POST-TEST

Vocabulary. Match the words in Column 2 with the meaning or phrase in Column 1.

Column 1

_____ 1. The body without head and extremities

_____ 2. Attaches bone to bone.

_____ 3. One of a pair of muscles, each having an action opposite from that of the other

_____ 4. The arms and legs

_____ 5. Attaches muscle to bone

_____ 6. A simple sugar, or fuel

_____ 7. Not likely to tip or fall

_____ 8. Formed by the gluteal muscles

_____ 9. The relationship of movable body segments to other segments of the body

_____ 10. A force that pulls toward the earth

Column 2

a. Body alignment

b. Gravity

c. Glucose

d. Hormones

e. Stability

f. Trunk

g. Antagonist

h. Ligament

i. Buttocks

j. Extremities

k. Tendon

l. Thorax

Completion. Complete the following statements.

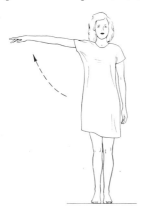

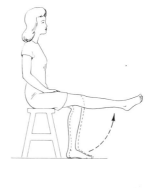

11. This movement is called _____ .

12. This movement is _____ .

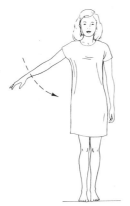

13. This movement is _____ .

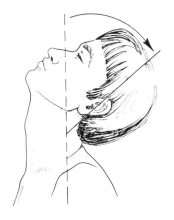 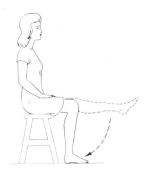

14. This movement is _____ .   15. This movement is _____ .

Matching. Select the muscle group from Column 2 that is used to produce the movement described in Column 1.

Column 1	*Column 2*
16. Flexion of the knee	a. Adductors—great, long, and short branches
17. Flexion of the elbow	b. Biceps
18. Extension of the hip	c. Triceps
19. Flexion of the hip	d. Quadriceps
20. Extension of the knee	e. Hamstrings
	f. Gluteus maximus

Multiple Choice.   Choose the best answer.

21. All but one of the following statements are characteristic of good body alignment and balance. The statement that is *not* characteristic is:

    a. The body is balanced over its base of support.

    b. Oxygen and glucose are used by muscles as "fuel."

    c. Segments of the body are in proper relationship.

    d. Strain on muscles and joints is minimized.

22. Balance of the body is *best* achieved by

    a. a low center of gravity, a narrow base, and the line of gravity passing through the base.

    b. a high center of gravity, a broad base, and the line of gravity passing outside the base.

    c. a high center of gravity, a narrow base, and the line of gravity passing through the base.

    d. a low center of gravity, a broad base, and the line of gravity passing through the base.

23. Balance of the body is maintained by

    a. the center of gravity passing through the base of support.

    b. a high center of gravity located outside a narrow base.

    c. a line of gravity passing through the base of support.

    d. a line of gravity passing outside the base of support.

24. The center of gravity in the body is a point

    a. around which the body weight or mass is centered.

    b. located and stabilized in the chest.

    c. that must lie outside the base of support.

    d. all of the above.

25. Low back strain in the hospital worker is most often caused by

    a. the carelessness of other people.

    b. lifting too heavy an object or person.

    c. using the back muscles to lift a weight.

    d. body segments aligned with one another.

26. The worker who suffers a muscle strain of the back or shoulder might

    a. have a lot of pain.

    b. lose a week or more of work.

    c. have prevented the injury.

    d. all of the above.

27. Movement of the body occurs

    a. where muscles are attached to bones.

    b. at joints that are acted upon by muscles.

    c. when bones are stimulated by nerves.

    d. at the immovable joints.

28. Ligaments are strong cartilage bands that

    a. connect muscles and tendons.

    b. connect muscles to muscles.

    c. connect bones to bones.

    d. connect tendons and bones.

29. The trunk of the body plays an important part in body alignment and balance. The "trunk" refers to

    a. the buttocks and the extremities.

    b. the thorax and the neck.

    c. the back and the extremities.

    d. the abdomen and the thorax.

UNIT 10

30. The palm of the hand is a subpart of the upper extremity and its surface is referred to as

    a. lateral.

    b. midline.

    c. posterior.

    d. anterior.

31. To ensure good stability of the base of support of the body, the feet should be positioned

    a. parallel and very close together.

    b. about 8 inches apart, one a little ahead of the other.

    c. about 8 inches apart, toes pointed laterally.

    d. parallel and at least 2 feet apart.

32. A person with sagging abdominal muscles often has a greater curve in the back, or a "swayback." This greater curve may cause

    a. less fatigue when doing heavy work.

    b. decreased strain on the backbone.

    c. uneven pressure on intervertebral discs.

    d. increased shock-absorber effect of the spine.

33. The large, strong muscle groups of the body include which of the following?

    a. The back muscles and the gluteals.

    b. The quadriceps femoris and the back muscles.

    c. The hamstrings and the adductors.

    d. The gluteals and the quadriceps femoris.

34. Muscles are frequently referred to by a name similar to the name of the movement produced by their action. Some of these muscles would be called

    a. flexion, extensors, and adductors.

    b. hyperextension, abduction, and extensors.

    c. flexors, adductors, and abductors.

    d. extension, hyperextension, and flexion.

35. Groups of muscles are usually found working in pairs to produce movement at the joints of the body, and are called antagonists. One example of antagonist muscles is

    a. flexor and adductor.

    b. quadriceps femoris and back muscles.

    c. abdominal muscles and diaphragm.

    d. extensors and hyperextension.

POST-TEST ANSWERS

1.	f	19.	a
2.	h	20.	d
3.	g	21.	b
4.	j	22.	d
5.	k	23.	c
6.	c	24.	a
7.	e	25.	c
8.	i	26.	d
9.	a	27.	b
10.	b	28.	c
11.	abduction	29.	d
12.	extension	30.	d
13.	adduction	31.	b
14.	hyperextension	32.	c
15.	flexion	33.	d
16.	e	34.	c
17.	b	35.	c
18.	f		

U
N
I
T
10

Unit 11

USING BODY MOVEMENT

GENERAL PERFORMANCE OBJECTIVE

You will demonstrate your knowledge of good body movement by taking the performance test.

SPECIFIC PERFORMANCE OBJECTIVES

Upon the completion of this unit you will be able to:

1. Stoop correctly using the large muscles of the thighs and buttocks and keeping the body balanced when performing activities below the level of your midthigh.

2. Reach and remove an object located at least 6 inches higher than you are tall without hyperextending or straining your back and without losing your balance.

3. Carry a heavy object for five minutes using techniques that will minimize fatigue and prevent straining muscles.

4. Push or pull a heavy object such as a wheelchair or a food cart by "setting" your muscles, using the leg muscles to supply most of the force needed and the body weight to assist the movement.

5. Turn or pivot by positioning your feet and body in such a way that you do not twist or strain muscles in your back or trunk.

6. State the five guidelines that permit good body alignment and efficient movement in the performance of your nursing skills.

VOCABULARY

contaminate—to soil or pollute; to render unclean or unsterile.
diaphragm—the musculomembranous wall separating the abdominal cavity and the thoracic (chest) cavity; a powerful muscle used in breathing.
friction—resistance to movement by two objects in contact.
fulcrum—the support (wedge or axis) about which a lever turns or moves.
lever—a bar with a fixed axis that is acted upon by an applied force at one end to move a resisting force at the other end.
leverage—the mechanical advantage gained by using levers.

INTRODUCTION

In "Body Alignment, Balance, and Movement" you learned how to position your body segments in proper alignment and balance for stability. This will serve as a "base position" or beginning point for all the movements you will make in the performance of your activities.

This lesson, "Using Body Movement," presents five guidelines to assist you in working with the natural laws of gravity, friction, and leverage, which will aid in giving patient care.

It will help you to use the muscles, ligaments, and joints that are best designed for safe and effective movements.

The movements of stooping, reaching, lifting and carrying, turning, pushing, and pulling will be explained in detail so that you can practice each one carefully.

BASIC MOVEMENTS FOR NURSING SKILLS

ITEM 1. GUIDELINES FOR BODY MOVEMENTS

The public expects those in nursing to be experts in the care of the sick and to know a great deal about health and the normal functioning of the body. The nurse who moves correctly and works efficiently serves as a model to others and is often regarded as more capable than those who do not. Although you have used these body movements most of your life, it is time to review the principles and steps involved in reaching, stooping, pushing, pulling, and pivoting so that these activities can be performed accurately and efficiently.

Our guidelines for performing body movements and work are as follows:

1. Maintain alignment and balance.

2. Work at a comfortable height.

3. Keep the work close to your body.

4. Use smooth, coordinated movements.

5. "Set" the muscles for action.

Guideline 1.   Maintain Alignment and Balance

You must start any body movement from a good base of support to provide stability. You can avoid twisting your back by keeping your feet pointed in the same direction as you will move and keeping your trunk aligned or in a straight position.

Before proceeding further, let's review the "key points" of our base position of good alignment and balance. These are the points to check when you assume a standing position.

1. A stable base of support with feet separated and one foot slightly ahead of the other.

2. Weight evenly distributed on both feet.

3. Both knees slightly flexed.

4. Buttocks tucked in.

5. Abdomen held up and in.

6. Rib cage raised.

7. Head held erect.

This standing posture, in good body alignment and balance, is the basis for all of the movements you will use in your work.

Guideline 2.   Work at a Comfortable Height

A comfortable working height for most people is between the waist level and a level about 6 inches below the hip joint. For most women, this level is about 30 to 32 inches from the floor. This working level minimizes muscle strain from reaching beyond the length of the arms, and allows the body to remain aligned and balanced. This working height allows us easily to flex the hip and knee joints and to apply leverage to our work.

Working at too low a level causes strain on muscles and produces fatigue. It is more difficult to maintain your balance within your base of support, and leverage may be poor. Avoid flexing your back to reach objects or to work at low levels, as shown in the figure below. In order to work at a low level, you may need to flex your knees and stoop so that the large thigh muscles are used rather than the weaker muscles of the back.

Working at too high a surface level adds to the demands on arms and shoulders, and this produces muscle strain and fatigue. Also, reaching a high work surface may cause hyperextension of the lower back, raises the center of gravity of your body, and results in a less stable position. Injuries such as low back strain may occur if you reach overhead incorrectly or stretch to perform work at too high a level.

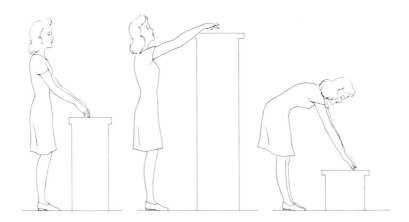

Correct work height.   Too high work level.   Too low work level.

All work should be performed at the proper height when possible. You may be able to change the level of the working surface; for example, most hospital beds today can be adjusted to a higher or lower position. In the high position, the bed is about 32 inches from the floor, a good working height to provide care for the patient. If you are unable to change the height of the work surface, you may need to use a stool to raise yourself to a more suitable level or you may have to stoop down, keeping your body in good alignment.

Guideline 3.   Keep the Work Close to Your Body

You can perform tasks more easily and with less strain or fatigue if your work is close enough to your body to avoid stretching or reaching. You apply this principle when you move the patient to the side of bed nearest you before giving a bath; or when you go around to the other side of the bed rather than reach or stretch across it and hyperextend your back or lose your balance.

Carrying an object is easier if the object's line of gravity falls within your base of support. The additional weight of the object may alter your center of gravity slightly, but the stronger muscles of your thighs and buttocks will help support the weight. If the object's line of gravity is outside your base of support, the muscles of your arms or shoulders must support the weight of the object and overcome the force of gravity. One point of caution: Carry objects close to the body, but do not contaminate your uniform or clothing by carrying *soiled* articles next to you.

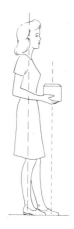

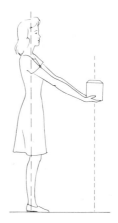

Object carried within base of support.   Object carried outside base of support.

We can summarize the first three guidelines that have been presented so far:

Maintain alignment and balance.

Work at a comfortable height.

Keep work close to the body.

U
N
I
T
11

‖‖

1. Pick up your heaviest book or a similar object and hold it out at arm's length for at least 30 seconds. Now bring it close to your body for the same length of time.

   a. What difference did you notice in its apparent weight?

   _____

   b. Explain why this is so. _____

   _____

2. List three methods you might use in order to work at a comfortable height.

   a. _____

   b. _____

   c. _____

3. How might you avoid hyperextending your back if you were asked to support a patient's leg in a cast while the doctor adjusted the cast?

   _____

‖‖

Guideline 4. Use Smooth, Coordinated Movement

Smooth, coordinated movements utilize the muscle contractions efficiently. The movements flow from one to the other in a rhythmic and graceful way, avoiding jolting and jarring that might cause discomfort, pain, or injury. The use of smooth, coordinated movement is especially important for nurses, who will be more competent and efficient, and appear more attractive when performing any task.

Smooth movements are safer for you as a worker and also for the patient. Uncoordinated movement produces sudden, jerky motions that may cause discomfort or injury. This is to be avoided, especially with patients with fractured bones, recent surgery, wounds, or other conditions in which movement might cause unnecessary pain. Before moving your patients, explain what you are going to do so that you may gain their cooperation and tell them what they should do.

Often you will be working with another person in order to lift or move patients or objects safely. When you have a helper, one person should give the signals for moving or lifting and thus coordinate the teamwork.

Guideline 5. "Set" or Prepare the Muscles for Action

Have you ever noticed that when you prepare to move a heavy object you take a deep breath and tense your muscles, and that you let your breath out slowly as you move the object? If you have done this, you have utilized several principles of body alignment and movement: (a) You have taken in a larger supply of oxygen in the deep breath; (b) you have "set" or tensed the abdominal muscles, which are antagonists of the diaphragm muscle; and (c) as the diaphragm relaxes in releasing the breath, you have caused the abdominal and gluteal muscles to do more of the work. You have made use of the "corset muscles" or the "living girdle" to lift, pull, or push a heavy object. "Setting" the muscles, or tensing them for action, helps to distribute the workload over a larger number of muscles and to decrease the load for any one muscle. This stabilizes the muscles to protect ligaments, joints, and muscles from sudden jerking and strain.

‖‖

4. Give two reasons for using smooth, coordinated movements in caring for the sick.

    a. _____

    b. _____

5. Why is it best to "set" or prepare the muscles before performing a strenuous activity?

    _____

‖‖

ITEM 2. LEVERAGE AND FRICTION

Knowledge of two physical forces is helpful before you study body movements in more detail. One of these forces, leverage, can make your movements easier. The other one, friction, makes your work more difficult. We will not go into detail about the physics involved in these two forces, but will describe them in simple terms.

If you tried to slide a heavy box across a damp wooden floor, friction would result from the contact between the box and the floor. This friction would make it difficult for you to slide the box. If the floor were clean, dry, and waxed, friction would be reduced and you could slide the box more easily. We can define friction as the resistance to movement by two bodies in contact with each other.

Leverage is used often in nursing to increase the amount of work that we can do and also to make it easier. A simple illustration of leverage is that of a child on a teeter-totter raising a heavier child at the other end of the board. In nursing, we often brace a knee against the side of the bed in order to pull a drawsheet tight and taut under the patient. Mechanical lifts to raise or transport patients are another form of lever. Your arms act as levers when you cradle a patient or child in them in order to lift him further up in bed. In simple terms, a lever is a

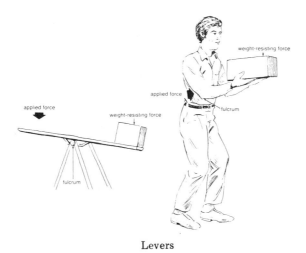

Levers

bar with a fixed axis or fulcrum acted upon at one end by an applied force, or power, and at the other by a resisting force, or weight.

6. Why is leverage important? _____

7. What causes resistance to movement? _____

8. When you reach out and pick up several school books from the desk, you are using leverage. For this movement, identify the parts of the body corresponding to the bar,

   the applied force, and the resisting force: _____

ITEM 3. THE MOVEMENT OF REACHING

You are to study five body movements in detail: reaching, stooping, turning, carrying, and pushing or pulling. These movements are basic to the performance of your hospital skills. When coupled with the five guidelines of movement you have just learned, you should be able to work with physical safety and with minimal fatigue.

Frequently, nurses must reach for objects that are stored on shelves, in cabinets, or in closets. When reaching for items, the nurse should observe the following principles:

1. Reduce the distance to reach across. Position yourself close to the object to avoid stretching and being off balance. If you have to rise up on your toes, or raise your foot from the floor while reaching, you are reaching too far.

2. See most or all of the object before reaching for and removing it from the shelf. Avoid reaching for things that are higher than your eye level. Accidents have occurred when smaller objects were lying unseen on the larger object and fell or caused injury when moved.

3. Use a stool, chair, or ladder to provide a firm base when you need to see and reach items stored in high places. Position it so you will not need to hyperextend your neck to see the entire object to be reached. Use your hand to support yourself when stepping up or down as needed to maintain your balance. Be sure to look down to see that the floor is clear before stepping down. You may not have noticed a spill or foreign object on the floor earlier.

In the skill laboratory, practice reaching to place or to remove an object from a shelf that is higher than your head without hyperextending or straining your back or without losing your balance.

Important Steps	Key Points
1. Start with the basic position and stable base of support.	Check your body alignment.
2. Stand on a footstool, if needed.	Check the distance to be reached. Avoid reaching above your shoulder level when possible because this tends to hyperextend the lower back and may cause strain. A ladder may be needed if the object is in a very high place.
3. Stand with your feet apart.	This broadens your base and provides better lateral stability.
4. Advance one foot forward in the direction of the reach.	This provides a stable stance by broadening the anterior-posterior base of support. The toes should be parallel to the direction of the body movement in order to prevent twisting of the trunk.
5. Look and reach in front of you rather than overhead.	The stool should be placed slightly away from the area of the high shelf so that when standing on the stool you can look and reach forward. Reaching or looking overhead hyperextends the neck and spine and makes you less stable, so that you may lose your balance.
6. Stabilize your body by "setting" your muscles.	"Setting" distributes the workload over many muscles, and the tensing or contracting prepares the muscles for further action. It protects the joints and ligaments from strain or injury.
7. Lower the object with smooth, coordinated movements.	Smooth movements prevent jarring or jolting of the body.
8. Look down; then step off the stool or ladder.	Step *carefully*. Watch where you are going. Deposit the article in the appropriate place.

To place an object on a high shelf, you would use the same procedure except to reverse steps 5 and 6, so that you would "set" your muscles, then reach in front of you to place the object on the shelf using smooth, coordinated movements.

Fill in the blanks.

9. In reaching, the goals are to do it in such a manner that we prevent hyperextension of

the _____ and we maintain _____ .

10. Why is the use of a footstool advisable when reaching?

_____

11. How do you provide lateral stability while reaching?

_____

ITEM 4. THE ACTION OF STOOPING

It is often necessary for us to stoop in the course of our work and everyday lives. Many objects and activities may be beyond the reach of our hands when are are in a standing position. A good many people stoop incorrectly to reach these objects or perform these activities. Incorrect bending over hyperextends the knees, curves the back, and forces the weaker back muscles to pull the trunk of the body upright again.

To stoop correctly, the back must be kept as straight as possible and the stronger gluteal and thigh muscles are used to return the body to an upright position.

Practice stooping correctly in the skill laboratory. Perform an activity at floor level, such as wiping up spilled water or obtaining supplies from a shelf near floor level.

Important Steps	Key Points
1. Start with a stable base of support.	Use good body alignment and place your feet apart with one foot advanced.
2. Advance one foot forward and lower the body by flexing the hip and knees.	This action is *controlled* by using the thigh and leg muscles, and keeping your trunk in an upright position. Gravity also pulls the body downward.
3. Balance your weight on the advanced foot and the ball on the back foot.	The heel of your rear foot will be off the floor. This relieves the tension on the tendons of the rear foot and helps to maintain body alignment and balance.
4. Keep back straight and bend from the hips.	Wipe the spill, or remove the item from the shelf.
5. Raise your body to standing position.	This takes advantage of the large, stronger extensor muscles of the hip and thigh. You can use your hands to steady yourself or assist yourself to stand if extensor muscles are weak. You should be able to feel your heavy thigh muscles working as you rise to the standing position.
6. Handle or dispose of the object in the appropriate way.	

U
N
I
T
11

||||||||||||||||||||||||||||||||||||||||||||||||||||||||||||||||||||||||||||||||||||||||||||||||||||||||||||||||||||||||||

Circle the best response among the italicized word or words.

12. The body is lowered by *(flexing)* *(extending)* the *(hip and knee joints)* *(trunk)*.

13. *(Leverage)* *(Gravity)* pulls the body downward.

14. In the stooped position, the *(rear)* *(advanced)* foot has its heel raised.

15. To rise from the stooping position, the large strong muscles of *(the back)* *(buttocks and thighs)* are used.

||||||||||||||||||||||||||||||||||||||||||||||||||||||||||||||||||||||||||||||||||||||||||||||||||||||||||||||||||||||||||

Stooping with the back held straight is difficult when you try to lift a heavier or bulky object from the floor or a low position because it is hard to keep your balance. This results in people lifting incorrectly or keeping their legs straight and flexing their backs, and it frequently leads to a back injury.

Some authorities now state that efficient and safe lifting of heavy objects is best achieved using the lumbar muscles along with the coordinated leverage provided by the leg and gluteal muscles. Balance is better maintained by some flexion of the back, and the upward thrust supplied mainly by the stronger leg muscle groups, with some help from the lumbar muscles. The steps recommended for lifting items weighing 10 pounds or more are as follows:

1. Reach for the object with the back, hips, and knees flexed.

2. Begin lifting by straightening the knees and hips.

3. Lift the object by flexing the arm muscles and bring it closer to the body. Flex the knees again for more thrust, and begin to straighten the back.

4. Keep knees and back in a slightly flexed position, not rigidly straight in the final position.

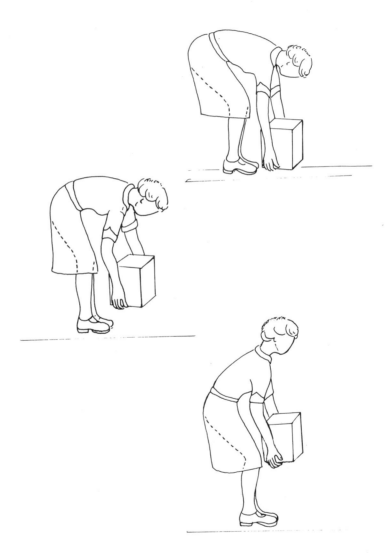

ITEM 5. THE PIVOTING TURN

A pivoting turn is used when changing direction, when assisting a patient from the bed to a chair, or when trying to avoid hitting some object. Also, a worker who is seated in a chair frequently turns to reach a file cabinet or drawer. A pivoting movement is used to change position and to avoid twisting the body.

When performing a pivoting turn correctly the entire body moves and turns as a *single unit*. The trunk of the body should be like a log — not twisting, turning, or bending. The upper and lower extremities should move in the same direction and at the same time as the trunk. Later on, you may help in caring for a patient when it is vital for him to be "turned like a log" in his bed, in order to avoid injury or damage to his neck, back, or hip.

Caution: An incorrect turning movement twists the trunk, and when the trunk or spine is twisted, even a relatively minor activity such as opening a drawer can cause muscle strain or injury. The body is not properly aligned if the trunk is rotated or twisted.

In the skills laboratory, stand in place and practice making a pivoting turn until it seems natural and comfortable. Then practice pivot turns when walking.

Important Steps	Key Points
1. Start with a stable base of support and good body alignment.	Stand with your feet apart and your knees slightly flexed. This allows you to use the leg muscles and avoid "locking" or hyperextending the knees.
2. Stabilize or "set" the trunk and leg muscles.	The "setting" of the muscles makes it easier to turn the body as a single unit and prepares the muscles for action.
3. Shift your weight to the ball of each foot.	The shifting of weight allows the heel to lift very slightly, making the turn easier.
4. Pivot, or make a rotating turn of about 90 degrees on the balls of your feet in the direction you wish to turn.	Move your feet and body *as a single unit.* Use a smooth, coordinated movement to prevent twisting of the trunk.
5. When the turn is completed, distribute your weight equally on each foot.	This provides a stable base of support and balance for further movements.

U
N
I
T
11

To make a walking pivot turn for a right turn (reverse directions for left turn):

1. Step forward with left foot.

2. Follow steps 3, 4, and 5 above.

3. Continue walking.

||||||||||||||||||||||||||||||||||||||||||||||||||||||||||||||||||||||||||||||||||||||||||||||||||||||||||||||||||||||||||||||||||

16. Why would you shift your weight to the ball of each foot before making the pivoting turn?

_____

17. List two nursing activities in which a pivoting turn could be used to prevent twisting the trunk of the body.

a. _____

b. _____

||||||||||||||||||||||||||||||||||||||||||||||||||||||||||||||||||||||||||||||||||||||||||||||||||||||||||||||||||||||||||||||||||

ITEM 6. LIFTING AND CARRYING OBJECTS

The availability of mechanical aids and other devices now makes it less likely that you will have to lift heavy objects, but hospital workers still must lift and carry frequently. You need to use good judgment in deciding which objects you can lift and carry alone. If you are in doubt, don't attempt to lift or carry any item by yourself; leave it or get others to help you.

In the skill laboratory, practice lifting and carrying an object weighing 10 to 15 pounds for 5 minutes in such a manner as to minimize fatigue and prevent strain.

Important Steps	Key Points
1. Start with the stable base position.	This ensures good body alignment and balance for further movements.
2. Grasp the object firmly on either side of its approximate center of gravity.	To lift an object weighing 10 to 15 pounds, you should use both hands, grasping the object near its center of gravity; this helps to balance it. For example, if you are lifting a square box, place your hands near the middle of the lateral sides.
3. "Set" your abdominal and arm muscles, then lift the object and bring it close to your body.	This acts to stabilize the muscles and to prepare for the action of lifting.
4. Carry the object as close to the midline of the body as possible.	When the object's line of gravity falls within your base of support, the large, stronger muscles of the buttocks and thighs help to support the additional weight.
5. Shift the object occasionally during the 5-minute period.	This relieves strain on certain muscles by rotating their activity.
6. Put the object down periodically.	This reduces the length of time the object must be supported and also allows the muscles a short period of rest.

||||||||||||||||||||||||||||||||||||||||||||||||||||||||||||||||||||||||||||||||||||||||||||||||||||||||||||||||||||||||||||||||||

18. When carrying an object, why is it best to hold it close to your body?

_____

19. List three ways to reduce strain if you must lift and carry heavy objects.

a. _____

b. _____

c. _____

||||||||||||||||||||||||||||||||||||||||||||||||||||||||||||||||||||||||||||||||||||||||||||||||||||||||||||||||||||||||||||||||||

ITEM 7. PUSHING AND PULLING MOVEMENTS

Pushing and pulling are frequently involved in the activities of hospital workers. They push or pull stretchers, food carts, housekeeping carts, beds, X-ray machines, wheelchairs, tables, therapy machines — the list seems endless. When we push or pull, we avoid carrying an object, an effort that is more tiring.

When we push or pull objects in the hospital, we are guided by the "rules of the road." Move your equipment down one side of the corridor so that other traffic can pass. Watch carefully when going around corners or approaching an intersection with another corridor. When you have pushed or pulled your equipment to its place of use, "park" it near the wall to avoid obstructing the hallway.

The decision of whether to push or to pull an object (or a patient in bed) depends on the size and weight of the object (or patient). Pulling involves primarily the muscles of the arms and the shoulders, so that lighter objects and patients may be pulled toward us. Pushing is used for heavier objects, since this movement utilizes the stronger muscles of the legs and hips and takes advantage of body weight.

In the skill laboratory, practice the movements of pushing and pulling an object such as a utility cart or a stretcher using your body weight, trunk muscles, and extensor muscles of the leg.

Important Steps	Key Points
1. Start with a stable base of support.	Check your position for good alignment and balance. Position your feet at least 8 inches apart, with one advanced forward in the direction you are working.
2. Stand close to the object to be pushed or pulled.	This keeps the work close to the body and also encourages good alignment by reducing distance of reach.
3. "Set" the trunk and leg muscles.	By now this should be familiar as a guideline to stabilize the body and prepare for action.
4. To push: *Lean toward* the object to be moved.	The body weight adds greater force to the muscular action and helps to move an object.
5. To pull: *Lean away* from the object to be moved.	This is done to apply as much force as possible in the direction of the movement by using the body weight.
6. Push or pull by letting your arms, hips, and thighs do most of the work.	The large muscles of the thigh and the leg do the work. Efficient use of these muscles conserves energy and prevents strain.

UNIT 11

20. List two safety precautions to observe if you are pushing or pulling a large object in the hospital corridor.

    a. _____

    b. _____

21. What do you do in pushing an object that utilizes your body weight as an additional force?

_____

_____

ITEM 8. CONCLUSION OF THE UNIT

You have now completed this lesson on body movements. You may need to practice some of the movements in the classroom or laboratory to be sure that you can do them correctly and know the reason for each step. When you feel confident that you have learned the body movements and related information, contact your instructor and arrange to take the performance test.

WORKBOOK ANSWERS

1. a. It seems lighter when held close to the body.

   b. The center of gravity of the book falls within my base of support. (Any similar answer.)

2. Any three of the following:

   a. raise or lower the work surface

   b. raise or lower yourself

   c. use stool

   d. stoop

   e. ladder, etc.

3. Stand on the same side of the bed as the leg with the cast, then move the patient to the near side of the bed.

4. a. Avoid injury or pain to the patient.

   b. Avoid strain or injury to the worker. (Any order.)

5. It stabilizes the muscles and joints, prepares the muscles for action, lessens danger of sudden movement or stress causing injury. (Any similar answer.)

6. Leverage makes work easier and increases the amount of work we can do.

7. Friction

8. The arm is the bar, the applied force is supplied by the flexor muscles or biceps as they contact, and the resisting force is the weight of the books.

9. back; balance

10. It decreases the distance to be reached.

11. Spread feet apart to broaden base of support.

12. flexing; hip and knee joints

13. Gravity

14. rear

15. buttocks and thighs

16. It allows the heels to lift slightly so that a pivot turn is easier.

17. a. Assisting the patient from bed to chair.

    b. Turning to answer the phone, pick up a chart, etc. (Any answer appropriate for your job.)

18. It is more stable to carry if its center of gravity falls within your base of support.

19. a. Don't lift more than is safe; get help; use mechanical lifters.

    b. Shift your load occasionally.

    c. Put the load down occasionally.

    d. Use proper body mechanics or movements.

    e. Hold the object as near the midline of your body as practical. (Any three of these, or similar answers.)

20. a. Watch carefully when going around corners.

    b. Approach intersections carefully.

    c. Move equipment down one side of the hall or corridor.

    d. "Park" equipment close to the wall to avoid obstructing the corridor.

    e. Use care not to bump into anyone. (Any two of these, or similar answers.)

21. Lean toward the object being pushed.

PERFORMANCE TEST

In the skill laboratory or your classroom, your instructor will ask you to demonstrate your skills in performing body movements and to state the reasons for each step in the movement. This is to be done without reference to your workbook, notes, or other source materials.

1. Perform an activity at floor level, such as wiping up some water or putting a slipper on a patient's foot, stoop, keeping the body aligned and balanced and using the large muscles of the thighs and buttocks to return to an upright position.

2. Given an object, such as a heavy book, located on a surface at least 6 inches above your head, reach and remove the object without hyperextending or straining your back, or losing your balance.

3. Given a box of books or similar object weighing 10 to 15 pounds and located on a surface about 32 to 36 inches high, lift and carry the box for 5 minutes using techniques that minimize fatigue and prevent muscle strain.

4. Push or pull a utility cart or similar object utilizing your body weight to assist in the movement.

5. Perform a pivoting turn in a way that would avoid straining your back or trunk muscles.

PERFORMANCE CHECKLIST

STOOPING

1. Assume a stable base of support.

2. Place feet apart, one foot slightly advanced.

3. Lower your body to stooped position by flexing your hip and knee joints.

4. Shift weight to the advanced foot and ball of the rear foot.

5. Keep your back straight and bend from the hips.

6. Raise your body to a standing position: Keep your back straight; initiate the move by extending your hip and knee joints.

7. Work your extensor muscles to bring your body upright.

REACHING

1. Start with a stable base of support and your body in good alignment and balance.

2. Check the distance to be reached to obtain the object. Use a footstool if necessary.

3. Stand with feet apart and one foot ahead of the other in the direction of the reach.

4. Look and reach in front, rather than stretching overhead.

5. Set your muscles to prepare for movement.

6. Lift the object from the shelf using good alignment procedures.

7. Lower the object with smooth, coordinated movement.

8. Look before stepping down from the ladder or footstool, if used.

9. Place the object on a shelf at working height, or stoop and lower it to the floor, observing good principles of body alignment.

LIFTING AND CARRYING

1. Start with a stable base.

2. Grasp the object to be lifted and carried in a balanced position; state the rationale for lifting the box at its center of gravity.

3. Set your abdominal and arm muscles for action: lift a box of books; bring it close to your own line of gravity.

4. Carry the box near the midline of your body for a period of approximately 5 minutes.

5. Shift the box from side to side as required during the period of support.

6. Place box on a counter or chair for short periods of time during which you rest.

7. Complete the performance by lifting and carrying the box for a period of time not to exceed 5 minutes.

PUSHING AND PULLING

1. Start your action with a stable base of support.

2. Position yourself.

3. Position your feet at least 8 inches apart with one foot slightly advanced.

4. Set your trunk and leg muscles.

5. Lean toward the utility cart in order to push.

6. Lean away from the utility cart in order to pull. Observe the principles of good body alignment, keeping your back straight and erect.

7. Move the utility cart using the large muscles of your leg and thigh.

PIVOTING

1. Stand with your feet slightly apart, knees slightly flexed.

2. Explain how this allows a stable base of support for use of the leg muscles.

3. Set your trunk and leg muscles for action.

4. Shift your weight to the ball of each foot.

5. Pivot or make a 90 degree turn on your feet.

6. Move your body simultaneously with your feet so that there is no twisting of your lower back.

7. Distribute your weight equally on each foot following the turn.

POSITIONING
THE BED PATIENT

GENERAL PERFORMANCE OBJECTIVE

Upon completing this lesson, you will be able to position the bed patient in good body alignment, using various aids for support or immobilization of various body parts, as well as protective aids to reduce pressure on skin areas.

SPECIFIC PERFORMANCE OBJECTIVES

After you have completed this lesson, you will be able to:

1. Provide support for or immobilize various parts of the body with the use of aids such as pillows, footboards, sandbags, hand rolls, and trochanter rolls.

2. Reduce and prevent formation of pressure areas by using protective aids such as pillows, synthetic lamb's wool pads, foam rubber pads, overbed cradle, protective heel (Posey), or flotation as with the alternating air-pressure mattress pad.

3. Place the helpless bed patient in the basic supine position according to the principles of positioning and in the variations of this position, including the Fowler's, semi-Fowler's, and Trendelenburg positions.

4. Place the helpless bed patient in the basic lateral position according to the principles of positioning and in the Sims' variation of this position.

5. Place the helpless bed patient in the basic prone position according to the principles of positioning.

6. Move the bed patient toward the head of the bed by using good body movements to prevent strain or injury to the patient or to yourself.

VOCABULARY

Some of the words used in this lesson may be new or unfamiliar to you. These have been listed below with their meanings. Go over this list several times, and when you see the word used in the lesson, refer to this section unless you are sure of its meaning.

alternating air-pressure pad—a plastic pad with rows of air cells that alternately fill slowly with air, then deflate.
alveoli—air sacs in the lung.
contracture—the permanent contraction of a muscle due to spasm or paralysis that leads to "freezing," or immobilization, of the affected joint(s).
decubitus (pl. decubiti)—a bedsore caused by reduction in circulation due to pressure on the affected part of the body.
deformity—an unnatural alteration; a misshapen or disfigured part of the body.
femur—the thigh bone, the longest and strongest bone in the body, extending from the hip to the knee.

flotation—the state of floating or buoyancy.

footboard—a board placed vertically at the end of the mattress to support the sole of the foot and to help prevent foot drop.

foot drop—hyperextension of the foot with permanent contracture of the calf muscles and tendons.

Fowler's position—a sitting position in bed with the backrest raised, usually to a 45 degree angle, and the knees kept flat.

fracture—a broken bone.

intravenous (IV)—within or into the vein, such as injection of fluids or puncture to obtain blood specimens.

overbed cradle— a device made of metal or wood placed over the patient's body or lower extremities to prevent the top bed covers from causing pressure.

paralysis—the loss of sensation or voluntary muscle movement in a part of the body.

pressure—the force caused by the weight of one object in contact with another.

prone—lying on the stomach, face downward.

sacrum—the flat triangular bone at the base of the vertebrae; it is composed of five fused vertebrae.

semi-Fowler's position—a reclining position with the backrest elevated, usually to 45 degrees or more, and the knee rest elevated to 15 degrees.

Sims' position—lying on one side with uppermost leg moderately flexed so it does not rest on the lower leg.

supine position—lying on the back with face upward; also referred to as dorsal recumbent position.

Trendelenburg position—the reclined position in which the head and chest are lower than the hips and lower extremities.

trochanter roll—a cylindrical cloth roll used to support the lateral hip joint or trochanter of the femur.

U
N
I
T
12

POSITIONING THE BED PATIENT

ITEM 1. WHY IS POSITIONING IMPORTANT?

One of the basic procedures that nursing workers perform most frequently is that of changing the patient's position. Any position, even the most comfortable one, will become unbearable after a period of time. Whereas the healthy person has the ability to assume any of a great variety of positions, the sick person's movements may be limited by disease, injury, or helplessness. It is the responsibility of the nursing worker to position the patient and to change his position frequently. Changing the patient's position accomplishes four things: (a) it contributes to the patient's comfort; (b) it relieves pressure on various parts of the body; (c) it helps prevent the formation of contractures or deformities; and (d) it improves circulation.

In this lesson, you will learn how proper body alignment contributes to the patient's comfort and helps prevent the occurrence of decubiti and contractures. You will be introduced to the various aids that you can use to support the body part in good alignment or to immobilize a part when it is necessary to limit its movement. The importance of reducing pressure on parts of the body and preventing the formation of pressure areas will become familiar to you as it is emphasized over and over again.

||||||||||||||||||||||||||||||||||||||||||||||||||||||||||||||||||||||||||||||||||||||||||||||||||||||||||||||||||||||||||||||

1. Four reasons for changing the position of the patient are:

    a. _____   b. _____

    c. _____   d. _____

2. When the bed patient is positioned by the nurse, it is necessary to maintain _____

_____ .

3. The ability of a patient to change position may be limited by:

_____ , _____ , or _____ .

―――

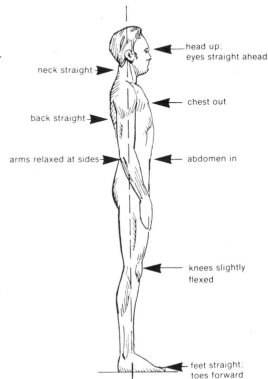

Good body alignment.

ITEM 2. PRINCIPLES OF BODY ALIGNMENT

Before we discuss the subject of how to turn and position the bed patient, we will review body alignment briefly. You may remember that alignment refers to the relationship of the movable segments of the body to one another. Good alignment is achieved when there is no undue stress placed on the muscles or skeleton.

The *checkpoints of good body alignment* are shown in the accompanying sketch.

―Head up, eyes straight ahead.

―Neck and back straight.

―Arms relaxed at sides.

―Chest up and out.

―Abdomen tucked in.

―Knees slightly flexed.

―Feet slightly apart, toes pointing forward.

There are several principles that guide the nurse in positioning the patient in good alignment. Each will be presented in more detail.

1. Good body alignment of patients is maintained at all times.

2. Body parts are supported in good alignment to promote comfort and to prevent undue muscle strain.

3. The position of the helpless patient must be changed at least every 2 hours to avoid prolonged flexion of any one body segment.

4. Pressure caused by body weight on another body or object can be reduced by changing position or by using protective aids.

PRINCIPLE 1.   GOOD BODY ALIGNMENT OF THE PATIENT IS MAINTAINED
AT ALL TIMES.

Good body alignment of the patient should be maintained from side to side (laterally) as well as from front to back (anterior-posterior).

Problems of Poor Body Alignment. Examples of poor alignment of the bed patient are shown in the adjoining figures. In the first, the patient's neck and back are flexed so that chest expansion for breathing is reduced, and the feet are hyperextended, which may lead to foot drop and interfere with later ambulation, or make ambulation impossible.

The second sketch shows the patient lying on his arm while on his side. The blood circulation is impaired in that arm. The other arm and leg are lying unsupported behind the patient, causing strain on the shoulder joint and inward rotation (turning) of the hip joint. The pull on the muscles makes this position very uncomfortable for the patient.

Avoid Muscle Strain. When the patient is supine (lying on the back), the pull and weight of the extended arms and legs cause strain on the muscles of the back, the abdomen, and the extremities themselves. Muscle strain in the supine position is most commonly felt in the neck, small of the back, elbow, wrist, knee, and foot. These areas are shown in the next illustration. Even the top covers of the bed put strain on the foot and toes of the patient when bedding is tucked in tightly or consists of heavy blankets, or when the patient is weak and unable to move alone. Although modern mattresses used in hospitals may reduce the strain felt in the small of the back, some patients still experience discomfort in this area.

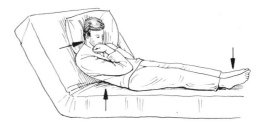

Poor body alignment: neck and back flexed, feet hyperextended.

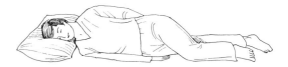

Poor body alignment: patient lying on arm, other arm unsupported.

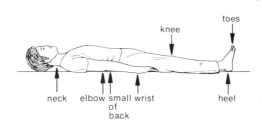

Supine Position: points of muscle strain.

U
N
I
T
12

4. The discomfort felt by the patient when lying in one position for a long period of time is the result of _____ .

5. Name four of the areas where discomfort may be felt when a person is lying in the supine position.

    a. _____ b. _____

    c. _____ d. _____ .

ITEM 3. SUPPORTIVE AIDS

> PRINCIPLE 2. BODY PARTS ARE SUPPORTED IN GOOD ALIGNMENT TO PROMOTE COMFORT AND TO PREVENT UNDUE MUSCLE STRAIN.

The patient's body alignment can be maintained and discomfort from muscle strain can be relieved by your use of *supportive aids.*

Pillows are most commonly used to support various parts of the body because they are soft and thus help reduce pressure; they can be folded over or rolled; and they can also be tucked firmly against the body to maintain its position. The footboard, sandbags, hand rolls, and trochanter rolls are also used to keep the body in alignment, to provide support for body parts, or to restrict movement of certain parts.

Pillows. Let us look at some of the ways that pillows may be used to support the patient's body. The helpless or weak patient who is turned onto one side may be unable to stay in this position and tends to roll onto the back again. A pillow placed lengthwise along the patient's back with one edge tucked under the side and the rest of the pillow rolled under (toward the surface of the bed) and tucked firmly against the back will support the patient leaning against it.

A pillow may also be used along the abdomen of the patient in Sim's position to prevent strain of sagging abdominal muscles. When a patient is lying on the side, a pillow placed between the knees helps reduce pressure on the knee joints and keeps the hip joint from rotating inward.

Pillows are used to support the neck and should be placed under the patient's head and shoulders to prevent flexion of the neck, which can interfere with breathing and swallowing. Strain on the muscles in the small of the back can be reduced by placing a small pillow or folded towel under the curve of the back. Avoid hyperextending the back. Hyperextension of the back causes strain on the abdominal muscles and some compression of the large blood vessels in the torso (trunk). Instead of using a pillow, which may be too large or bulky, it would be better to turn the patient to another position.

You will often find it necessary to support the patient's upper extremities. When a patient's arm is immobilized because of an IV or a cast, the pulling strain on the shoulder muscles can be relieved with a folded towel placed under the upper arm and a pillow placed to support the forearm and hand. Patients who are totally helpless or who must avoid all exertion should have their arms supported by pillows whenever they are in a sitting position. The positioning of pillows used to support the arm is shown.

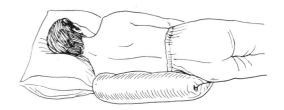

Pillow support of back.

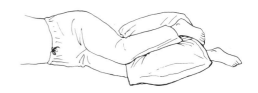

Pillow support of knee.

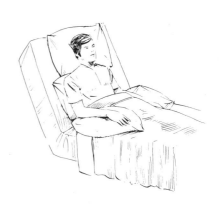

Pillow support of arms.

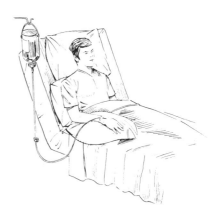

Pillow support with IV running.

6. Two reasons for using aids in positioning the patient are

   a. _____   b. _____ .

7. Underline your answers in the following statement: A pillow placed between the knees of a patient lying on his side will *(increase) (decrease)* the pressure on the knee joint and keep the hip joint from turning *(inward) (outward)*.

ıı

Hand Rolls. The hand roll is used to keep the fingers of the hand from being held in a tight fist, which could cause a flexion contraction. It provides some extension for the fingers and keeps the thumb in opposition to the fingers. It is used for the patient whose upper extremity is paralyzed, or who is unable to move his hand because of injury or disease.

The hand roll is a simple device and can be made by the patient's family or by volunteers if the hospital does not have an adequate supply. It is made of firmly woven cloth that is rolled into a cylinder about 4 to 5 inches long and 2 to 3 inches in diameter and is then stuffed firmly. It should fit into the palm of the hand, with the thumb curved on one side of the roll and the fingers flexed along the other side. A cloth loop or loose elastic band on one side for the fingers and on the other side for the thumb helps to hold them in position on the roll. (A rolled washcloth can be used temporarily.)

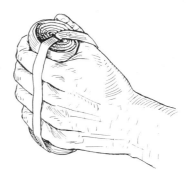

Footboards. To help keep the bed patient's feet in good alignment, you should place a footboard between the end of the mattress and the foot of the bed. The common type of footboard is made of wood and is L-shaped so that one end can be slipped under the mattress to hold the board in a firm upright position; it should be covered with a cloth pad or sheet.

The patient should be in a supine position so that the bottoms of the feet rest flat against the surface of the footboard. The top bedding is brought over the top of the footboard so that it will not cause pressure on the toes. The position of the feet on the footboard and the top bedding over it are shown in the drawing.

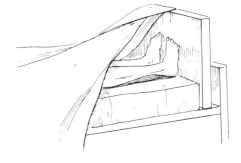

A footboard.

Sandbags. Sandbags are just that — canvas, rubber, or plastic bags filled with sand so that they are heavy in weight yet slightly flexible in use. Common sizes are 1 pound, 5 pounds, and 10 pounds. They are used to immobilize a part of the body by providing firm support that limits movement. You simply place the sandbag snugly next to the part that is to be supported. You will use sandbags on either side of the head following certain types of eye surgery when it is essential to prevent the patient from turning the head. Frequently, you will use sandbags to maintain the position of the feet on the footboard, especially when the foot tends to turn outward or inward. Sandbags are used as a temporary measure to immobilize a bone that has been fractured.

Trochanter Rolls. The trochanter roll should probably be used more often than it now is to support the hip joint and thigh. The trochanter roll prevents the hip and thigh from rotating outward and helps keep the foot in better alignment. Patients who have been paralyzed as a result of a stroke or other injury, those who have had a fracture of the femur, or those who have had surgery on the hip could benefit from the support given by the trochanter roll.

To make a trochanter roll:

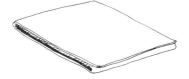

a. Fold in thirds.

a. The roll is made by folding a light bath blanket or a sheet to the desired length of 2 or 3 feet.

b. It is then rolled into a tight cylinder.

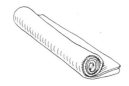

c. The loose end of the roll is placed under the patient's hip and thigh, with the roll under the flap end.

b. Roll up.

d. The roll is then tucked snugly along the hip and leg.

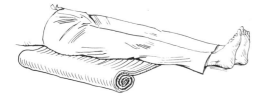

c. Place flap under patient.

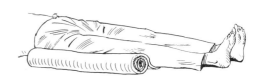

d. Roll in place.

ITEM 4. USE OF FLEXION IN POSITIONING

Our third principle for positioning the patient is concerned with nursing diligence to prevent the formation of contractures.

PRINCIPLE 3. THE POSITION OF THE HELPLESS PATIENT MUST BE CHANGED AT LEAST EVERY 2 HOURS TO AVOID PROLONGED FLEXION OF ANY ONE BODY SEGMENT.

A more comfortable position for the bed patient is produced by flexing (bending) segments of the body. The patient will feel better with some flexion of the elbows, hips, and knees while the alignment of the rest of the body is maintained. Those parts that are flexed may need to be supported to keep them in good alignment as well. Most of the positions in which you will place the bed patient will allow flexion of some part of the body.

Although the flexion position may be comfortable for the patient, the flexed body segment must be straightened after no more than two hours. In the helpless or weak patient, a position of prolonged or habitual flexion may result in *contractures.*

Contractures or the "freezing" of a joint, is caused by muscles that are permanently shortened. The joints of the upper and lower extremities are most likely to be affected by contractures. Failure to exercise or to change the position of the patient regularly will cause contractures and even greater immobility. The patient who recovers from a serious disease or injury only to be hopelessly crippled by contractures represents a tragic result of inadequate nursing care.

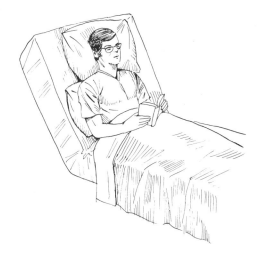

Positions of comfort involve alternating periods of flexion and extension of body parts.

ITEM 5. WHAT IS PRESSURE?

The final principle of positioning the patient can be stated as follows:

PRINCIPLE 4.   PRESSURE CAUSED BY BODY WEIGHT ON ANOTHER BODY OR OBJECT CAN BE REDUCED BY CHANGING THE POSITION OF THE BODY OR BY USING PROTECTIVE AIDS.

Perhaps the most important of all the reasons for changing the position of the patient is to reduce pressure on the various body parts and to prevent the formation of pressure areas. Now let us see why it is so important to reduce pressure by changing the patient's position frequently.

You already know that the body has weight and that every part of the body also has weight. The arm has weight. The eyelid has weight. The liver, blood, hair, and nails all have weight. The weight exerts a force when it comes in contact with another body or object, and this force is called pressure.

The weight of the patient's body in contact with the bed causes pressure both on the body and on the bed. (We won't worry about the bed at this point.) The longer the patient

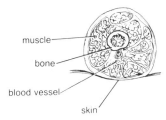

Initial Contact:
muscles, blood vessels, skin.

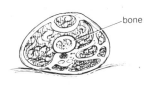

Continued Pressure:
muscles, skin, blood vessels.

remains in one position, the more the continued weight of the body presses down on the skin, blood vessels, and muscles on which the body rests. Since the skin, blood vessels, and muscles are not rigid enough to counteract this force, the pressure of the body weight makes them flatten out and become more compact.

Organs of the body are also affected by the force of pressure, and the lungs are extremely susceptible to it. As the patient's body remains in one position, the weight of the lung presses down on the rest of the lung beneath it and makes it more dense and compact. The air is squeezed out of the air sacs by the weight of the lung. The next two sketches show the lung changes produced by pressure.

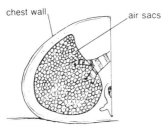

Initial Contact: lungs.

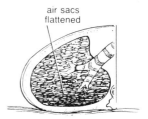

Continued Pressure: lungs.

The effects of pressure on the lungs can be very serious, even fatal, for the bedridden patient. As a result of lying still, the person tends to take very shallow breaths and take in less air. The alveoli, or air sacs of the lung, do not expand fully and there is less oxygen available for the body to use. Decreased oxygen affects every body tissue and system, making them less efficient. With less air to expand the lungs, the flattened alveoli are dark, warm, and moist — an ideal medium for the growth of bacteria. This often leads to pneumonia, a common complication of bed rest. Despite the use of antibiotic drugs, pneumonia is still the fifth leading cause of death in this country. Pneumonia due to lack of movement by the bed patient can be prevented by efficient nursing measures to (1) change the patient's position frequently and (2) ask the patient to cough and breathe deeply every hour in order to give the lungs regular opportunities to expand fully.

⸻

8. When a body comes in contact with another body or object, what causes the force known as pressure?

9. Prolonged pressure causes the skin, blood vessels, and muscles to become _____ _____ in shape.

10. The effects of pressure on the lungs lead to the complication of _____ .

⸻

ITEM 6. PRESSURE ON THE SKIN

Although we cannot see the effect of pressure directly on the organs of the body (like the lungs), it can be observed in the skin. The skin areas most commonly affected by pressure are those located over bony prominences. They are the back of the head, the shoulder blades, the elbows, the sacrum, the trochanter of the femur, the knees, and the heels.

The continued weight of the body on these areas produces a reddening of the skin from the pressure. The blood circulation to the skin area is impaired because the blood vessels are flattened out and carry less blood. The skin and muscle tissues are also flattened, becoming more dense and compacted, further slowing down the flow of blood to the part. The slowdown of the blood flow away from the pressure area causes the redness of the skin. With continuing pressure, the skin and muscle tissues are deprived of the oxygen and foods carried by the blood cells, and so they begin to die. When this happens, the skin forms a pressure sore. Other names for a pressure sore are bedsore and decubitus (plural, decubiti).

Pressure areas may develop within a period of a few hours on an undernourished patient and on the helpless or aged patient. Once a pressure area has broken down into a pressure sore it will take much time and effort to heal it. Some pressure sores take years of hospitalization to treat, cost thousands of dollars, and still never heal completely. *Prevention is the best cure.* Most often, pressure sores are the result of poor nursing care: not enough attention and care were given to turning the patient and preventing the development of pressure areas.

---

11. A pressure area that breaks down into a sore is called a _____

    or a _____ .

12. Pressure areas of the skin most often develop over _____ of bones.

13. The first sign of pressure usually noticed by the nurse is _____

    of the skin.

ITEM 7.   PROTECTIVE AIDS TO PREVENT PRESSURE

The primary method of preventing pressure areas is to change the patient's position at least every 2 hours. However, other aids are available for reducing pressure.

Flotation Pads.   In recent years, new products have become available to help reduce pressure for people confined to bed, and for treating patients with decubitus ulcers. Some products with promise are the flotation-type mattresses and pads. All flotation devices are based on the principle of distributing the body weight over a larger area than the areas in contact with one another. The water-filled mattress of a waterbed is a flotation device that produces less pressure on the body than most other types in use today. Use of water flotation pads and mattresses can have disadvantages, however, such as their weight, the need to control the water temperature, and possible damage from flooding should the plastic pad be punctured.

Flotation devices that utilize air as a method of displacing part of the body weight include air cushions, alternating air pressure pads, and air jets. All of these are designed to reduce pressure on the body and prevent the formation of decubiti. Although air flotation is less efficient than water flotation in reducing pressure, it is more convenient and has fewer disadvantages. Silicone gel pads, developed to protect delicate instruments in space flights,

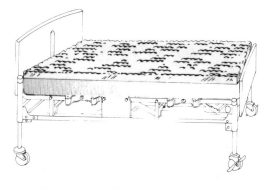

Eggcrate pad placed over the mattress.

have been effective in preventing pressure sores, but they are expensive and quite heavy to handle.

Thick foam pads are available commercially that resemble the inside of an egg carton. The full-length pad is placed on the bed mattress with the projections extending upward and covered with a sheet. The weight of the patient's body flattens the projections somewhat, but the trapped air in the foam acts like a flotation pad to reduce pressure.

Alternating Air-pressure Pads. The alternating air-pressure pad is currently a widely used flotation method for alleviating pressure in bedridden patients. The air pad is made of heavy vinyl plastic and has both an odd and an even set of vertical fingers or air chambers that alternately inflate and then deflate. The two sets of air chambers in the pad are connected by plastic tubes to a motor that cycles the air into the chamber. This produces a slight shifting motion that continually changes the pressure caused by the weight of the body.

To use the alternating air pad, place it on top of the bed mattress. Attach the tubes to the pump, plug the cord of the motor pump into an electric outlet, turn on the motor, and check to see that it is working. Cover the pad with the bottom sheet and then make the bed as usual. Do not put thick pads under the patient, since that would reduce the kneading action of the alternating air pad. Even with the alternating air pad in use, the patient should be positioned in good body alignment and turned every 2 hours or more often, unless prohibited by the doctor's orders. When using the alternating air pad, you should (1) avoid kinking the tubes and (2) avoid puncturing the plastic pad with pins or other sharp objects.

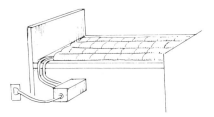

Alternating pressure mattress on bed,
attached to electrical outlet.

Antidecubitus Pads. The sacrum and the bony prominence of the hip joint (the trochanter of the femur) are frequent sites of pressure areas in the helpless bed patient. A synthetic lamb's wool pad, often referred to as a decubitus pad, may be placed under the patient's hips from the waist to the knees to reduce the pressure. Patients generally find these pads comfortable. They have a deep pile that resists matting and traps air between the fibers, thus forming a soft support for the body. Most of these pads can be laundered and dried by machine, then fluffed by a gentle shake so that they can be used for more than a year. The pads can also be used to turn or lift the patient, thereby avoiding the friction of sliding the patient's tender skin areas on the bed linen.

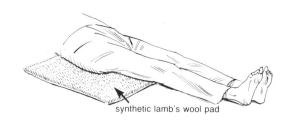

synthetic lamb's wool pad

Foam padding about 1/2 inch thick can be used to reduce pressure over any bony prominence. The sheet of padding can be cut to any size to fit under the body or protect the elbows, ankles, or heels. Specially designed heel pads are available, made of synthetic lamb's wool inside a sturdy cloth covering that is shaped to fit the heel.

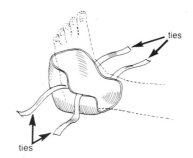

Heel protector

Overbed Cradle. The overbed cradle is a device used to prevent the weight of the top bedding from causing pressure on the patient's toes and feet. The cradle is placed over the bottom linen on the bed, and the top bedding is then brought over the cradle. Many overbed cradles are semicircular in shape. They may be made of wood and metal or constructed entirely of metal tubing or slats, as shown.

Some overbed cradles contain a light bulb which is used to supply dry heat to the extremities as part of the medical treatment. The heat (or light) cradles are ordered by the physician and are not used without an order.

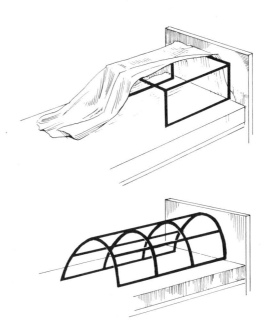

U
N
I
T
12

A Word of Caution. The inflated rubber rings and round donuts, frequently used in the past by nurses to ease pressure areas on the sacrum or the heel, are not recommended for use. Donuts made of absorbent cotton, shaped in a circle, and wrapped with gauze or other similar material tend to be too firm. They cause additional pressure around their circumferences that further decreases the blood flow to and away from the part already suffering from the effects of pressure.

Prevention of Pressure Areas. Although there are many devices to assist in preventing pressure sores, the key to their prevention is the nurse. Nothing can substitute for your personal, active attention on the patient's behalf. Correct positioning of the patient, frequent changing of position by turning, maintaining a clean and dry bed, and protecting body parts against pressure are important skills to use for the prevention of pressure areas and decubiti.

14. The primary method used by nursing workers to prevent the formation of pressure

   areas in the bed patient is _____ .

15. In addition to the primary method, what other two methods might you use for the patient who shows signs of pressure on the skin over his sacrum?

   a. _____   b. _____ .

ITEM 8.   BASIC BODY POSITIONS AND THEIR VARIATIONS

We have now identified four principles to remember in the positioning of the helpless patient in bed. They are

1. *Good body alignment of the patient is maintained at all times.*

2. *Body parts are supported in good alignment to promote comfort and to prevent undue muscle strain.*

3. *The helpless patient's position is changed at least every 2 hours to avoid prolonged flexion of any one body segment.*

4. *Pressure caused by body weight on another object or body can be reduced by changing the position of the body or by using protective aids.*

These principles form the guidelines for the skills you will use to position the bed patient.

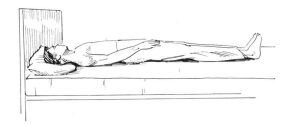

Supine position.

Basic Positions

There are three basic positions for the patient to assume while in bed. These are

a. the supine position, in which the patient lies on his back;

b. the lateral position, in which the patient lies on one side; and

c. the prone position, in which the patient lies on his stomach.

These positions are shown in the accompanying sketches. All other positions that you will use for your patients are variations of these three.

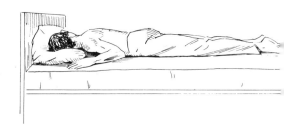

Prone position.

Fowler's Position. Fowler's position, a variation of the supine position, is produced when the head of the bed is elevated, placing the patient in a sitting position. The usual angle of elevation is 45 to 60 degrees, although it may be as little as 10 degrees or as great as 90 degrees.

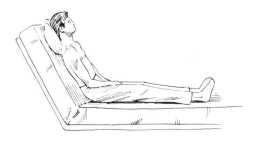

Fowler's position.

Semi-Fowler's Position. To produce the semi-Fowler's position, place the bed in Fowler's position, then raise the knee rest of the bed about 15 degrees. Patients often find this position comfortable because it reduces strain on abdominal and leg muscles and helps prevent the patient's sliding down in bed. *Caution:* Patients should not be placed in semi-Fowler's position following abdominal surgery unless it has been authorized by the physician. Elevation of the knees in postoperative patients is associated with decreased circulation in the legs and the formation of blood clots, a serious complication.

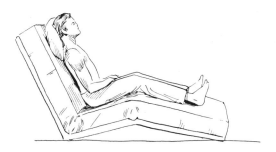

Semi-Fowler's position

Trendelenburg Position. Another variation of the supine position is the Trendelenburg position, in which the patient's feet are elevated and the head is lowered. This position is used mainly for patients who are victims of shock, although it may also be used in certain surgical procedures. There is a tendency for patients who are in this position to slide toward the head of the bed; to prevent this, sandbags should be placed against the patient's shoulders, and a pillow should be placed at the head of the bed for safety.

U
N
I
T
12

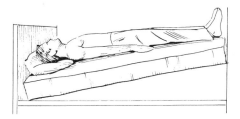

Trendelenburg position

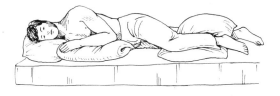

Sims' position.

Sims' Position. Sims' position is a variation of the lateral position. The uppermost leg is sharply flexed so that it does not rest upon the lower leg.

||||||||||||||||||||||||||||||||||||||||||||||||||||||||||||||||||||||||||||||||||||||||||||||||||||||||||||||||||||||||||||||||||||||||||

16. The four principles used in positioning the helpless bed patient are:

a. _____

b. _____

c. _____

d. _____

Please match the following definitions to the basic positions of the bed patient.

Definitions		*Positions*	
17.	head elevated, hips and knees flexed.	a.	Fowler's
18.	lying on one side with one leg resting on the other.	b.	Prone
19.	lying with face and feet upward.	c.	Lateral
20.	lying with feet elevated and head lowered.	d.	Sims'
21.	lying with foot of bed level and head elevated.	e.	semi-Fowler's
		f.	Trendelenburg
		g.	Supine

ITEM 9. PLACING THE PATIENT IN THE SUPINE POSITION

In the skill laboratory, practice placing the patient in each of the three basic positions and the four variations while using the principles of positioning to keep good body alignment, support parts of the body, and reduce pressure. One of the other students, or someone else, should play the part of the patient for your practice session. (Remember to use good body alignment principles for yourself.)

Given a bedpatient who became paralyzed on his right side two days ago, place him in a supine position using the principles of positioning as your guidelines and following the principles of good body movement to prevent injury or strain to yourself.

Supplies Needed

Adjustable hospital bed	Sandbag
Synthetic lamb's wool pad	Pillows
Heel protector	Footboards
Foam rubber pads	Trochanter roll
Hand roll	

Important Steps	Key Points
1. Wash your hands.	Universal Steps A, B, C, and D. See Appendix.
2. Approach and identify the patient and explain what you are going to do.	
3. Provide privacy.	
4. Position the bed.	Place the bed in a flat or level position at working height, unless contraindicated. Lower the siderails on the proximal side, if they are being used. (The proximal side is the side on which the patient is paralyzed.)
	Common contradictions for bed position change are severe cardiac (heart) or respiratory (lung) disease; brain injury or surgery; and some types of traction or cast. Be sure to obtain this

Important Steps	Key Points
	information from the nurse when you receive your assignment or refer to the patient's nursing care plan in the Kardex.
5. Move patient from a side position to the supine position.	For patient lying on one side, remove any supportive pillows, fold the top bedding back to the hips, and avoid any undue exposure of the patient's body. With one hand on patient's shoulder and one on the hip, roll body in one piece (like a log) over onto the back. Always avoid twisting the back by moving the torso (trunk) of the body as a unit.
6. Use protective aids to reduce pressure on bony prominences.	The paralyzed patient may not be aware of any discomfort caused by pressure, so you must be alert to prevent and reduce pressure, especially on any paralyzed parts.
	a. Place a synthetic lamb's wool pad under the patient's hips and thighs. With one hand on patient's shoulder and one on the distal hip, roll the patient toward you; continue to support shoulder and chest with one hand and place the pad along the hips and thigh, with one half of the pad tucked close to patient's side and the bed. Roll the patient onto back, reach under proximal side, and pull the remainder of pad into place. Be sure to reposition the patient's body parts.
	b. Place a piece of foam rubber padding under the patient's right heel, or use a protective heel of synthetic lamb's wool.
7. Align the patient's body in good position.	The head, neck, and spine should be in a straight line. The arms and legs should be parallel to the body. The hips, knees, and feet should be in good alignment.
8. Support the body parts in good alignment for comfort.	Place a pillow under the head and shoulders to prevent strain on neck muscles. Support the small of the back with a folded bath towel or small pillow. Since this patient is paralyzed on the right side, it will be difficult to keep the right led in good position. You should put a footboard at the foot of the bed and place the feet flat against it. Arrange a sandbag along the outer portion of the right foot to keep the foot upright. Now make a trochanter roll and arrange it along the right hip and thigh to keep the hip joint from rotating outward. Place a pillow under the right forearm so that the arm is at least 6 inches from the body and place a hand roll in the paralyzed right hand. Use the loops of a slightly loose bandage to keep the fingers flexed and the thumb in opposition on the roll; otherwise the roll will slip out of place.

UNIT 12

Important Steps	Key Points

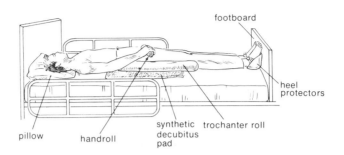

Patient in supine position with supportive
aids to maintain body alignment and protective
devices to reduce pressure.

Important Steps	Key Points
9. Provide for the patient's comfort.	Universal Steps Y and Z. See Appendix.
10. Report and record as appropriate.	10:00 A.M. Turned to supine position; no reddened areas observed on back; moves easily without pain or dyspnea. J. Jones, LVN

ITEM 10.   PLACING THE PATIENT IN FOWLER'S POSITION

Given a patient with paralysis of the right side who is in a supine position, place in Fowler's position.

▪▪

Supplies Needed

Adjustable hospital bed	Sandbags
Synthetic lamb's wool pad	Footboard
Heel protector	Trochanter roll
Foam rubber pads	Hand roll
Pillows	

▪▪

Important Steps	Key Points

Carry out Universal Steps A, B, and C. See Appendix.

Important Steps	Key Points
1. Elevate the head of the bed.	Elevate the head of the bed to an angle of approximately 45 degrees. (Note that Fowler's position can require the angle of elevation to be anywhere between 15 and 60 degrees.) The head of the bed is not brought to the full upright position (90 degrees) for weak or helpless patients who may be unable to maintain their balance.

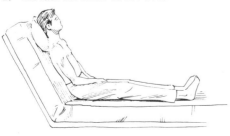

Fowler's position.

Important Steps	Key Points
2. Use aids to reduce pressure on bony prominences, if indicated by the condition of the patient.	You should prevent or reduce pressure by placing a synthetic lamb's wool pad or foam rubber pad under the hips and a protective heel or pad on the right foot.
3. Place the patient in good body alignment.	See that the head, neck, and back are all straight. The weight of the body should be supported at the point where the hips are flexed in the sitting position. See that the feet are straight and the toes are pointing in an upright position.
4. Support the body parts in good alignment for comfort.	The body parts should be supported in Fowler's position as they were in the supine position. Place the pillow under the head and shoulders, the trochanter roll along the right hip and thigh, the footboard at the foot of the bed, a sandbag along the outer part of the right foot, and a pillow under the right forearm to reduce the pulling drag on the shoulder joint. The hand and thumb should be supported on a hand roll.
Carry out Universal Steps Y and Z. See Appendix.	Charting example: 12:10 P.M. Position changed to Fowler's. Is in good spirits today, moving easily, without pain. J. Jones, LVN

ITEM 11.   PLACING THE PATIENT IN SEMI-FOWLER'S POSITION

Given the same patient who has paralysis of the right side and who is lying in a supine position in bed, place in semi-Fowler's position. Follow the same procedure as outlined in Item 10, except that you will add the following as Step 2, then carry out the remaining steps.

Important Steps	Key Points
2. Elevate the knee rest of the bed approximately 15 degrees.	Slight flexion of the knees gives more comfort by reducing strain on the patient's abdominal muscles and helps patient maintain a sitting position without sliding down in bed. It also prevents hyperextension of the knees. Charting example: 12:10 P.M. Placed in semi-Fowler's position. Says this is the most comfortable. J. Jones, LVN

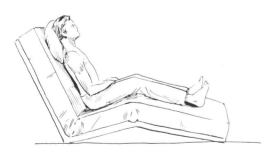

Semi-Fowler's position.

ITEM 12.   PLACING THE PATIENT IN LATERAL AND SIMS' POSITIONS

Given an elderly patient who is extremely weak and unable to turn without assistance, position in a lateral and then in Sims' position using the principles of positioning.

Important Steps	Key Points

Carry out Universal Steps B and C. See Appendix.

1. Position the bed.

Lower the head and foot of the bed so that it is level or flat. Then lower the siderail on the proximal side where you are working, if it was in use.

2. Turn the patient onto the side toward you. (Obtain assistance, if needed.)

Fold the top bedding back to the level of patient's hips, avoiding undue exposure of the patient's body, which may cause embarrassment.

To turn the patient onto the side toward you:

a. Flex the distal knee and place the distal arm across the chest.

b. "Log-roll" the body toward you by placing one hand on shoulder and the other on the distal hip and pulling without twisting the patient's torso.

c. Reach behind the patient's back with both hands, placing one on the proximal shoulder and one on the hip, and lift slightly outward to roll the body toward you.

Remember to use good body movements so that your back is straight and your knees are flexed.

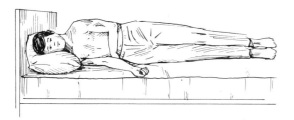

Lateral position.

To turn the patient onto the side away from you:

a. "Log-roll" the patient's body away from you by putting one hand on the proximal shoulder and the other on the hip and rolling patient to the distal side.

b. Lower your hands to the distal shoulder and hip, then pull them toward you to stabilize the patient in the lateral position.

Note that when the patient is large or extremely helpless, this procedure requires less effort than does turning patient toward you. Again, you must use good body movement to avoid possible strain or injury to yourself.

3. Align the patient's body in good position.

Make sure that the patient is not lying on his arm. See that his head, neck, and back are in a straight line and that his legs are parallel, with the knees slightly flexed. The patient's uppermost arm may be flexed across his abdomen or supported on his body and hip.

Important Steps	Key Points
4. Place the patient in Sims' position.	Flex the uppermost leg so that it does not rest upon the lower leg. The lowermost arm may be at the patient's back. To obtain this position, place this arm parallel to the body as the patient is being turned. Then, after you have turned the patient, support and slightly lift the shoulder from the bed with one hand and, with the other, grasp the elbow and draw the arm smoothly from under the patient toward the back.
5. Support the body in good alignment for comfort.	Place a pillow under the patient's head and neck to prevent muscle strain and maintain alignment. Put a pillow under the uppermost leg so that it is supported from the knee to the foot. Another pillow may be placed firmly against the patient's abdomen to support the back and hip in better alignment.
6. Use aids to reduce pressure over bony prominences.	You may need to use a foam rubber pad or a protective heel to prevent pressure on the ankle of the lowermost leg. Also, a synthetic lamb's wool pad or foam rubber pad should be used under the patient's hip and thigh to reduce pressure on the trochanter at the hip joint. Many elderly patients who are thin tend to show signs of pressure in this area.
Carry out Universal Steps Y and Z. See Appendix.	Charting example: 4:00 P.M. Placed in left Sims' position. Seems more alert this P.M. No complaints.

J. Jones, LVN

U
N
I
T
12

ITEM 13. PLACING THE PATIENT IN PRONE POSITION

Given a patient who is being treated for a draining wound of the sacral area, place the patient in a prone position using the principles of positioning.

Patients who are accustomed to sleeping on their abdomen would probably welcome such a change; others may resist, especially if they fear it will be painful. Some patients must be reassured that you will turn them back whenever the position becomes uncomfortable.

Important Steps	Key Points
Carry out Universal Steps A, B, and C. See Appendix.	
1. Adjust the bed.	Lower the headrest and knee rest so that the bed is in a flat position. Raise the bed to working height. Lower the siderails on the side where you are working. Fold the top bedding down to the level of the patient's hips. Avoid undue exposure of the patient's body, which may cause embarrassment.

Important Steps	Key Points
2. Position the patient in bed.	When there is room between the mattress and the foot of the bed, the patient should be moved down in the bed so that the feet will extend over the edge of the mattress. Remove the footboard, if one is present.
3. Turn patient on his side and onto stomach.	Turn the patient onto his side according to the procedure given in Item 12. It is preferable to roll patient toward you so that you can observe him closely. Continue to roll the patient over until he on his stomach.
4. Align the patient in good position.	The patient's head should be turned to one side; the neck and back should be in a straight line. The arms may be parallel to the body in a slightly flexed position, or the arm on the same side that the head is turned can be flexed sharply at the elbow so that the hand is near the head. The legs should be straight and the feet extended over the edge of the mattress to avoid hyperextension of the foot. If this is not possible, place a pillow under both ankles to prevent foot drop as a result of prolonged hyperextension.

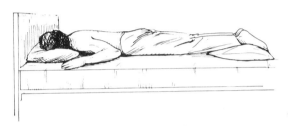

Prone position with foot positioned in good alignment to avoid hyperextension.

5. Support the patient's body in good alignment.	A small pillow or folded towel under the head may be used if the patient requests it. Generally, it will not be needed for comfort.
6. Use aids to reduce pressure on any bony part.	For the woman patient in a prone position, pressure on the breasts is relieved by placing a pillow under the chest and abdomen, below the breasts. A pillow placed under the lower abdomen of the male patient relieves pressure on the genital organs. Many infants and restless patients will develop reddened skin areas on the knees when in the prone position. The use of a synthetic lamb's wool pad or a foam rubber pad under the knees will reduce pressure and friction.

Carry out Universal Steps X, Y, and Z. See Appendix.	Charting example:
	
	6:00 P.M. Placed in prone position. No redness noted on bony prominences. Back massaged.
	          J. Jones, LVN
	
	6:20 P.M. Sleeping quietly.
	          J. Jones, LVN

ITEM 14.   PLACING THE PATIENT IN TRENDELENBURG POSITION

Given a patient going into shock as a result of possible internal bleeding, immediately place in Trendelenburg position.

Important Steps	Key Points

Carry out Universal Steps A, B, and C. See Appendix.

1. Position the bed.

If possible, place the head of the bed touching the wall. Lock the brakes on the wheels at both the head and the foot of the bed. Remove the pillow from under the patient's head and place it upright against the head of the bed. Lower the head of the bed.

2. Elevate the foot of the bed and place the patient in Trendelenburg position.

For automatically adjustable beds (electric or manual), disengage the headrest hold and raise the foot of the bed. The head of the bed will decline as the foot of the bed is elevated, so that the bed remains flat although on an incline.

For gatch adjustable beds, elevate the knee rest, then raise the footrest and engage the metal support in the ratchet on either side of the bed.

Alternative methods of raising the foot of the bed:

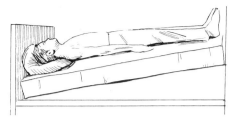

Trendelenburg position.

a. a hydraulic bed lifter may be used to elevate the foot of the bed;

b. two people may manually lift the foot of the bed while a third person places wooden "shock blocks" under the wheels at the foot of the bed;

c. two people may lift and support the foot of the bed on two chairs.

3. Align the patient's body in good position.

The patient should always be in good alignment: head, neck, and back straight, legs and arms should be parallel to the body. The weight of the arms on the chest or abdomen could restrict breathing movements.

4. Support the body in good alignment for comfort.

Use small pillows or folded bath towels to support the neck and the small of the back in order to relieve muscle strain. Since the patient in this position will tend to slide toward the head of the bed, place a sandbag above the shoulders to help maintain position.

5. Use aids to reduce pressure over bony prominences.

The initial use of the Trendelenburg position is generally required during a medical emergency, so other life-supporting treatment is carried out first. When time allows, you must reduce pressure because the patient's movements may be severely limited. Provide padding under the hips and heels as needed. The back of the head and the elbows may need to be padded as well.

Carry out Universal Steps Y and Z. See Appendix.

The patient must be observed closely during the emergency period and early convalescence.

Charting example:
2:00 PM B/P 88/40, P 132 R 20. Placed in Trendelenburg position per order. Skin cool and clammy, color pale. IV infusing in L arm.
D. Carmen, RN

UNIT 12

ITEM 15. MOVING THE PATIENT TOWARD THE HEAD OF THE BED

Given a patient who had abdominal surgery yesterday and who has slipped down toward the foot of the bed, move him toward the head of the bed with help from the patient, while following methods of good body movement.

Important Steps	Key Points
Carry out Universal Steps B and C. See Appendix.	
1. Adjust the bed.	Place the bed in a flat or nearly flat position. Lower the siderail on the side on which you are working.
2. Tell the patient how to help move up in bed. 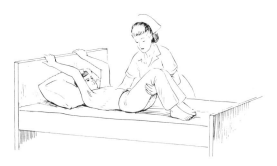	Ask the patient to flex both knees, then to push down on the bed with both feet to help move the hips upward in bed when you give the signal. If possible, the patient reaches up, holds the head of the bed with one or both hands, and pulls the body upward on signal as you assist moving the upper portion of the body.
3. Move the patient toward the head of the bed.	When the patient is in position with hands reaching the head of the bed and knees flexed, place one hand under his shoulder and across his back and support his head with the other hand. If there is no need to support the head, place the other hand under the hips to help move them. Upon your signal, both of you should move simultaneously toward the head of the bed.

Carry out Universal Steps X, Y, and Z. See Appendix.

ITEM 16. CONCLUSION OF THE LESSON

You have now finished the lesson on positioning the bed patient. When you have practiced the procedures sufficiently to gain some skill in aligning and moving the patient and using the appropriate supportive and protective aids, arrange with your instructor to take the performance test.

ADDITIONAL INFORMATION FOR ENRICHMENT

Positioning the bed patient is a basic skill that you will use daily in the care of all of your patients. Positioning is also an important part of the therapeutic treatment for many disease conditions. You may want to learn more about how positioning is used to meet a patient's special needs. Medical and surgical nursing textbooks are a rich source of information about the use of positioning in the treatment of various conditions. For example, the postoperative patient usually can be placed in Fowler's position but not in semi-Fowler's position. The right lateral position is used to advance the Miller-Abbott intestinal tube, whereas the left lateral position is best for giving an enema. You will be better able to help the patient cooperate with the treatment if you understand the conditions for the use and purposes of positioning.

In view of the importance of this aspect of nursing care, you may wish to read more about patient positioning. Much has been written about the effect of pressure on the body. Several articles are listed on page 161. The articles include references that will provide additional information and sources of material.

WORKBOOK ANSWERS

1. a. to increase patient's comfort

    b. to relieve pressure

    c. to prevent contractures

    d. to improve circulation

2. alignment of the body

3. disease, inability to move about, helplessness

4. strain on muscles

5. Any four of the following: neck, small of the back, elbow, wrist, knee, ankle; also (not mentioned in the text), shoulder, abdomen, hip.

6. Any two of the following: to keep the body in alignment; to provide support for body segments; to immobilize or prevent movement in a part

7. decrease; inward

8. weight

9. flattened (dense, compacted, etc.)

10. pneumonia

11. bedsore; decubitus ulcer

12. prominences

13. redness

14. to turn the patient frequently

15. Any two of the following: synthetic lamb's wool pad, foam rubber pad, alternating air-pressure pad

16. a. Good body alignment of patient is maintained at all times.

    b. Body parts are supported in good alignment to prevent undue muscle strain.

    c. Helpless patient's position is changed every 2 hours to avoid prolonged flexion of any part.

    d. Pressure caused by body weight on another object or body can be reduced by changing the position of the body or by the use of protective aids.

17. e

18. c

UNIT 12

19. g

20. f

21. a

PERFORMANCE TEST

In the skill laboratory, your instructor will ask you to demonstrate your skill in carrying out two of the following procedures without reference to source material. For these activities, you will need another person to play the part of the patient.

1. Given a patient in a lateral position with paralysis of both legs, place the patient in a supine position, using the principles of positioning to provide good alignment, support, and protection from pressure.

2. Given a patient in a supine position who has paralysis of both legs, place the patient (1) in Fowler's position, (2) in semi-Fowler's position, and (3) in Trendelenburg position.

3. Given a patient who had abdominal surgery yesterday, place the patient in Sims' position, using the principles of positioning to provide good alignment, support, and protection from pressure.

4. Given an adult woman patient with a disease that limits her movement, place her in a prone position, utilizing the principles of positioning.

5. Given a patient with a high fever who has slipped down in bed while in a supine position, assist to move toward the head of the bed, using principles of good body movement.

PERFORMANCE CHECKLIST

1. SUPINE POSITIONING OF PATIENT

1. Wash your hands.

2. Approach and identify the patient.

3. Explain the procedure to the patient.

4. Provide privacy.

5. Place the bed in flat position, at working level.

6. Lower the siderails on the proximal side.

7. Remove supportive pillows from patient's back and from between the knees.

8. Move the patient from side to back by placing your hands on patient's shoulder and hip and log-rolling the body.

9. Move and align the legs so that the hips, knees, and feet are parallel.

10. Provide protection against pressure points:

    a. Place a decubitus pad under the hips.

    b. Use heel protectors for both feet.

    c. Use a bed board or a cradle to keep the bedding off the feet.

11. Use supportive aids to maintain good body alignment:

    a. Place a pillow under patient's head and shoulders.

    b. Place a small pillow or towel at the small curve of the back.

    c. Use a trochanter roll along the hip and thigh of both legs.

    d. Support the position of the feet with sandbags, if necessary.

12. Provide for the patient's safety and comfort. Leave the call signal and bedside stand within easy reach.

13. Chart the change of position and observations of the patient's condition.

2. POSITIONING THE PATIENT

— IN FOWLER'S POSITION

Steps 1 through 5: Same as for supine positioning above.

6. Elevate the head of the bed to approximately 45 degrees.

7. Check the alignment and support of the patient.

8. Use protective aids to reduce pressure, as needed.

— IN SEMI-FOWLER POSITION

Steps 1 through 5: Same as for supine positioning.

6. Elevate the head of the bed to approximately 45 degrees.

7. Raise the knee gatch or the foot of the bed so that the knees are flexed approximately 15 degrees.

8. Check the patient's alignment and support.

9. Use protective aids to reduce pressure, as needed.

— IN TRENDELENBURG POSITION

1. Wash your hands.

2. Approach and identify the patient.

3. Explain the procedure.

4. Lower the head of the bed.

5. Elevate the foot of the bed by using the automatic controls or hydraulic lifter. Obtain assistance if the foot of the bed is to be placed on "shock blocks" or chairs.

6. Check the alignment and support of the patient.

7. Use protective aids to reduce pressure, as needed.

3. POSITIONING THE PATIENT IN SIMS' POSITION

1. Wash your hands.

2. Identify the patient.

3. Explain the procedure to him.

4. Adjust the bed to working height.

5. Prepare the patient for movement.

6. Place the patient in Sims' position.

    a. Place one hand on patient's distal shoulder and the other on the hip and draw the patient's body toward you, then adjust position when patient is lying on side.

    b. Flex the upper leg so that it does not rest on the lower leg.

    c. Position the lower arm to the rear.

7. Support the body for good alignment.

    a. Place a pillow under the head and neck.

    b. Place a pillow under the uppermost leg so it is supported.

    c. Put pillow against the abdomen to support the trunk and uppermost arm.

8. Use protective aids to reduce pressure, if required.

9. Provide for the patient's comfort.

10. Chart the procedure.

4. POSITIONING THE PATIENT IN A PRONE POSITION

1. Wash your hands.

2. Identify the patient and explain the procedure.

3. Adjust the bed to working height.

4. Position the patient in bed with patient's feet extended over the edge of the mattress, if possible.

5. Turn the patient onto stomach by placing one hand on the proximal shoulder and the other on the hip and rolling body away from you.

6. Adjust the patient's body alignment.

    a. Turn the head to one side.

    b. Position the arms for comfort.

    c. Place a pillow under the abdomen to relieve pressure on the breasts.

    d. Align the feet and avoid hyperextension by (1) extending the feet over the mattress or (2) supporting the ankles with a pillow.

7. Use protective aids to reduce pressure, as required.

8. Provide for patient's comfort and safety; state when you will return.

9. Chart the procedure.

5. MOVING THE PATIENT TOWARD THE HEAD OF THE BED

1. Wash your hands.

2. Identify the patient.

3. Explain the procedure to the patient.

4. Adjust the bed to working height.

UNIT 12

5. Instruct the patient to assist by:

   a. flexing both knees, placing the soles of his feet on the mattress;

   b. grasping the headboard with his arms;

   c. on command, pulling with his arms and pushing with his feet.

6. Initiate the procedure by:

   a. supporting the head;

   b. supporting the hips to assist in movement;

   c. coordinating the patient's efforts with your own.

7. Check patient's alignment and support.

8. Use protective aids to reduce pressure.

9. Provide for the patient's comfort; indicate when you will return.

10. Chart the procedure.

POST-TEST

Multiple Choice. Select the one best answer.

1. The force called pressure is the result of

    a. congestion with redness of the skin.

    b. having bony prominences.

    c. weight of one object pressing down on another.

    d. lack of friction when moving.

2. Prolonged pressure on the sacrum causes the skin, blood vessels, and muscles to

    a. become compact and flattened out.

    b. swell up and become larger.

    c. turn pale in color.

    d. receive too much oxygen and too many nutrients.

3. One organ of the body is quickly affected by pressure from lying in one position for a long period of time. This organ is

    a. the kidney.

    b. the stomach.

    c. the brain.

    d. the lung.

4. The nurse should see that the position of the bed patient is changed at least

    a. once every shift.

    b. every 2 hours.

    c. every hour.

    d. every ½ hour.

5. Jane has an injury to her arm and has kept her elbow flexed continually for several days. This flexion could result in

    a. a decubitus.

    b. a contracture.

    c. pressure.

    d. swelling.

6. Mr. Rose had a stroke several days ago and is now paralyzed on the right side of his body. When positioning him in good alignment, you place a hand roll in his right hand. The purpose of the hand roll is

    a. to encourage him to exercise his hand and fingers.

    b. to keep the palm of his hand warm and dry.

    c. to keep the fingers and the thumb flexed.

    d. to extend the fingers and keep the thumb in opposition.

UNIT 12

7. (See question 6.) A footboard is placed at the end of the mattress of Mr. Rose's bed. The purpose of the footboard is to

   a. keep the mattress from sliding toward the foot of the bed.

   b. support Mr. Rose's feet when lying in bed.

   c. keep the top bedding off the foot end of the mattress.

   d. prevent muscle strain in Mr. Rose's back.

8. All but one of the following are reasons for using aids in positioning the patient. Which one does not apply?

   a. To provide support of a body part.

   b. To improve elimination of wastes.

   c. To relieve pressure.

   d. To maintain the body in alignment.

POST-TEST ANSWERS

1. c	5. b
2. a	6. d
3. d	7. b
4. b	8. b

PATIENT MOVEMENT
AND AMBULATION

GENERAL PERFORMANCE OBJECTIVE

Upon completing this lesson, demonstrate your ability to assist the patient (or another person) to move his various joints through the range-of-motion exercises, to dangle his feet at the side of the bed, to stand, and to walk in a safe manner without causing additional pain or injury.

SPECIFIC PERFORMANCE OBJECTIVES

When you have completed this lesson you will be able to:

1. Assess the patient's physical and mental condition regarding aspects that may interfere with his ability to exercise his joints or to ambulate, and your own ability or limitations in carrying out the procedures.

2. Explain the need for exercising all of the joints to the patient who has limited or no motion in the joints on one side of the body. Show how to exercise the joints on the unaffected side and carry out the range-of-motion exercises for the affected joints. In performing the range-of-motion exercises, you will

   a. provide support for the body part that is distal, or away from, the joint being exercised.

   b. avoid forcing movement in the joint to the point at which it causes pain.

3. Assist the patient in bed in dangling both feet over the side of the bed by positioning on the proximal side of the bed, bringing patient to a sitting position, pivoting the body, and swinging the feet over the side of the bed in smooth, flowing motions, using principles of good body alignment and movement.

4. Assist the patient in standing, in balancing, and in walking safely, using principles of good body alignment, balance, and movement.

5. Assist the patient (whether a youth or an adult) who has lost his balance and begun to fall by slowing the rate of descent, and easing to the floor or ground. This will prevent injury both to the patient and to yourself.

VOCABULARY

active exercise—movement performed by the person without assistance from another.
axilla (pl. axillae)—under the arm at the shoulder; the armpit.
circumduction—the circular motion of a limb or body part in which the limb forms the side of a cone and the joint nearest the body forms the apex or tip of the cone.

immobility—the inability to move a part or all of the body.

infiltration—seepage of fluid into the skin tissue that causes blanching (turning pale) and swelling.

pace—the distance covered in one step, or the number of steps per minute.

passive exercise—the moving of parts of a person's body by another person.

physiological changes—alterations in body function due to disease or injury.

pneumonia, hypostatic—an inflammation of the lungs caused by lack of movement (by remaining in the same position).

pronation—the rotation of the palm of the hand so that it is facing downward (thumbs pointed medially).

rehabilitation—the process of restoring to a good condition, or an improvement in the state of one's efficiency or health.

rotation—the process of turning, or movement about an axis.

spasm—an involuntary, sudden movement or muscle contraction.

supination—the rotation of the palm of the hand so that it is facing upward toward the head (thumbs pointed laterally).

thrombus (pl. thrombi)—a blood clot that obstructs a blood vessel.

unconscious—the state of being insensible or without conscious experiences; in deep stupor; unresponding.

vertebra (pl. vertebrae)—the name for each of the 33 bones forming the spinal backbone in man.

PROMOTING PATIENT MOBILITY

ITEM 1.   THE IMPORTANCE OF MOVEMENT

Can you imagine what it would be like not to be able to move at all? Without movement, you would be a prisoner in your own body. How would you feel if you were unable to scratch your nose when it itched? Or to blink your eyelid when a speck of dirt irritated your eye? Or to walk, play, or participate in the many activities that make up your everyday life?

Movement is so important to the human being that most of our infancy and early childhood is devoted to learning and coordinating body movements. This task takes years to master. The infant must learn to focus and follow an object with the eyes, hold up the head, balance the body, and coordinate hand and eye movements before more complex movements involved in sitting, walking, grasping a cup, catching a ball, or dressing can be learned. As the child grows, he or she learns to perform progressively complex movements.

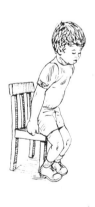
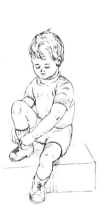
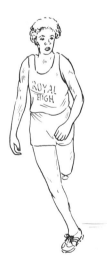

The health and well-being of a person is related to the ability to move the body and its various parts. Movement promotes more efficient functioning of all body parts. For example, movement enhances the firmness, tone, and elasticity of the muscles and promotes the elimination of waste products from the body. It is essential for the strength and hardness of the bones, helps maintain the blood pressure and efficient blood circulation, stimulates the appetite, and reduces fatigue through good posture and change of position.

Under conditions of illness or injury, the patient's ability to move part or all of the body may be impaired. In such situations, the patient must have exercise in order to regain health. When the patient is unable to move to get the exercise needed, the nurse must move and exercise the body parts. It is only in recent years that emphasis has been placed on range-of-motion exercises as a basic nursing skill. You will meet experienced nurses who know the importance of exercise for patients with limited movement but who may not know the range-of-motion exercises.

1. List at least four ways in which exercise promotes the functioning of the body.

    a. _____   b. _____

    c. _____   d. _____ .

ITEM 2. HOW DOES THE BODY MOVE?

The muscular and skeletal systems of the body provide support for the body structures, the means for movement and locomotion, and protection for the soft tissues of the body. The skeletal system is composed of a framework of bones. All movement of the body occurs through the action of the muscles on the skeletal bones. Muscles are attached to the bone by connective tissue and usually work in pairs.

The movement of bones by the muscles occurs at the joints. A *joint* is a junction between (or an articulation of) two or more bones. Joints are classified according to the amount of movement they permit. A *fixed* or *immovable* joint allows no movement of the bones, as exemplified by the bones of the skull. A *slightly movable* joint allows limited movement; examples are the spinal vertebrae and the joints of the pelvis and sacrum. *Freely movable* joints are the most common and can be found in the extremities and the lower jaw.

Joints allow movements that are classified as flexion, extension, abduction, adduction, circumduction, and rotation. In *flexion* the angle between the parts is decreased. *Extension* straightens the part by increasing the angle. In *abduction* the body part moves away from the midline of the body, and in *adduction* the part moves toward the midline so that the distance from the midline is decreased. *Circumduction* occurs when a part is moved like the side of a cone in a circular manner, with the joint acting as the point of the cone, such as when you swing your arm in a circle. *Rotation* is the circular or turning motion that occurs when you turn your head from side to side. When the palm of the hand or the sole of the foot is rotated to an upward position, it is called *supination*. When the palm or the sole is in a downward position or toward the back of the body, it is called *pronation*. Supination of the foot may be referred to as dorsiflexion; pronation of the foot may be referred to as plantar flexion.

The amount of movement allowed at the joint is termed its range of motion. Forcing movement beyond this range of motion will cause pain.

U
N
I
T
13

2. Movement is the result of action by _____ .

3. Movement occurs at the _____ of the body.

Please indicate in the adjoining sketches the type of movement allowed in the parts of the body, i.e., whether it is fixed, slightly movable, or freely movable.

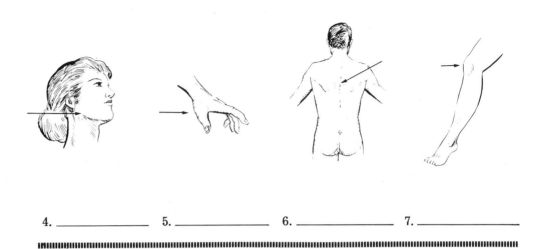

4. _____   5. _____   6. _____   7. _____

ITEM 3. HOW DO CONTRACTURES DEVELOP?

As stated before, the muscles usually work in pairs. The paired flexor and extensor muscles found in the arms, legs, and trunk of the body are important for body movements used in walking, working, playing, and other activities. The flexor muscles are among the strongest ones of the body, and when they are contracted, the body is shortened and curls up in the fetal position. The extensor muscles are relaxed and stretched when the flexors are contracted, but when extensors contract, they straighten the body parts that allow us to stand erect and walk on two feet.

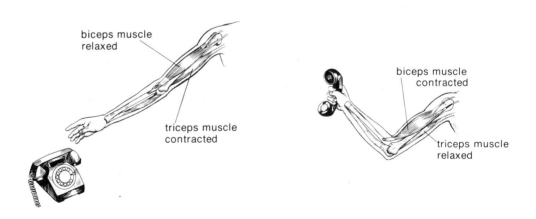

Work of opposing muscles of the arm: The biceps are strong flexor muscles, and the triceps are extensor muscles.

The prolonged flexion of muscles may result in common deformities that are painful and unattractive and that limit movement. These deformities are called *contractures.* A permanent contracture of the muscles "freezes," or locks, the joint so that the part cannot be extended. This results from the inability of the extensor muscle to overcome the strength of its flexor partner.

Contractures can occur in a period of less than three weeks and result in permanent deformity of the joint. Those who develop contractures are people with a severe limitation of movement involving one or more joints. Conditions that cause limited movement include fractures, severe burns, paralysis following a stroke, serious injuries, and states of coma. Contractures most frequently develop in the joints in the shoulder, elbow, wrist, hand, hip, knee, and ankle (where they cause foot drop).

Contractures can be prevented by exercise and by putting the joint through the range of motion several times daily. If the patient is unable to do this, it is essential for the nurse to take over this activity. Once a contracture has occurred, the normal and full use of the joint will seldom, if ever, be completely regained. Even slight improvement in the extent of joint movement may require months or years of intensive, often painful treatment.

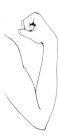

Contracture of the hand, wrist, and elbow. The joints are rigid and can only be moved slightly.

|||||||||||||||||||||||||||||||||||||||||||||||||||||||||||||||||||||||||||||||||||||||||||||||||||||||||||||||||||||||||||||||||||||||

8. The powerful muscles that contract and bend a part are called _____ .

9. Contractures are caused by the muscular action of _____ .

10. Permanent "freezing" of a joint has been known to occur in _____ time.

|||||||||||||||||||||||||||||||||||||||||||||||||||||||||||||||||||||||||||||||||||||||||||||||||||||||||||||||||||||||||||||||||||||||

U
N
I
T
13

ITEM 4.   PASSIVE AND ACTIVE EXERCISE

During illness, patients need some exercise. When they are unable to move a part independently, it becomes the responsibility of the nurse worker to exercise the joints, unless there are medical orders not to do so. The movement performed by the nurse worker or therapist with no help from the patient is called *passive exercise*. However, the patient should be encouraged to perform the movement when at all possible; this is called *active exercise*.

Passive and active exercise should begin as soon as possible after onset of the patient's illness. You should begin a program of passive exercise as soon as you see that the patient is incapable of moving parts of the body without your assistance. The patient should be involved in planning the exercise program and be shown how to exercise the joints. The best time for the patient to exercise joints through the *range of motion* is at bath time. Range-of-motion exercise should be done at least once every eight hours, and some joints may need to be exercised every hour or so in order to keep them flexible.

The patient who has an intravenous infusion (IV) for more than a few hours will often have stiffness and discomfort of the shoulder caused by the restriction of movement. Range-of-motion exercises often relieve the discomfort. You should use slow and smooth movements and support the arm when exercising the shoulder. The movements of lateral and upward abduction and adduction are most beneficial and should be followed with light massage to stimulate the circulation. Make sure that the IV tubing is long enough to permit movement of the shoulder, that the needle is not dislodged from the vein, and that the IV fluid does not infiltrate (seep into) the tissues. Notify the nurse immediately if there is a problem with the IV.

Principles related to carrying out range-of-motion exercises for your patient can be stated as follows:

1. Move the body part to stretch the muscles and keep the joint flexible, but avoid moving it to the point of causing pain.

2. Range-of-motion exercises of the joints of helpless or immobile patients are performed at least once every eight hours to prevent contractures from occurring.

3. Support the extremity when giving passive exercise to the joints of the arm or leg.

4. Each exercise should be performed a minimum of three times, and preferably five times, each time the joints are put through their range of motion.

5. Involve the patient in planning the program of exercise and encourage his or her active performance of the exercises and other activities to keep the joints flexible and movable.

||||||||||||||||||||||||||||||||||||||||||||||||||||||||||||||||||||||||||||||||||||||||||||||||||||||||||||||||||||||||||||||||||||||||||||

11. Mr. Hammer was admitted to the hospital after having a stroke that left him paralyzed on the left side of his body. The following day, you are assigned to give him morning care and a bath. His vital signs have stabilized. When should you begin to exercise his joints? _____ .

12. Which joints should be exercised? _____ .

13. When the patient needs the assistance of the nurse to exercise the joint, it is called _____ exercise.

14. When the patient is able to do it without help, it is called _____ exercise.

||||||||||||||||||||||||||||||||||||||||||||||||||||||||||||||||||||||||||||||||||||||||||||||||||||||||||||||||||||||||||||||||||||||||||||

ITEM 5. THE ROLE OF THE REHABILITATION TEAM

Patients who have limited movement in one or more joints may have many emotional needs related to their inability to move. They may be concerned about depending on others for help; they may be depressed about the nature of their disability, which could require a long convalescence; and they may have feelings of uncertainty or fears of being unable to resume normal activities. You will need to show patience and understanding by accepting their right to feel as they do, but you must emphasize what can be done and encourage their cooperation in exercising, moving about, and using the abilities they still have.

Often the patient will receive care and services toward rehabilitation from others, such as a physical therapist, an occupational therapist, a speech pathologist, family members, and, of course, the physician. The goal of all the specialists is improvement in the patient's condition. The physical therapist provides treatment aimed at restoring the use of muscles and helping the disabled person to relearn how to perform essential activities such as walking or climbing stairs. Exercise, heat, water, and massage are commonly used in physical therapy. Occupational therapists concentrate on helping the patients regain the use of the upper extremities so that they can carry out their daily living and recreational activities. Speech and hearing therapists work with patients who have difficulties communicating as a result of physical or mental disorders. You should learn as much as possible about the therapy recommended for your patients, as well as the short- and long-term goals of the therapy. Then you can better coordinate your care of patients with that scheduled by other members of the rehabilitation team.

As a nurse worker, you are a very important member of the team because you will be with the patient for long periods of time during his illness.

||||||||||||||||||||||||||||||||||||||||||||||||||||||||||||||||||||||||||||||||||||||||||||||||||||||||||||||||||||

15. Mr. Hammer is 49 and had a stroke several days ago. He is now conscious but has slurred speech and is paralyzed on his left side. He had done plumbing work, and two of his five children are still in school. Now he seems irritable and upset. What might be some of the reasons for his feelings?

_____

_____ .

16. Some of the persons who would be involved in the rehabilitation of the patient described above are:

a. _____ b. _____ c. _____

d. _____ e. _____ f. _____ .

||||||||||||||||||||||||||||||||||||||||||||||||||||||||||||||||||||||||||||||||||||||||||||||||||||||||||||||||||||

ITEM 6. ACTIVE RANGE-OF-MOTION EXERCISES

If possible, view a film or filmstrip showing how to perform range-of-motion exercises of the various joints. You will note that several types of movement occur at a joint. For instance, the muscles acting on the shoulder joint allow for all types of movement — abduction, adduction, flexion, extension, hyperextension, circumduction, and rotation. The range-of-motion exercises for this joint include all of these movements.

It is now time to see how well you understand how to do the range-of-motion exercises. Assume a standing position and carry out these movements. You will be performing active exercise.

1. Abduction and adduction of the shoulder: Raise your arm forward, up over your head, and return it to your side. Now, raise your arm to the side so it is straight with the shoulder and return it to your side. Both exercises moved the arm away (abduction) from the midline and back again (adduction).

2. Flexion and extension of the elbow: Bend your elbow, touch your shoulder with your finger tips, and straighten your arm. Flexor muscles bring body parts closer together and extensors straighten out body segments.

3. Rotation of the shoulder: External (outward) rotation — flex your elbow, bring your elbow up to the level of your shoulder, and reach the back of your neck with your fingers. Internal (inward) rotation — flex your elbow, draw your arm across your chest, and place your hand on your distal shoulder.

4. Flexion and extension of the spine: Reach down, try to touch your toes without flexing your knees, and then straighten up. Can you feel the muscles working in your back? Put your hand against the small of your back as you bend over and straighten up. You will be able to feel the muscles move.

5. Abduction and adduction of the thumb and fingers: Spread your fingers and thumb far apart like a fan (abduction), then bring them together again (adduction).

6. Flexion and extension of the thumb and fingers: Flex your hand at the knuckles, keeping the fingers straight, then bend the fingers and thumb to make a fist, and straighten them again.

7. Rotation of the neck: Turn your head to the left side, then to the right side.

UNIT 13

Lie down in a supine position (flat on your back) and practice these movements of the lower extremities.

1. Abduction and adduction of the hip: With your legs straight and toes pointed upward, move a leg to one side as far as possible (abduction) and return it to the original position (adduction).

2. Flexion and extension of the hip and knee: Bend your knee (flexion) and bring it up toward your chest as far as possible, then straighten your leg to the original position (extension).

3. Rotation of the hip: To rotate externally, or outward, flex your hip and knee so that your knee is parallel to the bed and turn your foot outward. To rotate internally, flex your hip and knee so that your knee is elevated and parallel to the bed and turn your foot inward.

4. Flexion and extension of the ankles: Bend your toes upward as far as possible so that your foot is supinated (dorsiflexion), then extend your toes downward as far as possible so that your foot is pronated (plantar flexion).

|||||||||||||||||||||||||||||||||||||||||||||||||||||||||||||||||||||||||||||||||||||||||||||||||||||||||||||||||||||||||||||||||

17. Which of these movements would you use to do the following?

    a. Brush your teeth? _____ .

    b. Wash the back of your neck and shoulders? _____ .

    c. Comb your hair? _____ .

|||||||||||||||||||||||||||||||||||||||||||||||||||||||||||||||||||||||||||||||||||||||||||||||||||||||||||||||||||||||||||||||||

ITEM 7. PASSIVE RANGE-OF-MOTION EXERCISES

In the skill laboratory with another student or someone else playing the part of a patient who is paralyzed on his left side, you will provide passive range-of-motion exercise to the joints of his neck, left shoulder, arm, hand, hip, knee, ankle, and foot while supporting the dependent part of the extremity and avoiding range-of-motion exercise beyond the point of pain.

Important Steps	Key Points
1. Wash your hands.	Universal Steps B and C. See Appendix.
2. Approach and identify the patient, explain the procedure, and gain cooperation.	
3. Prepare the patient.	Go to the side of the bed so that the paralyzed side is nearest you in order to prevent straining. Place bed in high position to prevent stooping and drape the patient with bath blanket or top bedding.

Important Steps	Key Points

4. Perform passive range-of-motion exercises of the neck and upper extremity.

   a. Flex and extend the neck.

Support the head with your hands and bring the head forward until the chin touches the chest. Extend the neck by elevating the chin and looking upward. Return the head to a neutral position. Repeat three to five times.

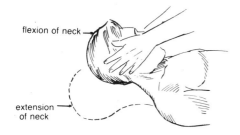

   b. Rotate the head.

Support the head with your hands, turn it toward the right shoulder, and then toward the left shoulder. Repeat three to five times.

   c. Flex and extend the left shoulder and elbow.

Support the elbow with one hand and grasp the wrist with your other hand. Bring the arm up straight, then bend the elbow and move the arm up over the head. This exercise involves flexion and extension of both the elbow and the shoulder. Return the arm to the patient's side. Repeat three to five times.

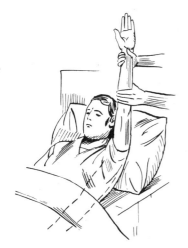

Extension of shoulder and elbow.

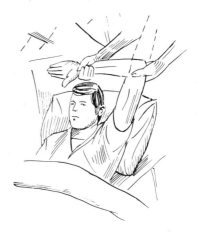

Flexion of elbow.

   d. Internal and external rotation of the shoulder.

Place one hand on patient's left arm above the elbow and grasp patient's hand with your other hand. Lift the arm and move it across the chest toward the right side and return to the original position. Repeat three to five times.

To rotate externally, move the arm out from the side in abduction, flex the elbow, and move the forearm over the head. Return the arm to the original position. Repeat three to five times.

U
N
I
T
13

Important Steps	Key Points

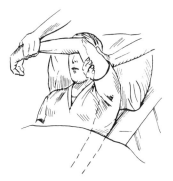

Internal rotation of shoulder.

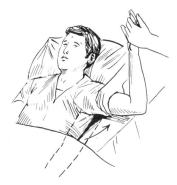

External rotation of shoulder.

e. Exercise the wrist and hand.

Rotate the wrist by grasping the wrist in both of your hands and turning the palm toward the face for supination and then toward the feet for pronation. Repeat three to five times.

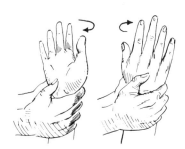

Rotation of wrist.

Hold the wrist with one hand and the palm of the hand with your other hand while keeping the patient's fingers straight. Hyperextend the wrist by bending it backward, extend it by straightening it, and flex the wrist by bending the hand forward and closing the fingers to make a fist. Repeat three to five times.

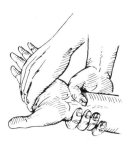

Hyperextension of wrist.

f. Exercise the thumb.

Hold the patient's hand with your hand, then grasp the thumb with your other hand, flex it into the palm, extend the thumb by moving it away from the hand, and rotate it in a circular movement. Repeat three to five times.

Contractures of the upper extremities most often occur in flexion position (internal rotation of shoulder and flexion of elbow, wrist, and hand).

Important Steps

Key Points

5. Perform passive range-of-motion exercises of the hip and lower extremity.

    a. Flexion and extension of the hip and knee.

Place one hand under the knee to support the leg and cup the heel in your other hand. Lift the leg up, bend the knee, and move the leg toward the chest as far as it will go without causing pain. Straighten the leg by lifting the foot upward and lower the leg to the bed. Repeat three to five times.

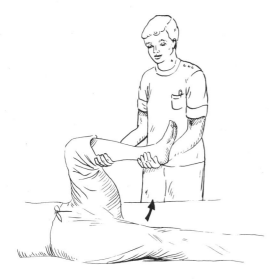

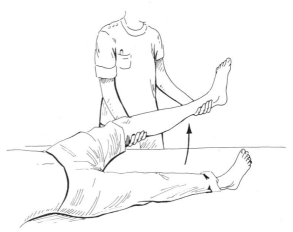

    b. Abduction and rotation of the hip.

To abduct the hip joint, place one hand under the patient's knee and the other hand under the heel. Keep the leg straight and slowly move it toward you. Then adduct the leg by moving it back to the original position. Repeat three to five times.

The hip joint is rotated in the following manner: Place one hand under the patient's left knee, the other under the heel; lift the leg and flex the knee at right angles. Without moving the knee, pull the foot slowly toward you for external rotation, then move the foot away from you and over the other leg for internal rotation. Repeat three to five times.

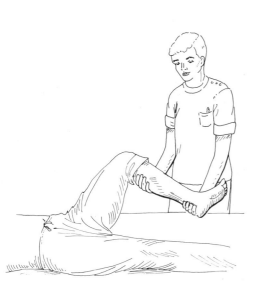

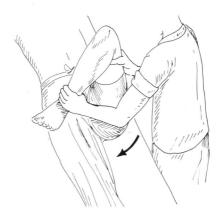

U
N
I
T
13

Important Steps	Key Points

c. Flexion and extension of the ankle.

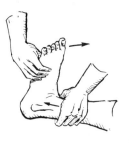

Dorsiflexion

To flex and extend the ankle, hold the patient's heel in one hand and place your other hand over his foot. Pull the foot forward and push down on the heel at the same time to flex the foot in supination (dorsiflexion). Then push on the foot to extend it in a "point-the-toes" position and push up on the heel at the same time to hyperextend the foot in pronation (plantar flexion).

d. Rotation of the ankle joint.

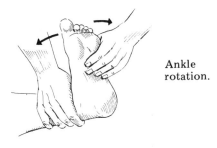

Ankle rotation.

To rotate the ankle, hold the ankle with one hand; with the other hand, turn the whole foot outward, then turn it inward. The patient can be taught and should be encouraged to use the stronger extremity (arm or leg) to move the weaker extremity in the range-of-motion exercises to flex, extend, abduct, and rotate the part.

6. Provide for the patient's comfort.

Universal Steps Y and Z. See Appendix.

7. Report and record as appropriate.

0945. Unable to move left arm or leg. Range of motion given to left upper and lower extremity. Unable to extend elbow or shoulder more than 60 degrees. Given instructions on how to do own exercises.

J. Jones, SN

ITEM 8.   EFFECTS OF IMMOBILITY

The patient needs rest to facilitate the repair of damage by injury or disease. When at bed rest, the patient can use more of his energy to combat the causes of the damage and to rebuild his defenses. However, total rest or prolonged bed rest also produces harmful effects when the body does not receive enough exercise to promote good functioning of its systems. The patient's body at total rest undergoes physiological changes in body chemistry and sometimes develops hypostatic pneumonia, pressure sores, contractures, constipation, urinary retention, insomnia, diminished appetite, and tendency to form thrombi (blood clots). Good nursing helps combat some of these changes, but the most important measure is early ambulation of the patient.

The patient who has been in bed for several days or more, or who may have had surgery just a few hours before, will need your assistance the first time he gets up. Even minor surgery produces circulatory, chemical, and emotional disturbances in the patient. When the physician has written an order allowing the patient to get up, the first step toward ambulation is for the patient to "dangle his feet" at the bedside. In dangling his feet, the patient has time to adjust to the change in position, recover from any dizziness, and adjust to a need for deeper breathing.

18. One advantage of bed rest for the patient with an injury or a disease is _____

_____ .

19. Which of the following are some of the hazards or dangers of bed rest? Place a check mark in front of your answers.

_____ a. Postoperative pain   _____ b. Blood clots

_____ c. Dizziness   _____ d. Pneumonia, hypostatic

_____ e. Altered body chemistries   _____ f. Contractures

ITEM 9. ASSISTING THE PATIENT TO DANGLE HIS LEGS

In the skill laboratory, practice the steps in the procedure of assisting a patient to dangle his legs at the side of the bed. One of your fellow students, or some other person, will be needed to play the part of the patient.

Supplies Needed

Patient's robe and slippers.

Important Steps	Key Points
Carry out Universal Steps A, B, and C. See Appendix.	
1. Position the patient.	Move the patient to the near side of the bed. If the patient has limited movement in an arm or leg, you should work on that side of the bed. You will not need to reach or strain as much, since the patient may be able to help move the stronger extremity from the far side of the bed.
2. Adjust the position of the bed.	Place the bed in a low position and elevate the head 45 degrees or more. This helps patients to adjust to the change of positions and makes it easier for you to bring them to a sitting position. Lower the siderail on that side of the bed.
3. Assist the patient to sit at the side of the bed and dangle his feet. 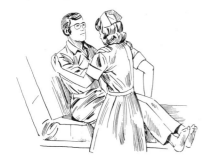	Place one hand on the patient's near shoulder and the other under the distal axilla. Have the patient hold onto your shoulders and pull to a sitting position. Continue to support patient with your one hand, then reach behind the far knee with your other hand and swing the legs off the bed while pivoting the body in the same direction. Use smooth and coordinated movements.

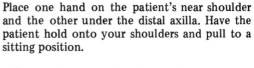

U
N
I
T
13

Important Steps	Key Points
4. Provide for patient's comfort.	Assist the patient to put on robe, slippers, or shoes, or place a blanket over the lap to prevent exposure and to provide extra warmth. Many patients will feel chilly after getting out of a warm bed. The patient's feet should be flat on the floor or on a footstool for proper support. Observe him closely and, if the patient is doing well, you could fluff up his pillows and replace them.
5. Assist the patient to return to bed.	Help the patient back to bed at the end of the specified period for dangling, or if the patient is unable to tolerate sitting up and dangling. Remove robe, slippers or shoes, or the lap blanket. Support the patient at the shoulders with one hand; with the other hand under both ankles, swing the legs up onto the bed while pivoting the body at the same time so that he is facing the foot of the bed. Ease the patient back onto the bed in a supine position.
Universal Steps X, Y, and Z. See Appendix.	9:30 A.M. Patient dangled for first time. Became cold, clammy, and pale. Returned to supine position. P88, R20. J. Jones, SN

ITEM 10. MECHANICS OF WALKING

How do you walk? Most of us would reply that you stand up and step forward on one foot, then on the other foot, and that is how you walk. We will now consider the mechanics of walking in more detail in order to assist the patient in walking.

Posture is important in walking. The body should be in good alignment, with the head up, shoulders back, spine straight, buttocks tucked in, knees slightly flexed, and feet slightly apart with the toes pointed forward. Poor body alignment will produce strain on the muscles, loss of balance, poor coordination, and a jerky and jolting rhythm with unnecessary motion which wastes energy. Good posture in walking allows a more attractive and energetic appearance, as well as the more efficient functioning of the parts involved.

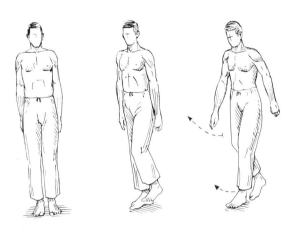

Double stance.   Single stance.   Swing.

In the walking cycle, the person stands with both feet on the ground in the double stance position. The body weight is shifted to one foot in the single stance phase as the other foot moves forward in the swing phase. The swing phase is completed as the heel of the foot strikes the ground. In the swing phase, the body twists inward slightly. To counteract this twisting movement, the person swings the arm on the opposite side. The single stance phase includes shifting the body weight to the heel that is striking the ground, and moving the weight along the outer edge of the foot to the ball of the foot, and then to the toes, as they "push off" in the swing phase for the next step.

The distance covered in each step is called a *pace*. "Pace" may also refer to the number of steps taken per minute. A normal pace for walking is 70 to 100 steps a minute, and a fast pace would be over 120 steps per minute. Most patients will walk at the slow pace of less than 70 steps per minute until they recover their physical strength.

In assisting patients in walking, you should attempt to have them walk as normally as possible. In other words, they should stand and walk with the body in good alignment or the best alignment they can achieve. The soreness and pulling of stitches may prevent some surgical patients from standing erect. They often are fearful that the stitches will break open, but you can assure them that the sutures are strong and that the body has already begun to repair or heal the incision. When the patient steps forward in the swing and especially in the single stance phases, your assistance may be needed to provide balance and support. Patients should be encouraged to step normally, striking the ground with the heel first, transferring the weight to the ball of the foot, and then "pushing off" with the toes, instead of shuffling, sliding forward, or letting the toes strike the ground first.

Patients who have had prolonged bed rest may be apprehensive about walking because of extreme weakness or fear or falling. Other patients may be so eager to get out of bed and walk that they may overestimate their strength and ability. You will need to caution them against overdoing it by instructing them to walk slowly at first and to gradually increase the distance walked.

20. The most stable phase of the walking cycle is the _____ .

21. In walking, a person swings the arm that is opposite the forward-moving foot in order

    to _____ .

22. Which portion of the foot should strike the ground first when walking?

    _____ .

ITEM 11.   ASSISTING THE PATIENT TO WALK

In the skill laboratory, practice helping the patient to walk and use the principles that are related to body alignment, balance, and movement. Ask another person to play the part of the patient for this practice session.

Supplies Needed

Patient's robe and slippers

Important Steps	Key Points
Carry out Universal Steps A, B, and C. See Appendix.	
1. Position the bed.	Place the bed in the low position and elevate the head of the bed 30 degrees or more to make it easier to bring the patient to a sitting position. Fold the top bedding back toward the foot of the bed.
2. Assist the patient to a dangling-feet position at the side of the bed.	Follow the instructions for dangling given earlier in this lesson. Assist the patient in putting on the robe and slippers.
3. Help the patient to stand.	Place patient's feet firmly on the floor, put your hand under the proximal axilla, and pull patient to a standing position. Stand at the side and provide support as the patient stands and balances before beginning to walk.
4. Assist the patient to walk.	Check posture and encourage patient to walk with the head up, eyes looking forward, and back straight. Provide support by walking at patient's side.
	a. For *minimal support*, the patient holds your elbow or hand;
	b. For *moderate support*, hold the patient's arm with your hand;
	c. To provide *more than moderate support* (to prevent the patient's loss of balance or falling), you should have another person help you so that support can be provided at each side.
5. Assist the patient to return to bed.	Have the patient walk to the side of the bed, pivot so that his back is to the edge of the bed, and reach for the mattress with his hands for support. With your hand under the axilla, help him to a sitting position. Remove the robe and slippers. Help swing the feet onto the bed as in the instructions given for dangling.
Universal Steps X, Y, and Z. See Appendix.	10:15 A.M. Patient ambulated the full length of the hall. Tolerated well. Returned to bed quite tired.
	J. Jones, SN

ITEM 12. WHY PATIENTS FALL AND WHAT TO DO

Basically, there are two reasons why a standing person will fall: (1) as the result of the collapse of the lower extremities or (2) through the loss of balance. In the collapse type of fall, the muscles of the legs lack the strength needed to support the body weight. The extensor muscles of the knees give way to gravitational pull so that the knees "buckle under" the person, resulting in a fall. In the collapsing fall, the safest method of assistance is to try to "break the fall" and ease the patient slowly to the floor. You should be walking alongside or slightly behind the patient when helping to walk, so that you can grasp the body firmly at the waist or under the axilla and ease the patient down to the floor if a fall should occur. It is necessary for you to keep your body in good alignment, with your line of gravity within your base support, and to lower your own body by stooping correctly.

Remember that stability is maintained when one's line of gravity and center of gravity are within the base of support. When the patient loses balance and begins to fall, his line of gravity and center of gravity are outside the base of support.

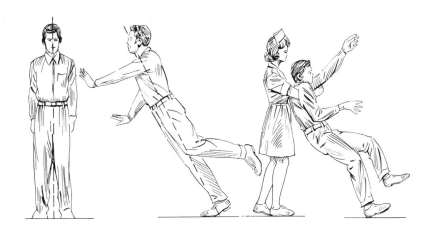

Stable balance.   Loss of balance.   Breaking patient's fall.

Unless you can bring the patient's line of gravity and center of gravity within the base of support, the patient will continue to fall. In order to help someone to regain balance, you need to be large enough and strong enough to overcome the force of the patient's body weight moving downward. Once an adult patient has started to fall, the amount of force that is needed is more than you can safely provide. You should then attempt to break the fall, slow the rate of descent, and ease the patient to the floor in order to avoid possible injury to him or to yourself. Remember, it is easier to guide the patient slowly down to the floor than it is to lift him up.

You may have an urge to try to hold up or to lift the falling patient. If you act on this impulse, you risk losing your own balance and falling, or straining or injuring your muscles. The most common disabling injury of hospital workers is muscle strain, usually of the lower back. Many of these injuries could be prevented through the use of good body alignment, proper movement, and safer methods of work.

Any patient who has fallen or who has been eased to the floor should be examined by a doctor or a nurse for possible injury before being moved. You should stay with the patient to provide comfort and reassurance and have additional help to get the patient up or return him to bed after the examination.

U
N
I
T
13

23. When a person loses balance and begins to fall, the center of gravity is (select the best answer)

a. too high from his base of support.
b. too close to his base of support.
c. inside his base of support.
d. outside his base of support.

24. The best method of helping a patient who has started to fall is to _____

_____ .

Why would you use this method? Explain. _____

_____ .

25. You are helping a patient to walk who weighs about 200 pounds and now has begun to fall. If you try to prevent this fall, what possible effect might this action have on you?

_____ .

‖‖

ITEM 13. PREVENTION OF PATIENT FALLS

Patient falls are the most common accidents that occur in the hospital, the extended-care facility, or the home. As in every type of accident, the major factors involved in patient falls are (1) the physical and mental condition of the victim, (2) conditions that are unsafe or pose a hazard in the environment, or (3) unsafe acts by an individual. Certain patients are more at risk of having accidents and falling than others because of their condition. You should be aware that the following groups of patients are just as much at risk as those with problems involving the musculoskeletal system:

1. Those with a disease or condition that reduces the amount of oxygen available for use in the body. These conditions include anemia, hemorrhage, congestive heart failure, pneumonia, and other diseases of the heart or lungs that interfere with the transport of oxygen to the brain and other body tissues.

2. Those who are elderly. Age produces changes such as decreased ability to see and hear well, less acute perception and balance, and deterioration of the muscles and bones, which can affect balance and the stable base of support.

3. Those who are receiving narcotics and other medications for pain, sedatives to promote sleep, tranquilizers, and other agents that dull the senses and make the person less alert.

4. Those with acid-base or electrolyte imbalances. One of the more frequently seen conditions is a low level of serum potassium, which results in soft, mushy muscles; this has led some nurses to compare the patient's strength to that of a "limp noodle."

5. Those who are highly anxious or in a state of confusion. Such emotional states distract one from paying attention to potential hazards in the environment and from taking the usual precautions to prevent accidents.

It is essential that the nurse evaluate the patients' ability to balance and to support their body weight when ambulating and provide adequate assistance or mechanical aids.

Unsafe acts involve individuals who bump into patients or push them out of the way, and patients who walk too fast, in crowded areas, on wet surfaces, or without adequate light.

The physical and environmental hazards that contribute to falls should be eliminated as much as possible. Anything spilled on the floor should be wiped up promptly, and foreign objects should be picked up. During the mopping or waxing of floors, the area should be posted with a warning sign and preferably roped off so that no one walks on the wet surface. Floor wax should be of the non-slip type. Electric cords should be shortened and not allowed to lie loose on the floors. Small objects or equipment should be removed from areas where patients walk. To assure additional safety for patients, siderails should be used on the bed for restless, aged, confused, or sedated patients.

In spite of all these precautions, the patient may lose balance when walking and begin to fall. The help that you can provide will depend on the size of the patient, whether the center of gravity is still within the base of support, and your own size.

ITEM 14. COMPLETION OF THE LESSON

You have now completed the lesson on patient movement and ambulation, which has included range-of-motion exercises, dangling, walking, and patient falls. Please make an appointment with your instructor to take the post-test.

INFORMATION FOR ENRICHMENT

Since exercise and ambulation are so important to the patient, you may be interested in reading more about the role of movement in nursing care. Patients with orthopedic, neurological, or cardiovascular problems may have limited movement and special needs related to their diseases. You will add more skill to your care of these patients as you learn more about their special needs. Much has been written about nursing care of specific diseases and to start you off, a few articles are listed on p. 161. Many of the articles have references at the end that you can use to find other related articles and books.

WORKBOOK ANSWERS

1. Any four of the following (among others): promotes firmness, tone, and elasticity of muscles; promotes elimination of waste products; strengthens and hardens bones; maintains blood pressure; promotes blood circulation; stimulates the appetite; reduces fatigue; promotes respiratory action.

2. muscles

3. joints

4. freely movable

5. freely movable

6. slightly movable

7. freely movable

8. flexors

9. flexion

10. less than three weeks

11. Exercises should start as soon as possible and you could give them during the bath.

12. All of his joints should be exercised.

13. passive

14. active

15. Some of the feelings the patient may have relate to his inability to speak clearly, inability to move his left side, worry about his role as a father and husband, concern about his ability to return to work and provide for his family, and so forth.

16. The rehabilitation team could consist of:

    a. nurse

    b. physician

    c. speech and hearing therapist

U
N
I
T
13

      d. physical therapist

      e. occupational therapist

      f. family

17. a. internal rotation

      b. external rotation

      c. internal and external rotation

18. so that healing or the rebuilding of body defenses can take place

19. b, d, e, and f

20. double stance

21. counteract the twist of the body

22. the heel

23. d

24. Ease the patient to the floor. This method provides more safety for the patient and the worker by breaking the force of the fall and working with gravity rather than trying to lift against gravity, and prevents possible injury to patient and worker.

25. You may lose your balance and fall, strain your muscles, or injure yourself.

PERFORMANCE TEST

In the skill laboratory, you will be asked to perform the following activities for your instructor without reference to any source material. You will need another person to take the part of the patient.

1. Given a patient with limited or no motion in the joints on one side of the body, explain the need for exercising all the joints and put the affected joints through range-of-motion exercises. In ranging the joint, support the part distal to the joint and avoid movement to the extent that it causes pain.

2. Given a patient who has been on bed rest and must be gotten up to dangle his feet at the side of the bed, assist to a sitting position, pivot the body, and swing the feet off the bed, using smooth flowing motions and principles of good body alignment and movement.

3. Given a patient who has been on bed rest and is to get up to walk, assist in dangling his feet at the side of the bed, help him to stand and balance at the bedside, and then to walk, using principles of good body alignment, balance, and movement.

4. Given a patient who has begun to fall, assist by grasping him firmly, slowing the rate of descent, and easing him slowly to the floor, using principles related to gravity to avoid possible injury to the patient or yourself.

PERFORMANCE CHECKLIST

RANGE-OF-MOTION EXERCISES

1. Wash your hands.

2. Identify the patient and explain the procedure.

3. Move the patient to the proximal side of the bed (on the affected side).

4. Perform passive range of motion of the neck and upper extremity.

    a. flexion and extension of the neck

    b. rotation of the head

    c. flexion and extension of the shoulder and elbow

    d. internal and external rotation of the shoulder

    e. exercise the wrist and hand

    f. exercise the thumb

5. Perform passive range of motion of the lower extremity.

    a. flexion and extension of the hip and knee

    b. abduction and rotation of the hip

    c. flexion and extension of the ankle

    d. rotation of the ankle joint

6. Throughout the procedure be careful not to cause pain to the patient.

7. Support the distal and proximal ends of the limbs during the exercise.

UNIT 13

8. Provide for the patient's comfort.

9. Report and record as appropriate.

DANGLING

1. Wash your hands.

2. Identify the patient and explain the procedure.

3. Move the patient to the proximal side of the bed.

4. Adjust the bed to the low position. Raise the headrest to approximately 45 degrees.

5. Raise the patient to a sitting position.

6. Continue supporting the shoulder and swing the legs off the bed while pivoting the body.

7. Dress the patient in robe and slippers.

8. Fluff the pillow while the patient is dangling feet over the side of the bed.

9. Remove his slippers and robe when patient is ready to lie down.

10. Return the patient to the supine position.

11. Swing the legs up onto the bed while pivoting the body.

12. Maintain principles of good body alignment while completing the motion. Patient movement should be slow, smooth, and steady.

ASSIST PATIENT TO WALK

1. Wash your hands.

2. Identify the patient and explain the procedure.

3. Move the patient to the proximal side of the bed.

4. Adjust the bed to the low position.

5. Raise the patient to a sitting position.

6. Assist the patient in putting on robe and slippers.

7. Continue supporting patient's shoulder and swing the legs off the bed while pivoting the body.

8. Help the patient to stand at the bedside, using good body alignment.

9. Walk with the patient:

   a. to give minimal support: the patient holds your arm or hand.

   b. to give moderate support: you hold the patient's arm with your hand.

   c. to give maximal support: obtain assistance by having another health worker walk on the other side of the patient.

10. Assist the patient back to bed.

11. Provide for the patient's comfort.

12. Report and record as appropriate.

The health worker must maintain good body alignment and balance throughout the procedure.

SAFEGUARDING THE FALLING PATIENT

1. Explain the rationale for breaking the patient's fall rather than trying to catch and raise him.

   a. Injury to the patient.

   b. Injury to yourself.

   c. Abrupt change in movement.

2. As the patient begins to fall, the worker takes a position to the rear of patient, attempting to break the fall by grasping him under the armpits.

3. Once contact is made, the health worker flexes her legs to lower the patient gently to the ground.

4. Ease the patient to a sitting or lying position on the floor.

5. Remain with the patient, reassuring and providing warmth until required help arrives.

6. Examine the patient for possible injury.

7. Prepare an accident report.

POST-TEST

Matching. For each of the figures shown, select the type of movement from the terms given.

a. abduction

b. adduction

c. rotation

d. circumduction

e. flexion

f. extension

g. supination

1.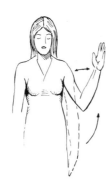

2.

3.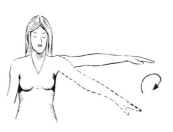

4.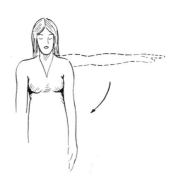

5.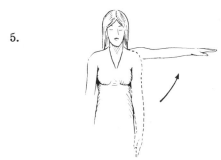

6.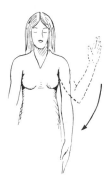

Matching.   Select the word from Column B that best fits the description in Column A.

Column A	Column B
7. Turning the sole of the foot upward.	a. pronation
8. Turning the palm of the hand downward.	b. dorsiflexion
9. Moving of one's joints or limbs by another person.	c. active exercise
10. Moving away from the midline of the body.	d. passive exercise
11. Decreasing the angle between two parts.	e. flexion
	g. abduction
	h. adduction

Multiple Choice.   Several questions are presented based on the situation described here. Select the one best answer for each.

Mr. Bond is a 67-year-old man in Bigtown University Hospital who had a stroke three days ago. He has been in the Intensive Care Unit until one hour ago, when he was transferred to the Medical floor. He is one of the patients assigned to you for care. When you first meet Mr. Bond, you notice that his mouth droops on one side, that his speech at this time is limited to "boler," "soup," and "no," and that his left arm and leg are paralyzed. He is conscious but seems quite depressed.

12. Later that morning, you return to Mr. Bond's bedside and explain that you will give him his bath and exercise his paralyzed arm and leg. He sobs and says "Boler, boler, boler." You don't understand what he is trying to say. What would you do now?

   a. Report to the team leader that he is crying and might be having pain or discomfort.

   b. Ask the patient to nod his head for "yes" and shake his head for "no," then explain again and ask questions to see if he understands what you mean.

   c. Go ahead and carry out the bath and exercises, since he must be confused.

   d. Tell Mr. Bond not to cry, and reassure him that everything will be all right.

13. Mr. Bond's tray arrives with his lunch. As you feed him, you hand him a piece of bread, which he holds in his unaffected hand. As he moves his hand to his mouth to eat, what movement does he use?

     a. flexion of the wrist

     b. external rotation of the shoulder

     c. internal rotation of the shoulder

     d. pronation of the wrist

14. When feeding Mr. Bond from a position on the left side of his bed, you notice that he doesn't seem to be able to see your hand and the food until it is near his mouth. In order to see more on his left side, he raises his head slightly from the pillow and turns his head in order to look straight at you. The movements of his neck are

     a. flexion and abduction

     b. flexion and rotation

     c. hyperextension and rotation

     d. extension and adduction

     e. none of these

15. The exercise program you have planned with Mr. Bond includes the range-of-motion exercises during his bath time. He has become interested in exercising the joints of his right side but needs you to exercise his affected side. When performing the range-of-motion exercises, you

     a. place several pillows under the affected knee to support it.

     b. support the part proximal to the joint being ranged.

     c. avoid moving the paralyzed joints.

     d. avoid moving beyond the point of pain.

16. Mr. Bond's rehabilitation includes physical therapy and speech therapy. He has been making a lot of progress since his stroke. His doctor has written an order allowing Mr. Bond to get up and walk with assistance. Before you assist him to walk for the first time, you help him to dangle his legs. The reason(s) for this could be:

     a. to strengthen his leg muscles before he stands.

     b. to improve the circulation of the paralyzed leg and foot.

     c. to help him adjust to the change of position and recover from any dizziness.

     d. to prevent contractures of the paralyzed arm and leg.

17. The weak or unsteady patient, like Mr. Bond, will require most of your assistance when walking during the

     a. swing phase.

     b. single stance phase.

     c. double stance phase.

18. Let us assume that Mr. Bond is now ready to walk with assistance. You and Miss Jones will help him walk in his room for the first time. Which of the following will you do?

   a. Provide support by having one walk in front of the patient and the other behind him.

   b. Make sure his bedroom slippers have a soft sole so his left foot will bend it easier.

   c. Have him hold his head up, look forward, and walk at a pace of about 80 steps per minute.

   d. Encourage him to walk as normally as possible and have his right heel strike the ground first.

19. Suppose that Mr. Bond has made progress in walking. You later assist him by yourself in walking to the bathroom. He has taken about ten steps when suddenly his left knee buckles and he begins to fall. You have been walking on his left side. What should you do?

   a. Grasp him firmly at the waist and chest to keep him from falling to the floor.

   b. Use your right thigh and foot to brace his buckling knee and foot to help him regain his balance.

   c. Hold onto him to slow his rate of descent and ease him to the floor.

   d. Brace your feet firmly to overcome the force of his fall and call for help.

20. If Mr. Bond should fall, the probable reason for this would be:

   a. His line of gravity and center of gravity are outside his base of support.

   b. His line of gravity and center of gravity are inside his base of support.

   c. His unaffected right leg is unable to support the weight of his body.

   d. His affected left leg is unable to support the weight of his body.

UNIT 13

POST-TEST ANSWERS

1. e	11. e
2. c	12. b
3. d	13. c
4. b	14. b
5. a	15. d
6. f	16. c
7. b	17. b
8. a	18. d
9. d	19. c
10. g	20. d

Unit 14

GENERAL PERFORMANCE OBJECTIVE

Upon completion of this lesson, you will demonstrate your ability to assist the patient (or another person) to use the common mechanical aids for ambulation or movement in a safe and effective manner.

SPECIFIC PERFORMANCE OBJECTIVES

When this lesson is completed you will be able to:

1. With assistance, transfer a helpless patient from the bed to a stretcher by positioning the stretcher, using a sheet to lift and move the patient, and using safety belts or siderails to protect the patient from falling.

2. Assist the patient (one who is able to stand) to transfer from the bed to a wheelchair and back to bed.

3. With assistance or the use of a mechanical lifter, transfer a patient (one who is unable to stand) from the bed to a wheelchair.

4. Instruct the patient in the use of a wheelchair when one is required as a means of locomotion.

5. Assist the patient in bed to transfer into and out of a walker safely and adjust the walker to the height best suited to patient's use.

6. Measure and adjust a pair of crutches to the proper length needed by the patient and adjust the hand-bar.

7. Demonstrate two-point, three-point, and four-point crutch-walking and explain the conditions related to each type.

8. Explain the principles of crutch-walking and the cause of "crutch palsy."

9. Apply a strap-on type of back brace for the patient and explain how to check for proper fit and possible pressure areas.

10. Apply a short leg brace to the patient's leg and explain the care of the brace and how to check for proper fit and possible pressure areas.

VOCABULARY

axillary bar—the upper crosspiece of a crutch that fits under the armpit.
brace—an appliance made of fabric, leather, plastic, or metal that supports a specific portion of the body.
crutch—a staff or support used in walking, usually with a crosspiece to fit under the armpit (axilla).

crutch palsy—a condition caused by pressure on nerves in the axilla that results in weakness of the forearm, wrist, and hand.

four-point, three-point, two-point gaits—methods of walking with crutches.

locomotion—the process of moving from place to place.

mechanical lifter—a device utilizing hydraulic principles so that a small force can lift a heavy weight.

orthopedics—the science of prevention, diagnosis, and treatment of diseases and conditions related to the musculoskeletal system.

pallor—lack of color, paleness.

self-esteem—the respect and value with which a person regards himself or herself.

therapeutic—pertaining to the treatment or cure of a disease.

walker—a metal rectangular frame with wheels used to assist a person in walking.

wing screws—adjustment screws that have two thumbpieces, or wings, for tightening; used on walkers, crutches, and other devices.

ITEM 1.   WHY DO YOU NEED TO KNOW ABOUT MECHANICAL AIDS?

Movement is one of the primary functions of the body. The heart muscle contracts to move the blood through the body, the chest wall moves to allow the lungs to draw in and expel air, the eyelids blink to protect and lubricate the eyes, the jaws move so that the teeth may chew food, and so forth. The muscles, bones, and joints work together so that a person may move from one position to another. For patients, the ability to move about or to walk during illness or convalescence decreases dependence on others, and increases self-esteem. It also improves the patient's mental outlook and widens the world beyond the patient's bed or the four walls of the patient's room. The general functioning of all body systems is enhanced through movement.

In order to move about or to walk, the patient may need to use a mechanical aid, such as a wheelchair, walker, crutches, or braces, as either a temporary or permanent measure. In general, when such an aid is needed permanently, the patient is taught how to use it by a physician, a physical therapist, or a member of the rehabilitation team. However, when the patient requires the use of a wheelchair, walker, or crutches on a temporary basis, teaching often becomes the responsibility of the nurse. You must know how to use the mechanical aid safely and effectively before you can teach the patient how to use it.

ITEM 2.   TYPES OF MECHANICAL AIDS

The type of mechanical aid that is selected for the patient's use will depend on the patient's physical condition and the degree of support that is needed. General support for the body is provided by the stretcher, wheelchair, walker, and crutches, with the stretcher furnishing the greatest support. Braces support specific portions of the body. Some patients with orthopedic (bone) problems may progress from one aid to the next, but most patients may need the general support of a wheelchair for a short time until they can walk unassisted. The pictures on the next page show how a patient may progress toward walking unaided.

Not all patients regain the strength and ability needed to walk unaided. Certain patients, like some of the elderly, become weaker and need progressively more support until the only way they can get about may be in a wheelchair. It is important that you remember to encourage patients to do what they can for themselves and to provide support for the motor abilities that they lack.

The patient's physician orders the level or the degree of ambulation desired for the patient. This level of ambulation may be the goal for the patient to achieve or the limitation of the amount of freedom allowed because of the condition. Generally, you may use the mechanical aids for the patient that are *below* the level ordered by the doctor, but *not those above* this level. An example: The doctor said, "Use crutches for walking." The patient should be encouraged to use crutches for some walking, but you may provide a wheelchair

U
N
I
T
14

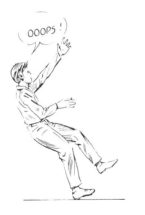

Person falling.

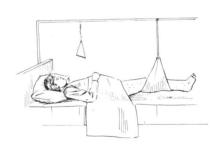

Patient in bed — maximum support.

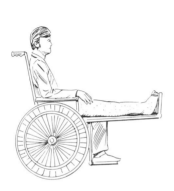

In wheelchair —
intermediate support.

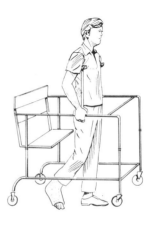

Use of walker —
intermediate support.

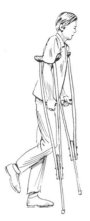

Patient
with
crutches.

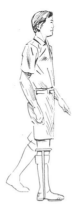

Support
with
leg
brace.

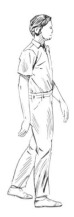

Walking
unassisted.

Progressive levels of patient movement and ambulation, from the total support provided by bed or stretcher to walking without assistance.

or a walker when the patient is tired, becomes weak, or has to travel a longer distance than usual. However, you should not allow the patient to walk without crutches, because this would be ambulation at a higher level than allowed by the doctor's order.

||||||||||||||||||||||||||||||||||||||||||||||||||||||||||||||||||||||||||||||||||||||||||||||||||||||||||||||||||||||||||||||||||||||||||||||||

From the information given, you should be able to answer these questions.

1. Mrs. Jay had an abdominal operation three days ago and now must be taken to X-ray. The doctor has written an order for Mrs. Jay to be up in a chair four times a day. Which of the mechanical aids would you use to take Mrs. Jay to X-ray?

_____ .

2. Mr. Zee came to the hospital several days ago for various tests. He is 68 years old, and the doctor has prescribed ambulation as desired. He feels weak today following extensive laboratory tests but would like to go to the patients' solarium to visit with his wife. What kind of supportive aid would you provide for Mr. Zee, and why?

_____ .

||||||||||||||||||||||||||||||||||||||||||||||||||||||||||||||||||||||||||||||||||||||||||||||||||||||||||||||||||||||||||||||||||||||||||||||||

ITEM 3. TRANSFERRING A HELPLESS PATIENT ONTO A STRETCHER

Frequently, you will be asked to help move a patient onto or off a stretcher. The stretcher is used to transport the bed patient to another area or department in the hospital, such as surgery or X-ray. Patients who are moved in this manner are usually more seriously ill, more limited in their movements, and consequently in greater need of support and assistance. Although some may be able to move freely from the bed to a stretcher, most of these patients will require help.

The stretcher is a type of bed that is made of metal; it is lightweight, with wheels that make it easy to roll. It is equipped with a pad for comfort and a safety belt or siderails to protect the patient from falling off.

In the skill laboratory, practice the procedure of assisting the transfer of a helpless patient from the bed to a stretcher. Ask one of your classmates to serve as a patient, and others to help you move the patient.

U
N
I
T
14

||||||||||||||||||||||||||||||||||||||||||||||||||||||||||||||||||||||||||||||||||||||||||||||||||||||||||||||||||||||||||||||||||||||||||||||||

Supplies Needed

Stretcher with pad and clean sheet   IV standard, if needed
Bath blanket or sheet to cover patient

||||||||||||||||||||||||||||||||||||||||||||||||||||||||||||||||||||||||||||||||||||||||||||||||||||||||||||||||||||||||||||||||||||||||||||||||

Important Steps	Key Points
1. Obtain the stretcher from storage.	Universal Steps A, B, C and D. See Appendix.
2. Wash your hands.	
3. Approach and identify the patient, explain what you are going to do, and secure his cooperation.	
4. Provide for privacy.	

Important Steps	Key Points
5. Position and prepare the patient.	Adjust the bed to the high position (flush with the height of the stretcher). Loosen the top bedding from the foot of the bed, remove the overbed cradles, excess pillows, and other things that might be in the way. Check all tubes that might be attached to the patient; make sure that they are free of the bedding and long enough to permit movement. Loosen the drawsheet and use it as a "lifting" sheet. Cover the patient with the bath blanket or sheet and remove the top bedding, which you leave on the bed.
6. Position the stretcher next to the bed and transfer the patient onto it. 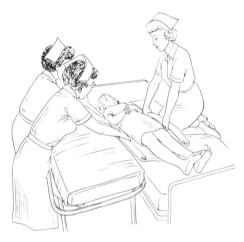	Station two workers next to the stretcher and lean across to reach the patient. The worker on the far side of the bed may have to get up and kneel on the side of the bed in order to avoid stretching and losing balance. All three then grasp the "lift" sheet and, on signal, move the helpless patient onto the stretcher. Place a pillow under the patient's head, and raise the siderails or fasten the safety belt.
7. Transfer the patient from stretcher to bed.	Reverse the procedure. Have the top bedding fan-folded to the side or the foot of the bed so that it is out of the way when moving the patient. You may find that it is easier to pull the patient onto the bed by having two workers on the distal side of the bed and one worker on the stretcher side.
8. Provide for the patient's comfort.	Universal Steps X, Y, and Z. See Appendix.
9. Return the stretcher to storage.	

10. Report and record as appropriate.	Charting example:
	 9:30 A.M. To X-ray per stretcher.
	             L. Smith, NA
	
	 10:35 A.M. Returned from X-ray per stretcher. Complains of pain in incision. IV running in left arm.
	             L. Smith, NA

ITEM 4. THE WHEELCHAIR

The wheelchair is the most commonly used mechanical aid for moving a patient safely from one place to another. It provides a great degree of general support for the entire body when the patient is out of bed.

A wheelchair consists of a seat on a frame suspended between two large rear wheels and two small front wheels. It has a turning rim on the large wheels, pushing handles behind the seat back, footrest pedals, and brakes. Most wheelchairs are constructed so that they can be folded for storage and transportation. The seat and back are usually made of a heavy-duty plastic material, which is easily cleaned with a damp cloth.

In order to be transported in a wheelchair by another person, the patient must be able to sit in an upright position. To move about independently in a wheelchair, the patient must be able to sit upright, support the upper body and head, and have the use of at least one arm in order to turn the wheel or set the brakes. The patient who must propel himself or herself should be instructed in the techniques of using the chair, such as how to set the hand brakes, transfer into and out of the chair, raise or lower the footrests with the foot, and propel the chair.

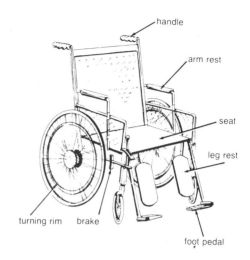

3. In order to propel himself in a wheelchair, a patient needs to be able to

    a. _____ .

    b. _____ .

    c. _____ .

ITEM 5. WHEELCHAIR TECHNIQUE

Let us now consider some of the elements of wheelchair technique. Before instructing a patient in this technique, you must first learn to do it yourself.

Supplies Needed

Wheelchair with brakes

Set Brakes. The large wheel of the wheelchair should be equipped with a brake that is operated by a hand lever. The accompanying figures show the hand brake in a set, or locked, position and in a released, or unlocked, position. Locate the hand brake levers on your wheelchair and set the brakes on both wheels.

Set, or locked.   Released, or unlocked.

U
N
I
T
14

Adjust Foot Pedals. With the brakes in the set position, locate the footrest pedals. Notice that each pedal can be swung upward to provide a clear entry to the chair and can be swung downward to serve as a footrest for the person in the wheelchair.

Now raise the foot pedals and sit in the wheelchair. Raise one foot and use it to swing the foot pedal down for that foot; repeat, using the other foot. Now remove one foot from the footrest, use the toe to swing the footrest pedal upward, and place your foot on the floor. Repeat, using the other foot. You should practice lowering and raising the foot pedals, using both feet. Now try lowering and raising the pedals by using only one foot.

Pushing and Turning. Pushing a patient in a wheelchair requires equal pressure on both handles for straight-ahead motion. To make a left turn with the wheelchair, your left hand on the handle should move just slightly or not at all, and you must exert more push on the right handle as the right portion of the chair moves a greater distance to make the turn. To make a right turn, the pressure would be reversed.

Passing Through Doorways. When approaching a closed door with a patient in a wheelchair, turn the wheelchair around so that its back is toward the door. You can then use one hand to open the door; pull the chair through as your body continues to force the door open wider. Turn the wheelchair around to a forward direction after you have cleared the door. This method prevents possible injury to the patient's feet or arms, damage to the finish of the door, and awkward or jerky movements of your body that may cause injury. You should practice pushing another person in the wheelchair, making several left and right turns, and going through a door.

Propelling Yourself. To propel yourself in a wheelchair, sit in the chair, place your feet on the footrests, and release the brakes on both wheels. Place your hands on the turn rim of the large wheels. For a straight-ahead movement, roll the rims forward with equal force on both rims. Turn to the left or to the right in the same manner as when you push the wheelchair by the handles, only now use the turning rim. Practice propelling yourself in a wheelchair and making right and left turns.

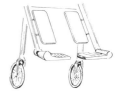

Footrest pedals in
down position

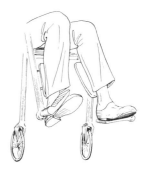

Raising footrest pedal
with foot.

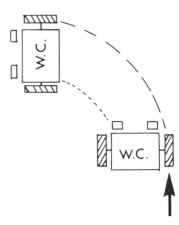

To make left turn, apply more
force at point of arrow.

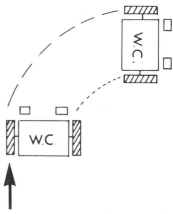

To make right hand turn, apply
force in direction of arrow.

You have practiced those steps of wheelchair technique that relate to using the hand brakes and the footrest pedals and to the propelling or pushing of the chair. Now we will go on to the procedure of transferring the patient into and out of the wheelchair.

ITEM 6.   TRANSFERRING THE PATIENT TO A WHEELCHAIR

In the skill laboratory you are to practice the procedure of transferring a patient (who can stand) into and out of a wheelchair. Have one of your fellow students play the role of the patient. A bed should be available for use by the "patient."

Supplies Needed

Wheelchair with brakes   Patient's robe and slippers

Important Steps	Key Points
Carry out Universal Steps A, B, and C. See Appendix.	
1. Position the wheelchair at the side of the bed near the patient.	Position the chair parallel to the side of the bed. Place the back of the chair even with the foot of the bed; the seat will be facing the head of the bed. Set the brakes on both wheels. Raise both footrest pedals.
2. Assist the patient to a "dangling-feet" position at the side of the bed.	Place the bed in the low position. Assist the patient to dangle according to instructions in "Patient Movement." Help patient put on robe and slippers.
3. Help the patient to stand up.	Have the patient rise from the bed or clasp your hands, arms, or shoulders to rise to a standing position. Use principles of good body alignment and movement to prevent injury to yourself.
4. Assist the patient into the wheelchair.	Direct the patient to pivot so that his back is toward the seat of the chair, then to reach down, grasp the arms of the chair, and sit down. Place both of the patient's feet on the footrests, then disengage, or release, the brakes.
5. Transfer from the wheelchair to the bed.	Reverse the procedure used to transfer patient into wheelchair. Position the side of the wheelchair parallel to the side of the bed, set both brakes, and raise the footrest pedals. Have the patient push up from the armrests to a standing position, then pivot so that his back is toward the bed and ease himself into a sitting position on the side of the bed. Remove the robe and slippers, and swing both the feet onto the bed.
Carry out Universal Steps X, Y, and Z. See Appendix.	Charting example: 1330. Up in wheelchair since 0945. Watching TV and visiting with others in lounge. No complaints. J. Jones, SN

U
N
I
T
14

ITEM 7.   USING A MECHANICAL LIFTER

A mechanical lifter should be used whenever a helpless or very heavy patient is to be transferred out of bed and into a chair, a wheelchair, or a tub. It is the safest method for moving the patient and avoiding injuries to health workers. Although not every nursing unit is equipped with a mechanical lifter, most hospitals have at least one. A variety of lifters are on the market; some of them, such as the Hoyer lift, are operated with hydraulic pressure.

Two workers are needed to transfer the patient safely from the bed to a wheelchair when using the mechanical lifter. One worker guides the patient into the sling while the other operates and rolls the lifter.

In the skill lab, practice transferring a helpless patient from the bed to a wheelchair, using a mechanical lifter similar to the Hoyer. One of your fellow students can play the role of the patient. Ask how it feels to be suspended by the lift and find out how you can reassure the patient.

Supplies Needed

Mechanical lifter with chain hooks and canvas belts or slings
Wheelchair with brakes

Important Steps	Key Points
Carry out Universal Steps A, B, and C. See Appendix.	
1. Position the wheelchair and set the brakes.	Allow enough space between the bed and the chair so that you can maneuver the mechanical lifter.
2. Position the mechanical lifter.	Place it with the base wheels under the bed and at right angles to the length of the bed. Adjust the level of the lifting bar over the bed and close the hydraulic pressure valve.
3. Place the patient in the sling of the lifter.	With a worker on each side of the bed, pass a sling strap under the patient's shoulders and another under the thighs. Fasten the strap to the corresponding hooks on the lifting bar.
4. Operate the lifter and, with assistance, move the patient to the wheelchair.	Close the pressure valve and pump the handle to raise the lifting bar with the patient in the sling straps so that his body clears the bed. Roll the lifter to the wheelchair while the other worker guides the patient into position over the chair seat. Release the pressure valve to lower the sling. Unhook the straps after the patient is in the chair, leaving them in place; then move the lifter out of the way.

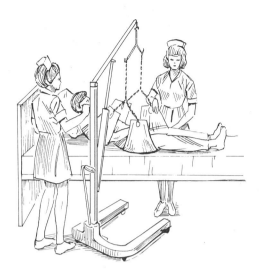

Transfer of patient from bed . . .

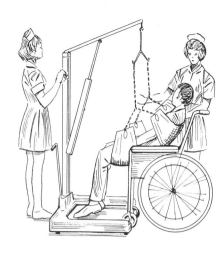

to wheelchair using
mechanical lift.

5. Return the patient to bed.

Reverse the procedure when getting the patient back into bed.

Carry out Universal Steps X, Y, and Z. See Appendix.

ITEM 8.   TRANSFERRING A HELPLESS PATIENT TO A CHAIR

Often you will be called upon to get a helpless patient out of bed and into a chair when a mechanical lifter is not available for the transfer. Avoid the method of lifting or swinging the patient from the bed to a wheelchair placed parallel to the side of the bed. Although this method is frequently used, many workers are injured by twisting and bending their backs and lifting the patient's body weight while off-balance.

You will need another person to assist you in transferring the helpless patient from the bed to a wheelchair. In the skill laboratory, practice the procedure until you feel at ease with it and confident of your ability to perform it with an actual patient.

Supplies Needed

Chair, or wheelchair with brakes   Patient's robe and slippers

Important Steps	Key Points
Carry out Universal Steps A, B, and C. See Appendix.	
1. Position the chair.	Place the chair at right angles to the bed and at about the level of the patient's hips. Put the bed in a low position — or even with the seat of the chair. Set brakes if a wheelchair is used.

U
N
I
T
14

Important Steps	Key Points
2. Position and prepare the patient.	Move the patient to the proximal side of the bed. Dress him in robe and slippers, if appropriate, and bring him to an upright sitting position.
3. With assistance, transfer the patient into the chair.	With one worker on each side, pivot the patient's body so that it is now positioned across the bed, then place one arm around the shoulders and one under the hips. Some patients may be able to sit erect and put their arms around the workers' necks and help support their weight, but weaker patients cannot do this. On signal, the workers slide the patient back into the seat of the chair. One worker then moves the chair away from the bed. The other worker supports the patient's feet and lowers them onto the floor.

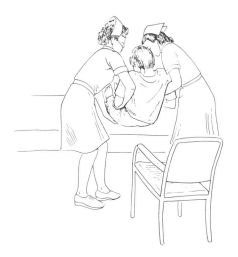

Using form of chair carry to transfer patient
to chair or wheelchair.

4. Return the patient to bed.	Reverse the procedure. The use of a trapeze for the patient to grasp is especially helpful for moving him back onto the bed.

Carry out Universal Steps X, Y, and Z. See Appendix.

ITEM 9.   USE OF WALKERS

Another mechanical aid that provides support for the patient in moving about from place to place is the *walker*, a waist-high tubular metal frame constructed in a rectangular shape with wheels attached to its legs. The preferred model has a movable swing-up seat and removable backrest that allows for easy entry and exit to and from the frame. The seat can be put down for use when the patient becomes tired.

The walker should be adjustable in height because it is used to provide support and stability for the patient who is learning to walk again. Any patient who has been confined to bed for a long period of time, or who has had fractures of the hip or bones in the lower extremity and must restrict weight bearing on the affected part, can use a walker. It is also employed to prepare the patient for the use of crutches or braces.

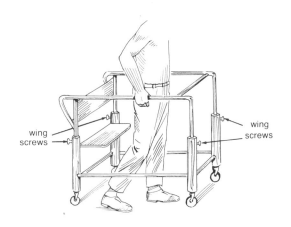

In order to use a walker, the patient must be able to bear weight on one foot, balance in an upright position, and have the use of the hands and arms. The walker should be adjusted to a height in which the upper rail fits the palm of the patient's hand with the elbow flexed or bent at a 30-degree angle.

4. In order to use a walker, the patient must be able to do three things:

   a. _____ b. _____

   c. _____ .

5. When using the walker, you noted that the patient's elbows were flexed (or bent) at a 90-degree angle and were resting on the upper rail of the walker. This would indicate

   that the height of the walker was too _____ .

6. Another patient was observed using a walker with his upper back and shoulders flexed and his arms extended straight down to reach the upper rail. The height of the walker

   was too _____ .

7. The recommended degree of flexion, or bend, of the elbow is _____ when using a walker.

ITEM 10. ASSISTING THE PATIENT WITH A WALKER

In the skill laboratory, practice the following steps in the procedure of assisting a patient into and out of a walker. Have someone play the part of the patient.

Supplies Needed

Walker   Patient's robe and slippers

Important Steps	Key Points
Carry out Universal Steps A, B, and C. See Appendix.	
1. Assist the patient to a sitting position.	Place the bed in the low position and assist patient to a dangling position at the side of the bed (see "Patient Movement and Ambulation"). Help patient to dress in robe and slippers.
2. Position the walker at the bedside.	Raise the seat; remove the back support, or move it to one side of the walker, and place the open back end of the walker in front of the patient. Securely hold the walker in place with one hand and use one foot to block one of the rear wheels.

Important Steps	Key Points
3. Adjust the height of the walker hand rail for patient.	Ask the patient to grasp the upper frame of the walker on each side and rise to a standing position. Have patient flex elbows about 30 degrees and measure the height needed to bring the upper rail of the walker to the level of the palm of the hands. If adjustment is needed, have the patient sit on the side of the bed while you loosen the screws and bolts on each of the four legs of the walker and refasten them at the adjusted height.
4. Assist the patient into the walker.	After adjustment, have the patient stand and step forward into the walker. Use your foot in front of the rear wheel to assist in holding the walker steady. Then lower the seat and replace the back support. Caution the patient to take small steps and to avoid going too fast or bumping into the front frame of the walker.

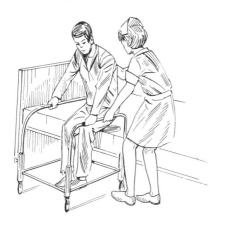

Assisting patient in and
out of walker.

Important Steps	Key Points
5. Assist the patient out of the walker.	Instruct the patient to approach the side of the bed, turning the walker around so that the back end is against the bed or chair. Remove the backrest or move it to one side and swing the seat up and out of the way. Hold the walker securely with one hand, use one foot to block one of the rear wheels, and instruct the patient to hold onto the upper rail while he steps back one or two steps to the edge of the bed, reaches for the bed with one hand, and eases himself to a sitting position. Remove the robe and slippers after pushing the walker to one side and help patient to swing the legs onto the bed.
Carry out Universal Steps X, Y, and Z. See Appendix.	10:10 A.M. Ambulated for first time in walker. Tolerated procedure well. Returned to bed in good condition in 15 minutes. Seems pleased with his progress. J. Jones, SN

ITEM 11. CRUTCH-WALKING

For some patients, crutch-walking is a difficult skill that requires careful supervision and practice. Crutch-walking is literally learning to walk with your hands. To use crutches, the patient must be able to balance the body in an upright position, have adequate strength in the arm and shoulder muscles to support much of his weight with the hands, have control of hip and knee joints to keep them from buckling, and be able to bear partial weight on both legs or full weight on one leg.

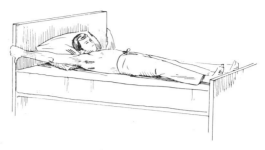

Arm exercises.

The physical preparation for crutch-walking can be started early, when the patient is still confined to bed or in a wheelchair. The patient should be encouraged to perform exercises that will help strengthen the muscles, particularly those of the arm and shoulder. Some of the exercises include lifting sandbags while lying flat in bed, grasping the head of the bed with the hands and pushing the body down in the bed, and alternately "setting" or contracting the muscles of the arm and leg without moving the joint, then relaxing them. When able, the patient should practice using his hands to push himself up to a sitting position in bed. While sitting in a chair or in bed, he should place his hands on the seat and push his body upward so that his buttocks clear the seat.

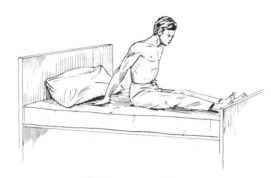

Sitting-up exercises.

8. In crutch-walking, much of the weight is supported by the patient's _____ .

9. It is essential that the patient have at least _____ weight bearing on both legs

or _____ weight bearing on one leg in order to learn crutch-walking.

ITEM 12. MEASURING CRUTCHES

Types of Crutches. There are many types of crutches. The most commonly used is the axillary crutch. It is adjustable in length, has a movable hand bar, and may be constructed of wood or aluminum. The top of the crutch has a crossbar, called the "axillary bar," which may or may not be padded. Some believe that padding reduces the pressure on the rib cage or the axillae.

A special feature of the Canadian type of crutch is that it lacks the axillary crossbar support but has a piece or cuff that fits around the upper arm. When using this crutch, the patient must support the body weight with the hands. All types of crutches should be equipped with heavy rubber suction tips to decrease the danger of slipping.

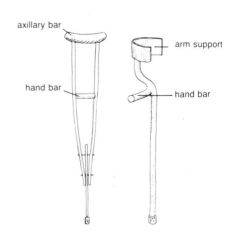

axillary bar

arm support

hand bar

hand bar

Axillary crutch.

Lofstrand or Canadian crutch.

Crutch Palsy. The pressure of bearing the body weight on the axillae may cause extreme weakness and tremor of the forearm muscles, wrist, and hand, a condition called "crutch palsy." Crutch palsy has been known to occur within four hours of leaning on the axillary bar and totally supporting the weight of the body without using the hands to bear any of the weight. This causes pressure on the nerves and blood vessels of the arm. Tissues are deprived of an adequate amount of oxygen and nutrients by the reduced blood flow. As a result, there is a loss of function and weakness of the muscles, which persists for days and even weeks. Not padding the axillary bar may discourage the patient from leaning so heavily on it and thus bearing the body weight solely from the axillae.

Adjustment of Crutches. Crutches may be measured and adjusted to the proper length for the individual patient. An easy method of measuring for crutches is to have the patient lie in bed, place a crutch alongside the leg on the bed, and measure from the axilla to a point six to eight inches out from the side of the heel. Adjust the crutches to this length, using the wing nuts and bolts. The hand bar should be located at a point equivalent to the distance from the axilla to the middle of the palm of the hand, with the wrist slightly hyperextended and the elbow flexed 30 degrees. Adjust the hand bar as needed; this allows the arms and hands to bear more of the body weight through the slight lifting of the body when the arms are straightened.

Crutches can be checked for proper fit by passing two fingers between the axillary bar and the axilla when the patient is in a standing position. The elbow should be bent about 30 degrees, with the hand gripping the hand bar and the axillary bar resting firmly against the patient's chest wall.

Using Crutches. The principles of crutch-walking are as follows:

a. The head is held up and the eyes look ahead, as in normal walking.

b. The crutches are placed slightly ahead of the patient's feet and to the outside of each foot.

c. The hands, not the axillae, are used to support the body weight.

d. The back should be kept in straight alignment and the patient should bend at the hips.

e. The crutches and affected foot should be moved forward together at the same time.

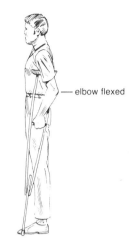

Crutch-walking — standing position.

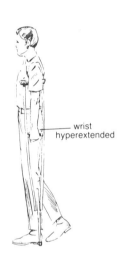

Crutch-walking — weight-bearing position.

f. A smooth, easy rhythm should be achieved in shifting the weight from the crutches to the good or unaffected leg and then to the crutches again.

g. The crutches should be of proper length and equipped with heavy rubber suction tips to prevent slipping.

h. The gait used will depend on the weight-bearing status of the lower extremities and the patient's ability.

You should be able to answer these questions about crutches.

10. Why is the elbow flexed about 30 degrees when measuring or fitting crutches?

_____ .

11. In the figures shown in the text, in which position is the elbow extended?

_____ .

In which position is the wrist hyperextended? _____ .

12. In crutch-walking, the patient should keep his back straight and bend from the

_____ .

13. The patient should look _____ when walking on crutches.

ITEM 13.   GAITS USED IN CRUTCH-WALKING

The type of gait used in crutch-walking depends upon the amount of weight the patient is able to support with one or both legs. The three-point gait is used more often in temporary crutch situations by patients with one affected leg, such as those with a fracture of the bones of one leg, knee or hip surgery, or paralysis of one leg. The four-point and two-point gaits are used by patients who can bear partial weight on both legs, such as those with cerebral palsy or arthritis.

In the skill laboratory, measure a pair of crutches and adjust them to the length you need for a good fit. Then practice the three-point, four-point, and two-point gaits of crutch-walking until you are familiar with each one. Remember to keep your head up, look forward (not down), keep your back straight, and bear your weight on your hands, not on your axillae.

U
N
I
T
14

Supplies Needed:

Pair of crutches

Three-Point Gait

Full weight bearing on one leg and partial or no weight bearing on the other.

Sequence of the gait: (1) Advance both crutches forward with the affected leg and shift weight to crutches then (2) advance the unaffected leg and shift the weight onto it.

Advantage of the three-point gait: It allows the affected leg to be partially or completely free of weight bearing.

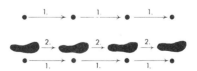

Three-point gait with the two crutches advanced first and then followed by the unaffected leg.

Four-Point Gait

Partial weight bearing on both legs is necessary.

Sequence of the gait from standing position: (1) Advance the left crutch, then (2) advance the right foot, (3) the right crutch, and finally (4) the left foot.

Advantage of the four-point gait is: It is the most stable.

Two-Point Gait

Partial weight bearing on both legs is necessary.

Sequence of the gait from standing position: (1) Advance left crutch and right foot, and then (2) the right crutch and the left foot.

Advantages of the two-point gait: It is a faster version of the four-point gait and is a more normal walking pattern, with the opposing arm and leg traveling forward at the same time.

Many patients are taught a swing-to and swing-through gait for rapid walking. However, you are not required to learn this gait in this lesson.

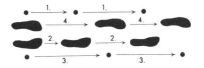

Four-point gait.

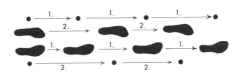

Two-point gait most nearly resembles the normal walking pattern.

ITEM 14. ASSISTING WITH THE USE OF CRUTCHES

In the skill laboratory, with another person playing the role of the patient, practice the steps of the procedure for assisting the patient with no weight bearing of one extremity to use crutches and the three-point gait.

||||||||||||||||||||||||||||||||||||||||||||||||||||||||||||||||||||||||||||||||||||||||||||||||||||||||||||||||||||

Supplies Needed

    Crutches   Patient's robe and slippers
    Walking belt (optional)

||||||||||||||||||||||||||||||||||||||||||||||||||||||||||||||||||||||||||||||||||||||||||||||||||||||||||||||||||||

Important Steps	Key Points
Carry out Universal Steps A, B, and C. See Appendix.	
1. Measure the patient and adjust the crutches to the proper length.	Have the patient lie supine in bed, in good body alignment. Measure the distance from the patient's axilla to a point 6 to 8 inches from the side of the heel. Loosen the wing screws and bolts of the crutches, adjust the length, and refasten. Measure the distance from the axilla to the palm of the hand with the elbow flexed at the 30-degree angle and the wrist slightly hyperextended; then adjust the hand bar. It is better to have the crutches an inch or so too short than to have them too long; this ensures weight bearing on the hands rather than on the axillae.

Important Steps	Key Points
2. Position the patient.	Assist patient in putting on pajamas, robe, and shoes (or street clothing). Place bed in low position and assist patient in sitting at side of bed with feet dangling. (See lesson on "Patient Movement and Ambulation.")
3. Demonstrate the crutch-walking gait the patient is to use.	The demonstration and explanation will show the patient how to use the crutches to walk. Emphasize these points:

a. Stand on unaffected leg and place each crutch 4 to 6 inches to the front and side of each foot.

b. Support the body weight with hands on the hand bars.

c. Move the crutches and affected foot 12 to 15 inches directly forward, all at the same time.

d. Move the unaffected foot up to the level of the crutch tips and support weight with hands during this brief period.

e. Continue steps c and d.

Important Steps	Key Points
4. Assist the patient to use the crutches and learn the crutch gait.	Help patient to stand at the side of the bed and balance on both crutches. Check the fit of the crutches. If the patient is unsteady in balancing, report this to your team leader before proceeding any further. When the patient is learning crutch-walking, walk behind him and hold onto the walking belt, the pajama waistband, or the ties of the drawsheet in order to provide support. Have another person walk at the side or in front of the beginner to help give additional support when needed.
5. Help the patient return to bed.	Keep practice sessions short to avoid strain and muscle fatigue. Ask patient to walk to the side of the bed using crutches and to turn so that his back is toward the bed. Ask the patient to set the crutches aside with one hand and, with the other, to reach down for the side of the bed to lower himself to a sitting position. If the patient is unable to use crutches without assistance, place them where they can be reached. Help the patient remove robe and slippers, take off walking belt or drawsheet if used, and swing patient's legs onto bed.
Carry out Universal Steps X, Y, and Z. See Appendix.	Charting example: 3:10 P.M. Instructed in the use of crutches. Ambulated 20 paces down the hall, and returned, using crutches and no weight-bearing on the left leg. Returned to bed. Resting. J. Jones, SN

UNIT 14

The procedure for assisting the patient in and out of bed with crutches is easily adapted to instructions for using crutches to sit in and rise from a chair. This is shown in the accompanying sketches.

Patients who use crutches must learn the skills of opening doors and going up or down steps. To open a door, the patient on crutches approaches the door, reaches out with one hand to unlatch the door, pushes it open and then holds the door open with the tip of his crutch and proceeds through the door.

Sitting
down
in chair.

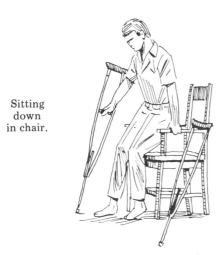
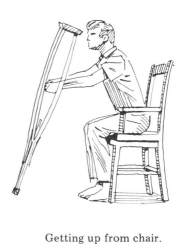

Getting up from chair.

The rule to remember when instructing the patient in going up and down steps is "angels go up and devils go down." When going up steps, the good leg ("angel") is advanced to the next step because it will support the weight. It is followed by the crutches and the affected leg. In going down steps, the crutches and the affected leg ("devil") lead off to the next step as the good leg again supports the weight until it can be shifted to the crutches.

Points to emphasize when instructing the patient on how to go up stairs:

a. Stand with no weight bearing on affected foot, crutches at the side.

b. Support body weight with hands on hand bars of crutches and advance unaffected foot to next step.

c. Transfer weight to unaffected leg and move crutches and affected leg up to same step riser.

d. Continue steps b and c up the stairs.

In going up or down a flight of stairs some patients may use only one crutch — but take the other along — and rely on the handrail or bannister for support. Caution the patient to take both crutches for use after negotiating the stairs.

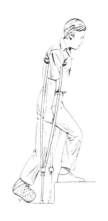
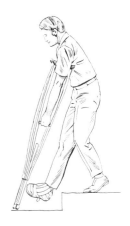

"Angels" go up . . .   "devils" go down.

The unsteady patient or the one who may be too weak to lift his body weight up or down steps on crutches could manage steps in this manner, sitting on step after step and dragging the affected leg along, if it were necessary. But don't forget the crutches.

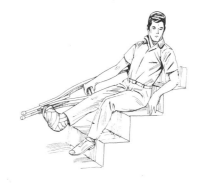

Even this works!

ITEM 15. USE OF A CANE

Canes are another mechanical aid for patient ambulation. Most people need little or no instruction in how to use a cane; however, the cane should be of proper height for the patient. When the patient's elbow is flexed at a 30-degree angle, the curve or handle of the cane should fit the palm of his hand and extend to the floor at a point about 6 inches out from his foot. The cane should have a good rubber suction tip to prevent slipping. There are many varieties, including crab canes, tripod canes, and others.

ITEM 16. WHAT ARE BRACES?

Braces provide specific support for weakened muscles and joints or provide immobilization of the injured part. Braces are ordered by the physician, and the cost of the brace is charged to the patient. Almost all braces are custom-made and fitted to the individual patient. Since the brace is the patient's property, it is generally kept at the bedside or with his or her belongings. The most common types of braces are those for the neck, the back, the arm, and the leg.

The most common complaint of a poor-fitting brace is caused by putting them on wrong. No brace will fit properly or be effective if it is put on upside-down or backwards. The well made and well fitted brace should not cause pressure at any point on the patients body. Patient may resist wearing braces that cause pain, pressure, or more discomfort.

Time, however, is required for the patient to adapt to the support of the brace, and even the best-fitting brace may cause slight pressure or soreness on the bony prominences or at the upper and lower cuffs of the brace. When there is irritation at these areas, thin layers of sponge rubber or folded layers of soft linen may be used to pad the area. Cotton batting should not be used because it has a tendency to become compacted and uneven.

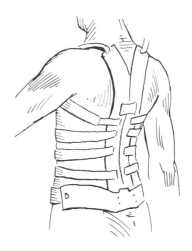

Back brace.

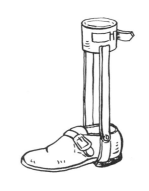

UNIT 14

There are many types of braces, and it would be impossible to describe them all. Most are made of various combinations of metal, leather, and cloth. Some braces, especially those for the arm or leg, have a hinge to allow movement at the joint. The hinges should be oiled every six weeks, and the metal lubricated to prevent rust. Lubricate hinges slightly with cup grease or silicone grease. The use of vaseline or light household oils is not advised because they are too thin, tend to run, and could stain clothing. Cloth braces should be hand-washed, and the leather portions cleaned periodically. Almost all leg braces are attached to the patient's shoe.

||||||||||||||||||||||||||||||||||||||||||||||||||||||||||||||||||||||||||||||||||||||||||||||||||||||||||||||||||||

After reading this section on braces, you should be able to answer the following questions.

14. A brace is used to provide _____ or _____ for weakened muscles or joints.

15. The most frequent cause of poor fitting braces is putting the brace on _____

or _____ .

16. The moving metal parts and hinges of braces should be oiled every _____

weeks.

17. The patient who is wearing a brace may develop pressure areas or soreness over _____

_____ or _____ .

||||||||||||||||||||||||||||||||||||||||||||||||||||||||||||||||||||||||||||||||||||||||||||||||||||||||||||||||||||

ITEM 17. ASSISTING WITH A BACK BRACE

In the skill laboratory, you are to practice the procedure of assisting to put on a back brace. Ask another person to play the part of the patient for your practice period.

||||||||||||||||||||||||||||||||||||||||||||||||||||||||||||||||||||||||||||||||||||||||||||||||||||||||||||||||||||

Supplies Needed:

Brace

||||||||||||||||||||||||||||||||||||||||||||||||||||||||||||||||||||||||||||||||||||||||||||||||||||||||||||||||||||

Important Steps	Key Points
Carry out Universal Steps A, B, and C. See Appendix.	
1. Position the patient.	Place patient in supine position on the proximal side of the bed.
2. Put the back brace on the patient.	Keep patient's back and neck in straight alignment and log-roll patient toward you. Place the top of the brace over the upper back and the bottom cuff or edge of the brace over the hips and lower back. The brace should slip readily into place and follow the contour of the patient's back. Gently roll patient from side position to his back. Reach under near side of patient and draw straps of brace through. Bring straps over from far side of brace and fasten them together snugly in front.

Important Steps	Key Points
3. Check for pressure points caused by the brace.	With the brace snugly fastened, assist the patient to a sitting position at the side of the bed. Check for possible pressure areas over the bony prominences of the hips, over the ribs, over the breastbone (sternum), and at the upper and lower edges of the brace. You should be able to slip your finger between the brace and the flesh at these points. If the brace fits properly and still causes some soreness in these areas, pad them with sponge rubber or soft cloth.
4. Assist the patient as needed for comfort and safety.	Help patient to put on robe and slippers or to dress in street clothing. Generally, the patient may walk or sit in a chair with back brace on. Some patients who have had recent surgery on the spine may begin wearing a brace while still on bed rest and would not be allowed in a sitting position to undergo a check for pressure areas.
5. Remove the back brace from the patient.	Assist the patient to lie flat in bed. Unfasten the straps in the front of the brace and push the proximal side straps down close to the side. Keep back and neck in straight alignment and log-roll the body toward you. Grasp the brace and remove it. Then position the patient for comfort.
Carry out Universal Steps X, Y, and Z. See Appendix.	Charting example: 6:10 P.M. Back brace applied for first time. Brace fits well, no pressure areas noted. Remained in chair throughout evening meal. In good spirits.

J. Jones, SN

or

6:10 P.M. Back brace applied for first time. Brace fits well except for pressure over right iliac crest. Area padded with foam rubber, with no relief. Brace removed. Reported to doctor.

J. Jones, SN

U
N
I
T
14

ITEM 18. ASSISTING WITH A SHORT LEG BRACE

As with other types of braces, long and short leg braces are fitted for the individual patient and are usually attached to a shoe. The brace and shoe provide support for the leg. The short leg brace is used for those who can control movement in the knee joint but need support for the lower leg and ankle.

You should now practice assisting the patient to put on a short leg brace, if one is available for your use.

Supplies Needed

Short leg brace with shoe   Patient's robe and other shoe

Important Steps	Key Points
Carry out Universal Steps A, B, and C. See Appendix.	
1. Position the patient.	Assist to a dangling or sitting position at the side of the bed. Most short leg braces are attached to a shoe and are easier to put on in a sitting position.
2. Put the leg brace on the patient.	Loosen the laces of the shoe if it is a laced type. Make sure the cuff of the brace is untied or unfastened. Slip the patient's foot (of the affected leg) into the shoe attached to the brace. Make sure that the toes are not curled under the foot. Tie the laces of the shoe. Slip the upper cuff of the brace around the calf of the affected leg and tie or fasten it snugly, but do not fasten so tightly that it interferes with the blood circulation.
3. Check the brace for pressure areas.	Have the patient stand at the bedside and check the areas around the upper cuff of the brace and the bony prominences just below the knee and around the ankle. You should be able to slip your finger between the brace and the flesh underneath it. Check the function of the hinge at the ankle (if the brace has one) by having the patient take one step on it. It should keep the toe of the shoe slightly upward to prevent the toe from dragging.
4. Provide for the patient's comfort.	Assist the patient in putting on robe and other shoe or to dress in street clothing. Most patients are permitted to be up in a chair or walk with a brace on. Stay nearby to give assistance if this is the first trial.
5. Assist the patient to remove the short leg brace.	While patient is sitting at the side of his bed, untie or unfasten the upper cuff of the brace and then untie the laces of the shoe. Slip the shoe and the brace off the affected leg.

Carry out Universal Steps X, Y, and Z. See Appendix.	Charting example:
	4:30 P.M. Applied short leg brace to left leg for first time. Tolerated well. No pressure areas observed or reported.
	                              J. Jones, SN
	6 P.M. Short leg brace removed. Tolerated well.
	                              J. Jones, SN

ITEM 19. ASSISTING WITH THE NECK BRACE

Neck braces are used frequently to support and to immobilize the neck following an injury. Generally, the neck brace is applied while the patient is in a sitting position. It is slipped under the chin and fastened at the back of the neck. You will not be expected to demonstrate the application of a neck brace in the performance test for this lesson.

ITEM 20. CONCLUSION OF THE LESSON

You have now completed the lesson on assisting the patient to use mechanical aids for ambulation and movement. When you have had sufficient practice in using these aids correctly, make an appointment with your instructor to take the post-test.

WORKBOOK ANSWERS

1. Wheelchair or stretcher

2. Wheelchair or walker — to provide support

3. a. sit upright

   b. support neck and head

   c. use at least one arm

4. a. balance in upright position

   b. bear weight on one foot

   c. have use of arms and hands

5. high

6. low

7. 30 degrees

8. hands

9. partial; full

10. When arm is straightened using the crutch, it will lift the body slightly.

11. weight bearing; weight bearing

12. hips

13. straight ahead

14. support; immobilization

15. backwards; upside down

16. six

17. bony prominences; around edges or cuffs of the brace

PERFORMANCE TEST

In the skill laboratory, your instructor will ask you to perform four out of the seven activities listed below without reference to any source material. For several of the activities you will need another person to take the part of the patient.

1. Given a patient sedated for surgery, you will obtain assistance from other workers and transfer the patient from the bed to a stretcher without causing discomfort or injury.

2. Given a patient who can stand on one or both feet, you will transfer the patient from the bed to a wheelchair.

3. Given a patient who cannot stand, you will use a mechanical lifter or obtain assistance from other workers to transfer the patient from the bed to a wheelchair, using good body alignment and movement to prevent strain and observing the principles of balance and lifting to prevent the patient from slipping or falling.

4. Given a patient who is capable of operating the wheelchair, you will demonstrate and explain the wheelchair technique for operating the brakes, using the footrest pedals, propelling the chair, and making a turn.

5. Given a patient who needs the support while walking, you will adjust a walker to the proper height and transfer the patient into the walker in a safe manner to prevent slipping or falling.

6. Given a patient who needs the support of crutches for walking, you will measure the crutches to the proper length for the patient, adjust them to this length, and adjust the hand bar.

7. Given a patient who is beginning to learn crutch-walking, you will demonstrate one of the following gaits and state the weight-bearing condition related to that gait: (a) four-point gait, (b) two-point gait, or (c) three-point gait.

8. Given a patient who needs a brace for support of a specific portion of the body, you will apply one of the following braces and state the possible areas of pressure that could result from wearing the brace.

    a. Back brace

    b. Short leg brace

PERFORMANCE CHECKLIST

TRANSFERRING THE PATIENT FROM THE BED TO THE STRETCHER

1. Obtain a stretcher.

2. Wash your hands.

3. Identify the patient and explain the procedure.

4. Provide for privacy.

5. Position and prepare the patient.

    a. Put the bed in high position.

    b. Loosen the top bedding.

    c. Check all tubing.

    d. Loosen the drawsheet for use as a "lifting" sheet.

6. Position the stretcher next to the bed and obtain two or more helpers.

7. With helpers on each side of the patient, transfer patient onto the stretcher by using the "lifting" sheet.

8. Make the patient comfortable.

   a. Place a pillow under patient's head.

   b. Cover with a blanket or sheet.

   c. Remove the top bedding.

   d. Raise the siderails or fasten the safety belt.

   e. Check and provide for tubes and tubing.

9. Report and record the procedure as appropriate.

TRANSFERRING THE PATIENT FROM THE BED TO THE WHEELCHAIR

1. Obtain the proper equipment.

2. Wash your hands.

3. Identify the patient and explain the procedure.

4. Position the wheelchair and set the brakes.

5. Position and prepare the patient.

   a. Place bed in the low position.

   b. Assist patient to sit on the side of the bed and dangle both feet.

   c. Help patient to put on robe and slippers.

6. Assist the patient into the wheelchair.

   a. Have the patient stand and walk to the chair.

   b. Direct patient to pivot and sit down in the chair.

   c. Place patient's feet on the footrest pedals.

   d. Release the brakes and transport.

7. Record and report as necessary.

TRANSFERRING A HELPLESS PATIENT BY USING A MECHANICAL LIFTER

1. Obtain the mechanical lifter and wheelchair.

2. Wash your hands.

3. Identify the patient and explain the procedure.

4. Position the wheelchair and set the brakes.

5. Position the mechanical lifter.

6. Place the patient in the slings.

   a. Put one sling under patient's shoulders at the level of the axillae and the other under the thighs.

   b. Attach the hooks of the slings to the lifting bar.

7. Operate the mechanical lifter.

    a. Release, or open, the hydraulic pressure valve to raise or lower the lifting bar and the patient in the sling.

    b. Close the hydraulic pressure valve to stabilize the position of the lifting bar.

    c. Use the handle pump to increase hydraulic pressure when the valve is open.

    d. With assistance in guiding the patient in the sling, roll the mechanical lifter to the wheelchair.

8. Place the patient in the wheelchair by lowering the lifting bar.

    a. Position in good alignment.

    b. Support with a pillow and safety belt, as needed.

    c. Put the feet on the footrest pedals.

    d. Release the brakes and transport.

9. Record and report as appropriate.

INSTRUCTING THE PATIENT IN USE OF A WHEELCHAIR

1. Obtain the appropriate equipment.

2. Check the equipment for proper working condition.

    a. Brakes.

    b. Wheels and tires.

    c. Upholstery.

3. Wash your hands.

4. Identify the patient and explain the procedure.

5. Demonstrate and describe the correct techniques for using the wheelchair to the patient.

    a. Proper use of brakes (setting and releasing).

    b. Positioning the footrest.

    c. Propelling the chair in a straight line.

    d. Turning corners.

    e. Passing through an ordinary doorway or one equipped with an automatic closing device.

6. Provide the patient with an opportunity to practice under supervision the techniques of propelling wheelchair.

7. Encourage patient to utilize the proper method of manipulating the wheelchair.

8. Report and record.

TRANSFERRING THE PATIENT FROM THE BED TO THE WALKER

1. Obtain the proper equipment.

2. Wash your hands.

3. Identify the patient and explain the procedure.

4. Adjust the bed to the low position.

5. Assist the patient to dangle feet and dress in robe and slippers.

6. Prepare the walker for occupancy and position it in front of the patient.

    a. Raise the seat.

    b. Remove the back support.

7. Secure the walker in place with one hand and use foot to block a rear wheel.

8. Help patient to stand and step into walker frame.

    a. Check and adjust the height of the walker as required.

    b. Be sure that patient's elbows are flexed approximately 30 degrees.

    c. Lower seat and replace the back support in the walker.

    d. Caution patient to take small steps and to avoid going too fast.

9. Chart the procedure.

ADJUSTING CRUTCHES

1. Obtain the proper equipment.

    a. Crutches should have no splinters, breaks, or bends.

    b. The crutch tip must be in good condition.

    c. The axillary pad bar should be installed, if required.

2. Wash your hands.

3. Identify the patient and explain the procedure.

4. Ask the patient to lie flat on the bed.

5. Measure to determine the length of crutch required.

    a. The crutch tip should be approximately six to eight inches from the side of the heel.

    b. There should be approximately two fingers' distance between the axillary bar and the axilla.

    c. The elbows should be flexed approximately 30 degrees.

6. Adjust the position of the hand bar and the height of the shaft as required.

7. Tell the patient when the crutch-walking lesson will be given.

8. Chart the procedure.

GAITS USED FOR CRUTCH-WALKING

1. Identify two-, three-, and four-point gaits.

2. Perform the three-point gait. Condition for use: full weight bearing on one leg, partial or no weight bearing on the other.

3. Perform the four-point gait. Condition for use: partial weight bearing on both legs.

4. Perform the two-point gait. Condition for use: partial weight bearing on both legs.

UNIT 14

APPLYING A BRACE

1. Wash your hands.

2. Identify the patient.

3. Review the procedure with patient.

4. Obtain the proper brace.

5. Position the patient appropriately.

6. Apply the brace correctly.

   a. Observe the principles of body alignment when moving the patient.

   b. Prepare the brace for application.

   c. Position the brace on the patient's body.

   d. Secure the brace correctly.

7. Adjust the brace for correct support and fit.

8. Check for pressure points.

9. Provide for the patient's comfort by assisting in dressing or moving to a chair, and so forth.

10. Report and record the procedure.

POST-TEST

Multiple Choice. Select the one best answer for each of the following questions.

1. A weak or helpless patient who is in need of the maximum amount of support is transported by means of

   a. a wheelchair.

   b. a patient lifter.

   c. a walker with a seat.

   d. a stretcher.

2. When patients need to use mechanical aids on a temporary basis to move about, the person most often responsible for teaching them how is

   a. the physician.

   b. the nurse.

   c. the physical therapist.

   d. the occupational therapist.

3. When transferring the helpless patient from the bed to a stretcher, nurses make use of

   a. the draw sheet as a "lifting sheet."

   b. pillows to make the stretcher level with the bed.

   c. air flotation pads to reduce pressure.

   d. the siderails to pull the patient to the side of the bed.

4. In order to use a wheelchair independently, the patient must be able to do all *except*

   a. bear full weight on one foot.

   b. support the head and upper body in an upright position.

   c. push the big turning wheels and move forward.

   d. set and release the brakes as needed.

5. When the patient propels the wheelchair alone, where is pressure exerted in order to make a left hand turn?

   a. On the left turning wheel.

   b. On the right turning wheel.

   c. On the right handle.

   d. On the left handle.

   e. Equally on both foot pedals.

6. The greatest advantage in using a mechanical lifter to move the helpless or heavy patient is that

   a. only one person is needed to move the patient.

   b. the sling helps to prevent patient falls.

   c. injuries to the health workers are reduced or avoided.

   d. it saves time.

UNIT 14

7. The height of the lifting bar of the mechanical lifter is adjusted by means of

    a. opening and closing a hydraulic valve.

    b. varying the length of the straps between the sling and the bar.

    c. moving the lifter closer to the patient's bed or chair.

    d. positioning the base wheels of the lifter under the bed.

8. In order to use a walker, the patient must be able to do which of the following?

    1. Bear weight on at least one foot.

    2. Balance in an upright position.

    3. Have strong spinal muscles.

    4. Be able to do quadriceps exercises ("quad sets").

    5. Have the use of the arms and hands.

        a. 3, 4, and 5   b. all   c. 1, 2, and 5   d. 2, 3, and 4

9. When using the walker, the height of the frame is adjusted so the patient's elbow flexes at

    a. 30-degree angle.

    b. 45-degree angle.

    c. 90-degree angle.

    d. 120-degree angle.

10. Crutch palsy occurs when the patient

    a. walks too far and for too long a period of time.

    b. supports the body weight by resting on the axillary bar.

    c. is unable to balance the upper torso.

    d. uses the Canadian type of crutch for walking.

11. Crutch palsy affects the forearm, wrist, and hand by causing primarily

    a. swelling of the wrist and fingers.

    b. soreness in all of the joints.

    c. painful rash of the skin.

    d. extreme weakness and tremor of muscles.

12. In order to use the three-point gait in crutch-walking, the patient must be able to do which of the following activities?

    a. Bear full weight on both legs.

    b. Shift body weight to the affected leg.

    c. Support the upper torso with one arm.

    d. Have full weight bearing on one leg.

13. The patient using crutches is instructed to observe all of the following principles *except* which one?

    a. Allow hands on the hand bars to support the body's weight.

    b. Take frequent rests by leaning on the axillary bar.

    c. Keep the spine straight and look ahead when walking.

    d. Move both crutches and the affected leg forward at the same time.

14. Your patient has been fitted with a lumbar brace but now complains that it rubs and doesn't fit well. What is the *first* action the nurse should take?

    a. Send the brace back to the manufacturer or fitter.

    b. Reassure the patient that it just takes time to get used to wearing it.

    c. Notify the doctor of the patient's complaints.

    d. Inspect the brace to see that it was put on correctly.

15. Most braces for the lower extremity have hinges that should be oiled

    a. every six months.

    b. only when needed.

    c. every six weeks.

    d. only by the physician.

POST-TEST ANSWERS

1. d		9. a	
2. b		10. b	
3. a		11. d	
4. a		12. d	
5. b		13. b	
6. c		14. d	
7. a		15. c	
8. c			

UNIT 14

Unit 15

GENERAL PERFORMANCE OBJECTIVE

Upon completion of this unit, you will be able to set and operate the Circ-O-lectric bed and the Foster or Stryker turning frame correctly, efficiently, and safely.

SPECIFIC PERFORMANCE OBJECTIVES

When you have finished this lesson you will be able to:

1. Set up a Stryker (or Foster) frame and assist in transferring the patient onto the frame in an accurate, efficient, and safe manner.

2. Turn the patient on a Stryker (or Foster) frame safely from the supine to the prone position with the use of the anterior frame.

3. Set up and operate the Circ-O-lectric bed and assist in transferring the patient onto the bed in an accurate, efficient, and safe manner.

4. Operate the Circ-O-lectric bed correctly and safely rotate the patient from a supine to a vertical standing position and then to a prone position, using the anterior frame.

VOCABULARY

paraplegia—paralysis of the lower portion of the body and both legs.
perineal—refers to the perineum, located between the vulva and the anus of the female, and between the scrotum and the anus of the male.
pubis—the lower anterior part of the innominate bone in the pelvis.
quadriplegia—paralysis of all four extremities (arms and legs).
vertigo—dizziness.

INTRODUCTION TO SPECIAL TURNING FRAMES

As you know, any position that is maintained for a long time becomes unbearable. In the hospital, however, patients with certain orthopedic conditions (disease, surgery, or fracture of bones or joints) must be kept immobilized in order that healing may take place. Other patients may be immobilized or unable to move because of their disease or physical condition. For example, the patient with a fracture or injury to the spinal column may need to be immobilized so that the spine can heal. At the same time, the patient needs to change position at frequent intervals to relieve pressure, to promote circulation, and to be more comfortable.

In order to maintain the immobilization of part of the patient's body and yet provide for turning, various types of turning frames or beds may be used. The more common types that you may see or use are the Stryker frame, the Foster frame, or the Circ-O-lectric bed.

Patients who may need to use these special turning frames include those who have paraplegia, quadriplegia, spinal fusion, multiple fractures of the spine or long bones, acute arthritis, severe dermatitis, genitourinary disorders, and other diseases that cause immobility or paralysis.

In this unit, you will become familiar with the various types of turning frames and the way to set them up and operate them in order to provide care for the patient.

TURNING IMMOBILIZED PATIENTS

ITEM 1. THE PSYCHOLOGICAL NEEDS OF THE IMMOBILIZED PATIENT

Immobilized patients have psychological needs as well as extensive need for physical care. These psychological needs are expressed in terms of emotions, such as fear, apprehension, anger, hopelessness, and withdrawal. Think how you might feel if you were unable to move or turn yourself and had to be confined to a narrow bed for days, weeks, or even longer.

Let us consider a few of the psychological needs that patients have, especially patients who are immobilized. First, they are concerned about their illness or injury itself and the effects it may have on their future. Second, because their movement is restricted by their medical treatment, they become, quite literally, prisoners of their bodies. This makes them dependent on others for everything they want or need to do, from getting something to eat or drink to turning off a light that may be shining in their eyes. Finally, this dependence affects their lives in more general ways; even such matters as what time they wake up in the morning are out of their control.

The concern and dependence just discussed are only two of the psychological stresses felt by patients. These can find expression in many different ways, one of the most common being hostility or anger directed at the nurse or some other person on the scene. It is important that nurses not take such aggressive feelings personally; rather, they should try to understand why the patients feel as they do. Even though the patient has angrily (and usually wrongfully) accused the nurse of neglect or error, it is more effective and beneficial for the nurse to respond empathetically — such as, "You seem to be very upset or angry about something. Can you tell me what happened?" — than to take an opposing point of view or to try to justify an action.

Another need patients feel when under medical care is the desire to know about their treatment and about certain equipment that applies to their condition, such as turning frames. It is not enough for the nurse merely to say that it has been ordered by the doctor or that "it is necessary in the treatment of your condition"; patients have a right to know the "why's." In the case of turning frames, an appropriate response to such a question might include the following points:

1. To change patient's position at frequent intervals with minimum of pain or discomfort.

2. To relieve pressure on parts of the body.

3. To increase circulation.

4. To maintain the immobility of the affected part so that healing can occur.

5. To increase comfort, well-being, and activity.

Each patient must be considered as a whole person. Even though the individual may be greatly restricted in physical activities and dependent on others for care, his or her mind may not be impaired. Such patients should be encouraged to use their intellectual abilities. The patient on a turning frame is not just a body to be looked after but a person who belongs to a family and to a community, one who has a purpose in life.

The immobilized patient needs safety and protection; moreover, he or she must be sure that those providing care know how to use the equipment correctly and safely. Apprehension and fear can be greatly increased by the groping and fumbling of workers who do not know how to operate the turning frames.

Finally, the patient should be given the opportunity to make decisions and have some control over events that concern him or her. Whenever possible, the patient should be involved in planning the nursing care, the time of the bath, menu selections, bedtime, and other activities that fall within allowable and recognized boundaries.

The psychological needs of the immobilized patient or the patient who must use a turning frame are very important. Usually such patients have serious injury or illness that requires a longer period of hospitalization than that required for most other patients. Thus, in addition to knowing how to set up and operate the equipment, you should understand how the patient might respond to these activities.

ITEM 2. THE STRYKER FRAME AND THE FOSTER FRAME

The Stryker frame consists of a cotlike frame with canvas stretched across it. This is attached at both ends to pivot joints on a large metal structure. When the patient lies on the cotlike frame, another similar frame is placed on top of the patient, who is thus sandwiched between the two with safety belts that hold the frames together. Owing to the pivot joints, the patient can then be turned from back to abdomen and vice versa on the cotlike frames.

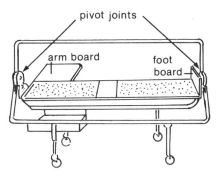

Stryker frame with posterior frame

The posterior frame on which the patient lies when in a supine position is prepared with padded sections: one that extends from the top of the frame to the pubis, a small middle section that can be removed for the use of the bedpan, and one that extends from mid-thigh to the foot end of the frame. The sections are covered with canvas and folded bath towels and drawsheets, which are pinned on the underside.

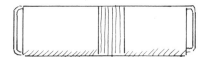

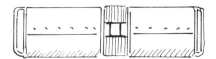

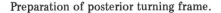

Preparation of posterior turning frame.   Underside of frame.

The anterior frame is usually prepared in a similar manner except that one section extends from the shoulders to the pubis in order to allow space for the head. The lower section extends only to the ankles so that the feet can be properly aligned when the patient is lying on his abdomen. A narrow section is used to support the forehead.

When the bedpan is needed, the small canvas section across the middle of the frame is detached and the bedpan is placed as shown. The fracture pan can be used for elimination if the lifting of the patient's hips is not contraindicated. (Refer to the unit on Urine Elimination.)

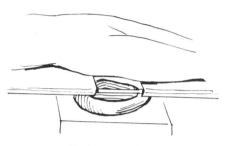

Perineal section
detached for bedpan use.

With the patient strapped securely between the anterior and posterior frames, the nurse can safely turn the patient in the Stryker frame by loosening a spring lock at either end of the frame. (Two nurses may be needed when the patient is heavy, or when required by hospital policy.) The frame will automatically trip the lock when it is turned and again be locked in place. After the patient has been turned, the upper frame is removed. Armrests can be attached to the sides of the frame when the patient is in a prone position. The sketch below shows the patient being turned to and in a prone position.

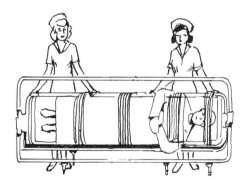

A. Turning patient.

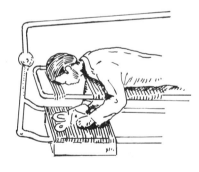

B. Patient in prone position.

The Foster frame is similar to the Stryker frame except that it is bigger, more stable, and more expensive. It is used for the same purposes and the procedure for setting it up and operating it is almost the same as that for the Stryker frame.

ITEM 3. SETTING UP AND USING THE STRYKER FRAME

||||||||||||||||||||||||||||||||||||||||||||||||||||||||||||||||||||||||||||||||||||||||||||||||||||||||||||||||||||||||

Supplies Needed:

Basic frame	Tray table
Anterior and posterior frames	Bedpan support
Four long-stem pins	Two safety straps (webbed) with
Canvas sections: two long, two short,	airplane buckles
and two narrow	Forehead strap or face mask
Sponge pads: two long, two short,	Cover for forehead strap or face mask
two narrow, two shoulder pads,	Spring clamps
and one abdominal pad	Covers for sponge pads, or linen and
Footboard and two armrests	safety pins to secure it

||||||||||||||||||||||||||||||||||||||||||||||||||||||||||||||||||||||||||||||||||||||||||||||||||||||||||||||||||||||||

Important Steps	Key Points
1. Prepare the posterior frame.	
a. Attach the canvas sections across the posterior frame and secure them with spring clamps.	Measure the canvas sections to fit the patient and fold the unneeded portion underneath.
	Top section — from the top of patient's head to the pubis.
	Middle section — (perineal section) from the pubis to the upper third of the thigh.
	Lower section — from the upper third of the thigh to the bottom of the frame.
b. Place sponge pads on the canvas sections and cover them with bath blankets or sheets.	Make sure that all ends of the linen coverings are secured (pinned) so they won't catch or interfere when the frame is turned.
c. Place the posterior frame on the basic frame.	Tightly latch or screw the nuts in place at the pivoting joint.
d. Attach the footboard in the slot at the bottom of the posterior frame.	
2. Wash your hands.	
3. Take the Stryker frame and its parts to the patient's room.	Universal Steps A, B, and C. See Appendix.
4. Approach and identify the patient, explain what is to be done, and enlist his cooperation.	
5. Transfer the patient to the frame.	A physician may be required to be present when a patient is transferred to the frame.
	Leave a folded bath blanket or sheet covering the patient to avoid exposing him.
	Move all furniture and equipment away to provide a clear path from the patient's bed to the frame. Reassure the patient during the transfer.

Important Steps	Key Points
a. Ask for additional help.	At least three or four people will be needed. Use at least a three-man carry, and another to support the head if needed. Use good body alignment and smooth, coordinated movements. Lift and move the patient on signal.
b. Lock the wheels of the frame.	
6. Position the patient in correct body alignment on the frame.	Usually no pillow is used, or a small one may be allowed. Avoid flexion of the neck.
	The arms should be alongside the body, or supported on the armrests attached to the sides of the frame.
	The feet should be in good alignment, placed against the footboard and supported laterally.
7. Place the top covers over the patient.	These covers may have to be folded so that they do not drag on the floor. Make sure that they cause no pressure on the toes or feet.
8. Provide for the patient's comfort and care.	Universal Steps X, Y, and Z. See Appendix.
9. Move the regular hospital bed and tidy the room.	
10. Record the pertinent information on the patient's chart.	Charting example: 1015. Transferred onto the Stryker frame under the direction of Dr. Jensen. Color good. Cardinal signs stable. No complaints. P. Shaw, RN

ITEM 4.   TURNING THE PATIENT ON THE STRYKER FRAME

Important Steps	Key Points
Carry out Universal Steps A, B, C, and D. See Appendix.	
1. Check or prepare the anterior frame for use.	The anterior frame should have its three canvas sections padded and covered. There should be space at the top for the head and the forehead support, and space at the bottom for the feet.
2. Remove the top covers and restraint or safety belt.	Pull the patient's gown down over the body to avoid undue exposure.
3. Attach the anterior frame in place over the patient.	Explain to the patient what you are doing as you go along.
a. Latch or screw the ends of the frame to the basic frame.	
b. Remove the armrests and place the patient's arms along the sides of the body.	
c. Adjust the forehead support or face mask to the proper position.	

U
N
I
T
15

Important Steps	Key Points
d. Wrap the safety belts around both frames and the patient: one around the chest and the other around the thighs.	
4. Turn the patient to a prone position.	The policy in many agencies requires that two people turn the frame for the patient's safety.
a. One worker stands at the head and the other at the foot of the frame.	
b. Each worker unlocks the safety lock at each end of the frame with one hand and, with the other hand, holds the same side of the frame.	Explain to the patient and your assistant that you will be turning the frame to the right on the count of three.
c. On a signal, such as "1, 2, 3, turn," quickly and smoothly turn the frame clockwise until it locks in position.	The patient will now be facing the floor, or in the prone position. Spend a few moments talking to and reassuring him or her.
5. Remove the posterior frame.	Place the frame so that it will be out of the way and will not tip over or interfere with work in the area.
6. Adjust the patient's body alignment.	Check for alignment and for pressure, particularly around the ankles, when the patient is in the prone position.

Carry out Universal Steps X, Y, and Z. See Appendix.

Note: To turn the patient from the prone to the supine position, a procedure would be used identical to that just described except that the posterior frame would be placed over the patient, and the turn would be made in the direction preferred by the patient (the frame can turn 360 degrees).

ITEM 5. PLACING THE PATIENT ON THE BEDPAN

Important Steps	Key Points
Carry out Universal Steps A, B, C, and D. See Appendix.	
1. Place the patient in a supine position.	Both male and female patients may be able to urinate while in the prone position, but need to be in the supine position for a bowel movement. (Some women patients find it difficult to urinate while in a prone position.)
2. Put the bedpan support on the proper inserts of the basic frame and place the bedpan on the support.	When the fracture pan is used, delete steps 2 and 3 and continue with steps 4 through 6.
3. Detach the perineal support (middle canvas section) and put it out of the way to prevent soiling.	

Important Steps	Key Points
4. Clean and dry the patient's perineum after use of the bedpan.	The immobilized patient is unable to do this, so you will therefore wipe him with tissue. If the patient is soiled, use soap, water, a washcloth, and a towel to clean and dry the skin.
5. Empty and clean the bedpan, then store it for later use.	The bedpan support may be left in place for future use but should be clean.
6. Reattach the perineal section to the frame.	

Carry out Universal Steps X, Y, and Z. See Appendix.

ITEM 6. THE CIRC-O-LECTRIC BED

The Circ-O-lectric bed is an electrically operated circular frame used to turn and position a patient who has restricted or limited body movement. The turning movement is in a vertical direction rather than from side to side as in the Stryker frame. It is used for patients who have severe circulatory conditions, orthopedic problems, or other conditions requiring specific treatment.

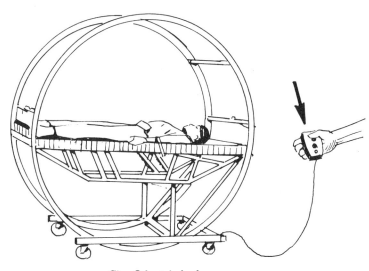

Circ-O-lectric bed.

The bed is operated by an electric motor that has hand controls and can be used by patients who are physically capable and alert. The worker can operate the bed by using a push-button on the control switch. The patient lies on a posterior frame that generally forms the diameter of the circular frame. Before the patient is turned, the anterior frame is placed over the patient's body and attached in place. The bed is then rotated forward to the "face" position until the patient is in a prone position. The posterior frame can then be raised in the frame so that it is not resting on the patient, as shown in the sketch.

U
N
I
T
15

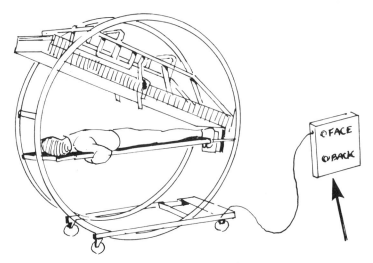

Face or prone position of Circ-O-lectric bed.

ITEM 7.   SETTING UP AND OPERATING THE CIRC-O-LECTRIC BED

Important Steps	Key Points
1. Order the Circ-O-lectric bed.	The bed is usually obtained from the storage area and delivered by the housekeeping department. The bed is set up before the patient is admitted to the room in order to lessen the number of times the patient is moved. The regular bed can be stored until it is needed.
2. Check the parts and accessories for the bed.	Follow the manufacturer's instructional manual. The parts of the Circ-O-lectric bed that should be checked are the basic frame, anterior frame, foam mattress, special sheet, safety or restraining straps, footboard attached to the frame, adjustable siderails, forehead and chin straps, and accessory parts such as traction bars, suspension, and exercise apparatus.
3. Prepare the bed.	Place the plastic cover over the posterior frame and use spring clamps to hold it in place. Place the foam mattress on the frame. (Note that the mattress has a circular section that can be removed when the bedpan is in place.) Use the special sheet that fastens to the mattress with elastic bands. Lock the wheels to stabilize the bed during the transfer.
Note: The nursing team may require practice in manipulating the bed, since it may have been some time since it was previously used.

Carry out Universal Steps A, B, and C. See Appendix.

Important Steps	Key Points
4. Transfer the patient to the Circ-O-lectric bed.	If at all possible, demonstrate the use of the bed for the patient before he or she is placed in it.
a. Move all furniture and equipment away to provide a clear path to move the patient onto the frame of the bed.	
b. Transfer the patient by using at least a three-man carry.	Three or four people will be needed for transferring the patient, and the presence of a doctor may be required.
	Use good body alignment and smooth, coordinated movements. Lift and move the patient on signal.
5. Position the patient in correct body alignment on the frame.	Follow steps 6 through 12 in Item 3 of the Stryker frame procedure.

ITEM 8.   TURNING THE PATIENT IN A CIRC-O-LECTRIC BED

Important Steps	Key Points
Carry out Universal Steps A, B, C, and D. See Appendix.	
1. Check or prepare the anterior frame for use.	Follow steps 1 through 3 in Item 4 of the Stryker frame procedure for turning patient to a prone position.
2. Remove the top covers and restraints or safety belt.	
3. Attach the anterior frame in place over the patient.	
4. Turn the patient to the prone position.	Set or press the "face" position button on the control and put the bed in motion. Turn the patient gradually and slowly to prevent vertigo and loss of consciousness.
5. Remove the posterior frame.	Release the locks on the posterior frame and push the frame upward at the head until it locks in position above the patient (see the sketch on page 300). Place the safety or restraining belts over the patient and hook them into the underside of the frame. These are used to prevent a possible fall because the siderails cannot be used in the prone position.

Carry out Universal Steps X, Y, and Z. See Appendix.

To turn the patient from the prone to the supine position, the same procedure is used except that the posterior frame is placed over the patient and secured in place and the "back" button is pressed on the control.

U
N
I
T
15

ITEM 9. USE OF THE BEDPAN IN THE CIRC-O-LECTRIC BED

Follow the same procedure as described in Item 5 for use of the bedpan on the Stryker frame except:

1. Remove the circular and metal plate and the circular mattress section under the perineal area.

2. Place the bedpan on the Evertaut fasteners so that it is held in place under the patient's buttocks.

3. The bed may be tilted slightly or the head elevated if the patient's condition permits.

4. The circular sections are replaced after the bedpan has been used.

5. Use the fracture pan for urine or bowel elimination unless it is contraindicated by the patient's condition.

ITEM 10. ADJUSTING THE POSITIONS OF THE CIRC-O-LECTRIC BED

When the patient is permitted unrestricted movements, the bed can be put in a sitting position. The hips should be centered over the point where the bed "breaks" for best body alignment when sitting.

Manual Gatching.   The posterior frame has a lever on each side within easy reach of the patient. When one or both levers are pulled, the head and foot sections adjust in relation to the amount of effort exerted to sit up when the levers are depressed. This action is similar to that of adjusting seats in a bus or an airplane. Releasing the pressure on the lever locks the posterior section to the desired degree of gatch.

Electrical Tilting.   After the bed is gatched, other positions can be obtained by tilting the bed forward or backward on the basic circular frame. When the bed is moving in the head-down position, automatic stops prevent it from going too far. The forward or "face" adjustments must be controlled by the patient or an attendant.

ITEM 11. CONCLUSION OF THE UNIT

You have now completed the lesson on the operation of patient turning frames. After you have had sufficient practice with the equipment to become familiar with it and learned some skills in performing the procedures, you should arrange with your instructor to take the performance test.

PERFORMANCE TEST

In your classroom or the skill laboratory, your instructor will ask you to perform the following skills accurately without any use of reference or source materials. You may need the assistance of other students in the procedures, and you may use the mannequin (Mrs. Chase) or another student to play the part of the patient.

1. Given a patient who is quadriplegic and paralyzed from the neck down, set up a Stryker frame and assist in transferring onto the frame so that the transfer is achieved safely and without injury to the patient or the workers.

2. Given a patient who had had spinal surgery and who is lying in a supine position on a Stryker frame, turn to a prone position.

3. Given a patient in a Circ-O-lectric bed, turn from a supine (back position) to a prone position and align the body properly. (If a Circ-O-lectric bed is not available for your use, describe the steps of the procedure to your instructor.)

PERFORMANCE CHECKLIST

SET UP AND TRANSFER A PATIENT TO A STRYKER FRAME

1. Obtain a Stryker frame.

2. Prepare the posterior frame.

   a. Measure and attach the upper, middle, and lower canvas sections to the frame.

   b. Place the sponge pads on the sections and cover them with linen so that all the ends are secure.

   c. Place the posterior frame on the basic frame.

   d. Attach the footboard.

3. Take the frame to the patient's unit.

4. Wash your hands.

5. Approach and identify the patient and explain the reasons for using the Stryker frame.

6. Obtain assistance to help transfer the patient.

7. Lock the wheels of the frame so that it will not move.

8. Clear the furniture and equipment away between the bed and frame.

9. Put a bath blanket or sheet over the patient during the transfer.

10. Use at least a three-man carry, lift on signal, and move the patient to the frame.

11. Position the patient in good alignment on the frame.

12. Replace the top covers on the patient.

13. Provide for the patient's comfort by giving him the signal cord and so forth.

14. Tidy the room.

15. Record the pertinent information on the patient's chart.

TURNING A PATIENT TO PRONE POSITION ON STRYKER FRAME

1. Wash your hands.

2. Approach, identify the patient, and explain what is going to be done.

3. Provide for the patient's privacy by pulling the curtains.

4. Check or prepare the anterior frame for use.

   a. Provide space for the patient's face.

   b. Provide support for the patient's forehead.

   c. Provide space for the bottom of the frame and the patient's feet.

5. Remove the top covers and the safety restraint and smooth down the patient's gown.

6. Place the anterior frame correctly over the patient's body.

7. Secure the ends of the frame to the basic frame.

8. Remove the arm supports if these have been used.

9. Apply at least two safety belts — one around the chest, another around the thighs; secure them snugly.

10. Have an assistant help to turn patient.

    a. One worker stands at the head and the other at the foot.

    b. Unlock the safety locks with one hand, hold the frame with the other.

    c. Both persons must turn in a clockwise direction smoothly until the frame is locked in place.

11. Remove the posterior frame.

12. Adjust the alignment of the patient's body.

13. Provide for the patient's comfort; leave the call signal within reach, and so forth.

14. Report or record the turning procedure.

TURNING AND ALIGNING THE PATIENT IN THE CIRC-O-LECTRIC BED IN THE PRONE POSITION

1. Wash your hands.

2. Approach and identify the patient and explain what is going to be done.

3. Provide for the patient's privacy by pulling the curtain and closing the door.

4. Check or prepare the anterior frame for use.

   a. Provide space for the patient's face.

   b. Provide support for the patient's forehead.

   c. Provide space for the patient's feet at the bottom of the frame.

5. Remove top covers and the safety restraint and smooth down the patient's gown.

6. Add the necessary padding for maximum body support.

7. Place the anterior frame correctly over the patient's body.

8. Secure the ends of the frame to the basic circular frame.

9. Apply safety belts and secure them snugly around the patient and both frames.

10. Turn the patient slowly by pressing the "face" button on the control.

11. Remove the posterior frame by pushing the head end up until it is locked in place on the frame.

12. Adjust alignment of the patient's body.

13. Provide for the patient's comfort, leave the call signal in reach, and so forth.

14. Report or record the turning procedure.

POST-TEST

Directions: Select the one best answer for each of the following.

1. Turning frames are used in the treatment of patients for all of the following reasons except

   a. to relieve pressure on parts of the body.

   b. to increase circulation to the back.

   c. to decrease the respiratory rate.

   d. to immobilize a part so healing can occur.

2. The patient's needs for nursing care should be based on consideration of the whole patient. These needs include all of the following except

   a. encouragement to use intellectual abilities.

   b. assurance that safety and protection needs are met.

   c. dependence on others for assistance.

   d. decisions made by others as to what to eat, when to sleep, and so forth.

3. The Stryker frame consists of all of the following parts except

   a. a canvas-covered frame for the patient to lie on.

   b. a second canvas frame placed on top of the patient.

   c. safety belts used to keep the patient securely in place.

   d. a metal frame that is attached securely to the wall.

4. When you transfer a patient from the bed to a turning frame, all of the following principles apply except for

   a. two people are needed to make the transfer.

   b. a physician may be required to be present.

   c. the patient is lifted and moved on a signal.

   d. at least three or four people are needed.

5. The most important safety measure to be taken when the patient is on a turning frame is

   a. taping the stop latch down for easier turning.

   b. keeping a restraint around the patient and the frame at all times.

   c. keeping the perineal section in place to support the sacrum.

   d. teaching the family and other visitors how to turn the frame.

6. The number of people required to turn the patient from the supine to the prone position on a Stryker frame is

   a. four.

   b. three.

   c. two.

   d. one.

7. Turning the patient on the Circ-O-Lectric bed from a supine to a prone position is done slowly and gradually to prevent

   a. nausea and vomiting.

   b. loss of bladder control.

   c. dizziness and loss of consciousness.

   d. distention of the abdomen.

8. The nurse provides for the patient's safety when turning the patient on the Stryker frame or the Circ-O-Lectric bed by following all of these steps except

   a. work rapidly in order to reduce the patient's apprehension.

   b. place safety straps around the patient and the frame.

   c. obtain assistance from another worker to help turn the frame.

   d. turn the patient on the frame on a signal.

POST-TEST ANSWERS

1. c   5. b

2. d   6. c

3. d   7. c

4. a   8. a

Section 3

SKILLS RELATED TO
PATIENT HYGIENE

INTRODUCTION

Patients who have limitations of movement due to their condition or to their medical therapy are often unable to perform all the activities of daily living. They rely on the nurse to bathe them, brush their teeth, and provide other related physical care that promotes health and cleanliness.

Although you have been able to dress yourself from an early age, it is a little more difficult trying to dress or undress a sick person lying in bed, or one who is unable to move about freely. Unit 16 describes various types of garments and efficient ways of dressing the patient. Procedures in Unit 17 describe how to perform A.M. and P.M. care, oral hygiene, back rubs, and the various types of baths. The bath time provides a special opportunity for nurses to assess their patients needs, observe the condition of the skin closely, and meet psychosocial needs of patients as well as merely cleansing the skin. The special attention given to the skin of the patients who have pressure areas, a cast, traction, or a colostomy or those who are incontinent is described in Unit 18. The methods of caring for hair, braiding, giving a shampoo, and the special care of extremely dry hair that many black patients have are dealt with in Unit 19, while Unit 20 provides information about perineal care for male and female patients.

DIRECTIONS FOR STUDENTS

The recommended approach for studying the units in this section is the same as that for Section 2. Read the objectives carefully to learn what you are expected to do, then review the words listed in the vocabulary. Proceed to study the items covered and read through the steps of the procedures and the accompanying key points. The first procedure in each chapter states each of the universal steps at the beginning and end of it, but the following procedures simply tell you to carry out the universal steps and then proceed with the steps of that procedure.

An essential part of your study of procedures is the practice period in the skills laboratory. During these sessions, practice your communication skills too. When working with a student partner who plays the role of the patient, greet your patient and give an explanation of what you plan to do. Ask yourself these questions: How much information is needed? Did the patient understand the words I used and what I tried to say? What should I talk about as I carry out the procedures? How do I communicate to patients that I am concerned about their welfare and about them as individuals? Think of what it would be like to be the patient and have a total stranger come in to give you a bath and not say a word or chatter constantly about personal problems.

When you feel that you can perform the skills accurately and completely, make arrangements with your instructor to take the Performance Test to demonstrate your ability to carry out the procedures. The written Post-Test will help you test your understanding of the rationale for the actions and the principles related to the procedures.

SELECTED REFERENCES

Unit 17: Baths and Back Rub

Bruya, Margaret A., and Madeira, Nancy P.: Stomatitis following chemotherapy. Am J Nurs 75:1349–1352 (August) 1975.
Gannon, Elizabeth P., and Kadezabek, Elizabeth: Giving your patients meticulous mouth care. Nursing 80 10:70–75 (March) 1980.
Howath, Helen: Mouth care procedure for the very ill. Nurs Times 73:354, 1977.
Michelsen, Dana: How to give a good back rub. Am J Nurs 78:1197–1199 (July) 1978.
Murray, Malinda: Fundamentals of Nursing. 2nd ed. Englewood Cliffs, NJ: Prentice-Hall, Inc., 1980.
Reitz, Marie, and Pope, Wilma: Mouth care. Am J Nurs 73:1728–1730, 1973.

Unit 18: Special Skin Care

Black skin problems. Am J Nurs 79:1092–1094 (June) 1979.
Brown, Sandy: Orthopedic nursing, part 1: Easing the burden of traction and casts. RN (February) 1975, pp. 36–41.
Gruis, Marcia, and Innes, Barbara: Assessment: Essential to prevent pressure sores. Am J Nurs 76:1762 (November) 1976.
Roach, Lora B.: Assessing skin changes: The subtle and the obvious. Nursing 74 4:64–67 (April) 1974.
Uhler, Diana: Common skin changes in the elderly. Am J Nurs 78:1342–1343 (August) 1978.

Unit 19: Special Hair Care

Davis, Mardell: Getting to the root of the problem: Hair-grooming techniques for black patients. Nursing 77 7:60–65 (April) 1977.
Grier, Marian: Hair care for the black patient. Am J Nurs 76:1781 (November) 1976.

DRESSING
AND UNDRESSING

GENERAL PERFORMANCE OBJECTIVE

You will be able to provide partial or total assistance, when needed by a patient, of any age, ranging from the newborn to the elderly in putting on or removing articles of clothing. You will provide assistance regardless of the physical or mental condition of the patient, and without causing additional discomfort or distress.

SPECIFIC PERFORMANCE OBJECTIVES

You will be able to:

1. Assess the patient's physical ability and willingness to dress or undress and your own ability or limitations in this aspect of the patient's care.

2. Demonstrate your regard for articles of clothing as the property of the patient or the hospital by carefully and neatly storing items not in use and by not cutting, tearing, or causing other damage to clothing.

3. Provide total assistance in removing the soiled gown of an adult bed patient and dressing him or her in a clean gown or pajamas in 5 minutes or less.

4. Provide partial assistance to the patient when removing the hospital gown and assist to dress patient in undergarments, street clothing, and shoes in 10 minutes or less.

5. Assist the patient to put on and remove robe and slippers.

6. Remove soiled gown from a patient who has an IV running and dress in a clean gown.

VOCABULARY

You will need to learn or review the meaning of the following words used in this lesson.

brain impairment—decreased function of the brain, damage to all or a part of the brain from any cause, e.g., mental retardation, tumor, injury, stroke.
distal—further away; the most distant.
maturation—the gradual process of growth, development, and integration of body structures.
mental retardation—the slower than normal development and maturation of the brain's intellectual functions.
monitoring device—a mechanical appliance that detects or measures one or more of the body functions, such as the vital signs of the heart action, respiratory rate, blood pressure, and temperature.
postoperative—happening or done following a surgical operation; commonly called "post-op."

preoperative—happening or done immediately before surgery.

proximal—the near side; closest.

stroke—a sudden, severe attack; usually refers to an accident in the circulatory system in the brain; also may be called apoplexy or cerebral hemorrhage.

ASSISTING WITH CLOTHING NEEDS

ITEM 1. WHY PATIENTS NEED HELP DRESSING AND UNDRESSING

Does it seem a little unusual to have a lesson on helping the patient to dress and undress? Didn't everyone learn how to put on and take off clothing as a young child? You have been doing this for so many years that it may seem like a simple procedure. As a young child learning to dress yourself, however, you had to practice how to get your arms into sleeves, how to fasten buttons, and how to tie your shoelaces. You had to learn all of the body movements that are involved in the process of dressing or undressing. You no longer consciously think of the movements that you perform in the process of dressing *except* where there is interference or restriction of your freedom of movement. Then dressing or undressing becomes complicated for you. And so it is with the patient.

Your help will be needed to dress or undress the infant or young child who has not reached the maturation level necessary to know and coordinate all the movements required in dressing. The older child or adult patient may need your assistance when movements are restricted as a result of illness or the type of treatment being received.

Your knowledge of how to help the patient dress or undress and your skill in performance will have an effect on the patient. The manner in which you assist may increase or decrease the patient's feelings of comfort, pain, trust, fear, confidence, acceptance, or rejection. By the time you complete this lesson, you should be able to recognize ways of helping the patient emotionally as well as assisting him to change clothing.

ITEM 2. LIMITATIONS OF BODY MOVEMENT

Physical Factors. Various conditions tend to limit movement. The patient's ability to perform movements required in dressing or undressing may be limited by one or more of the following conditions:

1. Lack of maturation, as in the case of infants and small children.

2. Brain impairment, as in mental retardation, injury, or coma.

3. Weakness.

4. Pain from any cause, such as disease or surgery.

5. Fractures.

6. Contractures.

7. Paralysis.

8. Special appliances or equipment, such as IV's, casts, braces, or monitoring devices.

9. Absence of a portion of a limb.

10. Lack of vision.

Psychological Factors. Some people may refuse to move or help themselves even when there seems to be no physical reason to limit their movement. Those who are unable or unwilling to move or dress and undress themselves will also need help and assistance from the health worker.

Psychological factors that may restrict movement include the fear of pain, discomfort, or possible harm resulting from the movement. The post-op patient is often afraid that moving will tear loose the sutures in the incision or dislodge the IV needle from a vein. Others may dislike being told what to do or being required to do something they feel is unnecessary. People who feel depressed or "blue," grief-stricken, worried, or tense often find it difficult to make decisions, even one as simple as to get out of bed and put on their clothes.

ITEM 3. CLASSIFICATION OF ARTICLES OF CLOTHING

Most of the clothing that we wear can be classified into several basic types. Although the styles may differ, each type requires similar movements in order to put on or remove the garment. The clothing you will be handling while assisting patients to dress and undress falls into these basic groups:

• cardigan-type — completely open from the neck to the lower edge in front or in back of the garment; examples are hospital gown, shirt, blouse, sweater, coat, jacket, vest, robe, pajama coat, and bra.

• Pullover-type — has a short or incomplete opening in the front, side, or back of the garment; examples include placket style of shirt, sweater, blouse, dress, skirt, slip, undershirt, and pajama top.

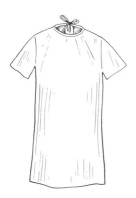

Typical hospital gown is cardigan-type garment with back opening. Gown is between knee and mid-thigh in length.

• pants-type — pulled up over the lower extremities and the hips, for example, trousers, slacks, shorts, pajama bottoms, panty girdle, and panty hose.

• diapers — similar to pants, but pinned or adjusted to fit around the hips.

• shoes and stockings — includes elastic hose.

• accessories — items such as belts, ties, hats, suspenders, and purses.

Loose-fitting clothing of the cardigan type is the easiest to put on the person who needs help in dressing.

ITEM 4. SOME GENERAL GUIDELINES

Clothing as Personal Property. The health worker should regard all clothing as the property of others, whether it belongs to the patient or to the hospital. Avoid cutting, tearing, or otherwise damaging it unless absolutely necessary. Even when the clothing appears worn and out of style, it should not be discarded because its replacement may cause a financial hardship to the owner.

Care of Clothing. Hospitals provide gowns and pajamas as part of the linen supply. These items can be obtained from the linen room or the linen cart. When soiled, they must be put into the soiled linen hampers; they are then laundered with the rest of the hospital linens.

Personal clothing belonging to the patient is usually stored in the patient unit. It should be neatly folded or hung on hangers in the closet. Soiled clothing should be set aside to be cleaned by the family. Soiled garments belonging to patients are not usually laundered by health workers; however, when the hospital provides for the cleaning of patients' clothing, follow the procedure for handling this responsibility.

Dressing an Affected Extremity. The patient who has limited movement in one or more extremities (either arms or legs) generally needs help to dress and undress. Select cardigan-type clothing or a pull-on garment with the largest possible opening. Pants-type clothing should be loose and easy to pull on.

When assisting the person to dress, start by putting the garment on the affected arm or leg; then slip on the rest of the garment. When undressing the patient, remove clothing from the unaffected limbs first, and then from the immobilized extremity. As described, the rule for the affected limb is to dress it first and to undress it last.

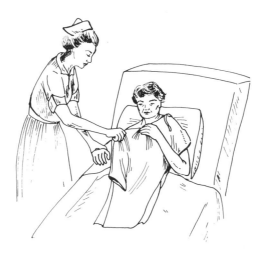

Diapering Practices. Many unthinking health workers have made it a practice to put diapers on adult or elderly patients who have lost control of their bowels or bladder. This is a practice that should be avoided. It does not remedy the patient's loss of control, but only serves to create more complex problems. Treating the older patient as an infant lowers self-esteem, the urine or feces in the diaper irritate the skin, and the diaper itself indicates lack of rehabilitation outlook on the part of the health worker.

You will learn more about the rehabilitation aspects of this problem in the units on elimination. Meanwhile, diapers are to be used solely for infants and young children who have not yet achieved control of bowel and bladder.

ITEM 5. CHANGING THE HOSPITAL GOWN

The hospital gown is an example of the cardigan type of garment that is open down the back.

In the skill laboratory, practice dressing and undressing the patient. One of your fellow students can play the role of the patient who needs help in dressing.

Given a helpless patient whose hospital gown has become wet, remove the soiled gown and replace it with a clean one in 5 minute or less.

Supplies Needed

Clean patient gown

Important Steps	Key Points
1. Wash your hands and obtain a clean hospital gown.	Universal Steps A, B, C, and D. See Appendix.
2. Approach and identify the patient.	
3. Provide for privacy.	
4. Position the patient.	Move the patient to the proximal (near) side of the bed. If the bed is an adjustable high-low type, it should be in the high position with the siderail lowered on the side of the bed on which you are working.
5. Avoid undue exposure of the patient's body.	Fold the top covers of the bed back to the patient's waist. Exposure of more of the body may cause chilling or may offend the patient's sense of modesty.
6. Untie or unfasten the gown and slip it off the patient's body.	With one of your hands, reach under the patient's neck, pull the neck fastening to one side, and unfasten. Free the sides of the gown from under the patient, and slip the arms out of the sleeves. Fold the top portion of the gown down to cover the chest.
7. Clean or dry the patient's body as needed.	Use a washcloth and towel to clean and dry the skin before putting on a clean gown.
8. Put a clean hospital gown on the patient.	Slip the patient's arms into the sleeves one at a time and pull the gown up over the shoulders. Reach under the patient's neck, grasp the other edge of the gown and tie, draw the tie through, and fasten or tie at the side of the neck. Smooth the gown over the shoulders, and down over the body.
9. Remove the used or soiled gown.	Reach under the clean gown and remove the soiled gown from the patient's chest. Place it in the linen hamper.
10. Provide for the patient's comfort.	Universal Steps X, Y, and Z. See Appendix.
11. Record and report.	

UNIT
16

ITEM 6. CHANGING A GOWN FOR A PATIENT WITH AN IV

You will find that many patients have restricted movement in one or both arms due to an IV running in a vein of the arm, to paralysis of the arm following a stroke, or to a cast applied to immobilize a fractured bone. Some hospitals provide a special IV gown for such patients, a cardigan type with a back opening and sleeves open from the neckline to the lower edge. Each sleeve can be closed with Velcro fasteners or ties. It is a simple matter to remove this type of gown and replace it with a clean one. However, it is frequently necessary to change the regular style of hospital gown or pajama top for a patient who is receiving an IV; this garment should be removed from the unaffected arm first, thereby allowing the patient more freedom of movement and better manipulation of the garment, which makes it easier to remove from the affected arm.

In the skill laboratory, given a patient with an IV running in one arm, remove the soiled hospital gown and put a clean one on, using a regular gown.

Supplies Needed

Clean patient gown

Important Steps	Key Points
Carry out Universal Steps, A, B, C, and D. See Appendix.	
1. Remove the soiled gown from the unaffected arm.	Untie or unfasten the soiled gown and slip it off the patient's unaffected arm.
2. Remove gown from affected arm by passing IV tubing and bottle through the sleeve.	Slide the sleeve down the affected arm, past the needle, and onto the tubing. Support the arm and tubing to avoid dislodging the IV needle. Now, slide the gown along the tubing, remove the bottle of fluids from the IV stand (holding it higher than the level of the arm to keep the blood in the vein from running into the tubing) and slip the gown over the bottle. Hang the bottle on the IV stand.

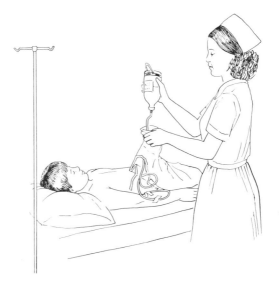

IV bottle and tubing are passed through the sleeve to remove soiled gown and to put on clean gown.

Important Steps	Key Points
3. Pass IV bottle and tubing through the sleeve of clean gown for affected arm.	Make sure that the IV is passed through the correct sleeve. Pass the IV bottle and tubing along the inside of the gown and through the sleeve. *Reverse* the procedure used in Step 2 and observe the same precautions. Fasten the gown at the neck and smooth it down over the body.
4. Put gown on the unaffected arm and tie.	

Carry out Universal Steps X, Y, and Z. See Appendix.

ITEM 7. ASSISTING THE PATIENT WITH ROBE AND SLIPPERS

In the skill laboratory, assist the patient to put on robe and slippers before getting out of bed to sit in a chair and, later, to remove the garments when returning to bed.

Supplies Needed

Patient's robe and slippers

Important Steps	Key Points

Universal Steps A, B, C, and D. See Appendix.

Important Steps	Key Points
1. Position the patient.	Adjust the bed to the low position for the patient's safety. Help to sit on the side of the bed and dangle legs. (For the helpless patient, keep the bed in a high position and the patient lying supine.)
2. Help the patient put on the robe.	Slip one arm into the sleeve, place the robe around the back, and guide the other arm into the other sleeve. Fasten the buttons and tie the belt if needed. For a helpless patient or a small child, run your hand through the proper sleeve of the garment, clasp the patient's wrist, and pull the arm through the sleeve. Put the robe over the back, roll the patient to the other side, and then pull the garment toward you. (Repeat the above procedure to put the other arm into the remaining sleeve.)

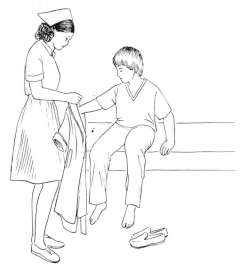

Assisting patient with slippers and robe.

U
N
I
T
16

Important Steps	Key Points
3. Assist the patient to put on slippers.	While the patient dangles his feet on the side of the bed, stoop down, using good body movements. Support the pateint's ankle and slide the slipper over the toes, foot, and heel. Make sure the toes are not curled under the foot inside the shoe, especially when the patient is a small child or an aged person. Finally, have the patient stand in order to position the foot better in the slipper or shoe.
4. Provide for the patient's comfort.	Help patient to stand up and straighten the robe. When patient is sitting in a chair, provide with a pillow, personal articles such as a comb or brush, or diversional items such as a newspaper or book.
5. When helping patient back to bed, remove the robe and slippers.	Stand the patient at the side of the bed, if patient is able to do so. Loosen the belt and unfasten the buttons. Pull the sleeve off one arm, slip the robe off the back, and then remove it from the other arm. While patient is sitting on the side of the bed, remove both slippers.

Carry out Universal Steps X, Y, and Z. See Appendix.

ITEM 8.   ASSISTING WITH PULLOVER GARMENTS

Pull-on garments include undershirts, sweaters, blouses, dresses, and skirts, many of which are pulled on or off over the head. The key points are described for the neck-opening type of pull-on garment.

Important Steps	Key Points

Undressing

1. Unfasten neck opening.

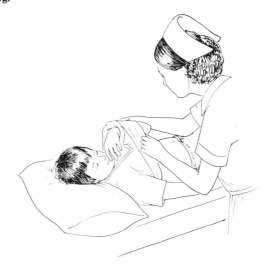

Assisting patient to remove a
pullover type of garment.

Important Steps	Key Points
2. Gather body of garment up to the level of the arms.	Ease garment down over the distal shoulder.
3. Remove garment from distal arm.	Grasp the sheeve at the lower edge, support the patient's arm, and remove the sleeve.
4. Remove garment from proximal arm.	Repeat the above to remove garment from the proximal arm.
5. Slip body of garment over the head.	Gather the front of the garment from hem to neckline and slip it smoothly over the head, reassuring the patient during the time the head is covered.
6. Remove the garment.	Support the patient's head and neck with one hand, reach under the neck with the other hand, grasp the garment, and remove it.

Dressing

IIIIIIIIIIIIIIIIIIIIIIIIIIIIIIIIIIIIIIIIIIIIIIIIIIIIIIIIIIIIIIIIIIIIIIIIIIIIIIIIIIIIIIIIIIIIIIIIIIIIIIIIIIIIIIIIIIIIIIIIIIIIIIIII

Supplies Needed

Pullover type of garment

IIIIIIIIIIIIIIIIIIIIIIIIIIIIIIIIIIIIIIIIIIIIIIIIIIIIIIIIIIIIIIIIIIIIIIIIIIIIIIIIIIIIIIIIIIIIIIIIIIIIIIIIIIIIIIIIIIIIIIIIIIIIIIIII

Important Steps	Key Points
1. Unfasten the neck opening.	
2. Put distal arm through sleeve.	Put your hand through the proper sleeve of the garment, clasp the patient's distal wrist, and pull it through the sleeve.
3. Put proximal arm through sleeve.	Repeat as above for the patient's proximal arm.
4. Slide the garment over the head.	Pull the garment up toward the shoulders. Gather the back of the garment from hem to neck in your hand, and with the other hand, stretch or shape the neck opening. Have the patient raise arms — or assist by pulling the garment up — and slide the neck opening smoothly over the head. Reassure the patient during the short time the head is covered.
5. Smooth garment over body.	
6. Fasten neck opening, if present.	

UNIT 16

ITEM 9.   ASSISTING WITH PANTS-TYPE GARMENTS

Both male and females wear a variety of pants-type garments, and pajamas are especially popular apparel for hospital patients. As a health worker, you need to know how to assist the patient with this type of garment. This section describes how to dress and undress the male patient in pajama pants.

Important Steps	Key Points

Undressing

1. Unfasten the pants closing.

Place a sheet or drape over the patient's lower abdomen and thighs.

2. Slide pants down over the buttocks.

Have the patient raise the buttocks and, with your hands at each side of the pants, slip them down over the buttocks to the thighs.

3. Pull the pants down over the ankles and feet.

Pull each pant leg down over the thighs and legs toward the ankles. Supporting the ankle with one hand, pull the pant leg off the foot, and repeat this step for the other foot.

4. Remove the pants.

Dressing

||||||||||||||||||||||||||||||||||||||||||||||||||||||||||||||||||||||||||||||||||||||||||||||||||||||

Supplies Needed

Pair of pants

||||||||||||||||||||||||||||||||||||||||||||||||||||||||||||||||||||||||||||||||||||||||||||||||||||||

Important Steps	Key Points

1. Position the patient.

Free the top coverings from the foot of the bed and fold them back to the patient's knees. Top sheet or blanket serves to drape patient and avoid undue exposure when putting on garments such as pajama pants. Position the patient on the proximal side of the bed so that his feet and legs can be reached without stretching.

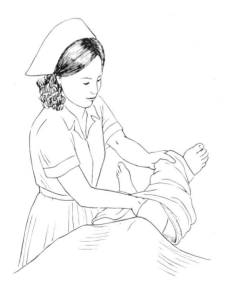

Top sheet or blanket serves to drape patient and avoid undue exposure when putting on garments such as pajama pants.

2. Put the distal foot through the pants leg.

Gather most of the pant leg of the garment in one hand, clasp the patient's distal ankle with the other hand, and guide the foot through the pant leg.

Important Steps	Key Points
3. Put the proximal foot through the pants legs.	Repeat the action just described for the other foot.
4. Pull pants up over the buttocks.	Have the patient raise the buttocks while you grasp the pants on each side, and pull them up to the waist.
5. Fasten the pants, if necessary.	

ITEM 10. USE OF DIAPERS

Diapers are used to collect the urine and stool eliminated by infants and small children who have not established control of their bowels or bladders. The diaper should be changed promptly when it is soiled. Prolonged contact of the wet, soiled diaper with the baby's tender skin can cause an irritation or diaper rash.

The use of disposable diapers has become increasingly popular in recent years. These diapers are prefolded and absorbent and are thrown away following use. Many have an adhesive tape fastening, which eliminates the need for safety pins. Reusable cloth diapers, however, are the most economical type. Large squares or rectangles of soft, absorbent material such as flannel or muslin are used to make the diapers. The material is then folded to fit the baby.

Many mothers use a rubber or plastic panty over the baby's diaper to protect other clothing and the bed linen from getting wet or soiled. You will recall, however, that bacteria thrive in warm, damp places, so it is important to keep the baby clean and dry when the plastic panties are worn.

Folding the Diaper. Disposable diapers are prefolded, but most reusable cloth diapers must be folded to fit the baby's lower trunk. The layers of absorbent material are usually folded in the shape of a rectangle or a modified triangle. Any excess material is folded inward to provide layers of extra absorbency. To adjust the fit and decrease the width of the diaper between the baby's legs, fold the sides inward.

For male babies and those infants who are placed on their stomachs to sleep, fold the excess material over in the front. For baby girls, the extra length of the diaper is folded down in the back of the diaper.

a. Disposable diaper with sealing tabs.

b. Modified triangular diaper.

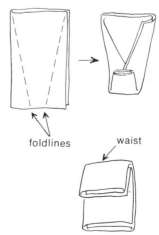

foldlines   waist

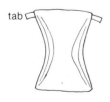

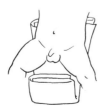

c. Extra-absorbent layers in front of diaper.

d. Folding diaper to provide extra layers at the back.

Methods of folding baby diapers.

Guidelines for Care of Infants.　When you are providing general care for infants, such as dressing, diapering, or bathing, there are several guidelines you should follow:

1. Do not leave the baby unattended. Raise the sides of the crib or carry the baby with you if you need to get other articles.

2. Close safety pins and keep out of the reach of the body. When using safety pins, place your hand under the area being pinned so that the baby will not be pricked or jabbed.

3. When dressing infants in shirts, sweaters, and other clothing, follow the steps of the procedures given in the preceding items for cardigan, pullover, and pants types of clothes.

Changing Diaper of an Infant

Supplies Needed

Diaper
Wash cloth and towel for cleansing
Powder, if used

Important Steps	Key Points
1. Position the baby.	Place the baby in a supine position on a flat, padded surface, such as bassinet, crib, or bed.
2. Unfasten the diaper at both sides.	Draw the front downward.
3. Raise the baby's buttocks and remove the soiled diaper.	Grasp the baby's ankles with one hand and raise the buttocks or roll the baby to one side. With the other hand, use the dry, clean portion of the diaper to gently wipe the urine and feces from the skin. Fold the diaper inward and remove.
4. Clean and dry the perineal area.	Clean the skin with a moistened washcloth and pat dry.
5. Put on clean diaper.	Lay a fresh folded diaper on a smooth surface. Place the baby on the diaper with the back edge at his waist level. Draw the front portion of the diaper between the baby's legs and up to the waist. 　　An alternative method is to grasp the baby's ankles with one hand, raise the buttocks, and with the other hand position the diaper underneath.
6. Fasten the diaper securely.	Fasten or pin the diaper securely at each side so that it fits snugly at the waist and thigh.

ITEM 11.　ASSISTING WITH ELASTIC STOCKINGS

Many patients in the hospital who have medical or surgical conditions are required to wear elastic stockings to prevent circulatory complications. Some brand names of these stocking include T.E.D. hose and the Jobst stocking. The stockings are generally removed during the bath so that the patient's legs and feet can be washed; they are reapplied before getting out of bed. The following method will help you avoid unnecessary struggling when putting elastic stockings on the patient.

Important Steps	Key Points
Remove the stockings.	Roll or pull the stocking down the leg to the ankle. Support the ankle with your hand and pull the stocking down over the heel and foot and off the toes. Repeat this procedure to remove the other stocking.
Put on the stockings.	Turn the leg part of the stocking inside out to the ankle portion just above the heel. Slip the foot portion of the stocking over the toes, foot, and onto the heel. Pull the everted leg portion of the stocking smoothly over the leg, avoiding wrinkles or folds in the elastic stockings. Ordinarily, garters are not used with elastic stockings but may be necessary with women's midthigh-length stockings.

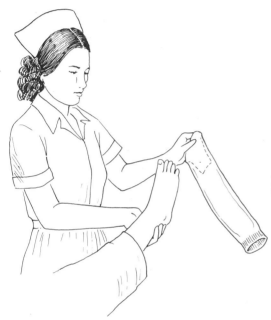

Elastic stocking is slipped on foot more easily by everting (turning inside out) leg of stocking down to foot part.

ITEM 12. CONCLUSION OF THE LESSON

You have completed the lesson on dressing and undressing the patient. After you have practiced the procedures to gain initial skills in assisting the patient to dress and undress, make an appointment with your instructor to take the performance test and demonstrate these skills. The performance test instructions follow.

U
N
I
T
16

PERFORMANCE TEST

In a performance testing situation in the skill laboratory, demonstrate dressing or undressing the patient by performing the following activities without reference to any source material.

1. In 5 minutes or less, give total assistance to a helpless patient by removing a hospital gown and replacing it with a clean one. Identify the conditions that limit the patient's movement.

2. Remove the soiled hospital gown from a patient receiving an IV and dress in a clean gown without disturbing the IV.

3. Give assistance as needed to the patient in putting on a robe and shoes or slippers preparatory to getting out of bed.

4. In 10 minutes or less, assist a newly admitted patient to remove street clothing and dress in a hospital gown or pajamas.

PERFORMANCE CHECKLIST

CHANGING THE HOSPITAL GOWN IN 5 MINUTES

1. Wash your hands.

2. Obtain the clean gown.

3. Approach and identify the patient.

4. Explain the procedure to the patient.

5. Place the patient on the proximal side of the bed in supine position, with the bed in the high position.

6. Fold back the top bed covers to the patient's waist.

7. Untie the gown, slip patient's arms out of gown, and fold it down over chest.

8. Clean and dry the patient's body as needed.

9. Take the clean gown and slip the patient's arms into the sleeves.

10. Pull the gown over the shoulders and tie at the side of the neck.

11. Smooth the gown over the shoulders and down the body.

12. Remove the soiled gown and put it into the linen hamper.

13. Provide for the patient's comfort by adjusting the linen, positioning in good alignment, and placing the bed in the low position.

14. Record and report as appropriate.

CHANGING THE GOWN OF THE PATIENT WITH AN IV

1. Wash your hands.

2. Obtain the clean gown.

3. Approach and identify the patient.

4. Explain the procedure to the patient.

5. Place the patient on the proximal side of the bed in a supine position, with the bed in the high position.

6. Fold back the top bed covers to the level of the patient's waist.

7. Untie the gown and slip the sleeve off the unaffected arm.

8. Remove the garment from the arm with IV running in it (affected extremity).

 a. Carefully slide the sleeve of the gown down the arm onto the tubing.

 b. Support the arm and tubing while removing the gown.

 c. Slide the gown along tubing and remove the IV bottle from the holder.

 d. Keep IV bottle above the level of the needle and slip the gown over the bottle; remove gown.

 e. Replace the bottle on the IV stand.

9. Put a clean gown on the patient by starting with the affected extremity.

 a. Remove the bottle from the IV stand.

 b. Slide the gown and the proper sleeve over the bottle.

 c. Replace the bottle on the IV stand and slide the gown over the IV tubing and the affected arm.

 d. Carefully support the arm and tubing during this step.

10. Slip unaffected arm into the other sleeve, pull the gown over the shoulders, and tie it at the neck.

11. Smooth the gown over the shoulders and down over the body.

12. Put the soiled gown into the linen hamper.

13. Provide for the patient's comfort by adjusting the linen, positioning in good alignment, and placing the bed in the low position.

14. Record and report as appropriate.

ASSISTING THE PATIENT WITH ROBE AND SLIPPERS

1. Approach and identify the patient.

2. Get the patient's robe and slippers.

3. Provide for privacy.

4. Position the patient, put the bed in the low position, and assist to dangle legs at the side of the bed.

5. Assist patient to put on the robe by slipping one arm into the proper sleeve, placing the robe over the back, and guiding the other arm into the other sleeve.

6. Stoop down and assist the patient to put on slippers.

7. Assist the patient to stand; adjust and button robe and tie the belt.

8. Provide for the patient's comfort while patient is sitting in a chair.

UNIT
16

9. Help return to the bed by removing robe and slippers.

    a. Have patient stand at the side of the bed if able.

    b. Unfasten and untie the belt of the robe.

    c. Slip the sleeve off one arm, slide the robe off back, and remove the other arm from its sleeve.

    d. Have the patient sit on the side of the bed; remove slippers.

10. Put the robe and slippers away in the proper place.

11. Record or report as appropriate.

ASSISTING THE PATIENT TO UNDRESS AND PUT ON HOSPITAL GOWN IN 10 MINUTES OR LESS

1. Approach and identify the patient; explain the procedure.

2. Obtain a hospital gown if not supplied in the admission pack.

3. Provide privacy.

4. Position the patient, either sitting on the side of the bed or lying down.

5. Remove shoes and stockings.

    a. Untie any shoelaces, supporting the ankle with one hand and sliding the shoe off the heel, foot, and toes with the other.

    b. Unfasten the stockings from their garters (if used), slide the stocking down the leg and over the heel, foot, and toes; remove.

6. Remove cardigan-type garments like coats, jackets, shirts, sweaters, blouses, dresses, or bras.

    a. Unbutton or open any fastenings.

    b. Slip the patient's arms out of the garment and remove it. If the patient is in the supine position, remove the garment from one arm, roll the patient to the distal side, tuck the freed portion of the garment along the side, roll the patient back, reach under the side for the garment, and remove it from the patient's other arm.

7. Take off pullover garments such as shirts, sweaters, blouses, skirts, or dresses. (Skirts are usually removed like pants.)

    a. Unbutton or open the neck or side fastenings.

    b. Gather the body of the garment up to the patient's arms.

    c. Remove the sleeve from one arm, then take off the other sleeve.

    d. Gather the front of the garment from the hem to the neckline and slip it smoothly over the patient's head.

    e. Remove the garment.

8. Put the hospital gown on the patient, avoiding unnecessary exposure of the body.

    a. Slip the patient's arms into the sleeves.

    b. Pull the gown over the shoulders and tie at the neck.

    c. Smooth the gown down over the body.

9. Remove the pants-type garments such as trousers, shorts, and panties.

    a. Loosen or open any fastenings.

    b. Have the patient raise the buttocks, if able, and slide the pants down over the hips.

    c. Pull the pants down over the patient's thighs and legs.

    d. Support the patient's ankle and slip pants off the foot. Repeat for the other leg.

10. Provide for the patient's comfort. Place in good body alignment, adjust the bedding, and leave the call light within reach.

11. Put the patient's personal clothing away in the proper place.

12. Report and record as appropriate.

Unit 17

BATHS AND
HYGIENE MEASURES

GENERAL PERFORMANCE OBJECTIVE

You will be prepared to meet the patient's hygiene and comfort requirements by giving A.M. care, mouth care, back rub, and various types of cleansing, medicated, or therapeutic baths.

SPECIFIC PERFORMANCE OBJECTIVES

Upon the completion of this unit you will be able to:

1. Provide mouth care as needed to the conscious or the unconscious patient.

2. Give a back rub that stimulates the circulation in the skin and is relaxing and enjoyable to the patient.

3. Give a complete bed bath to the patient confined to bed.

4. Describe the types of baths and be able to give any of the following as part of the performance test:

    a. a partial bath

    b. a medicated bath

    c. a sitz bath

VOCABULARY

caries—decay of teeth, causing a defect or hole in the tooth enamel.
perineal region—the area between the thighs at the lower end of the trunk of the body, including the rectum and the genitals.
perineum—the area between the anus and vulva in the female and between the anus and scrotum in the male.
sordes—a collection of brown, crusty material on the mouth and teeth of persons having fevers.
stomatitis—inflammation of the mouth.
suppuration—the formation of pus.
vaginal—relating to the genital canal in the female extending from the uterus (womb) to the external opening.

INTRODUCTION

Care of the person includes certain health measures whether or not there is acute medical or surgical illness, chronic disease, or mental deterioration. The extent to which these health measures can be carried out depends on the patient's physical condition as well as psychological state. The age of the patient is an important factor related to these health needs; for example, the older patient may not need a complete bath every day. A daily bath may result in excessively dry skin, with scaling and itching caused by loss of natural oils and decreased perspiration.

The general hygiene measures described in this unit on bathing include A.M. care, P.M. care, oral hygiene for conscious and unconscious patients, care of dentures, various types of baths, and the back rub. Oral hygiene and the back rub may be required several times a day, depending on the patient's needs. When patients are unable to carry out their own personal hygiene and attend to their appearance, the nurse does it for them. You therefore need to know how to proceed with these tasks to carry them out efficiently and with consideration for the patient's comfort and safety.

ASSISTING WITH PERSONAL HYGIENE

ITEM 1. A.M. CARE

This routine is usually performed early each morning before breakfast is served and the activities of the day are begun.

Supplies Needed

Basin of warm water	Bedpan or urinal
Soap	Toilet tissue
Towels and wash cloth	Emesis basin
Toothbrush and toothpaste	Mouthwash

Important Steps	Key Points
1. Wash your hands.	Universal Steps A, B, C, and D. See Appendix.
2. Approach and identify the patient, explain the procedure, and gain cooperation.	
3. Provide for privacy, as needed.	
4. Collect items and materials needed.	
5. Offer bedpan or urinal for elimination.	See Unit 24. If patient is able to get up with help, assist to the bathroom.
6. Provide water for washing.	Place on the overbed table and pull it across the bed so it can be easily reached. The hands and face are washed in preparation for breakfast.
7. Give oral hygiene.	The patient brushes own teeth if able. If not, the nurse may give oral hygiene now or later along with the bath.
8. Collect used items and dispose of them or store correctly.	Universal Steps X, Y, Z. See Appendix.
9. Provide for the patient's comfort.	Position the bed in Fowler's position for breakfast.
10. Record and report the procedure.	Charting example: 6:30 A.M. Early A.M. care given. J. Jones, NA

UNIT 17

ITEM 2. P.M CARE OR H.S. (HOUR OF SLEEP)

This routine is performed at bedtime:

||||||||||||||||||||||||||||||||||||||||||||||||||||||||||||||||||||||||||||||||||||||||||||||||||||||||||||||||||||||||||||||||||||||||||||||||||||||||||

Supplies Needed:

Basin of warm water	Bedpan or urinal
Towels and wash cloth	Toilet tissue
Alcohol or rubbing lotion	Soap

||||||||||||||||||||||||||||||||||||||||||||||||||||||||||||||||||||||||||||||||||||||||||||||||||||||||||||||||||||||||||||||||||||||||||||||||||||||||||

Important Steps	Key Points
Carry out Universal Steps A, B, C, and D. See Appendix.	
1. Offer the bedpan or urinal for elimination.	If the patient is able to get up with help, assist to the bathroom.
2. Provide basin of warm water for washing.	Pull overbed table over the bed, place water, soap, and towels on it and have patients wash own face and hands if able.
3. Wash and dry the back.	Patients often spend most of their time in bed, So back care should be done at least twice a day. Inspect the skin for redness and signs of pressure, especially over the sacrum.
4. Give a back rub.	See Item 6 for instructions.
Carry out Universal Steps X, Y, and Z. See Appendix.	Charting example: 2045. P.M. care given. Voided 300 ml. of yellow urine. Back rub given. Skin of back clear, no red areas noted.
	J. Ahmir, RN

ITEM 3. MOUTH CARE FOR THE CONSCIOUS PATIENT

Mouth care is as important as the bath for sick patients. If their condition permits, patients are encouraged to brush their own teeth, use floss, and cleanse the mouth as they normally do. For those patients confined to bed, however, the nurse must provide the supplies and the time for them to carry out oral hygiene several times a day. The purposes of cleansing the mouth are:

1. To remove trapped food particles and secretions. This helps to prevent bad breath, feelings of uncleanliness, and dental caries.

2. To prevent the lips from becoming dry and cracked. Cracked lips provide an opening for bacteria to enter the body.

3. To prevent sordes, stomatitis, and other disease conditions affecting the mouth.

Mouth care is extremely important for patients receiving chemotherapy for the treatment of cancer. The drugs are very potent and produce inflammation of the tissues of the mouth. They become bright red in color, very sore, and swollen, and the patient has little or no appetite because of the stomatitis. Often the strong antibiotics used in chemotherapy kill the bacteria normally found in the mouth and this permits the growth of yeast cells, which coat the mouth and tongue with a whitish and cheesy material. Your early observation and reporting of this condition is important so that treatment can be started with medications.

The items used in oral hygiene include a toothbrush, toothpaste or tooth powder, and mouthwash. Most patients bring these and other toilet articles to the hospital with them or have a member of the family bring them from home. These supplies may also be purchased or obtained from the hospital gift shop, pharmacy, or central supply. When no dentifrice is available, you can make up a mixture of equal parts of table salt and baking soda for brushing teeth. For cleaning the mouth of dried secretions and coating irritated tissues, a mixture of one half part milk of magnesia and one half part hydrogen peroxide is effective.

Supplies Needed:

Toothbrush	Emesis basin
Toothpaste or powder	Glass of water
Mouthwash	Face towel

Important Steps	Key Points
Carry out Universal Steps A, B, C, and D. See Appendix.	
1. Position the patient.	If allowed, raise the head of the bed to Fowler's position. If the patient is unable to sit up, turn him or her to the side facing you. Place the towel and curved basin under chin. Moisten toothbrush with water or mouthwash and spread toothpaste or toothpowder on it. Hand the toothbrush to the patient.

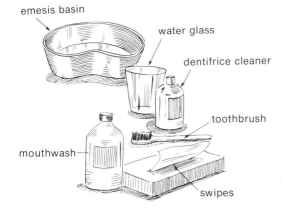

emesis basin
water glass
dentifrice cleaner
toothbrush
mouthwash
swipes

2. Assist the patient to brush teeth as needed.	Teeth should be brushed in this manner: downward on upper teeth and upward on lower teeth. This applies to both front and back teeth.

UNIT 17

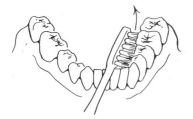

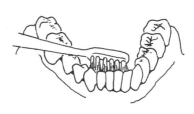

Brush teeth from gum-line up to edge of teeth.

Important Steps	Key Points
3. Rinse the mouth.	Have the patient use water or mouthwash to rinse the mouth and spit out the solution into the emesis basin. May repeat as desired. Wipe mouth when finished.

Carry out Universal Steps X, Y, and Z. See Appendix.

ITEM 4. MOUTH CARE FOR THE UNCONSCIOUS PATIENT

Whenever you provide nursing care to an unconscious patient, you should give good mouth care at least once every eight hours, and some patients may need oral hygiene as often as every four hours. The muscles of the face are slack and the mouth lies partly open, so patients often breathe through it. This causes dryness of the tongue and crusting from dried secretions. These need to be removed, as they cause a foul-smelling breath and may obstruct the air passages.

Supplies Needed

Applicators of lemon and glycerin	Petrolatum or lubricant
Emesis basin	Towel

Optional Supplies

4 × 4-inch sponge	Tongue blade

Important Steps	Key Points
Carry out Universal Steps A, B, C, and D. See Appendix.	
1. Position the patient.	Turn the patient's head to the side facing you and place the towel and curved basin under the chin.
2. Use applicator to cleanse the teeth and mouth.	Using a glycerin and lemon applicator thoroughly clean the inside of the mouth, the cheek sides, the roof of the mouth, the teeth, and the tongue. A 4 × 4-inch gauze wrapped around the index finger may be used instead of an applicator. Half-strength hydrogen peroxide and milk of magnesia make a good agent for cleaning the mouth.

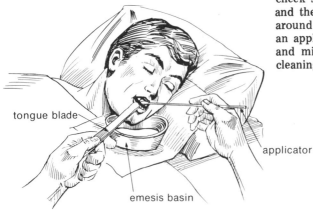
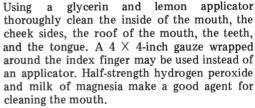

tongue blade

applicator

emesis basin

Oral hygiene.

Important Steps	Key Points
3. Rinse the mouth if needed.	Discard the applicators into the trash and rinse the patient's mouth with water. Very small amounts of liquid are used, since the patient is not able to spit it out. However, you must keep the teeth and tissues of the mouth clean and moist. Keep the patient's head in such a position that fluid drains out of the mouth by gravity.
4. Lubricate the lips.	Dry the patient's mouth and lubricate the lips to prevent cracking. Do not use mineral oil since it may drain down into the lungs and cause lipid pneumonia.

Carry out Universal Steps X, Y, and Z. See Appendix.

ITEM 5. CARE OF DENTURES

Comatose patients' dentures should be removed from their mouths and placed in containers.

‖‖‖

Supplies Needed

Denture brush or toothbrush   Denture paste or powder
Denture cup

‖‖‖

Important Steps	Key Points
1. Remove the dentures and put them into the emesis basin.	If the patient cannot remove them, you must do it. To remove the upper denture (it is held in place by a vacuum), grasp the front teeth with the thumb and index finger. Move the denture up and down slightly to break the vacuum seal. Slip it out of the mouth. The lower denture may be picked out of the mouth; exercise care to turn it slightly to prevent the discomfort of stretching the lips. Place the dentures in a basin and take them to the sink to wash. Dentures must be handled with care; dropping may cause breakage. When not in the mouth, they should be kept in a labeled denture box with water or normal saline to keep them moist.

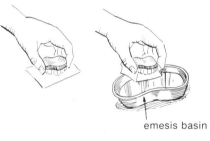

emesis basin

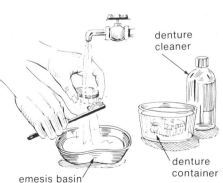

denture cleaner

emesis basin

denture container

Care of dentures.

U
N
I
T
17

Important Steps	Key Points
2. Clean the dentures.	Use a toothbrush and toothpaste or tooth-powder to clean by brushing motions. A commercially prepared material may be used for soaking the dentures. Rinse them with running water, exercising care not to allow the wet dentures to slip from your fingers.
3. Replace the dentures in the patient's mouth.	Return to the bedside and allow or assist the patient to put the dentures in his mouth. Dry the patient's mouth and hands.

ITEM 6.   THE BACK RUB

The back rub is an important procedure in your care of the patient. It involves the sense of touch and becomes a way of communicating a caring attitude to the patient, which helps foster trust in the nurse-patient relationship. Other benefits of the back rub are:

1. It provides an opportunity for you to observe the condition of the skin on the back and begin early treatment of any pressure areas.

2. It is a passive form of exercise for the patient confined to bed.

3. The rubbing action on the skin and the pressure on the back muscles stimulate circulation of blood to the area.

4. The rubbing reduces tension and promotes relaxation of the body.

Back rubs are given to patients confined to bed for the major part of the day as part of the bath and again as part of P.M. care. Rubbing alcohol, oils, lotions, or powder can be used, depending on the preference of the patient, the nurse, or the condition of the skin on the back. Alcohol is frequently used because it evaporates quickly and has a cooling effect. It is often used in sponge baths to reduce the body temperature when patients have fevers. Oils and lotions reduce the friction and serve to lubricate the skin as well. As you give the back rub, use more pressure on the upstrokes toward the head and less pressure on the downward strokes. The amount of pressure should provide a firm touch but should not cause tensing of muscles or discomfort for the patient.

Before giving the back rub, you need to prepare yourself as well as the patient. Minimize the noise and distraction in order to make the back rub a relaxing and enjoyable event. Use good body alignment and movement to prevent strain or tension in your muscles, which can be communicated to the patient. Good body alignment can be achieved by having the bed in a high position and the patient on the side near you and keeping the knees flexed and toes pointed toward the patient's head. Except when using alcohol, make sure that your hands are warm and relaxed; cool hands cause tensing and pulling away by the patient.

Supplies Needed

Rubbing alcohol, oil, lotion, or powder   Towel

Important Steps	Key Points
Carry out Universal Steps A, B, C, and D. See Appendix.	Back rub may also be included in the bath procedure or in P.M. care.
1. Position the patient.	If possible, have the patient lie on abdomen. Some patients may need to lie on their side. Put the bed in high position and have patient near the side so you can reach the back easily.
2. Uncover the back and hips.	If patient is prone, place the towel over the lower buttocks. Lay the towel along the back to protect the bed linens when the patient lies on the side.
3. Apply rubbing solution or powder to your hands.	Oils and lotions may be warmed before using; however, alcohol is used for its cooling effects.
4. Use several long superficial strokes. 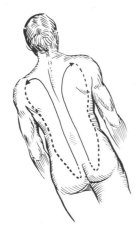	Start with hands on lower back with fingers pointed toward the head. Move hands straight up the back to the shoulders. Stroke each hand cupped over the shoulder, then over the shoulder blades and down along the sides to the lower back. Keep your hands in contact with the back at all times during the stroke.
5. Knead the thumbs along either side of the spine.	On each side of the spine, use your thumbs to make short, rapid strokes outward toward the side. Begin at the lower back and progress up toward the neck.
6. Use a criss cross movement over the back.	Place your hands on each side, then move each hand up and over the body with medium pressure to the opposite side. Continue from the hip level up toward the shoulders.
7. Use circular strokes up and down the back. 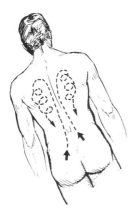	With hands at the waistline, make large circular movements over the buttocks and lower back. Then make a long stroke toward the neck and make broad circular motions down the back toward the sacrum. Repeat as desired.

UNIT 17

Important Steps	Key Points
8. Use feathering strokes to conclude the backrub.	You may use any combination of the strokes described and repeat those that seem pleasing to the patient. End the backrub by making a series of long superficial strokes (see Step 4), making each successive one lighter than the previous one.

Carry out Universal Steps X, Y, Z. See Appendix.

ITEM 7. TYPES OF BATHS

Nurses must pay careful attention to the patient's skin during illness. The intact skin provides the body with the first line of defense against invasion by pathogenic organisms. Many microorganisms normally found on the skin are relatively harmless, and the healthy person can combat and overcome them. The sick person, however, has lowered resistance and is much more susceptible to further infection. There are a number of other changes in the body's chemistry and function during illness that lead to the necessity for daily cleansing of the skin for patients who spend more than eight to ten hours a day in bed. Patients who have fevers perspire more than normal and the perspiration is slightly acidic. It is composed mainly of water but contains some salts and urea, a substance excreted by the body as a waste product. The skin sheds dead cells from the surface layers, and these are removed by bathing, as well as accumulations of dirt and bacteria.

Baths are given for a variety of reasons: (1) to cleanse the skin; (2) to stimulate the circulation of blood to all areas of the body; (3) to remove waste products excreted through the skin; and (4) to refresh the patient through the warm, soothing, and relaxing effect on the nerve endings in the skin.

A number of terms are used when referring to baths and bathing patients.

1. Complete bath: all areas of the body are washed.

2. Partial bath: there are two uses of this term, so find out which one is used in your agency.

   a. Only certain parts of the body are bathed; these usually include the face, hands, under the arms, the back, and the perineal area.

   b. A complete bath is done, part by the patient washing areas that can be reached, and the nurse who washes all of the other parts.

The Cleansing Bath

The most common type of bath is the cleansing bath. It may be a complete or partial bath and may be carried out by the patient alone, with some assistance by the nurse, or totally by the nurse. The bath may be given to the patient while in bed or taken by the patient sponging at the sink, in a bathtub, or in the shower. When bathing feet in a basin or immersing the patient in the bathtub, avoid filling the basin or tub too full, since the foot or body displaces an equal volume and the water may overflow. The temperature of the water should be 105° F (40.5° C).

The Medicated Bath

This type of bath may be administered as a tub bath or a sponge bath and is used to soothe or provide relief from the itching and irritation of various skin disorders. Following the bath, the skin is patted dry, not rubbed, since rubbing stimulates the nerve endings again.

Various substances may be added to the bath water for their soothing effects. The water temperature is 100 to 105°F (37.7 to 40.5°C).

Oatmeal Bath. The new instant oatmeal can be added directly to the bath water. Stir in the amount needed to make the desired consistency. Then proceed as with a regular tub bath.

To use regular oatmeal, add 3 cups of oatmeal to 2 quarts of water and cook until it has the consistency of paste. Place the cooked oatmeal in a cheesecloth bag and tie securely Twirl the bag in the bathtub of water until the water has a mucilaginous (or slippery) feel to it.

Sodium Bicarbonate Bath. The baking soda that is found in kitchens and used in baking is often used in sponge baths for its soothing effect on the skin. To make a 5 per cent solution, add one teaspoon of baking soda to 500 ml of water. Continue using this ratio and fill the basin one third to one half full. If using a bathtub, the same ratio calls for one ounce of sodium bicarbonate to one gallon of water.

Cornstarch Bath. Cornstarch is a smooth powder without grit that can be used as a dusting powder for the skin and in a soothing bath for irritated skin. To prepare the cornstarch, mix one pound with cold water. Then add boiling water to make a thin solution and boil for one or two minutes. Add to a bathtub half-filled with water and proceed with the bath.

Saline Bath. Bathing in salt water is invigorating and stimulating, as those who go swimming in the ocean can testify. A solution of saline is prepared by adding one teaspoon of salt to 500 ml of water, or one ounce of salt to a gallon of water. Continue to fill the basin or tub by adding more of the 1:500 ratio of salt to water. Temperature of the water is between 95 to 108°F (35 to 42.2°C).

Mustard Bath. Mustard has a stimulating effect on the skin and has been used to relieve muscle spasms and tense muscles associated with convulsions. Use a weaker solution when preparing the mustard bath for a child.

For adults, use one tablespoon of dry mustard per gallon of water. For children, use one half teaspoon of dry mustard per gallon of water. Dissolve the mustard in tepid water and add to the bath water. Temperature of the bath is 100°F (37.7°C).

Therapeutic Baths

Specific types of baths may be performed in order to achieve a desired effect. These include the cooling sponge bath, the relaxing bath, the whirlpool bath, and the sitz bath.

Cooling Sponge Bath. Generally, an order from the physician is needed before you give a cooling or alcohol sponge bath in order to bring down a fever. The patient's temperature is taken before the sponge bath and periodically during the bath, which is continued until the temperature falls. The body temperature decreases by the transfer of heat when water evaporates. To hasten the cooling process, add plain cool water or alcohol, which evaporates faster than water. With fevers over 103°F (39.4°C), you may need to continue the sponge bath for 30 minutes or longer. The temperature of the water should be 35 to 50°F (2 to 10°C).

Relaxing Bath. The relaxing bath is used to calm and sedate. The patient lies suspended in a tub of water with only the head above water. The bath may last for 20 minutes to an hour, and the temperature of the water is maintained at 105°F (40.5°C).

Whirlpool Bath. A bathtub with a whirlpool attachment is used to provide agitation of the water, which gently massages the skin and has a soothing effect. Tension and discomfort are relieved. Water temperature is 105°F (40.5°C).

Sitz Bath. The sitz bath is used to apply moist heat to the perineal or anal area to promote healing and to relieve pain and discomfort. Specially designed shallow tubs or basins are available for the patient to sit in. Fill only one third with water, because the immersed part of the body replaces the water and it may overflow. Temperature of the water is 95 to 105°F (35 to 40.5°C). The bath lasts about 20 minutes, and is commonly used after rectal or vaginal surgery and following the birth of a baby.

ITEM 8.   GIVING A BED BATH

Supplies Needed

Basin of warm water   Clean linen for bed
Soap   Clean gown
Towels and wash cloth   Toilet articles
Alcohol or rubbing lotion   Hamper or bag for soiled linen

Important Steps	Key Points

Carry out Universal Steps A, B, C, and D. See Appendix.

1. Offer the bedpan or urinal.

    See Unit 24.

2. Provide for the patient's mouth care.

    See Items 3 and 4 of this unit.

3. Replace the top linen with the bath blanket.

    Fan-fold the bath blanket and place it across the patient's chest. Ask the patient to hold the top edge of the bath blanket.

    Grasp the bottom edge of the bath blanket and the top of the covers and pull the covers and bottom edge of the blanket to the foot of the bed.

4. Remove the top bedding.

    Inspect the spread for soiled areas. If it appears clean, fold it in this manner:

    a. Bring the top edge to the bottom edge. The spread is now in half.

    b. Fold one side to the other side edge. The spread is now in quarters.

    c. Fold it again in half. Place it over the back of the chair.

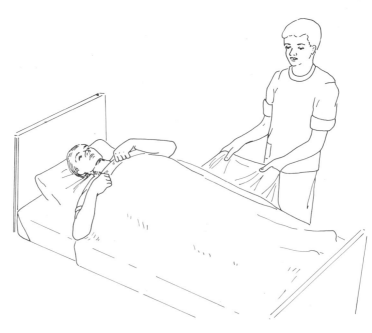

Important Steps	Key Points
	If the blanket is on the bed, remove it and fold as above.
	Discard the top sheet into the laundry bag. In some settings the top sheet, if clean, may be reused as the bottom sheet. In this case, fold and hang it on the back of the chair.
5. Prepare the patient.	Lower the siderail on the side near the bedside table. Remove the gown, being careful to keep patient covered with a blanket. If an IV is in place, see Unit 16, Dressing and Undressing.
	Remove the pillow unless the patient is more comfortable with it. Spread a towel across patient's chest.
6. Assemble the equipment on the bedside table.	Remove any items from the bedside table and place the bath articles on the table top.
	Prepare the bath water at 110 to 115°F (43.3 to 46.1°C) (water cools rapidly). Place the soap dish near the basin of water. Do not leave the soap in the bath water; the water becomes excessively soapy.
	Raise the bed to working level.

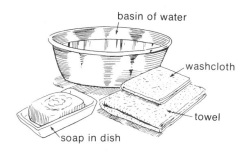

Bath equipment.

7. Make a bath mitt.	Grasp the washcloth at an edge and fold one-third over the palm of your hand. Bring the opposite edge across the palm of your hand and hold it with your thumb. Bring the extreme end of the cloth up to your palm and tuck the edge under the upper edge. You now have a bath mitt. This prevents loose ends of the washcloth from dragging across the patient. These tails become cool quickly and chill the patient.

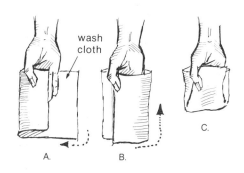

How to make a bath mitt.

8. Wash the patient's face and neck.	The patient may wash own face if able. Use soap only if the patient desires. If patient is unable to do this, moisten the bath mitt with water and wash one eye from the inner lid to the outer side near the ear. Rinse the cloth before washing the other eye. Dry well. Wash the forehead from center to side. Rinse and dry it well.

UNIT
17

Important Steps	Key Points
	Wash the cheeks from the nose to the side of face. Wash the bridge and tip of the nose. Wash the mouth area with a circular motion. Wash the neck. Rinse and dry the face and neck well.
9. Wash the arms.	If an IV is in place, take care not to disturb the needle. Place a towel under the distal arm, make a bath mitt, use soap, and wash the entire arm with long, sweeping strokes. Give special care to the armpit with extra soaping. Rinse and dry it well. Wash the hands and fingers, rinse, and dry. Dry well between the fingers. Wash the proximal arm and hand in the same manner and dry them well.

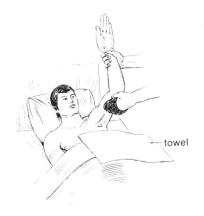

Wash arm with long, sweeping strokes.

10. Wash the chest and abdomen.	Place a towel over the patient's chest. Fold the bath blanket to the waistline. Make a bath mitt and wash under the towel to include the entire chest. Wash the breast with circular movements. Rinse and dry it well. Fold the blanket to the top of the pubic bone and wash the lower abdomen. Dry well.
11. Wash the feet and legs.	Expose only the leg being washed. Tuck the blanket around the patient to prevent draft. Flex one leg and place a towel lengthwise on the bed. Wash from the hip to the knee with long, sweeping strokes. Wash from the knee to the foot in the same manner. Rinse and dry the leg well. Place the bath basin on the towel. Lift the patient's foot, placing your hand under the heel, and put it into the water. This is very refreshing for the patient. Wash the foot and dry it. Dry each toe separately and place the leg and foot under the blanket. Wash the remaining foot and leg in the same manner.

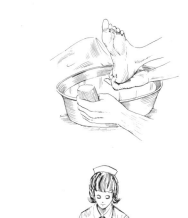

Place foot in water.

Important Steps	Key Points
12. Change the bath water.	Remove the bath water and obtain fresh bath water 110 to 115°F (43.3 to 46.1°C). Return to the patient, and prepare to complete the bath.
13. Wash the patient's back.	Turn the patient to the side. Wash the back with long, sweeping motions. Rinse and dry it well.
14. Give a backrub.	Refer to Item 6.
15. Wash the perineal area.	While the patient washes the genital area, the health worker may walk outside the unit but remain within hearing distance.
	If the patient is unable to wash the perineal area, the health worker does so. The genital area is washed thoroughly, rinsed well, and dried carefully.
	If the patient has a catheter in place, attention is given to washing around the catheter with soap and water to remove body secretions. Rinsing follows. Check with your health facility for special catheter care.
16. Put a clean gown on patient.	If the patient is unable to put on the gown or has an IV in place, proceed as described in Unit 16, Dressing and Undressing.
17. Complete the personal care.	Comb the patient's hair. Refer to Unit 19 for information on special hair care.
	Care for the fingernails and toenails. Take care not to break skin when doing the nails. Some agencies do not permit cutting the nails. Check with your agency procedure.
	Permit the male patient to shave. Assemble an electric shaver, a mirror, and the patient's shaving lotion. Provide warm water and shaving cream if the patient uses a safety razor. If he needs help, follow the hospital policy for shaving patients or calling the barber.
	Remove the bath basin. Clean, rinse, and return it to storage.
18. Make an occupied bed.	See Unit 9, Hospital Beds, and follow the directions given there.
Carry out Universal Steps X, Y, and Z. See Appendix.	Charting example: 0930. Complete bed bath given. Has reddened area 1 inch in diameter over sacrum. Back rub given. Turned on right side. Resting quietly.
	M. Victory, LPN

UNIT 17

ITEM 9. THE PARTIAL BATH

Partial baths may be given to convalescent patients who wash as much as they can reach but need help to complete the bath, or to those not in need of a complete bath. The partial bath includes the face, hands, armpits, back, and genital area.

Supplies Needed

Basin of warm water   Clean linen
Soap   Clean gown
Towels and wash cloth   Toilet articles
Alcohol or rubbing lotion   Hamper for soiled linen

Refer to these steps in the section on bed baths:

1.   Approach the patient.

2.   Offer the bedpan or urinal.

3.   Arrange the bath equipment.

4.   Perform mouth care.

5.   Position the patient for the bed bath.

6.   Assemble the equipment on the bedside table.

7.   Replace the top linen with the bath blanket.

8.   Prepare the patient.

9.   Make a bath mitt.

10. Wash the patient's face and neck.

11. Wash the arms.

12. Wash the back.

13. Give a backrub.

14. Wash the genital area.

15. Put a clean gown on the patient.

16. Complete personal care.

17. Make an occupied bed.

18. Chart.

Charting example:
9:30 A.M. Partial bath given. Is very restless and talkative. Complained of pain in upper right quadrant.

J. Jones, NA

ITEM 10.   THE TUB BATH

This procedure may be used for cleansing, medicated, or therapeutic baths.

Supplies Needed

Soap   Clean linen for bed
Towels and wash cloth   Clean gown
Bath mat

Important Steps	Key Points
1. Assemble the bath materials.	Before taking the patient to the bathroom, clean and prepare the bathtub and assemble equipment.

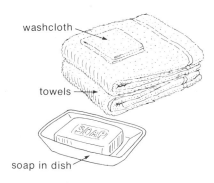

washcloth

towels

soap in dish

	Place a bath mat by the tub. Wash your hands, identify the patient, and explain the procedure.
	Accompany the patient to the bathtub. Seat your patient comfortably nearby, and fill the bathtub one half full. Check the temperature and adjust it to read 100 to 110°F (37.8 to 43.3°C).
2. Assist the patient to the tub.	Assist the patient into tub. If the patient does not require complete assistance, the bed may be changed during the bath. The bath should not exceed 15 to 20 minutes. Explain the system for signalling for help if needed. Hang the "occupied" sign on the door and return within a few minutes to see if the patient is satisfactory. Do not lock the door. If the patient appears weak, assist with the bath. (The male patient may use a towel for a sarong to provide privacy when a female worker cares for him.) Remain near the patient at all times. Ill patients frequently become weak and may faint.
3. Wash the patient's back.	
4. Assist the patient to get out of the tub and dry.	Have the patient use the side of the tub and grab bars to pull up to a standing position. Provide a bath mat outside the tub to stand on.
5. Return the patient to the room.	Assist the patient in drying and putting on a clean gown. Escort the patient back to bed. Give back rub.
6. Clean the tub and bathroom.	Return to the bathroom and wash the bathtub. (Use the scouring powder and disinfectant prescribed by your agency.) Remove the towels and soiled linen and prepare the facility for another to use. Remove the "occupied" sign.
7. Chart the procedure on the nurse's notes or check off sheet.	

ITEM 11. THE SITZ BATH

For the sitz bath, you may use the common bathtub or a tub specially designed for sitz baths that some agencies have. Plastic sitz bath kits are also available and are more convenient than the other forms. The basin fits over the toilet, and a bag with tubing is used to supply additional warm water to the basin during the procedure. The patient sits on the seat and the excess water in the basin drains down the toilet.

UNIT 17

Supplies Needed

Bath towels (2 or 3)   "Occupied" sign
Patient gown

Important Steps	Key Points
1. Prepare the equipment.	Wash your hands. Fill the tub about 1/3 full. Water temperature should be 100 to 110°F (37.8 to 43.3°C). Place a towel or folded bath blanket in the bottom of the tub. Hang "occupied" sign on the door.

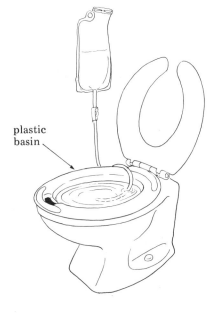

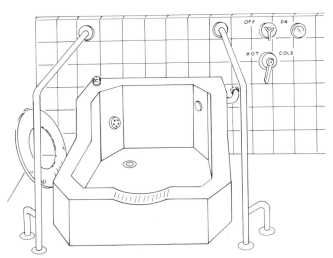

Sitz bath basin placed on toilet.

2. Assist the patient to the tub.	Check the patient's identification band and explain the procedure. Assist the patient to remove robe and sit in the tub with the hospital gown on for 20 to 30 minutes, or as ordered. *Check frequently* on the patient's condition and keep the temperature of the water even. When adding warm water, avoid burning the patient.
3. Remove the patient from tub.	Help the patient to remove gown, if wet, and to stand up and step out of the tub. Assist in drying the perineal area and putting on the hospital attire. Loosen the drain plug of the sitz bath so that the water can drain out.
4. Return patient to room.	Escort the ambulatory patient back to the room or use a wheelchair to transport, if necessary. You may have made the bed while the patient was in the sitz bath; if not, make the bed with clean linen at this time.
Carry out Universal Steps X, Y, and Z. See Appendix.	11:00 A.M. Sitz bath taken for 30 minutes. States there is less soreness in perineal area today. Redness 1 inch around the incision, no drainage. Dry dressing applied.

L. Gomez, SN

plastic basin

PERFORMANCE TEST

In the laboratory setting, with a student partner, you will give a complete bed bath, tub bath, or sitz bath. Keep in mind the supplies you will need and the major steps of the procedure.

You should be prepared to explain to your instructor the indications and procedure for the partial bath, the medicated bath, A.M. care, and h.s. care.

PERFORMANCE CHECKLIST

THE BED BATH

1. Wash your hands.

2. Select and assemble all needed materials before beginning the bed bath.

3. Identify the patient and explain the procedure to the patient.

4. Raise the bed to working height. Use good body alignment procedures.

5. Offer the bedpan or urinal to the patient.

6. Encourage the patient to give own mouth care. Remove, clean, and return the equipment to storage.

7. Apply the bath blanket.

8. Remove and dispose of the linen correctly by folding for reuse or put in soiled linen bag.

9. Remove the patient's gown, being careful not to expose the patient.

10. Wash and dry the face using a bath mitt.

11. Wash and dry the arms. Protect the bedding with a towel under the patient's arm.

12. Wash and dry the chest using circular motions. Put a towel across the upper chest; fold the bath blanket to the waist.

13. Wash and dry the abdomen. Fold the bath blanket to the pubis, with a towel across the chest.

14. Wash the legs with long, firm strokes, and dry them well.

    a. Put the towel lengthwise under the leg.

    b. Place the bath basin on the towel.

    c. Place the foot in the basin.

15. Wash and dry the feet and remove the basin.

16. Change the water when cool; water temperature should be 110 to 115°F (43.3 to 46.1°C).

17. Wash and dry the back.

18. Give backrub with special attention to bony prominences, scapula, and sacrum.

19. Wash, or permit the patient to wash, the perineal area.

20. Help the patient to put on the gown.

UNIT 17

21. Comb hair or provide assistance to the patient as needed (mirror, comb, brush, towel, covering, etc.)

22. Check nails; clean or cut them as needed.

23. Remove the soiled items; clean the equipment and return it to storage.

24. Make the occupied bed using good body movement and without raising dust. (Do not shake linens.) Carry the linens away from your uniform.

25. Leave the unit neat and tidy with the bedside stand and call signal within easy reach of the patient.

26. Chart the procedure.

THE TUB BATH

1. Wash your hands.

2. Assemble the supplies and equipment for use.

3. Check the tub and clean it if necessary.

4. Identify the patient and explain the procedure.

5. Assist the patient to the bathroom.

6. Fill the tub half full with water at 100 to $105°$F (37.7 to $40.5°$C).

7. Assist the patient into the tub.

8. Hang the "occupied" sign on the door.

9. Check on the patient frequently.

10. Wash and dry patient's back.

11. Assist the patient as needed to get out of the tub and dry the body.

12. Put a clean gown on the patient.

13. Return the patient to bed.

14. Give backrub.

15. Change the linen and dispose of the soiled linen in the designated manner.

16. Leave the room neat and tidy.

17. Return to the bathroom.

    a. Remove the soiled linen and equipment.

    b. Clean the tub.

    c. Remove the "occupied" sign from door.

18. Chart the procedure.

THE SITZ BATH

1. Wash your hands.

2. Prepare the equipment: fill the tub one-third full of water (100 to $110°$F (37.8 to $43.3°$C). Hang an "occupied" sign on the door.

3. Explain the procedure to the patient and check identification band.

4. Assist the patient to the tub and allow him to remain there for 20 to 30 minutes. Check frequently. Keep the water warm throughout the procedure.

5. Assist the patient out of the tub and in drying the area, if necessary.

6. Drain the water from the tub.

7. Help the patient back to bed.

8. Change the bed linens.

9. Leave the room neat and tidy.

10. Return to the bathroom.

    a. Remove the soiled linens and equipment.

    b. Clean the tub.

    c. Remove the "occupied" sign from the door.

11. Chart the procedure.

Unit 18

SPECIAL SKIN CARE

GENERAL PERFORMANCE OBJECTIVE

When you have finished this unit, you will be able to give special care to the geriatric or incontinent patients, to the patient in a cast or in traction, and to one with an ileostomy or colostomy, while maintaining a good body alignment both for the patient and yourself and providing a safe, comfortable environment.

SPECIFIC PERFORMANCE OBJECTIVES

On completion of this unit, you will be able to:

1. Identify specific skin indications that could lead to a breakdown and formation of a decubitus and begin appropriate preventive measures.

2. Prevent decubitus ulcers by examining the patient's skin, removing pressure from bony prominences, correctly changing the patient's position, and using appropriate supportive aids.

3. Detect signs of impaired circulation in an extremity of a patient who has a cast, and start appropriate nursing measures.

4. Change an ileostomy or colostomy appliance using clean technique, observing the skin condition, and applying the appropriate ointment, while reassuring the patient.

5. Clean and cut the patient's toenails or fingernails according to your agency procedure.

VOCABULARY

abrasion—a scraping of the skin, a minor injury.
compound fracture—a broken bone that has an accompanying skin wound, i.e., the bone protrudes through the skin.
cyanosis—bluish color caused by decreased oxygen content in the blood.
decubitus ulcer—a bedsore or pressure sore occurring over any bony prominence, caused by prolonged pressure on the skin covering that area, which decreases the circulation.
dermis—the second layer of the skin (commonly called the "true skin").
epidermis—the outer layer of skin.
evaporation—the changing of a substance from a liquid form into vapor (steam).
excoriation—damage or abrasion to skin caused by chemicals or burns, for example, diaper burn on an infant.
gangrene—death of tissues due to lack of circulation.
incontinence—inability to retain feces or urine; lack of voluntary control over anal or urinary sphincter.
necrosis—death of tissue from any cause.
orthopedics—treatment of abnormalities and diseases of the musculoskeletal system.
scapula— a large, flat, triangular bone of the shoulder.
sebaceous glands—oil-secreting glands of the skin.

simple fracture—a broken bone that does not have an accompanying skin wound.

sweat (perspiration) glands—glands in the skin that secrete a salty, colorless liquid; they keep the body cool by the process of evaporation.

traction—an arrangement of ropes, pulleys, and weights that exerts a pulling force on a part of the body that requires this type of treatment.

wound—a break in the continuity of soft tissues due to trauma (injury).

INTRODUCTION

Care of the skin is basic to all nursing care. It is not only a part of your daily routine but also a special procedure in certain cases such as newborn infants, geriatric patients, incontinent patients, and patients who are immobilized over a long period of time because of a cast, traction, or paralysis. Frequent bathing of all or parts of the body prevents skin irritation from perspiration, urine, feces, or drainage. Bathing should depend on the regular habits of the individual as well as the condition of the skin. Some people take daily baths; others bathe only once or twice a week because of excessive dryness of the skin. Of course, certain areas must be washed daily: groin, underarms, face, hands, perineum and body creases.

Structure of the Skin. Skin is a remarkable part of the body. Its condition provides us with one indicator of the general health of the patient. The outer layer of the skin, called the epidermis (often referred to as "false skin"), constantly sheds dead cells. It also acts as a barrier between the individual and the environment by protecting him against physical attack on the underlying tissues and preventing microorganisms and other foreign subtances from entering the body.

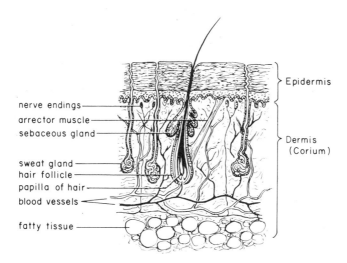

The dermis is the layer directly below the epidermis and is called the "true skin." This layer is made up of tissue that contains hair follicles imbedded in bundles of smooth muscle, sweat glands, sebaceous glands, blood vessels, and nerve endings. The skin has a sensory role in being sensitive to touch and temperature. The skin also acts as a regulator of body fluids and temperature. The sweat glands excrete waste products from the body, and the evaporation of these waste products has a cooling effect, thereby helping to regulate the body temperature.

The skin varies in thickness in different parts of the body; for example, the eyelid is paper thin, while the sole of the foot and the palm of the hand are very thick because they must withstand much abuse, wear, and tear.

UNIT 18

Functions of the Skin. To summarize, the skin serves several functions:

1. It acts as a protective barrier against microorganisms.

2. It is a sensory organ that enables the body to feel pain, pressure, and temperature.

3. It shields body tissue from injury.

4. It insulates against heat and cold.

5. It aids in elimination of waste products.

6. It helps produce vitamin D for body use.

Reasons for Skin Care. One route for the elimination of waste products from the body is provided by the sweat glands of the skin. Other routes are the urinary tract and the alimentary tract. The accumulation and decomposition of urine, feces, sweat, or drainage on the skin can cause chemical reactions and so must be washed away to prevent excoriation or burning of the skin.

Oil is secreted by the sebaceous glands in the skin and helps to prevent dryness. When the skin becomes excessively dry through the aging process, damage to the sebaceous glands, or excessive washing away of protective skin oils, it becomes chapped and may break open. Pathogenic organisms gain entry to the underlying body tissues and set up an infection.

Isopropyl alcohol in 70 to 95 per cent solution is used for disinfecting the skin, for back rubs, and for cooling sponge baths. Alcohol is an effective agent in reducing the bacteria normally found on the skin, and the longer the contact with the skin, the more bacteria are killed. It also evaporates rapidly at body temperatures, which produces a cooling effect. For this reason, it is often used in cool sponge baths to lower the body temperature when a patient is running a fever. These effects of alcohol have a drying effect on the skin, so lotions or oils are often needed to keep the skin soft and pliable.

NURSING CARE OF THE SKIN

ITEM 1. SKIN CARE FOR INCONTINENT PATIENTS

One of the early lessons we learn in childhood is "toilet-training." When adults, for any reason, cannot maintain their excretory control of urine or feces, they become embarrassed and lose their self-esteem. Loss of control occurs more often in patients who are elderly, paralyzed, or lacking full mental awareness. Chemicals in the urine and feces soon become irritating if left on the skin and lead to burned areas, or excoriation. It is essential that these patients be kept clean and dry at all times. This means that you will be checking them frequently for soiled skin and linen.

Patients who are incontinent must be treated with kindness and understanding. Assure the patients that you will help them regain as much control as possible. Use retraining methods and toilet them at regular intervals before the incontinence occurs. Your goal should be to toilet the patient before soiling occurs. Don't scold, threaten, or abuse the patient in any way. Avoid using a diaper on these patients: it is often demoralizing to the patient. In addition, a wet diaper causes skin irritation from the acid content of the waste products, and this leads very quickly to rashes, open sores, and decubiti.

In the clinical setting, after practice in the skills laboratory, cleanse the soiled skin, change linens, and provide for the comfort of an incontinent patient. You will assist the patient to take care of his excretory functions.

Supplies Needed

Clean linen (drawsheet, bottom sheet, gown)   Basin of warm water and soap
Washcloth and towel   Toilet tissue

Important Steps	Key Points
1. Wash your hands.	Universal Steps A, B, C, and D. See Appendix.
2. Approach and identify the patient and enlist his cooperation.	
3. Assemble the necessary supplies.	
4. Provide for privacy.	
5. Position the bed.	Place the bed in the working level position to avoid undue backstrain. Have the patient roll on the side away from you.
6. Remove the soiled linen and wash the soiled skin.	Wash the patient's skin gently with warm water and mild soap; rinse the soap off the skin thoroughly. Pat the skin dry carefully with the bath towel. Be sure that it is thoroughly dry. Inspect the skin carefully for evidence of beginning skin breakdown such as the development of an excoriated or reddened area. If incontinent of stool, use toilet paper to remove feces from the skin and discard in the toilet.
7. Give back care.	Give a backrub and massage *around* any reddened areas noted over the sacrum, shoulders, and hips. Use lotion or powder as recommended by your agency.
8. Put a clean gown on the patient and remake the bed.	Adjust the gown to keep wrinkles from gathering under the patient and to provide for free movement. Proceed to make an occupied bed.
9. Provide for the patient's comfort.	Universal Steps X, Y, and Z. See Appendix.
10. Remove the soiled materials.	
11. Report and record.	Charting example: 1110. Incontinent of urine. Back washed and rubbed. Skin color is pink, no broken areas noted. Turned to left Sims' position. J. Jones, SN

ITEM 2. CARE OF THE PRESSURE SORE

You will recall from the earlier unit on Positioning the Bed Patient that changing the patient's position will be one of your most frequent activities. Three reasons for positioning are (1) to relieve pressure, (2) to provide comfort, and (3) to prevent contractures. In this section we are particularly concerned with the effects of pressure on certain bony prominences due to the patient remaining in the same position, either lying down or sitting up, for a prolonged period of time.

Causes of Pressure

You will recall that every part of the body has weight. The weight exerts pressure when it comes in contact with another object, such as the bed. Remaining in one position over a prolonged period of time causes the body weight to exert pressure on the skin, blood vessels,

U
N
I
T
18

and muscles at the areas where the body is in contact with the bed or chair. The evidence of pressure can easily be observed by closely inspecting the skin over the bony prominences of the scapulas, trochanters, knees, elbows, heels, and sacrum.

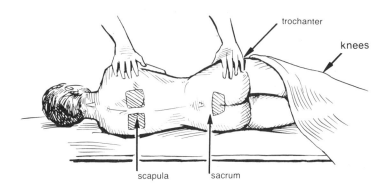

You will observe that the skin becomes reddened, often within 30 to 60 minutes. Because the blood vessels are compressed by the weight of the body pressing against the bed surface, the circulation slows down and the skin takes on a mottled dusky or bluish appearance. Continued compression of the blood vessels decreases the supply of oxygen and nutrients to the surrounding tissues, resulting in *necrosis,* or death of the tissue, which leads to the formation of a decubitus ulcer or pressure sore. Although a decubitus ulcer may develop after only a few hours, particularly in the aged or poorly-nourished patient, the process of healing often takes many weeks, months, and sometimes years of treatment. It is easier to prevent decubitus ulcers than it is to cure them.

The damage to the skin can be further aggravated by heat, soiled or wet bedclothes, and irritation from perspiration, urine, feces, or vaginal discharges. These environmental factors also provide breeding places for bacteria that cause infection in the broken skin area. Wrinkles in the bedding, crumbs and other foreign substances in the bed, and friction from restless moving about in bed can also lead to the development of pressure sores.

Prevention of Pressure Sores

The prevention of pressure sores is the responsibility of the nursing staff. When a patient develops a decubitus, it is often considered a sign of neglect and poor nursing care. You can prevent pressure sores by:

1. Carefully and frequently observing the color of the skin. Skin that is red, blue, or mottled signifies impaired circulation.

2. Changing the patient's position at least every 2 hours.

3. Restoring circulation to a deprived area by rubbing *around* a reddened area. Do not massage the reddened skin itself, because it has already suffered temporary damage. Use a circular motion, starting just outside the reddened area and moving outward in an ever-widening circle. This will rush the stagnant venous blood away from the affected area and replace it with fresh arterial blood. The friction causes the blood vessels to dilate and bring more blood to the area, and more nutrients and oxygen are delivered to the affected area.

4. Keeping the patient dry and clean at all times. The application of small amounts of powder helps to keep the skin dry.

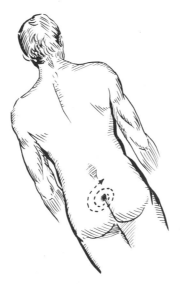

5. Avoiding any mechanical or physical injury to the skin from improper fitting of splints, braces, casts, and prostheses, or from burns caused by excessively hot or cold applications such as hot water bottles, ice bags, heating pads, heating lamps, and so forth.

Treatment of Pressure Areas

Specific treatments for the care of a decubitus ulcer are usually ordered by the physician, although nursing departments have developed nursing procedures that may be instituted when a decubitus is first discovered. When the decubitus is large and far-advanced, surgical intervention to remove necrotic tissue or to cover it with a skin graft may be indicated.

Given an elderly, severely undernourished, and emaciated (extremely thin) male patient who has been lying on his back for two hours, change his position to the left Sims' position using good body alignment principles for both yourself and your patient and observing the condition of the skin and taking appropriate steps.

Supplies Needed

Rubbing alcohol, lotion, or powder
Protective devices (antidecubitus pads, heel protectors, eggcrate mattress pad, Reston foam pads, and so forth)

Pillows

Important Steps	Key Points
Carry out Universal Steps A, B, C, and D. See Appendix.	
1. Place the patient in the Sims' position.	Inspect the bony prominences over the scapula, sacrum, elbows, and heels for redness.

UNIT 18

Important Steps	Key Points
2. Massage the back and bony prominences.	Frequent brief massages or backrubs with lotion or alcohol when changing your patient's position not only improve the circulation but also help to relax the patient. If you should find evidence of beginning pressure areas, start prompt action. Massage the area carefully to increase the circulation. Follow your agency's procedure for the use of special solutions to apply to the skin, foam padding around the pressure areas, or dry heat from an electric light.
3. Align and support the patient in good position.	See that the head, neck, and back are in a straight line. Place a pillow under the head and neck to prevent muscle strain. Put a pillow under the right leg for support from knee to foot.
4. Use protective aids to reduce pressure on the skin.	You will want to plan to turn patient frequently, give back care, and use antidecubitus pads, heel protectors, alternating air-pressure pads, and other protective devices.

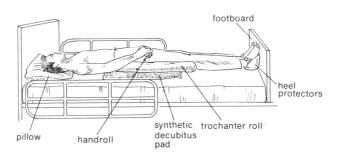

Patient in supine position with supportive
aids to maintain body alignment and protective
devices to reduce pressure.

Carry out Universal Steps X, Y, and Z. See Appendix.	**Charting example:** 0310. Position changed to left Sims'. Reddened area on sacrum massaged. Placed on antidecubitus pad. <div align="right">J. Jones, NA</div> 0345: Sleeping quietly. <div align="right">J. Jones, NA</div>

This can be one of your most important and satisfying procedures. You can be particularly pleased with your performance if you prevent bedsores from beginning or from advancing after they are discovered.

ITEM 3. SKIN AND CAST CARE

People with diseases or injuries involving the bones and joints generally require immobilization for long periods of time so that healing can take place. Fractures of bones must be immobilized in the correct position until they have healed. Casts, splints, surgical pinning or repair, and various types of traction are used to prevent movement in the bones or joints.

Those who have a simple fracture of a bone in an extremity may be able to resume many of their normal activities after a cast has been applied to the part. Healing can be expected to occur within four to six weeks. Serious or multiple fractures, however, may require months of hospitalization and different combinations of casts or traction. Because of such prolonged inactivity, it is vital that general hygienic care be carried out daily. This includes attention to diet, rest, cleanliness, elimination, alignment, care of the skin, and prevention of pressure.

Care of Newly Applied Casts

As a nurse, you need to become familiar with the general procedures of providing skin care and checking circulation while working with patients in casts and traction. After a brief explanation about casts we'll consider the patient who has just returned to the unit with a new cast.

There are a number of preparations used in making casts, but plaster of Paris has been the most widely used material. It is available in powder form or in specially prepared strips. When moistened with water, plaster can be shaped or molded into casts for any portion of the body. Various types of plastic or acrylic materials are also used in making casts. Purported advantages of these over the plaster cast include more rapid drying, better resistance to breaking or cracking, lighter weight, and greater porousness, which allows air to circulate more readily.

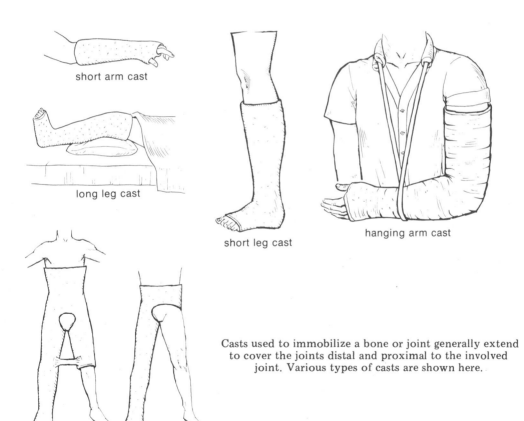

short arm cast

long leg cast

short leg cast

hanging arm cast

hip spica casts

Casts used to immobilize a bone or joint generally extend to cover the joints distal and proximal to the involved joint. Various types of casts are shown here.

U
N
I
T
18

Casts are applied, adjusted, split, or removed only by the doctor or a cast room technician working under the doctor's direction. When a cast is to be used, a length of stockinette material is put over the body part, which is then wrapped with soft wadding material; then the plaster or plastic cast is applied. After that procedure the nursing care of the patient begins as follows:

1. Check the circulation in the part every hour for 24 to 48 hours and at least every 4 hours thereafter, unless specified otherwise by the doctor's orders or agency policies.

2. Allow time for drying; plaster takes between 24 and 48 hours to dry, although the plastic casts may dry in a few hours. Some agencies permit the use of fans or hair dryers to hasten the drying of the cast, but you must avoid chilling the patient.

3. Support the casted portion of the body at all times until the cast is dry. If the cast is on an extremity, elevate the part above the level of the heart to reduce possible swelling.

4. Keep the cast whole and intact. Do not twist or apply pressure on the wet cast. Even finger print indentations on a cast may cause pressure on underlying tissues.

Check of Circulation

Nurses must frequently check the circulation of any body part to which a cast has been applied. You must do this deliberately and thoroughly, then record the information. Check the circulation every hour for the first 24 to 48 hours, and then at least once every four hours. Look for signs of impaired circulation and listen carefully to possible complaints of discomfort from the patient. Complaints of pain involving any area under the cast should never be taken lightly because the pain may be the only sign of pressure on a bony prominence or it may indicate impaired circulation. Unless you act promptly, the tissues will die, causing a condition called gangrene; this means that the cellular death has occurred because of poor or inadequate blood circulation to the body part in the cast.

Five specific areas must be checked for one or more of these cardinal signs of impaired circulation:

1. Temperature — coldness.

2. Color — paleness or cyanosis.

3. Movement — numbness or inability to move.

4. Pain — burning or tingling.

5. Edema or swelling.

First, feel the part to check its temperature, then ask the patient to move or wiggle the part. At the same time note the color of the skin and whether there is swelling. Even when the patient is asleep, check the circulation by observing the temperature, color, swelling, and movement of the part. If you find any of the signs of impaired circulation, notify the nurse at once. Delays in restoring adequate circulation to an extremity have led to nerve and tissue damage, and even to amputation. Remember that not all of the signs of impaired circulation need be present for severe damage to occur.

Skin Care and Cast Care

Immobilizing a body part with a cast often causes tightness or pressure after even the *slightest* change in position from the time the cast was first applied. The most common pressure areas are located around the top and botton edges of the cast and over any bony prominences. At the top or bottom edges, you may be able to rearrange some of the wadding to provide more room and relieve the pressure. If this doesn't work, tell the nurse, who may be able to try other methods before notifying the doctor. Pressure over bony prominences such as the ankle, knee, or wrist should be reported to the doctor, who will cut a window in the cast over the area, or bivalve the entire cast and secure the two halves in position with Ace bandages or tape.

When the plaster cast dries, small bits of plaster break off the cast or drop off the skin. If these crumbs fall inside the cast, they cause discomfort and irritate the patient's skin. Some of this can be prevented by washing the dried plaster off the skin and by covering the raw edges of the cast. You can fold the stockinette material down over the edges of the cast and secure it with adhesive tape. Small strips of adhesive tape can also be used to "petal" or enclose the raw, uneven edges. Long pieces of tape applied in a running manner usually do not cover tightly enough or remain in place for long.

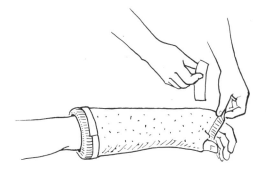

Pull stockinette over edge
and secure with tape.

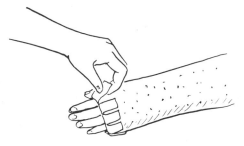

Use short strips of adhesive tape
to "petal" edges.

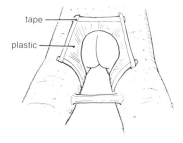

Methods of smoothing
rough edges of cast.

Line opening of spica and body casts with
plastic material to keep cast dry and clean.

Patients frequently complain about the skin itching under a cast after a week or so. A soothing lotion may help relieve itching near the edge of the cast where you can reach it. You must discourage the patient from using long objects to reach under the cast and scratch the itching area. This can easily break the skin, after which it can become infected. The warm, dark, and moist atmosphere under the cast can cause bacteria to flourish if once introduced.

When healing has occurred and the cast is removed, the underlying skin is dry, crusty, and flaking. Although the outer layer of skin is constantly being shed by the body, the dead skin cells accumulate on the skin when it is covered by a cast. You will have to soak off this layer of old, dead skin by using oil or lotion; do not just pull it off. Caution the patient not to scrub the area too vigorously, because this may damage the tender skin.

Given a patient with a long leg cast who is perspiring and in poor alignment, you are to provide care, position, and check the circulation in the casted leg.

UNIT
18

Items Needed

Basin of warm water and soap   Pillows
Towels and washcloth

Important Steps	Key Points
Carry out Universal Steps A, B, C, and D. See Appendix.	
1. Check the circulation of the part.	Check the circulation every hour: Note the color and temperature of the skin. Ask patient to move the part and observe for signs of swelling and pain caused by the cast. Elevate the casted extremity on pillows to reduce swelling.
2. Check the edges of the cast.	Inspect for rough or frayed areas around the edges of cast. When the cast is dry enough for tape to stick to it, smooth off its edges. Rough edges can cause pressure on the skin. Redness and discomfort are the first signs.
3. Check for dryness of the cast.	When the plaster of Paris cast is wet, it is shiny and white. When it dries, the cast becomes dull and gray. During the drying process, leave the cast uncovered so that the air can circulate fully to help it dry. It takes more than 24 hours for a cast to dry thoroughly.

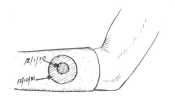

Short arm cast
with bloody seepage.

Elevate or support a wet new cast with pillows covered with plastic. If the fracture was repaired by a surgical operation (an open reduction), there may be some seepage of blood through the cast. Mark the extent of the seepage in pencil around the seepage area on the outside of the cast along with the date and time. If the area enlarges, report this at once to the doctor.

4. Check pressure areas.

Observe carefully to prevent pressure areas from developing. If the patient has a long leg cast, the cast should be supported so that the top of the cast does not cause pressure at the groin. You can do this by placing a pillow under the calf of the leg.

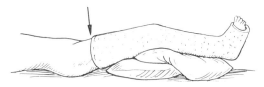

Long leg cast.

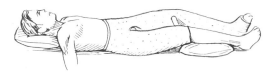

Body cast.

If the patient is in a body cast, you must make sure that his respirations are not obstructed. You will need additional pillows to minimize pressure on the skin at the edges of the cast.

Important Steps	Key Points
5. Bathe and dry patient's skin and provide dry linens.	Inspect the bed for dryness and cleanliness. Change linen as necessary. Since the patient is perspiring freely, you will need to bathe and dry the skin.
6. Have the patient assist you in shifting position.	This activity helps exercise the muscles. The patient can tell you if he is comfortable. During the moving and repositioning, the trapeze is especially useful. Pillows are helpful if properly placed when the patient is on a bedpan.

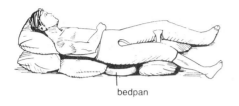

bedpan

You will need to keep all casts clean and dry. If the cast becomes soiled with urine or feces, it soon gives off a very offensive odor, which is not only embarrassing to the patient but also disagreeable to everyone. You can lightly sponge the cast with soap and water after it has become completely dry.

Carry out Universal Steps X, Y, and Z. See Appendix.

Charting example:
1045. Position and linen changed. Toes move and are warm to touch, and pink in color. No swelling and no complaints of pain.

J. Jones, L.V.N.

ITEM 4. TRACTION

Running Traction Versus Balanced (Suspension) Traction

Traction, the application of a pulling force, is employed to maintain parts of the body (bones, joints, body segments) in extension and alignment. In *running traction*, the pulling force is in one direction and is produced by weights that are attached by means of a rope passing over a pulley.

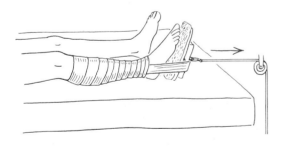

Buck's traction is an example of running traction, with force in one direction. It is also a type of skin traction.

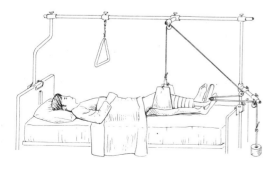

Russell's traction is an example of balanced traction in which force is exerted in several directions. Overbed frame and elevation of lower leg are required.

U
N
I
T
18

Balanced, or *suspension*, *traction* provides support for the extremity and exerts pulling forces in several directions through a system of balanced weights. In both of the foregoing types of tractions the weights are counteracted by the patient's own weight, and this provides the pulling force. The weights must be freehanging in order to exert the required force; check frequently to make sure that the weights are not resting on the floor or hooked under the bed frame. The patient's body should be lying free in bed, so that the feet do not rest against the foot of the bed if the force is in that direction.

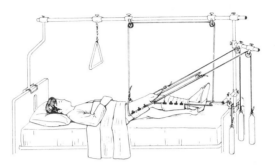

Balanced traction to align broken bone in thigh.
Pin is inserted in bone below knee for skeletal
traction. Note overbed frame and trapeze bar.

Skin Traction and Skeletal Traction

In *skin traction*, the pulling force is applied to the body surface. The part or extremity is wrapped in stockinette, moleskin, or some other type of material and attached to a footplate or spreader board by means of straps. This in turn is attached to weights through a rope and pulley arrangement. Slings, girdles, and elastic bandages work on the same principle as skin traction. Two examples of this are Buck's traction and pelvic traction.

In contrast to skin traction is *skeletal traction*, in which the pulling force is applied directly to the bone. This can be done by means of surgical pins or wires inserted through the bone or metal tongs anchored into the skull. Weights are attached via a rope and pulley.

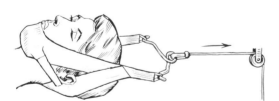

One type of skin traction
using head halter.

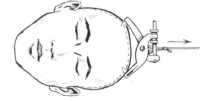

Skeletal traction with use of Crutchfield
tongs inserted in skull bone.

Like the patient in a cast, the patient who has traction on a portion of the body needs to have frequent changes of position. Skin care should also be given to prevent pressure areas from developing. Be sure to use aseptic technique to prevent infection at the sites where pins, wires, or tongs are inserted.

ITEM 5. SKIN CARE FOR THE PATIENT WITH A COLOSTOMY

As explained in Unit 25, Bowel Elimination, a colostomy is formed by bringing a segment of the colon through the abdominal wall and making a stoma through which fecal material is eliminated. The colostomy is often a life-saving procedure, but many patients have difficulties in coping with their feelings about this drastic change in the functioning of their bodies. When caring for such patients, you will have to be warm but matter-of-fact; you must listen when they express their feelings. As soon as they are able to look at the stoma and show an interest in how the colostomy works, you should teach them how to take care of the skin and change or empty the stoma bag.

As a beginning practitioner in nursing, you will not be expected to change the colostomy bag in the early postoperative care of patients who have colostomies or ileostomies. Once their bowel movements have become somewhat regulated, however, you may be expected to dispose of the collected drainage and to cleanse the skin around the stoma.

The skin must be carefully protected in patients who have had ileostomies or colostomies to avoid any excoriation of the skin by the digestive juices that are often present in the fecal drainage. The acid and enzymes in the digestive juices literally eat away the outer layer of skin. An area denuded in this way is painful and may easily become infected. The lower the location of the colostomy in the intestinal tract, the less the amount of irritating substances in the drainage.

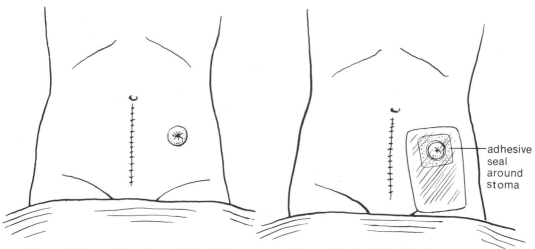

adhesive seal around stoma

Stoma of descending colon with healed midline suture lines.   Disposable plastic bag in place over stoma.

In the skill laboratory, become acquainted with the colostomy materials. Examine different types of collecting bags used on ileostomies, and the disposable stoma bags used for colostomies. Then practice the procedure of changing a colostomy bag, paying particular attention to the patient's skin around the stoma.

Supplies Needed

Disposable stoma bag   Toilet tissue
Medication, if ordered   Paper bag or newspaper
Basin of warm water   Towels and washcloth

Important Steps	Key Points
Carry out Universal Steps A, B, C, and D. See Appendix.	
1. Place the patient in a supine position and put the bed at a comfortable working height.	Fowler's position allows the patient to see more easily and become more involved. Fold the top bedding across the lower abdomen and expose only the portion where you will be working.
2. Remove the bag filled with drainage.	Most disposable plastic stoma bags are stuck to the skin with an adhesive. The adhesive may be part of the bag itself, or a gasket may be attached to a bag that can be hooked to a belt for added security. Use toilet paper to remove excess drainage from the stoma and skin surfaces. Put the soiled tissue on an old newspaper for later disposal. Empty the contents of the bag into the toilet and dispose of the bag.
3. Cleanse the skin and stoma.	Wash gently with soap and water and pat dry. Avoid using friction on the stoma. Inspect the skin areas; redness is the first sign of irritation.
4. Apply special powder or ointment around the stoma, if ordered.	Following surgery, many doctors order karaya gum powder or other medications such as Amphojel, zinc oxide, lanolin, or Vaseline to protect the skin from the drainage.
5. Apply a clean stoma bag.	The opening in the bag should be the correct size. If too large, it leaves skin surfaces exposed, and if too small, it puts pressure on the stoma. The stoma does shrink during the first few weeks and months, so it should be measured again for correct fit. The adhesive backing on the disposable bag sticks directly onto the skin. Fasten the belt to the gasket of the bag if a belt is used.
Carry out Universal Steps X, Y, and Z. See Appendix.	Charting example: 1410. Colostomy drainage bag changed. Moderate amounts of soft brown stool. Skin around stoma shows no sign of irritation. J. Jones, LPN

ITEM 6.   USE OF PERMANENT STOMA BAGS

Patients who have ileostomies or colostomies of the ascending or transverse colon commonly use the permanent stoma bag to collect the drainage that flows day and night. The continual flow requires frequent removal of the drainage to keep it from irritating the stoma and skin. Pulling off the disposable stoma bags with the adhesive backing irritates the skin and leads to severe excoriation by the drainage. This damage to the skin must be prevented if at all possible. The permanent, nondisposable stoma bag is one method used to reduce skin irritation, since it remains in place for days and even weeks at a time.

The permanent drainage collecting bag is firmly attached to the skin with a cement. It is removed only when the drainage seeps under the seal or if there is a need to deodorize or to replace the bag. An opening at the bottom of the bag can be unplugged or unclamped to allow the removal of the collected drainage. You can use an irrigating syringe and tap water to flush out the inside of the bag before reclosing it.

Directions for caring for the patient who has a permanent stoma appliance follow.

Remove the Drainage from the Bag

||||||||||||||||||||||||||||||||||||||||||||||||||||||||||||||||||||||||||||||||||||||||||||||||||||||||||||||||||||||||||||||||||

Items Needed:

| Disposable irrigating set with | Collecting basin |
| irrigating syringe | Toilet tissues |

||||||||||||||||||||||||||||||||||||||||||||||||||||||||||||||||||||||||||||||||||||||||||||||||||||||||||||||||||||||||||||||||||

Important Steps	Key Points

Carry out Universal Steps A, B, C, and D. See Appendix.

1. Unplug or unclamp the bottom of the bag and remove the drainage.

The bag can be drained into a plastic basin or bedpan. Measure the amount, record it on the output record, and flush the drainage down the toilet. Refer to Unit 25 for illustration of permanent stoma bag.

2. Rinse the inside of the bag.

Use tap water and an irrigating syringe. Instill the water into the bag. Then hold the end of the bag shut and swish the water around without pulling on the seal. Drain and use more clear water to rinse.

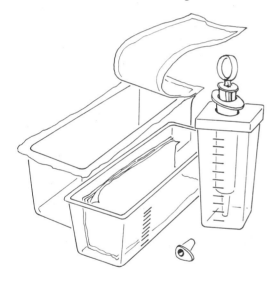

Typical disposable irrigation set

3. Close the bottom of the bag.

Carry out Universal Steps X, Y, and Z. See Appendix.

Apply the Permanent Stoma Bag

If possible, arrange to observe when the ostomy nurse specialist changes the permanent stoma bag for the patient. After the used bag is removed, the skin is thoroughly cleansed to remove the old cement and other material. Medication is used to protect any exposed portion of the skin and the stoma before a new bag is reapplied.

Supplies Needed

Stoma bag   Basin of warm water
Stoma adhesive or cement   Towel and washcloth

Important Steps	Key Points
Follow steps 1 through 4, Item 5.	
5. Apply the first coat of cement around the stoma and the ring or gasket of the bag.	Follow the directions on the appliance package for measuring the opening for the stoma. Use an applicator to apply the cement. Cover an area at least one inch larger than the ring or gasket will cover. Let the skin area and the gasket dry completely; allow 30 to 60 seconds.
6. Apply a second coat of cement.	Again cover both the skin area and the gasket or ring of the bag.
7. Place the ring or gasket on the skin covering the stoma.	Press it firmly to the cemented area of the skin. Hold it in place until the two are tightly stuck together.
8. Attach it to the belt.	Make sure the end of the stoma bag is secured to prevent leakage.

Complete and chart the procedure.

ITEM 7. CARE OF FINGERNAILS AND TOENAILS

This is one aspect of personal care that most patients can handle for themselves. However you may need to do it for patients who cannot because they are unconscious, blind, confused, unsteady, or in a cast or traction.

Usually nail care is accomplished at the time of the regular bath. The nails should be kept clean and trimmed according to your agency regulations. Do not cut the toenails or fingernails of a diabetic patient or one who has circulatory disease of the lower extremities until you have checked your agency's regulations.

Since nails frequently can become tough and thick, soak the hands and feet 5 to 10 minutes in warm, soapy water before attempting to cut the nails. The soaking will soften the nail and the cuticle (the outer portion of the skin surrounding the nail) sufficiently so that you can easily cut or file the nails and gently push back the cuticle with an orange stick.

Toe nails are cut straight across to prevent them from growing into the skin along the sides, which causes pain or infection and leads to a condition called ingrown nails. Ingrown toenails may require a surgical procedure to correct. Manicured cuticles prevent hangnails (a partly detached piece of skin at the base of the fingernail), which are painful and unsightly, and the source of possible infections.

If it is necessary for you to observe the color of a patient's nailbeds — for example, after surgery or cast application — it may be necessary to remove any colored polish on the nails. Well-cared for fingernails and toenails are an essential part of good grooming for your patient as well as for yourself.

PERFORMANCE TEST

In the skill laboratory or the classroom, your instructor will ask you to perform the following procedures without reference to any source material.

1. Given an elderly patient who has had surgical repair of a fractured hip, provide special skin care after the patient has been incontinent of urine.

2. Given a patient with a head injury who has been lying in one position for about two hours, provide care to prevent the formation of decubitus ulcers.

3. Given a young boy with a long leg cast applied three hours ago, check for signs of pressure or impaired circulation to the limb and describe how you would care for the drying cast.

4. Given an older woman who had a colostomy of the descending colon six days ago, remove the partially filled stoma bag and replace it with another.

PERFORMANCE CHECKLIST

SKIN CARE FOR THE INCONTINENT PATIENT

1. Wash your hands.

2. Approach and identify the patient and explain what you are going to do.

3. Pick up the required supplies: clean linen, soap, and water.

4. Provide privacy.

5. Adjust the bed to working height.

6. Assist the patient to turn onto side.

7. Remove the soiled linen.

8. Wash the urine from the skin, then dry it thoroughly.

9. Give patient a backrub and massage possible pressure areas.

10. Put a clean gown on the patient; remake the bed.

11. Provide for the patient's comfort, attach the signal light, and raise the siderails.

12. Remove the soiled materials.

13. Report and record.

SKIN CARE TO PREVENT DECUBITUS ULCERS

1. Wash your hands.

2. Approach and identify the patient; explain the procedure.

3. Provide privacy.

4. Adjust the bed to working height.

5. Turn the patient to Sims' position.

6. Align and support the patient in good position.

7. Inspect the skin of his back; give a backrub and massage over the bony prominences.

8. Use protective aids to reduce pressure.

9. Provide for the patient's comfort. Rearrange the bedding neatly, raise the siderails, and secure the call light within reach.

10. Report and record as appropriate.

CIRCULATION AND CAST CARE

1. Wash your hands.

2. Approach and identify the patient; explain the procedure.

3. Adjust the bed to working level.

4. Check the circulation in the toes.

   a. Note their temperature, color, and movement.

   b. Check for complaints of pain.

   c. Observe for signs of swelling.

5. Check the dryness of the cast.

6. Look for signs of pressure around the edges of the cast.

7. When the cast is drier, finish the rough edges with tape or stockinette.

8. Reposition the patient; support the cast when being moved.

9. Provide for the patient's comfort.

10. Report and record appropriate information.

CHANGING A COLOSTOMY BAG

1. Wash your hands.

2. Approach and identify the patient; explain the procedure.

3. Assemble the equipment needed.

4. Provide privacy.

5. Place the bed at a comfortable working height.

6. Have the patient in supine or semi-Fowler's position.

7. Remove the bag filled with drainage and discard it.

8. Cleanse the skin and stoma.

9. Apply medication or ointment if ordered.

10. Apply a clean bag to the stoma and attach it to the belt if one is used.

11. Provide for the patient's comfort.

12. Report and record appropriate information.

POST-TEST

Matching.   Select the phrase from Column 2 that best describes the words in Column 1. Write the letter designating that phrase in the blank space in Column 1.

Column 1	Column 2
_____ 1. necrosis	a. damage to skin from chemicals
_____ 2. dermis	b. excretion of perspiration
_____ 3. decubitus	c. the first, or outer layer of skin
_____ 4. abrasion	d. inability to control feces and urine
_____ 5. cyanosis	e. circulation of blood in arteries and veins
_____ 6. sebaceous gland	f. a pulling force on the body
_____ 7. incontinence	g. the second, or true, layer of skin
_____ 8. excoriation	h. excretes an oily substance
_____ 9. epidermis	i. damage to the skin by scraping
_____ 10. traction	j. death of tissues
	k. skin color change caused by insufficient oxygen
	l. damage to skin due to pressure

Multiple Choice.   Circle the letter of the best answer for each of the following questions.

11. When you give a bath or special skin care to a patient, the layer or structure of the skin that you touch is

   a. muscle.

   b. epidermis.

   c. dermis.

   d. follicles.

12. The nerve ending and the blood vessels of the skin are located in which layer or structure?

   a. muscle

   b. epidermis

   c. dermis

   d. follicles

13. When the continuous surface of the skin has been damaged or broken, as in an abrasion or decubitus ulcer, the body has lost some of its ability to

   a. resist infections.

   b. take in oxygen supply.

   c. eliminate waste products.

   d. maintain body alignment.

14. A possible disadvantage to the use of alcohol when giving a backrub is that

    a. it evaporates and cools the body.

    b. it removes oils and waste products from the skin.

    c. it toughens and dries out the skin.

    d. it coagulates blood in the tissues.

15. In some patients, pressure can cause the beginning of a decubitus within a matter of hours. When you observe the *first* sign of pressure, you should immediately do which of the following?

    a. Make sure that the skin is clean and dry.

    b. Turn the patient at least every two hours.

    c. Use padding or protective aids to reduce pressure.

    d. Massage around the reddened skin area to stimulate circulation.

16. In caring for the patient who is incontinent, you should keep the skin clean and dry and

    a. use padding or disposable diapers to catch the urine or feces.

    b. offer the bedpan or urinal frequently for retraining.

    c. check the bed linens frequently to see if they are soiled.

    d. remind the patient that soiling the bed made extra work for you.

17. For the bed patient, pressure over a bony prominence such as the sacrum can result in

    a. necrosis and formation of a sore or ulcer.

    b. reddening of the skin due to impaired circulation.

    c. decreased supply of nutrients and oxygen to the tissues.

    d. a, b, and c

    e. a and b

18. A patient has had a cast applied for a fracture of the leg and now complains of pain in the ankle area. The toes move, are warm to touch, and are of normal skin color. You would conclude that

    a. the patient is a complainer.

    b. the pain is normal because of the fracture.

    c. the cast may be causing pressure.

    d. the signs do not indicate impaired circulation.

19. A sharp object should not be used by the patient to scratch the itching areas under the cast because

    a. it may poke holes in the cast or damage it.

    b. infection may occur if the skin is broken.

    c. the itching is just caused by accumulated dead skin.

    d. it could cause injury that the person might not feel.

20. Excoriation often occurs in the skin around the stoma of an ileostomy or a colostomy as a result of

    a. excessive flatus and the odor of the drainage.

    b. decreased circulation of blood to the area.

    c. poor absorption of fluids in the colon.

    d. action of digestive juices in the drainage or feces.

21. The ointment used around the stoma of a colostomy

    a. cements the colostomy bag in place.

    b. lubricates the stoma for passage of the feces.

    c. provides a protective covering for the skin.

    d. allows easier cleansing of the skin.

22. Before trimming the nails of a patient who has diabetes or circulatory disease of the legs, you should

    a. check with your team leader for instructions.

    b. soak the patient's hands or feet in warm, soapy water.

    c. plan to do this task as part of the bath procedure.

    d. check for hangnails around the cuticles.

POST-TEST ANSWERS

1. j	12. c
2. g	13. a
3. l	14. c
4. i	15. d
5. k	16. b
6. h	17. d
7. d	18. c
8. a	19. b
9. c	20. d
10. f	21. c
11. b	22. a

Unit 19

SPECIAL CARE OF HAIR

GENERAL PERFORMANCE OBJECTIVE

When you have finished this unit, you will be able to demonstrate satisfactorily how to brush, comb, and shampoo a patient's hair without causing discomfort to the patient.

SPECIFIC PERFORMANCE OBJECTIVES

In the clinical setting or in the skill laboratory, you will be able to:

1. Brush, comb, braid, and arrange a patient's hair in accordance with recommended procedure.
2. Prepare and give a shampoo to a patient in bed or at the sink in the bathroom.
3. Care for the hair of members of the black race.

VOCABULARY

braiding (plaiting)—a method of hair styling frequently used for the hospitalized patient with long hair to keep the hair neat.

dandruff—fungus infection of the scalp in which the scalp becomes dry and scaly; daily hair care and frequent shampoos help prevent this condition; dandruff infections may be transmitted from one person to another by sharing a comb or brush.

nits—eggs of the louse (plural, lice).

pediculosis—the presence of the parasitic lice on the body, in the hair of the scalp, or in the hair of the pubic area.

INTRODUCTION

The condition of the hair is affected by the general health of the individual. In some cases, it is easy to note disease conditions by the appearance of the shaft of the hair. Coarse and dry hair may be associated with an underactive thyroid gland (hypothyroidism); hair falling out may be associated with the incidence of high temperatures lasting long periods of time.

The visible portion of the hair (shaft) is supplied with nutrients (food) through the roots, which are anchored in the scalp. The supply of nutrients is therefore very important to the health of the hair. It is important to brush and comb the hair, because this stimulates the circulation of the scalp, cleans the hair shafts of dirt particles and dead skin cells, and brings nutrients to the roots.

Hair care should be given regularly during illness just as it would be normally, usually with the morning care activities and throughout the day as needed. The morale of the patient is improved when his or her appearance is tidy. Neat, clean hair is particularly important to the female patient's sense of well-being. The best time to give hair care is after the morning bath or with the early A.M. care.

DAILY CARE OF HAIR AND SHAMPOOS

ITEM 1. PRINCIPLES OF HAIR CARE

Different types of hair are described in a number of ways. The shaft of the hair may be coarse and thick or thin and wispy. The amount of hair on the head may be thick and profuse or thin and skimpy. Hair is straight or may have some degree of curl to it. Very tightly curled hair may be called kinky, since it resists rearranging and tends to return to the coiled position. This is often seen in blacks, although not universally. It also occurs following the shampooing of a new permanent when the hair is allowed to dry without further styling. Finally, hair is referred to as normal, oily, or dry, depending on the amount of oil secreted by the glands in the scalp.

Care of Normal Hair

The hair picks up the same dirt and oils as the skin and should be washed at frequent intervals to remove these and keep it clean. Most people shampoo weekly, but during illness a longer period of time may elapse between shampoos. At other times, you may need to shampoo the hair of an accident victim or injured person with matted, snarled, and blood- and dirt-soiled hair as soon as it is permitted by the doctor.

The following principles can serve as guidelines for the nurse in caring for the hair.

1. According to the policy of most agencies, there must be permission of the doctor or a written order before hospitalized patients may be given a shampoo.

2. Hair is not cut without the patient's permission. When it is medically necessary to cut the hair or shave a portion of the head, most agencies obtain the patient's consent first, and in writing when possible. The consent given for emergency medical treatment and the consent for surgery on the head would cover cutting the hair in those cases when necessary.

3. Care of short hair is seldom a problem, as it is easier to manage, easier to brush and comb, and easier to arrange attractively. Long hair may need to be gathered together and secured neatly, or braided.

4. Bacteria can be carried on the hair, so nurses should avoid touching and brushing back their own hair when giving care to patients. Nurses should cover their hair when providing care to patients in reverse isolation, for skin and wound precautions, and in surgery and other areas where sterile technique is carried out. Shampooing removes bacteria, microorganisms, and oils and dirt that cling to the hair.

Special Care for Oily Hair

About the only care required when the patient has hair that is oilier than normal is more frequent shampooing. Some may require the use of more detergent-type shampoos in order to get the hair clean, and in some instances alcohol is used to help break down the oils.

Special Care for Dry Hair

People who have hair that is drier than normal need to take special care of their hair. They shampoo less frequently and may extend the period between shampoos to as much as two weeks. Gentle shampoos and soaps are used to remove the dirt and oils, then conditioners are used to restore oils to the hair shaft.

Many, but not all, blacks have very curly and dry hair that requires more complex care. Such dry hair tends to break off at the follicle, and the ends split very easily without the application of additional oils. Because the hair is fragile, and easily damaged, care must be

UNIT 19

used when combing and brushing it. Very wide-toothed combs and picks are used to remove tangles and separate the hair strands. The oils applied to combat the dryness also help to straighten out the curl and make the hair easier to manage. Popular hair styles are the natural curly look — the Afro style — and the use of braiding in many different ornamental and intricate ways.

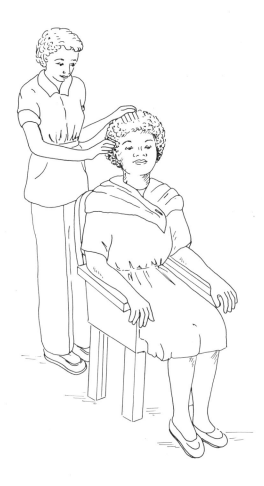

When black patients enter the hospital with bloody or dirty hair and scalp following an injury, shampooing the head with soap and water only makes the hair curlier and harder to comb than before. After the doctor has authorized cleaning the hair, talk to the patient or a family member about the methods used in caring for the hair. If special hair products are not available, the hair can be cleansed with a mixture of alcohol and mineral oil. The alcohol helps to dissolve the oils that have been used on the hair, and the mineral oil helps to cleanse and lubricate the shaft, straighten it out, and make it easier to manage. One method of cleaning the hair and scalp of the black patient follows.

Supplies Needed

Solution of 1 ounce alcohol and 4 ounces mineral oil	Towels (2 or more)
	Afro comb with wide-spaced teeth

Important Steps	Key Points

Carry out Universal Steps A, B, C, and D. See Appendix.

Important Steps	Key Points
1. Place towels under head and over chest.	Protect the bed linen by putting plastic under the towel, if available.
2. Hyperextend the patient's neck.	This position helps prevent the solution from running down the face or into the eyes.
3. Apply solution beginning at the front and side hairlines.	
4. Gently massage the solution into the hair, working toward the back of the head.	The alcohol and oil solution cuts through other oils used previously and helps to clean the hair and scalp.
5. Comb through the hair to remove tangles.	Hold the hair between the scalp and the ends to provide more support. Begin combing out snarls or tangles from the end and work toward the scalp.
6. Towel dry the hair.	This removes the loosened dirt and excess solution.
7. Shampoo hair with water, if necessary.	This may be necessary to remove sand from the scalp.
8. Apply oil or lotion to hair.	
9. Arrange the hair in a neat style.	
10. Carry out Universal Steps X, Y, and Z. See Appendix.	

The daily care of the hair of your black patient generally involves applying some oil or lotion to lubricate the dry hair, combing or brushing it, and arranging it in a neat style. Check with the patient to find out the preparation that is preferred for use. Daily care of your black patients' hair is essential in contributing to their health, appearance, and well-being.

Other Conditions of the Scalp

Special hair care may be needed to treat other conditions of the scalp. Various types of shampoos are used to treat scalps with dandruff, which is a fungus infection that causes the scalp to become dry and scaly. Other medicated shampoos are used to remove nits and pediculi. Pediculi are parasites called lice and are found on the hair of the scalp, body, and pubic area of infected persons. Nits are the eggs of the lice and must also be removed in order to prevent reinfection.

Care of Wigs

The use of certain drugs in the treatment of cancer leads to loss of hair and baldness. Hair may fall out by the handful when it is combed or brushed. These patients, especially women, often wear wigs to conceal their baldness. Generally, these wigs require little care by the nurse, as they tend to hold the hair style in which they were made. When a wig needs to be shampooed or styled, it should be done by a professional hairdresser.

ITEM 2.   COMBING AND BRUSHING HAIR

Given a female bed patient with long hair, you are to comb, brush, and arrange her hair in a becoming manner.

IIIIIIIIIIIIIIIIIIIIIIIIIIIIIIIIIIIIIIIIIIIIIIIIIIIIIIIIIIIIIIIIIIIIIIIIIIIIIIIIIIIIIIIIIIIIIIIIIIIIIIIIIIIIIIIIIIIIIIIIIIIIIIIIIIIIIIIIIIIIIIIIIIIIIIIIIIIIIIIIIIIIIIIIIIIIIIIIIII

Supplies Needed:

Comb and brush   Bath towel
Mirror   Hair spray or lotion

IIIIIIIIIIIIIIIIIIIIIIIIIIIIIIIIIIIIIIIIIIIIIIIIIIIIIIIIIIIIIIIIIIIIIIIIIIIIIIIIIIIIIIIIIIIIIIIIIIIIIIIIIIIIIIIIIIIIIIIIIIIIIIIIIIIIIIIIIIIIIIIIIIIIIIIIIIIIIIIIIIIIIIIIIIIIIIIIIII

Important Steps	Key Points
Carry out Universal Steps A, B, and C. See Appendix.	

1. Place a towel over the pillow.

   Put a clean towel over the patient's pillow to keep it from becoming soiled.

2. Turn the patient's head away from you.

   This will make it easier for you to comb and brush the back of the hair. It will also keep the hair from getting in the patient's face and eyes.

3. Part the hair.

   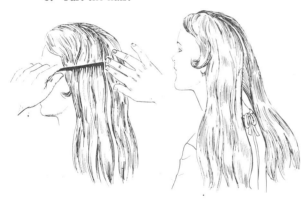

   It will be easier to handle if you part the hair from the front to the back. The hair is thinner in front and it will eliminate some of the pulling of the hair, thus making it more comfortable for your patient.
   The teeth of the comb should be dull so that they will not scratch the scalp. Stiff bristles on the brush are best for hair care. Brushes which have widely separated tufts (clumps) or bristles are the easiest to clean.

4. First divide the hair into three main sections; then, as you work, handle it in smaller subsections.

   This will make it simpler for you to proceed in a systematic way as you comb or brush. You will reach every portion of the scalp if you proceed in this manner.

5. Brush or comb the hair in an upward manner, starting near the scalp.

   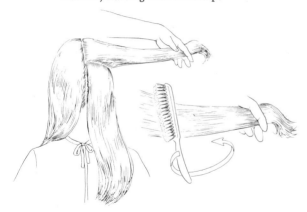

   Grasp a small section of hair between your index and middle fingers. Place the brush or comb near the scalp and use a rotating semi-circular wrist movement to push the brush or comb through the hair. This motion will not scratch the scalp or split the shaft of the hair. It stimulates circulation, massages the scalp, and loosens dry scales and dirt from the scalp and the hair. Remember that some people have very sensitive scalps and that during an illness the scalp becomes more sensitive to pressure; therefore, make every effort not to hurt the patient.

Important Steps	Key Points
6. Keep the hair between your fingers when brushing or combing matted or tangled hair. 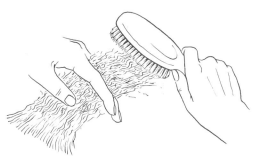	This provides a counterforce to prevent undue pulling on the scalp when you are brushing or combing matted or tangled hair. Alcohol, astringents, or water can be used to loosen hair strands when they are tangled or matted. *Do not cut* the hair to remove them. Daily and frequent brushing or combing prevents tangling and matting of the hair. Talk with the patient in a warm, concerned manner. Observe the patient's condition as you work. If she becomes unusually tired, complete the hair care later in the day.
7. Continue brushing or combing.	Finish all the sections on both sides.
8. Arrange the hair attractively.	The style should be simple and neat. You are not expected to be a professional hair stylist. The patient will probably tell you what is most comfortable. Short hair is the easiest to care for when a person must remain in bed for a long period of time. If the hair is long, you may want to braid it. The procedure for braiding is described later in this unit.
9. Spray the hair or apply hair cream.	Use as desired by the patient to keep the hair neat and in place.
10. Remove the towel. Clean and return the items to the bedside stand.	Universal Steps X, Y, and Z. See Appendix.
11. Provide for the patient's comfort.	
12. Record and report as appropriate.	Record any unusual observations about the condition of the scalp or hair. Usually the entry will be included as a part of the morning care.

ITEM 3. BRAIDING HAIR

Braiding is a method of weaving three strands of hair. Braids are sometimes used as a hair style for youngsters or for patients with long hair. This style is easy to maintain and comfortable, as it keeps the long hair from becoming matted or tangled, conditions that can be particularly painful when the hair is being combed.

Practice braiding in the skill lab on a classmate who has long hair (and is a willing subject) or with three strands of heavy knitting yarn or similar materials. When you are sure you can braid, ask your instructor to observe you in a test situation. You will be checked on the neatness of your finished product. The hair should be firmly anchored with a ribbon or a rubber band to prevent the braids from coming apart.

Supplies Needed

Comb and brush   Bath towel
Rubber bands (2)   Ribbons (optional)

Important Steps	Key Points
1. Explain the procedure to the patient.	You will be using this method as part of the basic hair care procedure. Position the patient's head on the towel-covered pillow with her face turned away from you. Part the hair in the center (from front to back) and work half of the head.
2. Brush or comb the hair and then divide it into three even sections on each side of the head.	Usually the hair can be handled in three large sections for the weaving process. Proceed with each of the sections in the following manner.

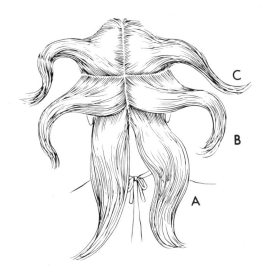

Hold the left (A) strand of hair in three closed fingers of your left hand.

Hold the center (B) strand between the index finger and thumb of your left hand.

Hold the right (C) strand in your right hand.

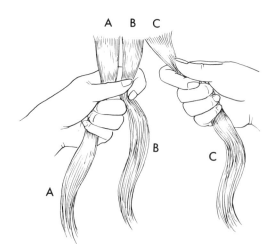

Bring the hair to the side of the patient's head, near the ear. As you entwine the hair, hold the strands taut so that the braid will be firm and will not loosen when the patient moves around. After practice you will learn the correct amount of "pull" that is needed to keep the strands taut.

Important Steps	Key Points

3. Cross the right strand (C) over the center strand (B).

Strand C becomes the new middle strand, and will be transferred to the left hand. The center strand (B) is transferred to the right hand.

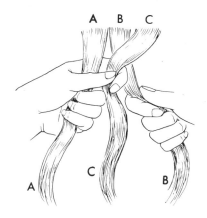

4. Cross the left strand (A) over the center strand (C).

Strand A now becomes the middle strand. Move it to your right hand.

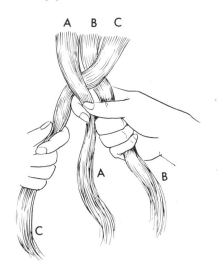

5. Cross the right strand (B) over the center strand (A).

Step 6 can start with the left strand over; step 7 would then be the right strand over the center, and so on.

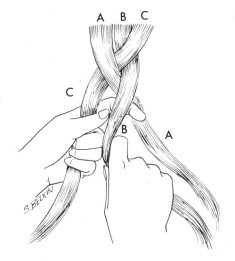

Important Steps	Key Points
6. Continue, repeating steps 3, 4, and 5.	Alternate crossing the left strand over the middle strand, then the right one over the middle strand, and so on until all of the hair is braided.

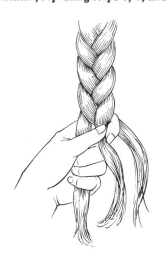

7. Secure the end of the braid.	Bind it with a rubber band looped several times around the tip end of the braid. This will keep the braid from becoming unwound.

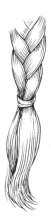

8. Move to the other side of the bed.	Proceed with the other side of the hair, as in steps 2 through 7. Tie with a bright-colored ribbon if available. This provides a touch of color for the patient and will often raise her spirits.

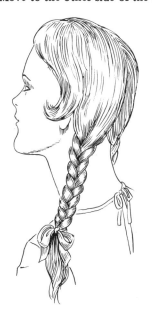

ITEM 4. SHAMPOO FOR THE BED PATIENT

Shampooing of the hair is done only upon the order of the physician. Shampoos may be given in bed with the patient in a sitting or recumbent position, in the utility room on a stretcher, or in the shower. The supine position is preferred for weak patients and by some nurses; however, patients with disease conditions such as asthma, certain heart diseases, and some lung diseases have difficulty breathing unless they are in a sitting position.

Be sure that your patient is well rested. Shampooing is a lengthy procedure that tires the patient a great deal. It is wise to consider a rest period for the patient after the shampoo is completed.

Today many patient rooms are equipped with showers, and the procedure of choice may be to assist the patient with the shampoo while he or she is in the shower. This, of course, will depend entirely upon the patient's general condition.

Supplies Needed

Pitcher	Plastic trough
Bath thermometer	Basin or pail for waste water
Liquid shampoo or soap	Bath towels (2 or more)
Rinse (1 cup of diluted lemon	Bath blanket
juice, vinegar, or commercial	Hair dryer
hair rinse)	Comb and brush

Important Steps	Key Points
Carry out Universal Steps A, B, C, and D. See Appendix.	
1. Prepare the patient for the shampoo.	Remove the pillow and move the patient toward the proximal (near) side of the bed. Have the bed at a convenient working height. Cover the patient with a bath blanket to keep her warm and to protect the bed linens from becoming wet. Fan-fold the top linen to the bottom of the bed. Put a towel around the patient's shoulders.
2. Prepare the equipment.	Place the chair at the head of the bed and put a basin or pail on it to collect the water. Place a trough under the patient's head with one end over the drainage basin.

Important Steps	Key Points
3. Moisten the hair with water (105°F [40.5°C]) and apply the shampoo.	Check the water temperature with a bath thermometer or pour over inner part of your wrist and, if hot, add more cool water. Pour a small amount of water through the patient's hair from the front hairline to the back to moisten the hair thoroughly. A folded washcloth placed over the patient's eyes will help to protect them from soap and water.

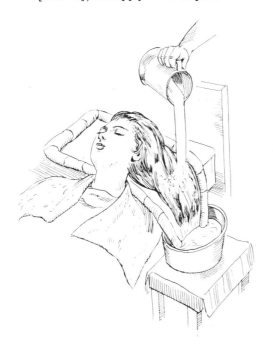

Work the shampoo into a good lather, using your finger tips to massage all portions of the scalp. The patient will tell you if the massage is uncomfortable. Start from the front hairline and proceed toward the back of the head, just as you shampoo your own hair. Add water as needed to keep the lather going.

Important Steps	Key Points
4. Pour water through the hair.	Rinse thoroughly with warm water.
5. Repeat steps 3 and 4.	Apply one more soaping if the hair is not "squeaking clean," and if your patient can tolerate the procedure. Work quickly so that your patient does not become excessively tired. Pour the water carefully as you rinse the shampoo out of the hair.
6. Test for clean, well-rinsed hair.	Continue rinsing the hair until strands pulled between your index finger and thumb produce a squeaking sound.
7. Apply the rinse solution.	It may be necessary to use a commercial rinse, lemon juice, or vinegar solution (1 ounce to 1 quart of water) to rinse the shampoo from the hair.
8. Dry the hair, ears, and neck.	Use a heavy bath towel to remove excess water from the hair. Dry the hair as thoroughly as possible. Keep your patient warm and dry throughout the procedure. Avoid drafts.
9. Arrange the hair.	Comb and brush the hair using a clean comb and brush. Arrange the hair in a neat, attractive way and allow it to dry. An electric hair dryer may be used if one is available in your agency.
Carry out Universal Steps X, Y, and Z. See Appendix.	Charting example: 1030. Bed shampoo given. Became very tired and weak. Stated it "felt very good to have clean hair again." Resting quietly. R. Ryan, LVN

Improvising a Trough

When a commercially made trough is not available in your agency, you can prepare one out of newspaper and plastic sheeting in the following manner.

Important Steps	Key Points
1. Spread six to eight sheets of newspaper on a flat surface.	Use several thicknesses of paper (six to eight sheets), spread out to the length of 3 feet on the bed or a table top.
2. Place plastic sheeting on top of the papers.	Sheeting should be about 36 inches long and 24 inches wide.
3. Roll the long sides of the paper and plastic sheeting toward the center.	Roll each side toward the center of the sheet, leaving the center third flat. This will form two rolled edges.
4. Place one end of the trough under the patient's head.	Place the center flat surface under the head, allowing the rolled edges to provide a channel for the water to run through.
5. Place the other end of the trough in a basin on the chair.	Put a rolled bath towel or small pillow under the trough so that it tilts in a gradual slope, causing the water to run from the patient's head to the side of the bed and into the basin.

ITEM 5. STRETCHER SHAMPOO

||||||||||||||||||||||||||||||||||||||||||||||||||||||||||||||||||||||||||||||||||||||||||||||||||||||

Supplies Needed

Stretcher with safety straps	Plastic trough
Spray attachment for faucet	Bath towels (2 or more)
Bath thermometer	Bath blanket
Liquid shampoo or soap	Hair dryer
Rinse (1 cup of diluted lemon juice, vinegar, or commercial hair rinse)	Comb or brush

||||||||||||||||||||||||||||||||||||||||||||||||||||||||||||||||||||||||||||||||||||||||||||||||||||||

Important Steps	Key Points
Carry out Universal Steps A, B, C, and D. See Appendix.	
1. Check conditions of the room where shampooing will be done.	Be sure that it is warm and free of drafts, and that there is enough space for you to move easily around the stretcher.
2. Bring the stretcher (guerney) to the bedside.	Lock the wheels of the stretcher and the bed to prevent them from rolling as the patient moves onto the stretcher.
3. Move the patient to the stretcher.	Place a bath blanket over the patient, and fan-fold the top linens to the bottom of the bed.

UNIT 19

Important Steps	Key Points
	Follow the procedure used in Unit 14, Item 3. Stand with your body bracing the stretcher against the bed. Ask the patient to move onto the stretcher, first the head and shoulders, then the hips and legs. Assist as necessary while keeping her covered with the bath blanket.
	Secure the safety belts firmly, one over the chest and one over the thighs, to prevent the patient from falling off the stretcher.
4. Transport the patient to the shampoo area.	Place the back wheels in the swivel position (labeled on the wheels) so you can control the stretcher as you move it down the corridor. Push the stretcher from the head end.
5. Place the head end of the stretcher against the sink.	Lock the wheels so that the stretcher will not move during the shampoo procedure.
6. Wrap a towel around the patient's shoulders and neck.	Secure the ends with a safety pin at the patient's chest to keep her warm and dry.
7. Position the patient's head for the shampoo.	If the sink is at or slightly lower than the level of the stretcher, the patient may lay with the head over the end of the stretcher and the rim of the basin. In other cases, the use of a trough is more comfortable and directs the water flow back into the sink.
	A small pillow protected with plastic may be placed under the shoulders if this position is uncomfortable.

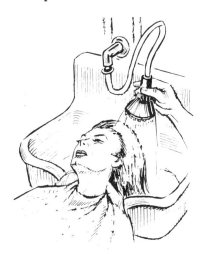

8. Attach the spray nozzle to the faucet and regulate a gentle flow of water until it is warm (105°F [40.5°C]).	Check the water temperature with a bath thermometer or test by running it over your wrist. Avoid splashing.
9. Shampoo the hair.	Use the procedure described for the bed shampoo, steps 3 through 9.
10. Comb or brush the hair.	Arrange it in a neat style. Wrap the hair with a clean, dry towel to keep from chilling the patient when you transport her back to her room.
11. Return the patient to her room.	Check that the safety belts are securely fastened. Push the stretcher from the head end so that you can see where you are going, and transport the patient to her room. Transfer patient from stretcher to bed.

Important Steps	Key Points
Carry out Universal Steps X, Y, and Z. See Appendix.	Charting example: 1030. Taken to bathroom per stretcher and given shampoo. Hair dried. Returned to bed with no complaints. R. Ryans, LVN

PERFORMANCE TEST

In the skill laboratory your instructor will ask you to perform three of the five activities listed below without reference to any of the source materials. For some of the activities you might have to ask another person to take the place of a patient.

1. Given a patient who has suffered a stroke and is unable to comb and brush his or her hair, explain and demonstrate daily care of the hair.

2. Given a female patient who has very long hair and is unable to braid it herself because the exertion would be too strenuous for her condition, braid the hair after the daily brushing and combing.

3. Given a person who is conscious but unable to leave the bed because of recent abdominal surgery, demonstrate giving a shampoo in bed.

4. Given a convalescing patient who is still on partial bed rest, explain and demonstrate how to wash her hair in the bathroom while she is lying on a stretcher.

5. Given a black patient with very curly, dry hair, provide daily hair care.

PERFORMANCE CHECKLIST

BRUSHING AND COMBING HAIR

1. Wash your hands.

2. Identify the patient and explain the procedure.

3. Assemble the correct equipment.

4. Prepare the patient properly, with the bath blanket in place, a towel over the pillow, and the patient's head turned away.

5. Part the hair in the center from the front to the back and divide into three sections on each side.

6. Grasp a small section of hair between your index and middle finger, place the brush near the patient's scalp, and use an upward rotating semicircular wrist movement to push the brush through the hair.

7. Hold the section between your index and middle finger, and in an upward motion, comb through the hair.

8. Perform all brushing and combing without pulling at the patient's scalp or otherwise causing her discomfort.

9. Finish the procedure by arranging the hair neatly and symmetrically.

10. Apply hair spray avoiding the patient's face.

11. Hold up a mirror for the patient to see her hair.

12. Remove the towel and bath blanket.

13. Replace the bed linen properly.

14. Tidy the area, returning all items to their proper places.

BRAIDING HAIR

1. Wash your hands.

2. Identify the patient.

3. Explain the reasons for braiding the patient's hair, such as comfort, neatness, and the prevention of matted hair.

4. Divide the hair into three sections on each side.

5. Begin braiding with the left and middle strands in your left hand and the right strand in your right hand.

6. Proceed by crossing the right and left strands alternately over the center strand.

7. Complete the braiding without losing hold of the strands or causing them to become partly unraveled.

8. Exert sufficient tension on the strands to form neat braids without pulling at the patient's scalp.

9. Bind the tips of the braids with ribbon.

10. Arrange the braids so that they fall at each side of the head.

SHAMPOO OF BED PATIENT

1. Assemble all material needed for the shampoo.

2. Identify the patient and explain the procedure.

3. Complete all preparations before beginning the shampoo.

   a. Place a drawsheet at the head of the bed to protect the linen.

   b. Prepare the patient in the correct position near the side of the bed with the pillow removed, bath blanket in place, and linen folded toward the foot of the bed.

   c. Place a towel securely around the patient's shoulders.

   d. Adjust the bed to a comfortable working position.

   e. Slip the trough under the patient's head, providing it with sufficient slope for drainage into the pail.

   f. Place a chair at the head of the bed, protect it with a plastic cover, and put a pail on the chair.

4. Fill pitcher with warm water ($105°F$ [$40.5°C$]), using a bath thermometer to measure the temperature.

5. Moisten the patient's hair with water before applying the shampoo.

6. Apply the shampoo and work it into the hair fron the front hairline to the back of the head, massaging the scalp firmly with your fingertips.

7. Rinse the hair, removing all shampoo and taking care that the water drains properly into the trough.

8. Repeat the cycle (steps 6 and 7) until the hair is clean, testing for a squeaky sound after each rinse.

9. Dry the patient's ears, neck, and hair thoroughly with the bath towel.

10. Brush the hair and comb out tangles, holding the strands correctly and not pulling at the patient's scalp.

11. Remove the towel and other materials from the bed and dispose of all soiled materials.

12. Restore the linen and bed to their original positions, put back the pillow, and remove the bath blanket, leaving the patient dry and comfortable.

13. Tidy the area, returning all articles to their proper places.

14. Record the time and method of the shampoo in nurses' notes.

STRETCHER SHAMPOO

1. Assemble all materials before moving the patient.

2. Identify the patient and explain the procedure to the patient.

3. Bring stretcher to bedside.

4. Move patient onto the stretcher. Refer to Unit 14, Item 3.

5. Transport the patient to the shampoo area.

6. Place the stretcher with patient's head near the sink and lock the wheels.

7. Place a towel around the patient's shoulders and neck.

8. Position the patient's head over the rim of the sink, or use a trough under the head with the end in the sink for the return flow of water.

9. Attach the spray nozzle to the faucet.

10. Regulate the flow of water and test the temperature with the bath thermometer. Use warm water: $105°$ F $(40.5°$C).

11. Shampoo the hair, following steps in the bed shampoo procedure.

12. Brush or comb the hair and arrange in a neat style.

13. Transport the patient back to the room without bumping or jolting, pushing the stretcher from the head end.

14. Record and report the procedure.

HAIR CARE FOR BLACK PATIENTS

1. Wash your hands.

2. Approach and identify the patient, explaining the procedure.

3. Confer with the patient and find out the type of lotions or oils used.

4. Place towel under the head to protect the bed linens.

5. Apply solution, beginning at the forehead and temporal hairline.

6. Massage into the hair.

7. Use wide-toothed comb to comb through hair.

8. Towel the hair dry to remove excess solution.

9. Arrange neatly or braid if preferred.

10. Remove towel and return items to their proper storage place.

POST-TEST

Multiple Choice. Choose one answer.

1. The reasons for daily brushing and combing of the hair include all of the following except

   a. to stimulate circulation of the scalp.   c. to stimulate the hair to curl.

   b. to clean her hair shafts.   d. to bring nutrients to the roots.

2. Water temperature for shampoos should be approximately

   a. 120°F.   c. 115°F.

   b. 85°F.   d. 105°F.

3. A style that is often used for keeping a patient's long hair neat and tidy is called

   a. braiding.   c. Afro.

   b. a finger-wave.   d. a shag.

4. A common fungus infection on the scalp is

   a. impetigo.   c. eczema.

   b. dandruff.   d. herpes simplex.

5. Parasites of the scalp are called

   a. impetigo.   c. pediculi.

   b. ascaris.   d. ringworm.

6. The hair of many members of the black race is characterized by being

   a. coarse and strong.   c. oily and straight.

   b. fine and shiny.   d. dry and very curly.

7. One of the most effective ways of cleaning dirt from the hair of a black accident victim is to use

   a. alcohol and mineral oil solution.   c. regular soap and water shampoo.

   b. detergent-type shampoo.   d. a lemon juice rinse.

8. The room environment for giving a patient a shampoo in bed should be

   a. warm and free of drafts.   c. at a temperature of 100°F.

   b. at a temperature of 68°F.   d. at a temperature of 95°F.

9. Illness often causes the scalp to become very

   a. sensitive.   c. colorful.

   b. shiny.   d. coarse.

10. Braided hair does not easily become

   a. damaged.   c. matted.

   b. stiff.   d. loose.

11. The hair should be brushed with

   a. an upward motion.   c. a stiff bristled brush.

   b. strokes toward the scalp.   d. A & D ointment.

12. Dandruff causes the scalp to become

    a. oily and scaly.   c. discolored.

    b. dry and scaly.   d. very sore.

13. A patient's hair should be shampooed only on the order of the

    a. patient.   c. physician.

    b. head nurse.   d. patient's family.

14. Each time a shampoo is given, it should be recorded on the

    a. progress sheet.   c. nurses' notes.

    b. physician's order sheet.   d. Intake and Output sheet.

15. After giving a shampoo in the bath or utility room, you should make sure that the area is cleaned

    a. before you return the patient to the room.

    b. after you return the patient to the room.

    c. before you put the patient to bed.

    d. after you put the patient to bed.

16. Wigs should be shampooed by the

    a. patient's family.   c. professional hairdresser.

    b. nurse.   d. orderly.

POST-TEST ANSWERS

1. c		9. a	
2. d		10. c	
3. a		11. a	
4. b		12. b	
5. c		13. c	
6. d		14. c	
7. a		15. d	
8. a		16. c	

PERINEAL CARE

GENERAL PERFORMANCE OBJECTIVE

As a health worker, you will be able to assist the patient with the care and cleansing of the perineal area, and to give perineal care as required. You will perform this task skillfully, effectively, and in a reassuring manner to reduce or avoid embarrassment to the patient.

SPECIFIC PERFORMANCE OBJECTIVES

Upon completion of this lesson you will be able to:

1. Approach the patient, explain the procedure in an objective and matter-of-fact way, and give reassurance in a nonjudgmental way in order to avoid embarrassing the patient.

2. Provide perineal care for the female or male patient by pouring warm solution over the perineal area, cleansing and drying the area properly, applying a dressing or pad, if required, and securing it in place.

VOCABULARY

genitalia—the reproductive organs of the male and female.
lochia—the discharge from the uterus consisting of blood, mucus, and tissue during the period immediately after the delivery of a baby.
perineum—the area between the vulva and the anus in the female, and between the scrotum and the anus in the male.
scrotum—the double pouch containing the testicles and part of the spermatic cord in the male.
uterus—the muscular, hollow, pear-shaped organ of the female, located within the abdomen; the womb.
vulva—the external female genitalia.

INTRODUCTION

Perineal care (often referred to in the hospital as "peri care") is the term applied to the external irrigation or cleansing of the vulva and perineum following voiding or defecation. The procedure is performed to prevent contamination or infection in the genital area and to remove drainage or odors through cleansing. The procedure is used following the birth of a child or following an operation involving surgery on the perineum, the vagina, the lower urinary tract, or the anus. Although the procedure is more commonly performed for the woman patient, it may be required for the male patient following surgery on the perineum or the anus.

You will find that some nurses use the term "peri care" to refer to the portion of the patient's bath when the genital area is washed and dried. Usually the patient is able to perform this part of the bath, but you may need to assist certain patients who are helpless. The use of the term "peri care" is correct in such a situation, but this lesson will be concerned with cleaning the perineal area by external irrigation, or the pouring of a solution.

PERINEAL IRRIGATIONS

ITEM 1. DEALING WITH PATIENT EMBARRASSMENT

The procedure of giving perineal care to the patient may cause him or her embarrassment as a result of the nurse's close contact with the genital area. Most patients will accept the nurse's assistance and make very little fuss about having the procedure done. A few, however, may find it very difficult to overcome their feelings of embarrassment and will try to avoid the perineal care, even when they know it might be necessary.

Why do patients become embarrassed and reluctant about using the bedpan or having perineal care? We all know some of the reasons. Until very recently, our cultural and social customs were such that certain parts of the body and their functions were not seen, discussed, or even acknowledged in public. The genital region was considered very private, and the person raised in this kind of culture and according to these customs regards it as so. When this person becomes a patient, his or her attitude about the privacy of the body does not change much.

As a nursing worker, how can you deal with this problem? First, you need to understand that *you* may have some embarrassment initially if you have been raised in a similar culture with similar customs. Your own embarrassment will be reduced if you remember that your purpose is to *assist the patient.* By regarding the patient as a whole person, you can develop a calm and matter-of-fact attitude, and a nonjudgmental manner while accepting the other's right to have and express his or her feelings. Explaining the need for perineal care and the reasons for it can reassure the patient and gain cooperation in the procedure without undue embarrassment. When performing the procedure, you should be matter-of-fact and objective and avoid any sexually suggestive conversation or actions.

ITEM 2. PERINEAL CARE FOR THE FEMALE PATIENT

Supplies Needed

Pitcher	Sterile forceps or gloves
500 cc water at 105°F (40.5°C)	Chux
Cotton balls or sponges	Bed pan
Sanitary belt	Bath blanket
Dressing or sanitary pad	

Important Steps	Key Points
1. Wash your hands.	Universal Steps A, B, C, and D. See Appendix.
2. Approach and identify the patient, explain the procedure, and gain cooperation.	
3. Provide for privacy.	
4. Provide the items and materials needed.	

Important Steps	Key Points
5. Drape the patient.	Drape the patient to avoid undue exposure. Put the bath blanket over her and have her hold the upper edge while you fan-fold the upper covers to the foot of the bed. Raise the lower edge of the bath blanket to her pubic area and place the lower sides of the blanket over each knee as shown in the sketch.

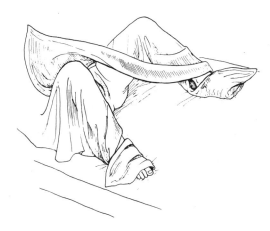

6. Remove soiled pads or dressings.	Remove the soiled pad or dressing. Observe the amount and type of drainage, then wrap it in paper for discarding.
7. Place on bedpan.	After slipping the Chux under her hips, place the patient on a bedpan.
8. Put on disposable gloves.	
9. Pour water over the perineum.	Pour warm (105°F [40.5°]) tap water or prescribed solution over the perineal area to rinse off urine, feces, or vaginal drainage.

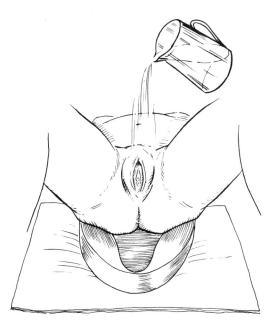

Important Steps	Key Points
10. Cleanse the perineum with moistened cotton balls or sponges.	Moisten several cotton balls or gauze sponges with the remaining solution. Use forceps or your fingers to hold the cotton ball, and wipe from the pubic area down toward the rectum. Make only one downward stroke with each cleansing cotton ball, then discard. Cotton balls and sponges clog the plumbing, so they should be discarded by wrapping them in paper and putting them in the trash container, not in the bedpan.

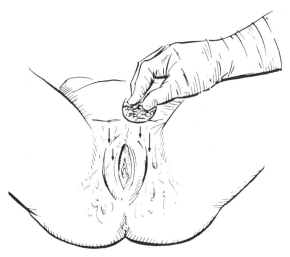

11. Remove bedpan.	Wipe the perineum dry with fresh cotton balls, gauze squares, or toilet tissues. Dry the lower perineum and the buttocks. Wrap soiled cotton balls or gauze before disposing of them in the trash. Remove and dispose of gloves.
12. Apply clean pad or dressing.	Apply the clean dressing or the pad. Fasten ends of pad to a sanitary belt. Use a T-binder to secure the dressings in place. (The crossbar of the T-binder is fastened around the waist; the tail of the T passes through the legs from the back and is fastened to the waist of the binder in the front.)
13. Replace the top covers and remove the bath blanket.	Fold it and return it to the bedside stand or the storage place. Remove the Chux.
14. Remove the equipment from the patient's unit.	Universal Steps X, Y, and Z. See Appendix.
15. Provide for the patient's comfort.	
16. Report and record.	Charting example: 1030. Perineal care given. Moderate amount of lochia, a few small clots. <div align="right">B. Olsen, NA</div>

ITEM 3. PATIENT SELF-CARE OF THE PERINEUM

When the patient is allowed up and is able to care for herself, she should be taught to perform the procedure herself. She can assemble the necessary materials, take them to the bathroom, pour the solution, cleanse and dry herself, and apply a clean pad or dressing.

The following points should be stressed when you give instructions to the patient:

1. Be sure to have a paper or brown bag in which to wrap the soiled pad or dressing and the cotton balls or gauze used to clean and dry the perineum. Wrap all soiled material securely before you dispose of it.

2. When cleansing or drying with a cotton ball or gauze, wipe once *from front toward the rectum* with each ball. Discard, and use a clean ball for the next stroke until the entire perineum has been cleaned and dried.

ITEM 4. PERINEAL CARE FOR THE MALE PATIENT

Perineal care may be ordered for the male patient following various types of perineal surgery. The steps of the procedure are the same as those listed in Item 2 for the female patient.

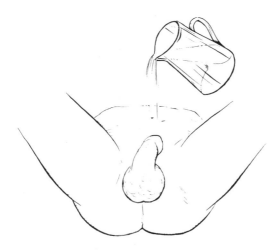

A sanitary pad would not be used for the male patient; his dressings would be held in place by a double-tailed T-binder, which allows for proper support of the scrotum as shown below. See application of T-binder in Unit 35, Bandages and Binders.

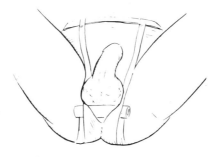

ITEM 5. CONCLUSION OF THE LESSON

After you have practiced the perineal care procedure until you are thoroughly familiar with it and can do it skillfully, arrange with your instructor to take the performance test. You should be able to demonstrate the procedure accurately.

PERFORMANCE TEST

In the classroom or skill laboratory, your instructor will ask you to demonstrate your skill in carrying out the following procedures without reference to your study guide, notes, or other source material. You are to use Mrs. Chase to simulate the patient.

1. Given a female patient who delivered a baby a few hours ago, you are to provide perineal care in order to cleanse the perineum of discharges and apply a clean sanitary pad without causing her embarrassment or discomfort.

2. Given a male patient who has had perineal surgery, you are to provide perineal care, apply clean dressings, and secure the dressings with a double-tailed T-binder in the proper way. State how you would attempt to reduce his embarrassment about this procedure.

PERFORMANCE CHECKLIST

PERINEAL CARE TO A FEMALE PATIENT

1. Wash your hands.

2. Obtain all needed supplies.

3. Identify the patient and approach her in a matter-of-fact, reassuring manner.

4. Provide for the patient's privacy by closing the door, pulling the curtain, or using screens.

5. Position the patient on her back with knees bent and elevated.

6. Drape the patient with a bath blanket to prevent undue exposure.

7. Remove the soiled dressing or pad.

8. Place the patient on a bedpan with a Chux under her hips and the pan.

9. Put on disposable gloves.

10. Pour water or a solution of 105°F (40.5°C) over the perineal area.

11. Use moistened cotton balls, one at a time, and stroke gently from the pubic area toward the rectum once with each to cleanse the perineum. Use gentle strokes to avoid causing discomfort.

12. Use dry cotton balls, gauze, or tissue to dry the perineum, stroking from the front to the rectum once with each ball. Remove gloves.

13. Remove the bedpan and apply a clean pad.

14. Discard all soiled dressings, pads, cotton balls, and so forth by wrapping them in paper before disposing of them.

15. Provide for the patient's comfort by removing the bath blanket, adjusting the top covers, placing the signal cord, and elevating the siderail.

16. Remove equipment from the bedside and clean it before returning it to storage.

PERINEAL CARE FOR THE MALE PATIENT

1. Wash your hands.

2. Obtain all supplies.

3. Identify the patient and approach him in a matter-of-fact, reassuring manner.

4. State ways in which you would attempt to reduce embarrassment, such as an explanation of the procedure and reasons for it, avoiding suggestive conversation or actions.

5. Provide for the patient's privacy by closing the door, pulling the curtain, or using screens.

6. Position the patient on his back with knees bent and elevated.

7. Drape the patient with a bath blanket to prevent undue exposure.

8. Remove the soiled dressing.

9. Place a Chux under his hips and place him on a bedpan.

10. Put on disposable gloves.

11. Pour water or a solution of $105°F$ ($40.5°C$) over the perineal area.

12. Clean the perineum by using moistened cotton balls and stroking gently from the pubic area toward the rectum once with each one.

13. Dry the perineum by using dry cotton balls, gauze, or tissue, wiping from the front to the rectum once with each one. Remove gloves.

14. Remove the bedpan.

15. Apply a clean dressing and secure it with a double-tailed T-binder. Apply a T-binder and dressing correctly to support the scrotum.

16. Discard all soiled dressings, pads, and cotton balls by wrapping them in paper before disposing of them.

17. Provide for the patient's comfort by removing the bath blanket, adjusting the top covers, placing the signal cord, and elevating the siderail.

18. Remove equipment from the bedside and clean it before returning it to storage.

POST-TEST

Directions. Mark the answer that makes the statement complete.

1. Perineal care is usually referred to as

   a. sitz care.   c. peri care.

   b. pedi care.   d. trach care.

2. The most prevalent feeling that patients receiving perineal care will need to overcome is

   a. anger.   c. indifference.

   b. embarrassment.   d. resentment.

3. The position of the patient when receiving perineal care is

   a. prone with legs extended.

   b. on the right side with knees flexed.

   c. on the left side with knees extended.

   d. lying on the back with knees flexed and draped.

4. The temperature of the solution used for perineal care is

   a. 105°F.   c. 212°F.

   b. 90°F.   d. 150°F.

5. The most important aspect of perineal care to be carried out by the nurse and the patient is using the following stroke:

   a. Start the cleaning stroke from the rectum to the pubic area.

   b. Use one cotton ball for each cleaning stroke.

   c. Use one cotton ball for each cleaning stroke, from front to back.

   d. Use one cotton ball for all the cleaning strokes.

POST-TEST ANSWERS

1. c.

2. b

3. d

4. a

5. c

Volume 2

Nursing Skills
for Clinical Practice

Section 4

SKILLS RELATED
TO OTHER BASIC NEEDS

INTRODUCTION

As a beginning level nurse, you need a number of skills to assist patients in carrying out activities that satisfy their basic needs. Nursing becomes more interesting and satisfying when you see how well patients meet these needs and the extent to which they need nursing assistance. By using skills to help meet these needs, you are doing more than merely getting a job done, giving a bedpan, or feeding a person; you are contributing to the patient's needs and welfare.

The basic needs of individuals were described in Unit 4 and form the basis of many activities of daily living. Everyone has to eat food, drink fluids, move about, and eliminate wastes from the body day after day. When patients are unable to do these activities without assistance, a number of procedures and skills are used by nurses to help them meet these needs.

Foremost of all the basic needs is the body's constant demand for oxygen. The periodic measurement of the vital signs provides the nurse with information about how the body is satisfying its oxygen requirements. Changes in temperature, pulse, respiratory rate, or blood pressure are often the first indication of problems in meeting the need for oxygen. Unit 21, The Vital Signs, describes the normal ranges, some of the problems that can arise, and the methods of measuring these signs of bodily functions. Complete failure to meet the oxygen needs through a breakdown in respiratory or cardiac function results in cardiac arrest. When this occurs, basic cardiac life support techniques are carried out. Unit 26 gives step-by-step instructions for CPR by one or two rescuers, as well as the recommended procedure for assisting the person who is choking because of an obstructed airway.

In many diseases, the fluid balance of the body is easily disturbed, which can lead to prolonged illness or severe complications. Nurses should focus attention on intake and output, not just because it was ordered by a physician, but because these records provide an indication of how well patients are meeting their fluid needs. The nurse is concerned about any patient with a decreased intake of liquids or an abnormal loss of fluid, as described in Unit 22.

It has often been said that patients are at risk of developing malnutrition during hospitalization because of the effect of illness on the appetite. When the disease affects the digestive system, the diet is part of the treatment as some foods may be restricted. And in order to be effective, the patient must eat the food so that it gets inside the body. The types of diets and ways to assist patients to eat are covered in Unit 23. The many procedures used to help patients meet their elimination needs are described in Units 24 and 25.

For many patients, not only the physiological needs but also spiritual needs are vitally important. Guidelines are given in Unit 27 for assisting the clergyman and understanding other religious beliefs and practices your patients may hold. These beliefs should be treated with respect even though they may differ from your own.

DIRECTIONS FOR STUDENTS

The recommended approach for studying the units in this section is the same as that for previous sections. Read the objectives through to learn what you are expected to do, then review the terms listed in the vocabulary. The items provide information about the purposes of the procedures, including the rationale and principles on which they are based, and describe briefly what is normal and what kind of problems might arise. Other items list the supplies needed to perform a procedure along with the steps and accompanying key points. The first procedure in the unit states each of the universal steps to be carried out for every procedure involving patients. (The Universal Steps are described in detail in Appendix I.) The procedures that follow will direct you to carry out the Universal Steps and will then list the steps for that specific procedure.

Be sure to practice in the skills laboratory whenever possible so that you gain a beginning level of competence before you attempt to perform the procedure in the clinical setting with patients. Continue to practice your communication skills with your fellow students as you explain the procedure, demonstrate the need for it, and seek to gain cooperation.

When you believe that you can perform the skills accurately and with a degree of competence, arrange with your instructor to take the Performance Test. Refer to the Performance Checklist when practicing, as it is a step-by-step guide to the procedure. The Post-Test contains multiple choice questions designed to test your understanding of the rationale, principles, and facts related to the procedures.

SELECTED REFERENCES

Unit 21: The Vital Signs

Abbey, June C., et al.: How long is that thermometer accurate? Am J Nurs 78:1874–1877 (August) 1978.
Adelman, Eleanore M.: When the patient's blood pressure falls. Nursing 80 10:26–33 (February) 1980.
Bangs, Cameron: Do's and don'ts of immediate treatment. RN 42:43–44 (November) 1979.
Baughman, Diane: The frozen patient: Handle with care. RN 42:38–42 (November) 1979.
Beaumont, Estelle: Blood pressure equipment. Nursing 75 5:56–62 (January) 1975.
Davis-Sharts, Jean: Mechanisms and manifestations of fever. Am J Nurs 78:1874–1877 (November) 1978.
DeLapp, Tina D.: Taking the bite out of frostbite and other cold weather injuries. Am J Nurs 80:56–60 (January) 1980.
Felton, Cynthia L.: Hypoxemia and oral temperatures. Am J Nurs 78:56–57 (January) 1978.
Gedrose, Judith: Prevention and treatment of hypothermia and frostbite. Nursing 80 10:34–36 (February) 1980.
Hill, Martha: What can go wrong when you measure blood pressure? Am J Nurs 80:942–946 (May) 1980.
Ozuna, Judith, and Foster, Charlene: Hypothermia and the surgical patient. Am J Nurs 79:646–648 (April) 1979.
Programmed Instruction: Patient assessment: Pulses. Am J Nurs 79:115–132 (January) 1979.

Unit 22: Fluid Intake and Output

Burgess, Audrey: The Nurse's Guide to Fluid and Electrolyte Balance. New York: McGraw-Hill Book Company, 1970.
Grant, Marcia, and Kubo, Winifred: Assisting a client's hydration status. Am J Nurs 75:1306–1311 (August) 1975.
Metheny, Norma M.: Water and electrolyte balance in the postoperative patient. Nurs Clin North Am 10:49–57 (March) 1975.

Metheny, Norma M., and Snively, Jr., W.D.: Nurses Handbook of Fluid Balance. 2nd ed. Philadelphia, J.B. Lippincott Company, 1974.

Murray, Malinda: Fundamentals of Nursing. 2nd ed. Englewood Cliffs, NJ: Prentice-Hall, Inc., 1980, pp. 481–497.

Unit 23: Assisting with Nutrition

Brody, Jane E.: How good are fast foods? Readers Digest, February, 1980, pp. 127–128.

Caly, Joan C.: Assessing adults' nutrition. Am J Nurs 77:1605 (October) 1977.

Cook, Kathleen: Diabetics can be vegetarians. Nursing 79 9:70–73 (October) 1979.

Dansky, Kathryn: Assessing children's nutrition. Am J Nurs 77:1610 (October) 1977.

Fleshman, Ruth: Eating rituals and realities. Nurs Clin North Am 8:91–104 (March) 1973.

Food and Nutrition Board: Recommended Dietary Allowances. 8th ed. Washington, D.C.: National Academy of Science, National Research Council, 1976.

Fulmer, Teresa T.: If elderly patients can't chew. Am J Nurs 77:1615 (October) 1977.

Guyton, Arthur: Textbook of Medical Physiology. 5th ed. Philadelphia: W.B. Saunders Company, 1976.

Hetrick, Ann, Gilman, Cyrena M., and Frauman, Annette C.: Nutrition in renal failure: When the patient is a child. Am J Nurs 79:2152–2154 (December) 1979.

Luke, Barbara: Nutrition in renal disease: The adult on dialysis. Am J Nurs 79:2155–2157 (December) 1979.

Oakes, Gary K., Chez, Ronald A., and Morelli, Irene C.: Diet in pregnancy: Meddling with the normal or preventing toxemia? Am J Nurs 75:1134–1136 (July) 1975.

Parker, Cherry: Food allergies. Am J Nurs 80:262–265 (February) 1980.

Price, Mary: Nursing diagnosis: The patient is starving . . . RN 42:49–56 (November) 1979.

Rose, James C.: Nutrition problems in radiotherapy patients. Am J Nurs 78:1194–1196 (July) 1978.

Salmond, Susan W.: How to assess the nutritional status of acutely ill patients. Am J Nurs 80:922–924 (May) 1980.

U.S. Department of Agriculture: Desirable weight ranges for adults. Calories and Weights: USDA Pocket Guide. (No. 364) Washington, D.C.: U.S. Printing Office, 1974.

Williams, Sue R.: Nutrition and Diet Therapy. 3rd ed. St. Louis, C.V. Mosby Company, 1977.

Unit 24: Urine Elimination

Brunner, Lillian S., and Suddarth, Doris S.: Textbook of Medical Surgical Nursing. 4th ed. Philadelphia: J.B. Lippincott Company, 1980, p. 905.

DeGroot, Jane: Catheter-induced urinary tract infections. How can we prevent them? Nursing 76 6:35, 1976.

Delehanty, Lorraine, and Stravino, Vincent: Achieving bladder control. Am J Nurs 70:312–316 (February) 1970.

Lundin, Dorothy V.: Reporting urine test results: Switch from + to %. Am J Nurs 78:878–879 (May) 1978.

Schumann, D.: Tips for improving urine testing techniques. Nursing 76 6:23–27 (February) 1976.

Tudor, Lea L.: Bladder and bowel training. Am J Nurs 70:2391–2393 (November) 1970.

Winter, Chester, and Barker, Marilyn R.: Nursing Care of Patients With Urological Diseases. 4th ed. St. Louis, C.V. Mosby Company, 1977.

Unit 25: Bowel Elimination

American Cancer Society: Care of Your Colostomy: A Source Book of Information. New York: American Cancer Society, 1964.

Bass, Linda: More fiber — less constipation. Am J Nurs 77:254–255 (February) 1977.

Beber, Charles: Freedom for the incontinent. Am J Nurs 80:482–484 (March) 1980.

Blackwell, Ardith, and Blackwell, William: Relieving gas pains. Am J Nurs 75:66–67 (January) 1975.

Broadwell, Debra, and Sorrells, Suzanne: Loop transverse colostomy. Am J Nurs 78:1029–1031 (June) 1978.

Gibbs, Gertrude, and White, Marilyn: Stomal care. Am J Nurs 72:268–271 (February) 1972.

Gutowski, Frances: Ostomy procedures: Nursing care before and after. Am J Nurs 72:262–267 (February) 1972.

Guyton, Arthur: Textbook of Medical Physiology. 5th ed. Philadelphia: W.B. Saunders Company, 1976.

Hogstel, Mildred: How to give a safe and successful cleansing enema. Am J Nurs 77:816–817 (May) 1977.

Hollister Ostomy Guide. Chicago: Hollister, Inc., 1972.

Jeffrey, H.C., and Leach, R.M.: Atlas of Medical Helminthology and Protozoology. London: E & S Livingstone, Ltd., 1968.

Kabeeb, Marjorie C., and Kallstrom, Mina D.: Bowel program for institutionalized adults. Am J Nurs 76:606–608 (April) 1976.

Watt, Rosemary C.: Colostomy irrigation — yes or no? Am J Nurs 77:442–444 (March) 1977.

Whitley, Nancy, and Mack, Esther: Are enemas justified for women in labor? Am J Nurs 80:1339 (July) 1980.

Unit 26: Cardiopulmonary Resuscitation

American Heart Association: Basic Cardiac Life Support: A Manual for Instructors. Dallas, Texas: American Heart Association, September, 1977.

Davis, A. Jann: Code 45! Am J Nurs 77:627–628 (April) 1977.

Gildea, Joan H.: Techniques of cardiopulmonary resuscitation in infants. Am J Nurs 78:265 (February) 1978.

JAMA Supplement: Standards for Cardiopulmonary Resuscitation (CPR) and Emergency Cardiac Care (EOC). Vol 227, No. 7, February 18, 1974.

Nussbaum, Gloria, and Fisher, John: A crash cart that works. Am J Nurs 78:45–48 (January) 1978.

Perro, Kathleen, Goetze, Carolynn, and Monaghan, Joan: Making every minute count with an esophageal gastric tube airway. Nursing 80 10:61–63 (August) 1980.

Unavarski, Peter, Argondizzo, Nona, and Boos, Patricia: CPR: Current practices revised. Am J Nurs 75:236–241 (February) 1975.

Unit 27: Assisting with Spiritual Care

Naiman, Harriet L.: Nursing in Jewish law. Am J Nurs 70:2378–2379 (November) 1970.

Pumphrey, John B.: Recognizing your patients' spiritual needs. Nursing 77 7:64–69 (December) 1977.

Stoll, Ruth: Guidelines for spiritual assessment. Am J Nurs 79:1574–1577 (September) 1979.

Unit 21

THE VITAL SIGNS

GENERAL PERFORMANCE OBJECTIVE

After completing this lesson, you will be able to obtain an accurate temperature, pulse, respiration, and blood pressure on adults and children and record readings correctly on the patients' charts.

SPECIFIC PERFORMANCE OBJECTIVES

Following this lesson you will be able to accurately carry out the following procedures within stated time limits:

1. Take and record the body temperature of an adult and a child at the oral, rectal or axillary site using a glass or electric thermometer.

2. Take and record an apical and radial pulse.

3. Count and record the patient's respirations.

4. Take and record blood pressure.

5. Recognize deviations from normal vital sign patterns.

VOCABULARY

1. **Temperature**

    axilla—the armpit.
    Celsius—a thermometer scale used to measure heat; it is divided into 100 degrees from the freezing point of water at 0°C at the bottom, to the boiling point at 100°C at the top.
    Fahrenheit—a thermometer scale used to measure heat; the freezing point of water is 32°F, and the boiling point is 212°F; and used chiefly in the U.S. (Medically, a thermometer is a glass or electric instrument used to measure the body temperature.)
    febrile—feverish, pertaining to fever.
    metabolism—all the chemical reactions needed to keep the body tissues living and functioning.
    mucosa—mucous membrane that lines body passages and cavities communicating with the air and secretes mucous.
    pyrexia—fever, or elevation of temperature above normal, which is 98.6°F (37°C.) for the average person.

2. **Pulse**

    arrhythmia—irregular heart beat.
    bradycardia—slow heart action; generally a rate below 60 beats per minute for an adult and below 70 per minute for a child; seen in cases of uremia, jaundice, fractured skulls, and stroke.
    bounding—a full, strong pulse.

tachycardia—abnormal rapidity of heart action, usually over 100 beats per minute for adults at rest, and over 200 in infants; seen in patients with heart disease or goiter, or those in shock.

thready—a pulse that feels weak and feeble; it can heardly be felt.

3. Respiration

apnea—absence of respirations.

Cheyne-Stokes—irregular or arrhythmic breathing in which periods of dyspnea last for 30 to 45 seconds, followed by periods of apnea.

diaphragm—a muscular wall separating the abdominal cavity from the thoracic (chest) cavity.

dyspnea—difficult breathing, as though one had just climbed a stairway; it is usually rapid, labored, and noisy; long periods of dyspnea are very tiring for the patient.

hyperventilation—excessively fast breathing.

Kussmaul's respirations—rapid, deep, panting type of breathing.

shallow breathing—small amount of air taken in.

4. Blood Pressure

aneroid manometer—a device for measuring blood pressure.

diastolic—the resting pressure of the heart between contractions; the last sound heard with the filling of the vein.

hypertension—blood pressure elevated above normal levels.

hypotension—blood pressure below the normal levels.

sphygmomanometer—device used to measure blood pressure.

stethoscope—instrument used to listen to sounds within the body.

systolic—the first sound heard as blood enters the collapsed vein; the force of the ventricular contraction of the heart.

INTRODUCTION

In Unit 4, we stated that healthy people were those who were able to meet their own basic needs. According to Maslow's hierarchy of needs, physiological needs are basic to all others; they must be attended to first and take priority over other needs. These basic needs are oxygenation, fluid and electrolyte balance, nutrition, elimination, rest, activity, and sensory regulation. These needs exist at the cellular and organ level as well as for the whole person. Even though infants and children depend on others to help them obtain or prepare food, for example, they are able to meet their nutritional needs within the body when healthy.

Whenever something interferes with these needs, internal changes occur. The organs and structures of the body require a fairly constant internal environment in order to carry out their normal functions. The cells must be kept at an optimal temperature as they go through a series of complex chemical reactions and rid themselves of waste materials. The chemicals that are needed must be in the proper amounts (neither too much nor too little), and the organs must have a time for rest, as well as periods of activity.

Nurses look for physiological changes in the patients, and the best early indicators are changes in the temperature, pulse, respirations, and blood pressure, commonly called the vital signs (or cardinal signs). Changes in the patient's vital signs most often provide the nurse with the first indication of either disturbances occurring within the body, or a return to a more stable condition. As important as the accurate measurement of the vital signs is the interpretation of what the changes indicate in the patient.

Temperature: Measures the balance between heat production and heat loss of the body. Disturbances in temperature are pyrexia, or fever, and hypothermia, or body cooling and freezing of body parts.

Pulse: Measures the rate at which the heart beats per minute. Disturbances cause the heart to beat too rapidly, too slowly, or at an irregular rate.

Respirations: Measure the rate of breathing and provide an indication of oxygen entering the body. Disturbances of the oxygen-carbon dioxide balance can be caused by difficulties in breathing, such as breathing too rapidly, or too slowly, or by obstructions of the air passages.

Blood pressure: Measures the force of the heart beat, that is, the pressure of the blood as it circulates throughout the body. Together with the pulse rate, it provides information about how effectively the heart is working.

In this unit, you will learn how to measure the vital signs of temperature, pulse, respirations, and blood pressure. Even more importantly, you will be able to compare the patient's vital signs with his or her normal range, detect deviations that signify a change in condition, and report these promptly so that appropriate treatment can be started.

MEASURING BODY TEMPERATURES

ITEM 1. BODY TEMPERATURE

Have you ever wondered how the body is able to adapt to wide ranges of external temperatures, which can vary as much as 30 to $40°F$ in a matter of hours in the course of a day? When it is near freezing outdoors, what keeps our body temperature in the same range as it is on a pleasant summer day? Although our extremities are able to temporarily withstand wide variations in temperature, our internal organs must be kept within narrow temperature limits if cellular life and functions are to continue.

Heat Production and Heat Loss

In healthy people, the body temperature remains fairly constant and when it fluctuates more than two or three degrees from normal, significant physiological changes take place. An increase above normal, or a fever, causes impairment of nerve fibers and increased metabolic rate, which leads to destruction of tissue proteins. A decrease of temperature below the normal range decreases metabolism, slows the pulse rate and the respirations, and lowers the blood pressure.

Body temperature is the balance between the heat produced and the heat lost by the body. Body heat is derived from ingested foods; adjustable heat is produced by physical exercise, by the tensing of muscles and shivering, by hormonal actions that lead to constriction of the blood vessels, and by any external application of heat, such as eating hot foods or drinks, wearing additional clothing, and so forth. Heat loss occurs through increases in the blood circulation through the skin and through sweating. The heat is dissipated by means of convection, radiation, vaporization, and conduction. Convection is the cooling of a heated surface by the movement of air over or around the body, while radiation is the direct movement of heat rays from the body. The temperature of a room filled with people increases as a result of the heat lost from their bodies by radiation. Other methods of dissipating heat are through vaporization of water from the lungs and the skin and through the direct transfer of heat by conduction when the body is in direct contact with a cooler object.

In summary, then, the temperature of the internal organs of the body is fairly constant and represents the balance between the heat produced and the heat lost.

Heat Production	Heat Loss

Heat Production

1. Cellular metabolism of nutrients
2. Shivering and increased muscular activity
3. Vasoconstriction of peripheral blood vessels (hormonal)
4. External sources of heat: clothing, hot foods, liquids, and so forth

Heat Loss

1. Vasodilation of peripheral blood vessels (hormonal)
2. Convection: air movement in the surroundings
3. Radiation: heat rays from the body
4. Vaporization of water from lungs and skin
5. Conduction: direct transfer of heat by contact

ITEM 2. NORMAL BODY TEMPERATURE

Two different scales are still commonly used in this country to measure temperature: the Fahrenheit and Celsius. Since either may be used in your agency, a short table of equivalent values is included here for your reference.

Common equivalent values:

Fahrenheit	Celsius	Fahrenheit	Celsius
95.0	35.0	100.4	38.0
95.9	35.5	101.3	38.5
96.8	36.0	102.2	39.0
97.7	36.5	103.1	39.5
98.6	37.0	104.0	40.0
99.5	37.5	104.9	40.5

The normal, or average, temperature of most people is 98.6°F or 37.0°C. It fluctuates within the normal range as the body adjusts to changes in the amount of heat produced or the amount of heat lost. Some people run a "low-normal" or a "high-normal" temperature consistently; this represents the normal body temperature for them. It is important to know what your patient's temperature usually is and then compare changes to that measurement.

	Fahrenheit	Celsius
Normal temperature	98.6°	37.0°
Normal range	97.0 to 99.6°	36.1 to 37.6°

Factors Influencing Temperature

The temperature reading that you will obtain will vary according to the site you used. Measurements can be made at a variety of body sites by placing thermometers or probes in the mouth, the rectum, the vagina, the axilla, or the groin or on the skin. Most temperatures are measured orally or rectally, however. Rectal temperatures are usually about one degree higher, and the axillary temperature is about one degree lower, than those measured orally.

Sometimes the doctor specifies the type of temperature to be taken, but when it is not, you follow these guidelines.

Oral temperatures are convenient for older children and adults and are the most commonly used. The glass clinical thermometer must be left in place under the tongue for at least 5 to 8 minutes in order to register the temperature, although newer types of electronic, chemical, and infrared thermometers register in much less time. If the patient has recently ingested hot or cold foods and liquids or has been smoking or chewing gum, wait 15 to 30 minutes for these effects to pass in order to get a more accurate measurement.

Rectal temperatures are taken when the accuracy of the oral method is questionable; when there is discomfort due to mouth breathing, nasal congestion, nasal or oral surgery, or the use of nasal tubes; or when the patient is unable to keep the mouth closed. Rectal temperatures are often required for infants, young children, and the aged.

Axillary temperatures are taken when oral or rectal temperatures are contraindicated. It is a less reliable measure and is not generally used.

Other factors influencing the body temperature are the time of day; the weather; exercise; the menstrual cycle; and the age, emotional state, and disease condition of the patient.

1. *The time of day.* The body temperature upon awakening is generally in the low-normal range owing to the inactivity of the muscles. Conversely, the afternoon body temperature may be high-normal, owing to the body's metabolic processes, the patient's activity, and the temperature of the atmosphere.

2. *Environmental temperature.* As you might expect, the body temperature is lower in cold weather and higher in hot weather.

3. *The age of the patient.* In old age, the loss of subcutaneous tissue (tissue directly under the skin) and decrease of blood flow due to arterial changes may cause the temperature to be lower and may cause less tolerance for cold weather. The muscle activity of older patients is limited, and therefore less heat is produced. At birth, heat-regulating mechanisms are generally not fully developed, so there may be marked fluctuations in body temperature occurring during the first year of life.

4. *The amount of physical exercise the patient performs.* Physical exercise calls for the use of large muscles, which create greater body heat by burning up the glucose and fat in the tissues. Muscle action generates heat. You know that when you are cold, you exercise to warm up. Also, chattering or shivering are ways in which the body tries to keep its temperature balanced. The reverse is true in hot weather; we tend to become inactive, since muscle exercise generates heat.

5. *The phase of the patient's menstrual cycle and pregnancy.* Body temperature drops slightly just before ovulation (the normal monthly ripening and rupture of the ovum) and then may rise to one whole degree above normal during ovulation. Within a day or two preceding the onset of the next menstrual period, the temperature drops again. During pregnancy, the body temperature may consistently stay at high-normal due to an increase in the patient's metabolic rate.

6. *The emotional status of the patient.* Highly emotional states cause an elevation in body temperature. The emotions increase the activity of secreting glands and thereby increase heat production.

7. *The disease condition of the patient.* Toxins from some infective agents, pathogenic diseases, or chemical reactions may produce elevated body temperatures or fevers. Fever is a protective defense mechanism that the body employs to fight germs and their toxins.

ITEM 3. PROBLEMS OF TEMPERATURE REGULATION

Elevated Temperatures

A condition in which the patient's temperature is above the normal range is called a fever, a febrile state, or pyrexia. A fever is usually a common symptom of disease, especially infection, in which the heightened temperature helps to destroy invading bacteria. Very high fevers, however, such as those above $105.8°F$ or $41°C$, cause damage to body cells, particularly cells of the central nervous system. Patients with temperatures above $107°F$ have only hours to live unless the temperature is brought down rapidly.

The body temperature is regulated by the temperature-regulating center located in the hypothalamus of the brain. In fever, this physiological thermostat is "set" at a higher level than normally, and the heat-producing mechanisms of the body elevate the body temperature to the new setting. The patient experiences chills, and the metabolic rate increases by about 7 per cent for each degree Fahrenheit (10 per cent for each degree Celsius) rise in temperature. The patient with a fever of $102°F$ has a fever of three degrees above normal; multiplied by 7 per cent, this yields a bodily demand for 28 per cent more energy than the patient normally uses. If this increase in energy is not provided by food and other forms of nourishment, the body turns to its own fat and muscle cells and metabolizes them to meet the energy need.

The course of a fever can be observed on the recorded temperature graph in the patient's chart. There are three distinct stages in a fever:

1. The onset, when temperature begins to rise. It can be sudden and violent, as in pneumonia, or it can be slow and gradual as in typhoid fever.

2. The fastigium or stadium. (Fastigium is a Latin word for roof; stadium is a Greek word for the distance in a race.) This is the period when the temperature remains at a high, constant level.

3. The subsiding stage is the period during which the temperature returns to normal. It can fall slowly over a period of days or abruptly; in the latter case it is called the crisis. The crisis used to be a very significant point in the recovery or death of a pneumonia patient. With the advent of powerful drugs to combat pneumonia, however, the temperature now drops more gradually.

Fevers are classed according to certain characteristics:

1. During constant fever the temperature is continuously elevated; usually there is less than one degree of variation within a 24-hour period.

2. Intermittent fever is the alternate rise and fall of the temperature, e.g., low in the morning, high in the afternoon, or low for two to three days followed by a high temperature for two to three days.

3. Remittent fever is the falling of a high temperature, usually in the morning, rising later in the day. The significant fact is that the temperature never falls to normal in this type of fever until recovery occurs.

The following nursing measures are used to reduce pyrexia.

1. Lower the room temperature, if possible, using the room thermostat.

2. Increase the rate of circulating air.

3. Reduce the amount of clothing or bed covers.

4. Control or reduce the amount of body activity.

5. Carry out the physician's orders for cooling measures and supportive treatment: alcohol or tepid sponge bath; high caloric diet and force fluids; medications to lower temperature and combat the cause.

Hypothermia States

A subnormal body temperature is called hypothermia. It refers to a lowering of the temperature of the entire body, not just a portion of it.

The thermal regulating center in the hypothalmus is greatly impaired when the temperature of the body falls below 94°F. At this level, the activity of the cells is reduced, less heat is produced, and sleepiness and coma are apt to develop. People at risk of hypothermia are postoperative patients who shiver in the recovery room, newborn infants who are exposed to room temperatures and a bath before their body temperature has stabilized, and elderly or debilitated patients.

People exposed to extremely cold weather often suffer "frostbite" of ears, hands and feet, where the surface areas freeze. If thawed immediately, there is little effect on tissues, but if frostbite is prolonged, it causes death of cells, necrosis, and loss of the frozen area.

Nursing activities for treating the patient with a below-normal body temperature should focus upon reducing heat loss and supplying additional warmth; these activities may include

(1) providing additional clothing or blankets for warmth (an electric blanket is most effective for raising temperature); (2) giving warm fluids, if permitted; (3) adjusting the temperature of the room to 72°F or above; (4) eliminating drafts; (5) increasing the patient's muscle activity; and (6) submerging frost-bitten areas in a warm bath, with water temperature no warmer than 110°F or 43.3°C.

Answer the following questions based on information about body temperature.

1. Why would you take the patient's vital signs at frequent intervals during a period of illness?

2. What is the normal temperature of a healthy person in degrees Fahrenheit?

3. What is the normal temperature in degrees Celsius?

4. Above what temperature is a person considered to have a fever?

Name at least four factors that influence body temperature:

5. _____   7. _____

6. _____   8. _____

List the three most common sites used for taking the body temperature:

9. _____   10. _____

11. _____

12. With a fever of two degrees (F) above normal, how much is the metabolic rate increased?

ITEM 4. TYPES OF THERMOMETERS USED

Thermometers are used to measure the body temperature, and there are a growing number of different types on the market today. The clinical thermometer made of glass with a mercury-filled bulb is familiar to most people, but other types are gaining popularity for hospital use. They include electronic thermometers, disposable single-use thermometers, and disposable temperature-sensitive tape applied to the skin.

Clinical Glass Thermometers

The clinical thermometer is a glass bulb containing mercury and a stem in which the mercury can rise. On the stem there is a graduated scale representing degrees of temperature, the lowest registered being 95°F and the highest 110°F because body temperatures below and above these points are rare. The range on a Celsius thermometer scale is 35° to 43.3°C.

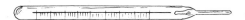

Glass oral thermometer.

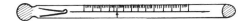

Rectal thermometer.

Oral thermometers have a bulb containing mercury. The mercury expands when the bulb is in contact with body heat and registers on the scale in the stem. The bulbs of oral thermometers may be long and slender or blunt like the short fat bulbs used for rectal thermometers. Rectal thermometers often have a red tip on the stem to signify that it is for rectal use only and should not be used orally. Oral thermometers may be used to take axillary temperatures, however. All clinical thermometers must have the mercury below the normal range before using, and this is done by "shaking down" the mercury.

Reading the Clinical Thermometer. The stem of the mercury-in-glass thermometer contains the scale for measuring the temperature. The scale may be calibrated in either Fahrenheit or Celsius degrees. The Celsius scale has long lines indicating the degree and short lines for each 0.1 of a degree. In contrast, the Fahrenheit scale has an arrow marking the normal temperature of $98.6°$. Long lines on the scale represent each degree, but only the even-numbered degrees are written as 96, 98, 100, and so on. Short lines between the degree lines represent 0.2 (two tenths) of a degree. All temperatures are recorded as ending in an even number when using this thermometer because it does not measure odd tenths of a degree. For example, you would read and record $99.2°F$ or $99.8°F$ but never $99.3°F$ or $99.7°F$.

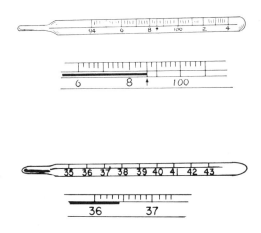

When clinical thermometers are used by the agency, patients are supplied with a thermometer for their individual use during the hospital stay; otherwise, a stock supply of thermometers is used and the thermometers must then be cleaned and resterilized before each use.

The method of cleansing of the thermometers is determined by agency procedure. If you are using an individually issued thermometer, the cleansing you give it after taking it out of the patient's mouth will be sufficient, since only one person is using it. If the agency returns thermometers to the processing area after each use, you will need to wash it in *cold* running water and soap before returning it to the stock tray for reprocessing.

Do not store oral and rectal thermometers together; they can easily be confused; It would be totally unsanitary to place a rectal thermometer in a patient's mouth by error!

Electronic Thermometers

The portable battery-operated electric thermometers register body temperature in 10 seconds or less. They usually have an "on-off" button or an area to be pressed in order to activate the battery. They may require a warming-up period, depending on the particular model that is used. The oral probe is placed in a plastic cover or sheath that is used one time and then discarded. The temperature is displayed digitally, in the actual numbers, on a small screen on the hand-held unit. The reading is in tenths of a degree, so temperatures taken with this unit may end in odd numbers, such as $99.5°F$.

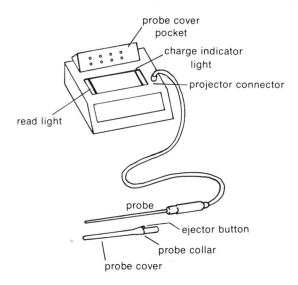

probe cover
pocket

charge indicator
light

projector connector

read light

probe

ejector button

probe collar

probe cover

Electric thermometer.

The method for taking oral temperatures follows.

1. Remove the probe from the unit and push down on the probe cover until it is firmly in place.

2. Insert the probe under the tongue and in contact with tissues.

3. Hold the unit steady and read temperature on the screen when the light stops flashing.

4. Discard probe cover by pressing ejector button.

5. Clear thermometer by returning the probe to its holder.

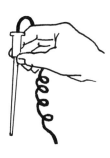

Grasp probe by probe collar.

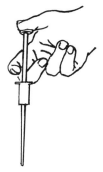

Eject the probe cover.

A special rectal probe is supplied with most units when rectal temperatures are required. A probe cover is used for rectal probes as well as for the oral ones.

Continuous monitoring of the patient's temperature is carried out when a hypothermia/hyperthermia machine is used. A rectal probe is inserted and attached to the control console at the bedside, where it then displays a continual reading of the body temperature.

Disposable Thermometers

Single-use, disposable thermometers are available. Among the various types available are temperature-sensitive tapes that are put on the abdomen and record the heat of the body. These are often used in newborn nurseries. Other types are the ready strip thermometers.* The sensor end of the shaft contains a series of dots arranged so that each one changes color at a different temperature from that of the preceding dot. To use this type of thermometer, (1) remove the sterile wrapper; (2) insert the thermometer under the tongue; (3) close the mouth and wait 45 seconds; and (4) remove and read the thermometer. The last colored dot represents the temperature.

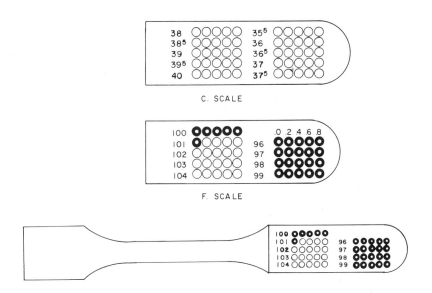

Rectal temperatures can be taken by using an adapter to hold the thermometer and leaving it in place in the rectum for 90 seconds. Read the thermometer, then dispose of it and the adapter.

ITEM 5. TAKING AN ORAL TEMPERATURE

Supplies Needed

Tissue   Oral clinical thermometer

Important Steps	Key Points
1. Wash your hands.	Universal Steps A, B, C, and D. See Appendix.
2. Obtain the equipment.	
3. Approach the patient and explain what you are going to do.	

*Tempa-Dot Ready Strip thermometer, manufactured by Organon Inc., West Orange, New Jersey.

Important Steps	Key Points
4. Rinse the thermometer in cool water if kept in antiseptic solution.	*Always rinse* under cold water to remove the solution before placing the thermometer in the patient's mouth. Remember, do not use hot water to rinse because it will cause the mercury to expand, which could break your thermometer.
5. Shake the mercury down. 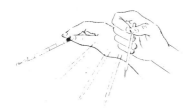	If the mercury is above the $96°F$ ($36.5°C$) mark, it will need to be shaken down. Hold the thermometer securely at the top end between your thumb and index finger. Shake the thermometer in a quick downward flip with a twisting motion of the wrist. (See the diagram). Usually this will take some practice. Shake down to $96°F$ ($36.5°C$) or lower.
6. Place the thermometer in the patient's mouth. 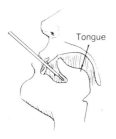 Tongue	Put the thermometer under the tongue deep in the mouth where it will be surrounded by tissue that is rich in blood supply, thus providing an accurate temperature reading. Remind the patient to keep the lips tightly closed; this will prevent the cooler outside air from affecting the temperature recording.
7. Leave the thermometer in place for an accurate recording.	When using the glass thermometer, leave it in place for 5 to 8 minutes. Be sure to warn the patient not to bite down on the glass thermometer; it might break. For oral reading by electronic thermometer, merely wait until the temperature registers on the display; the time required for the disposable thermometer is 45 seconds.
8. Remove the thermometer and read it. 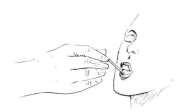	Again, hold the top end of the thermometer between your thumb and index finger. Wipe the thermometer off with tissue. Wipe from the top end to the bottom to avoid taking the patient's germs up to your fingers. Hold the thermometer at your eye-level. Rotate it toward you until you can clearly see the column of mercury. Remember, each of the long lines represents a full degree.
9. Replace the thermometer in its holder.	Universal Steps X, Y, and Z. See Appendix.
10. Record the patient's temperature.	

ITEM 6. TAKING A RECTAL TEMPERATURE

IIIIIIIIIIIIIIIIIIIIIIIIIIIIIIIIIIIIIIIIIIIIIIIIIIIIIIIIIIIIIIIIIIIIIIIIIIIIIIIIIIIIIIIIIIIIIIIIIIIIIIIIIIIIIIIIIIIIIIIIIIIIIIIIIIIIII

Supplies Needed

    Rectal thermometer or probe   Tissue
    Lubricant

IIIIIIIIIIIIIIIIIIIIIIIIIIIIIIIIIIIIIIIIIIIIIIIIIIIIIIIIIIIIIIIIIIIIIIIIIIIIIIIIIIIIIIIIIIIIIIIIIIIIIIIIIIIIIIIIIIIIIIIIIIIIIIIIIIIIII

Important Steps	Key Points
Carry out Universal Steps A, B, C, and D. See Appendix.	
1. Shake down the thermometer, if using a mercury-in-glass type.	Shake the mercury down to 96°F or below.
2. Lubricate the tip of the thermometer. 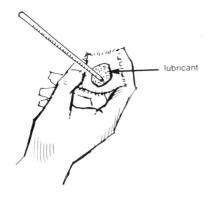	Lubricant makes it easier to insert the thermometer. Open the disposable packet of lubricant used by most hospitals today. If not available, remove a small amount from a jar with a tongue depressor, or squeeze a small amount from the tube onto a paper towel. Spread the lubricant over the thermometer tip.
3. Place the patient in Sims' position.	This will make the anal opening clearly visible for ease of insertion. Drape the upper bed covers to expose only the rectal area. Do not expose the patient unnecessarily.
4. Insert the thermometer in the patient's rectum. 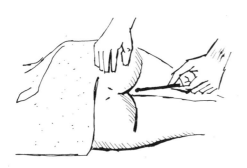	With your hand, lift the upper buttock slightly so that you can see the anus clearly. Insert the lubricated bulb end of the thermometer into the rectum about 1½ inches. Ask the patient to take a deep breath; this will relax the rectal sphincter and make for easier insertion of the thermometer.
5. Hold the thermometer in place.	If the patient is restless and you are not holding the thermometer securely, it could easily break off inside the patient's rectum and may even necessitate taking the patient to surgery. You must prevent this from happening.

Important Steps	Key Points
6. Leave the thermometer in for the required length of time to obtain an accurate reading.	Leave the thermometer in place for the proper length of time: a. glass: 3 to 5 minutes b. electronic: until registered c. disposable: 90 seconds.
7. Remove the thermometer and read it.	Wipe it clean with gauze or tissue. Read it in the same manner as you would an oral thermometer. The rectal temperature is usually ½ to 1 degree higher than the oral temperature.
Carry out Universal Steps X, Y, and Z. See Appendix.	When recording a rectal temperature, you chart this sign ® over the temperature reading to designate that it was taken rectally, as shown here:

$$\overset{\textstyle ®}{98.6°F}$$

ITEM 7. TAKING AN AXILLARY TEMPERATURE

Supplies Needed

Oral thermometer or probe

Important Steps	Key Points
Steps 1 through 5: Use the same procedure as for taking oral temperatures.	
6. Place the thermometer in the patient's axilla (armpit).	Be sure that the axilla is dry. If wet, pat it dry gently with a towel — excessive rubbing will generate heat. Place the thermometer in the center of the armpit. Have the patient hold his arm tightly against the chest; the arm can rest on the chest.
7. Leave the thermometer in place.	Leave the thermometer in place for the specified period of time: a. glass: 10 minutes b. electronic: until registered c. disposable: 90 seconds
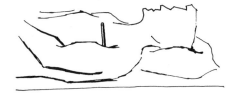	This is the least satisfactory way to take the temperature and is done when the temperature cannot be taken orally or rectally. The axillary temperature is about one degree lower than the oral temperature.

Important Steps	Key Points

8. Remove the thermometer and read it.

Carry out Universal Steps X, Y, and Z. See Appendix.

When charting an axillary temperature on the graphic record, write Ⓐ over the temperature reading to indicate that it was taken by the axillary method:

Ⓐ
97.6°F

MEASURING THE PULSE

ITEM 8. THE ARTERIAL PULSE

Each time the heart contracts to force blood into an already full aorta (artery leading from heart), the arterial walls in the blood system must expand to accept the increase in pressure. This expansion is called the *pulse*. By counting *each* expansion of the arterial wall, the *pulse rate* can be determined.

Common Pulse Points

The pulse can be felt wherever a superficial (lying just beneath the skin) artery can be held against firm tissue, such as a bone. The pulse is felt most strongly over the following areas:

1. Radial artery in the wrist at the base of the thumb.

2. Temporal artery just anterior to, or in front of, the ear.

3. Carotid artery on the front side of the neck.

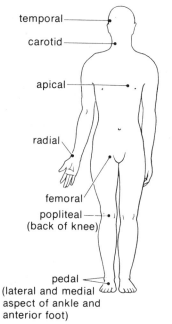

Locations where pulse can be taken.

4. Femoral artery in the groin.

5. Apical pulse over the apex of the heart. It is the actual beat of the heart.

6. Popliteal pulse behind the knee.

7. Pedal pulse of the posterior tibial artery at the ankle and dorsalis pedis on the arch of the foot.

The radial artery in the wrist is most often used to palpate the pulse when taking the vital signs. It is best found by placing the flat part of your first two fingers against the tendon, or cord, on the thumb side of the inner wrist and then rolling the fingers slightly into the little trough on the thumb side of the wrist. When it is difficult to find or to count the radial pulse, the apical beat of the heart is counted with the use of a stethoscope. The apical pulse is counted when it is important to have an accurate measure of the heart rate and may be ordered by the doctor for patients with heart diseases or other conditions or following heart surgery. Nurses routinely take apical pulse before administering heart medications of the digitalis family. One method of locating the apical heart sound is to place the bell of the stethoscope on a point midway between the imaginary line running from the breastbone or sternum to the left nipple. This point is approximately at the fifth intercostal space and 3 inches left of the midline.

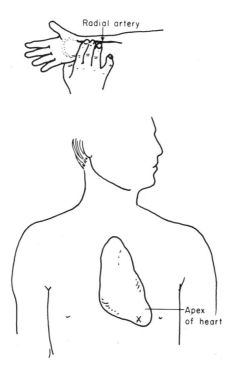

Occasionally you may need to take both a radial and apical pulse when the radial pulse is very irregular, skips beats, and is difficult to count. This requires two people who count the radial and apical pulses simultaneously in order to determine if there is a deficit in the radial pulse. Since the pulse originates with the heart beating, the radial pulse can never be more than the apical beat, except when the pulse wave is split into two or more impulses.

As the blood travels further away from the heart, the distinct wave of the pulse begins to fade, so that the pulse can be palpated at the ankle or top of the foot, but it may be more difficult to count. Pedal pulses are checked to determine if there is any blockage in the circulation in the artery up to that point, especially in patients who have had cardiac catheterization using the femoral artery for the insertion of the catheter. Most nurses mark an "X" on the skin over the spot where the pedal pulse is felt so that all use the same location.

The Pulse Rate

The pulse rate varies widely and is influenced by a large numbers of factors. Anxiety, fear, anger, excitement, pain, fever, hot weather, exercise, work, and muscular activity all increase the heart rate. Since the pulse rate is influenced so greatly by emotions and activity, it should be counted when the person is at rest.

Commonly Accepted Pulse Rates	Beats per Minute
Normal pulse range	60 to 100
Some athletes	45 to 60
Adult males	72
Adult females	76 to 80
Child, age 5	95
Child, age 1	110
Newborn infant	115 to 130

The term tachycardia is used to refer to a pulse over 100; bradycardia indicates a slow pulse that is less than 60 beats per minute. You should report these to the nurse or the physician since they are outside of the normal range. Medications may be prescribed to speed up the pulse if it is too slow or slow it down when it is too fast. Women have a slightly faster pulse rate then men, and the range may vary from seven to eight beats more per minute. Other factors that affect the pulse rate are:

Age:	The pulse rate gradually diminishes from birth to adulthood.
Body Build and Size:	Tall, slender persons may have a slower rate than short, stout persons.
Blood Pressure:	When the blood pressure rises, it causes a decrease in the pulse rate. When the blood pressure is lower, there is an increase in the pulse rate because the heart is attempting to increase the output of blood.
Drugs:	Stimulants increase the pulse rate. Depressants decrease the pulse rate.
Exercise:	Increases the pulse rate as the heart pumps faster to meet circulatory needs.
Foods:	Increase the pulse rate slightly as a result of metabolic processes.
Increased Body Temperature:	The pulse rate increases at the rate of 7 to 10 beats for each degree of temperature.
Pain:	Increases the pulse rate.

Characteristics of the Pulse

When the pulse is being counted, the rate, rhythm, and volume should be noted. An irregular pulse is one that has a period of normal rhythm broken by periods of irregularity or skipped beats. This can occur as a temporary condition of emotional stress or fright. An arrhythmia is indicative of heart disease and should be reported to the nurse or physician and recorded. Medication may be given to correct the irregular pulse, so it is important to record arrhythmias each time they occur.

According to the following graphs, the pulse rate and rhythm may be:

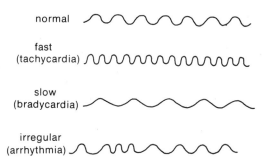

The volume or strength of the pulse is equally as important as the rate of the pulse. With moderate pressure of the first two or three fingers on the vessels, a strong pulse would beat regularly and with good force. There are several means of describing the strength of a pulse. Most of the common ways are:

1. Strong and regular—even beats with good force.

2. Weak and regular—even beats with poor force.

3. Irregular—both strong and weak beats occur within a minute.

4. Thready—generally indicates that it is weak and irregular.

The volume of the pulse cannot be measured directly, but a general idea of its strength may be found in thinking of blood flow as the flow of water from a faucet and relating this to the feel of the pulse.

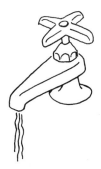

This volume indication is described as *feeble, weak,* or *thready.*

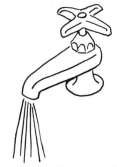

This volume indication is described as *full and bounding.*

13. What is the normal range for pulse in a healthy adult?

14. In addition to the rate, what characteristics of the pulse should you note and be able to describe?

15. List the points on the body where the pulse can be palpated.

16. What is the medical term used to describe a pulse of 48?

17. What is the medical term used to describe a pulse of 128?

18. Name at least six factors that might increase the pulse rate.

What are the three types of abnormal pulse that you would report to the nurse or to the physician?

19._____ 20._____ 21. _____

||||||||||||||||||||||||||||||||||||||||||||||||||||||||||||||||||||||||||||||||||||||||||||||||||||||||||||||||||||||||||||||||||

ITEM 9. MEASURING THE RADIAL PULSE

||||||||||||||||||||||||||||||||||||||||||||||||||||||||||||||||||||||||||||||||||||||||||||||||||||||||||||||||||||||||||||||||||

Supplies Needed

   Watch with a second hand   Paper and a pencil or pen

||||||||||||||||||||||||||||||||||||||||||||||||||||||||||||||||||||||||||||||||||||||||||||||||||||||||||||||||||||||||||||||||||

Important Steps	Key Points
Carry out Universal Steps A, B, C, and D. See Appendix.	
1. Locate the radial artery pulse with your three fingers.	Place the pads of your fingers lightly over the artery; the tips of the fingers are less sensitive in feeling the pulse wave and the nails could poke the skin. Do not use your thumb, because it has a strong pulse that could be confused with the patient's pulse.
2. Count the pulsations.	Count the pulse for 30 seconds by the clock, and multiply by 2 to obtain the rate per minute. As you count, note the regularity, any abnormalities, and the strength of the beat. If the pulse is irregular, too rapid, or too slow, take the pulse again for one full minute.

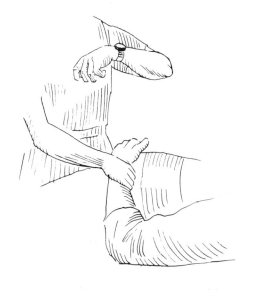

3. Record the pulse and report as appropriate.

ITEM 10. TAKING THE APICAL PULSE

Supplies Needed

Watch with a second hand   Alcohol sponge
Stethoscope   Paper, pencil or pen

Important Steps	Key Points
Carry out Universal Steps A, B, C, and D. See Appendix.	
1. Expose the chest over the apex of the heart.	Fold the top bedding to the bottom of the patient's rib cage. Fold the gown up toward the head, exposing an area of about 12 square inches.
2. Locate the apex of the heart.	Warm the diaphragm of the stethoscope for a moment if it is made of metal, then place it on a point midway between the left nipple and the midline of the body, or at the fifth intercostal space.
3. Listen to heart sounds with the stethoscope.	The heart makes a sound of "lup-dup" as it beats — this is one beat, not two. If you are unable to hear a beat, move the diaphragm around on the anterior, lower left quadrant of the left chest until you pick up the sound.

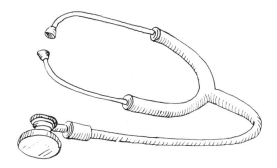

4. Count the number of beats for one minute.	Observe the second hand on your watch for the correct time. Note the rate, rhythm, and strength of the beat for the purpose of recording it later on the chart.
5. Wipe the earpieces and diaphragm with an antiseptic.	This will help prevent the spread of infection from worker to worker if the stethoscope is used by more than one person.
Carry out Universal Steps X, Y, and Z. See Appendix.	Record the apical pulse on the Graphic Record, TPR sheets, or Nurse's Notes, and indicate that it was measured apically. Charting example: 0800. P — 60^Ap irreg. J. Jones, SN

Measuring an Apical/Radial Pulse Rate

This procedure is ordered by the physician for patients with cardiac impairment or for those who are receiving medications to improve heart action.

||||||||||||||||||||||||||||||||||||||||||||||||||||||||||||||||||||||||||||||||||||||||||||||||||||||||||||||||||||||||||||||||||||||||||||

Supplies Needed

Stethoscope   Alcohol sponge
Watch with second hand   Paper, pencil or pad

||||||||||||||||||||||||||||||||||||||||||||||||||||||||||||||||||||||||||||||||||||||||||||||||||||||||||||||||||||||||||||||||||||||||||||

Important Steps	Key Points
(Refer to "Important Steps" for measuring radial pulse rate and measuring apical pulse rate. Follow the steps for each.)	Two nurses are required for this procedure. One nurse uses a stethoscope to measure the apical rate while another simultaneously measures the radial rate.
1. Place a watch conveniently so that both nurses can see it.	Each nurse listens to or feels the pulse beat for the best possible count.

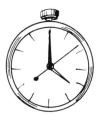

2. The nurse taking the apical pulse rate gives the signal to begin counting.	A time is decided upon to begin counting, for example, when the second hand is on the 3 or 6.
3. Count one full minute; end by saying "stop."	Return the patient to a comfortable position. Compare the pulse rate count with the other nurse later, when you are *out* of the patient's hearing.
4. Record the information on the patient's chart.	

MEASURING RESPIRATIONS

ITEM 11. THE RESPIRATIONS

Respiration is the process by which oxygen and carbon dioxide are interchanged. External respiration refers to the delivery of oxygen to the lungs so that it can be taken into the blood stream. Internal respiration is the process by which oxygen from the blood is taken to the cells in the body and carbon dioxide is removed from tissues and carried into the blood.

Exhalation is the process of expelling air from the lungs. Inhalation is the process of taking air into the lungs. Note that the chest circumference is greater during inhalation than it is during exhalation. During inhalation, the diaphragm descends as it contracts and the rib cage is lifted upward and outward, giving the lungs more room to expand and creating a slight negative pressure in the chest that helps draw air into the lungs. During exhalation, the diaphragm rises as it relaxes and the rib cage is drawn down and inward as air rushes out of the lungs.

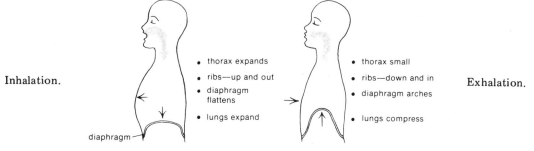

Inhalation.

- thorax expands
- ribs—up and out
- diaphragm flattens
- lungs expand

diaphragm

- thorax small
- ribs—down and in
- diaphragm arches
- lungs compress

Exhalation.

Rate and depth of respiration are controlled by the respiratory center in the brain.

The Rate of Breathing

A number of factors that affect the breathing rate are similar to those that affect the pulse rate, since the heart and lungs are intimately related in providing oxygen to sustain life. Although the rate and depth of respirations are controlled by the respiratory center in the brain, they are influenced by emotions, pain, the degree of activity, age, fever, drugs, and disease conditions. The respiratory center is more sensitive to changes in the carbon dioxide level in the blood, and, to a lesser degree in the oxygen level. Individuals can voluntarily control the rate and depth of respirations to a degree, as may happen when patients are aware that you are counting their respirations.

The respiratory rates vary according to age; these are commonly accepted as being the normal limits:

	Respirations per Minute
Healthy adult	14 to 20
Adolescent youth	18 to 22
Children	22 to 28
Infants	30 or more

The ratio of respirations (R) to the heart beat (P) is fairly constant at approximately 1 R to 4 P. In addition, the rate of respirations increases in fever as the body attempts to remove excess heat. Increased levels of carbon dioxide or lower levels of oxygen in the blood trigger an increase in the respiratory rate to restore the chemical balance and "blow off" the carbon dioxide.

Head injury or any increased intracranial pressure will depress the respiratory center and result in shallow or slow breathing. Certain drugs also tend to depress the respiratory rate. If an adult does not breathe at a minimal rate of 10 respirations per minute *and* in sufficient depth, you may note some of the following symptoms as a result of low oxygen supply in the blood:

1. Apprehension and restlessness.

2. Confusion, dizziness, and change in the level of consciousness.

3. Cyanosis or skin color changes, particularly around the mouth and in the nailbeds.

Patterns of Breathing

As you count respirations, observe for variations in the pattern of breathing. A normal, relaxed breathing pattern is effortless, quite evenly paced, regular, and automatic. Changes from this normal pattern are described in a variety of ways:

1. *Dyspnea:* Difficult and labored breathing, often with flared nostrils, anxious appearance, and even statements such as "I can't get enough air." It is very important to know how much exertion or activity causes the dyspnea: does it occur when walking down the hall, trying to eat a meal, or even when trying to talk?

2. *Increased or rapid breathing:* May be called by the medical term of tachypnea. This is seen in fevers and in a number of other diseases. Breathing rate increases about 4 breaths for each $1°F$ or $0.5°C$ increase in temperature.

3. *Slow and shallow:* There is a limited amount of air exchanged, and less oxygen is taken in. This type of breathing often leads to hypoxia, or decreased levels of oxygen in the blood. It is often seen in patients who are under medical sedation, recovering from anesthesia, following abdominal surgery, and in weak or debilitated condition.

4. *Cheyne-Stokes respirations:* A pattern of dyspnea followed by a short period of apnea. Respirations are rapid and gasping in nature for 30 to 45 seconds and are followed by a period of no breathing for 20 seconds, with continuation of this cycle. It is seen in critically ill patients with brain conditions, heart or kidney failure, and drug overdose.

5. *Hyperventilation:* A pattern of breathing in which there is an increase in the rate and the depth of breaths and carbon dioxide is "blown off," causing the blood level of CO_2 to fall. The condition is seen after severe exertion and during high levels of anxiety or fear and with fever and diseases such as diabetic acidosis.

6. *Kussmaul's respirations:* The increased rate and depth of respirations, with panting and long, grunting exhalation. It is seen in diabetic acidosis and renal failure.

Any change from the normal respiratory pattern of breathing should be reported to the nurse or physician so that appropriate treatment can be carried out. For more information on this subject, refer to Unit 31, Oxygen Therapy. As a rule of thumb, you should regard any noisy respirations as obstructed breathing. Some of the terms used to describe noisy respirations are:

1. Rales and rhonchi: rattling sound caused by secretions in the lung passageways.

2. Stertorous: a snoring sound produced when patients are unable to cough up secretions from the trachea or bronchi.

3. Stridor: a crowing sound on inspiration due to the obstruction of the upper air passages, as occurs in croup or laryngitis.

4. Wheeze: a whistling sound of air forced past a partial obstruction as found in asthma or emphysema.

llllllllllllllllllllllllllllllllllllllllllllllllllllllllllllllllllllllllllllllllllllllllllllllllllllllllllllllllllllllllllllllllllllll

22. The normal range of respirations for a healthy adult is _____ .

23. The respiratory center of the brain is more sensitive to changes in the _____ levels in the blood.

24. What is the ratio most often found between the number of respirations and the number of pulse beats?

25. The normal pattern of breathing is described as _____ .

26. Any type of noisy breathing should be regarded as _____ .

27. What is the term used to describe difficult and labored breathing?

28. What is the name of the breathing pattern that occurs in cycles with rapid, difficult breathing followed by a period of no breathing?

IIIIIIIIIIIIIIIIIIIIIIIIIIIIIIIIIIIIIIIIIIIIIIIIIIIIIIIIIIIIIIIIIIIIIIIIIIIIIIIIIIIIIIIIIIIIIIIIIIIIIIIIIIIIIIIIIIIIIIIIIIIIIIIIIIIIIIIIIIIIIIIIIIIIII

Measuring the Respirations

For an accurate accounting of the respirations, the patient should be at rest and unaware of the counting process. Since this is difficult to do with children who are hospitalized, their respiration rates are generally taken when they are sleeping. If adult patients are aware that you are counting their respirations, they may voluntarily breathe faster or slower. The most satisfactory time to count respirations is after the patient's pulse count.

Important Steps	Key Points
1. After taking the pulse, continue holding the wrist while counting respirations.	Do *not* tell the patient you are counting his or her respirations.
2. Observe the respiratory movements, rate, depth, pattern, and sounds.	One respiration includes both the inspiration and expiration.
3. Count the rate.	Count for 30 seconds by your watch and multiply by 2 to get the rate for one minute. If there is an abnormal rate or pattern, count for a full minute.

MEASURING THE BLOOD PRESSURE

ITEM 12. THE BLOOD PRESSURE

Blood pressure may be defined as the pressure exerted by the blood on the walls of the vessels. The pressure is the product of (1) the force of the contraction of the ventricles of the heart, (2) the amount of blood pumped out of the heart, and (3) the resistance of the blood vessels to the flow of the blood through them. By measuring the blood pressure, we obtain information about the effectiveness of the heart contractions, the adequacy of the blood volume in the system, and the presence of any obstruction or interference to flow through the blood vessels.

The blood pressure is abbreviated as BP and consists of two numbers: the systolic pressure written over the diastolic pressure. The systolic pressure represents the force of the contraction that empties the ventricles and pushes additional blood into the still-full aorta. Diastolic pressure is the lowest pressure in the vessel and occurs between heart beats while the heart is at rest. The difference between the two readings is the pulse pressure, or the force that causes the surge of blood in the artery that we palpate as the pulse.

The average blood pressure in a healthy young adult is considered to be 120/80 mm of mercury: 120 is the systolic pressure, 80 is the diastolic; the difference between the two, or 40, is the pulse pressure. As a result of the many factors influencing it, the blood pressure is a dynamic force that can vary from minute to minute as the heart adjusts to demands and responses of the body and mind. Infants have very low blood pressure, and the blood pressure gradually but steadily increases with increasing age.

It is important to know the usual range of pressures of your patient and some of the factors that may be influencing it, rather than to make judgments based on just one measurement. You can ask patients whether they have high or low pressure or look on the chart for other readings that have been recorded. A reading of 110/60 may be normal for a young man of 20, but low for someone aged 70 who has been averaging pressures of 154/90.

Factors Influencing Blood Pressure

Just as with the pulse and respirations, many factors exert an influence on the blood pressure. They include the following:

1. Age: Blood pressure is lower in children; it may be elevated in adults.

2. Sex: Blood pressure is higher for men than women of the same age level.

3. Body build: Obese persons usually have higher blood pressure than do those who are of average weight and build.

4. Exercise: Muscular exertion temporarily increases pressure.

5. Pain: Moderate and severe pain will usually elevate pressure.

6. Emotion: Fear, worry, or excitement will increase pressure.

7. Drugs: Vasoconstrictors elevate blood pressure. Vasodilators decrease blood pressure. Certain narcotics decrease blood pressure.

8. Disease: Any disorder affecting the circulatory or renal system may increase the blood pressure. Disease that weakens the heart may lower the blood pressure.

9. Hemorrhage: Decrease of blood volume lowers pressure and may lead to shock.

10. Intracranial pressure: Pressure in the space between the skull and the brain can elevate blood pressure.

A noisy environment and crowded conditions in the room may cause a temporary elevation of blood pressure. Take a person's blood pressure in a quite room with a relaxed environment.

Hypertension

Pressure elevated above the normal range is called hypertension. Anxiety, fear, and stress drive up the blood pressure. Hypertension is most often found in people living in urban areas, in blacks, and in those under emotional stress; it affects twice as many women as men. Exercise, strenuous work, and obesity cause an elevation in pressure. The danger of prolonged hypertension is that it causes permanent damage to the brain, the kidneys, the heart, and the retina of the eye. It is the cause of many cerebral vascular accidents (strokes).

Patients with an elevated systolic pressure and a normal diastolic pressure should have the blood pressure retaken every ten minutes or so until the systolic returns to the normal range. The temporary rise is related to anxiety when the body prepares for "fight or flight" and returns to normal as the anxiety state is reduced.

For the purposes of this unit, you should regard a systolic pressure above 140 and a diastolic pressure above 90 as being outside the normal range. Pressures higher than these should be reported to your nurse, as should low pressures that indicate circulatory collapse or shock.

Hypotension

Low blood pressure is called hypotension. Some people have a blood pressure that is normally below 95/60, but they are healthy with no other symptoms. However, hypotension with symptoms of shock or circulatory collapse is a dangerous condition that can rapidly progress to death unless treated. Shock is caused by hemorrhage, vomiting, diarrhea, burns, myocardial infarction, and other conditions. Symptoms include a fall in blood pressure, increase in pulse rate, cold and clammy skin, dizziness, blurred vision, and apprehension. Report such conditions to your nurse without delay and assist in treating the shock. See Unit 29, Postoperative Care, for information about shock and its treatment.

‖‖

Answer the questions and fill in the blanks.

29. The normal blood pressure in healthy young adults is _____ .

30. Systolic pressure refers to the (highest) (lowest) pressure caused by the contraction of the ventricles.

31. Which pressure reading is written below the line in BP?

32. How do you determine pulse pressure, the force we can feel when taking the pulse?

33. BP measurements above what level indicate hypertension?

Name at least five factors that cause an elevation in the blood pressure.

34. _____ 37. _____

35. _____ 38. _____

36. _____

39. Low blood pressures are dangerous when they occur with symptoms of _____ .

‖‖

ITEM 13. EQUIPMENT USED FOR MEASURING BP

The sphygmomanometer with an occlusive cuff and the stethoscope are the most commonly used pieces of equipment for measuring the blood pressure. Their continued popularity is due to their being economical, simple to use, and easy to handle and providing a reading quickly. Two types of manometers are generally used in clinical settings: the mercury gauge, when greater accuracy is needed, and the aneroid gauge, which is a smaller unit and easy to carry about but less accurate. Some hospitals have manometers attached to the wall in each patient room.

A new electronic sphygmomanometer now in use all but takes the blood pressure by itself. The cuff is placed on the arm and pumped up. As the air is released, the systolic and diastolic pressures are displayed on a screen in the unit. This model does not require the use of a stethoscope for listening to pressure sounds, but it is much more expensive than the traditional manometer.

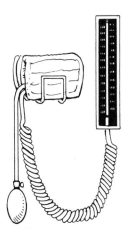 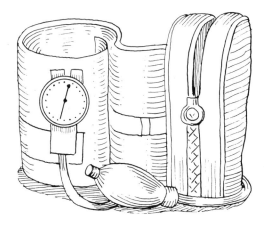

The manometer consists of a gauge for measuring the blood pressure sounds, tubing from the gauge to a cuff, which is wrapped around the arm or leg, and a control bulb that inflates and deflates the cuff.

The cuff must be the correct size in order to obtain an accurate BP. A narrow cuff is used for the small child and a wider cuff is needed for a muscular or obese person. The wrong size produces errors as great as 25 mm Hg. The proper width is 20 per cent wider than the diameter of the arm, and the inflatable bladder should go around at least half of the arm.

Many nurses buy their own stethoscope because they are used so frequently to assess the condition of patients. Many models are available, from low cost, plastic models to the expensive special electronic and Doppler ultrasound models. A standard acoustic stethoscope with a "Y" tubing, soft eartips, and diaphragm head is satisfactory for taking vital signs. The combination head is preferred, because the smaller bell head can be used to hear specific heart sounds.

ITEM 14.   PRINCIPLES RELATED TO BLOOD PRESSURE

In order to obtain an accurate reading and to avoid the pitfalls that lead to errors, follow these guidelines when taking blood pressures.

1. Have the patient lie down or rest for 5 minutes.

2. Use the brachial artery in the elbow joint of either arm. The arm should be supported on a surface about the level of the heart.

3. Check the condition of the equipment and position the manometer gauge so you can see it at eye level from a distance of 3 feet. The gauge indicator should be at zero when the cuff is deflated. Use the correct size of cuff.

4. Bare the arm and place the cuff and stethoscope directly on the skin. Bunched or wrinkled clothing prevents the correct placement of the cuff.

5. Palpate the brachial or radial artery before taking the blood pressure and then inflate the cuff about 30 mm. above the point where the pulse disappeared.

6. Make sure the diaphragm of the stethoscope is firmly but lightly over the artery. All surface edges should be in contact with the skin.

7. Once you begin to deflate the cuff to obtain systolic and diastolic readings, deflate all the way to zero. Do not stop midway and begin to inflate again, because this gives a false reading.

8. Listen for the different sounds while steadily deflating the cuff and identify the systolic and diastolic pressures. The first sound is the systolic pressure; the disappearance or 5th sound is the diastolic pressure. If the sound persists down to zero, then indicate the point at which the 4th sound occurred and record both as in this example: 130/62/0.

Korotkoff Sounds

While taking the blood pressure, you may hear certain sounds that relate to the effect of the blood pressure cuff on the arterial wall. These are known as Korotkoff sounds and are characterized by the following terms.

1. *Tapping:* Systolic pressure indicated by faint, clear tapping sounds that gradually grow louder.

2. *Swishing:* Murmur or swishing sounds increase as cuff is deflated.

3. *Knocking:* Louder knocking sound that occurs with each heart beat.

4. *Muffling:* A sudden change or muffling of the sound. Diastolic pressure in children and some adults.

5. *Silence:* Disappearance of sound. Diastolic pressure in adults.

Fill in the blanks or answer the questions.

Name two types of manometers most commonly used by nurses to take blood pressures.

40. _____

41. _____

42. The blood pressure is usually measured over an artery at what site?

43. Describe the sound that indicates the systolic pressure.

44. Describe the sounds that are associated with the diastolic pressure.

45. To avoid making errors in reading the pressure, where should the manometer gauge be located?

46. Why would you palpate the brachial or radial artery before taking the blood pressure?

ITEM 15. MEASURING THE BLOOD PRESSURE

Supplies Needed

Sphygmomanometer with cuff   Stethoscope

Important Steps	Key Points
Carry out Universal Steps X, Y, and Z. See Appendix.	
1. Position the patient.	The patient should be at rest and in a comfortable position sitting down or lying in bed. Support the arm you plan to use for measuring the BP.
2. Select the cuff and apply it.	Identify the bladder part of the cuff, fold it in half, and place the middle of the cuff 1 to 2 inches above the anticubital space. Wrap it smoothly and snugly around the arm, and fasten it.

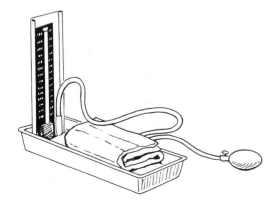

Important Steps   Key Points

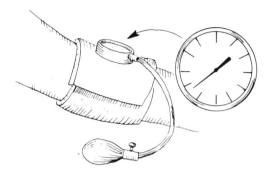

If there is a gauge attached to the cuff, be sure that it faces you so you can easily read it. Otherwise, place the gauge on a flat surface where you can clearly read the scale.

The aneroid sphygmomanometer gives blood pressure reading on dial indicator.

3. Attach the tubes from the BP cuff.

One tube goes to the air pump bulb, the other to the gauge tubing.

4. Close the valve of the air pump.

Turn the thumbscrew on the air pump bulb in a clockwise direction until it is closed, but not so tightly that it will be hard to open when deflating.

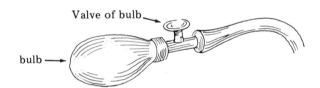

Valve of bulb

bulb →

5. Inflate the cuff and palpate the approximate systolic pressure.

Place your fingers on the radial or brachial pulse and inflate the cuff. Note the point at which the pulse disappears. This measure gives you an indication of the systolic pressure.

6. Deflate the cuff and wait 15 seconds.

Open the valve and quickly release all of the air from the cuff. Wait about 15 seconds and proceed to take the BP.

7. Position the stethoscope.

Make sure the ear tips are directed forward toward the nose when placed in the ear. Put the bell or diaphragm of the stethoscope over the brachial artery. It should be firmly pressed so that all edges are in contact with the skin. Avoid noises caused by contact of the stethoscope with the cuff, tubing, or clothing.

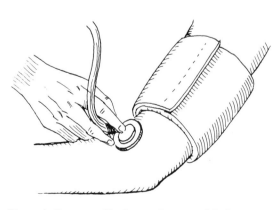

Place stethoscope diaphragm in antecubital space.

Important Steps	Key Points
8. Inflate the cuff.	The bladder of the BP cuff inflates as you pump. The column of mercury rises, or the needle of the aneroid gauge moves. Inflate at least 30 mm. higher than the palpated pulse.
9. Deflate and obtain systolic and diastolic reading.	Release the air at a steady rate of 2 to 4 mm. per second until the sound dies out; the rest of the air can be rapidly released. Note the point on the scale at which the first sound occurs — this is the systolic reading. As the sounds grow louder, note the point at which they disappear or change and become muffled if the sound continues down to zero. This is the diastolic pressure.

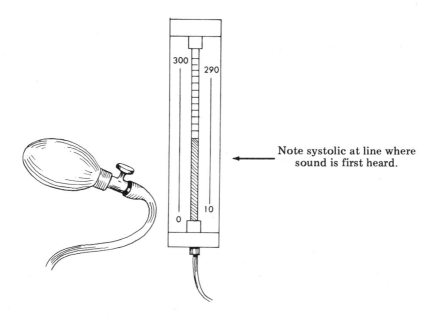

Note systolic at line where sound is first heard.

10. Remeasure as needed.	Repeat the process to check your accuracy. It is difficult to obtain blood pressure readings on some people. When you have trouble, *do not hesitate* to ask for assistance or confirmation of your reading. Even after you have been in the business many years, you may still find the need to have assistance occasionally. It is more important to get a correct reading to ensure that the patient can be correctly treated than for you to be embarrassed about asking for assistance.

Carry out Universal Steps X, Y, and Z. See Appendix.

ITEM 16. CHARTING VITAL SIGNS

The vital signs should be written down as soon as you obtain the measurements. It is easy to make errors or to forget the reading, especially when taking vital signs for more than one patient. Most nursing units record the vital signs on a TPR record or work sheet used as a quick reference by the nurses and doctors. Then the TPR vital signs are recorded on the patient's chart by the unit secretary or the nurse. In addition, you would describe any unusual or abnormal findings in the nursing notes, as they are important findings about the patient's condition. The method for charting vital signs is shown here.

Refer to the graphic sheet, which has space for recordings for several days. Each space is ruled into A.M. and P.M. columns, each of which is divided into three hourly columns for recording purposes. They are numbered for:

| 12 midnight (2400) | 4 A.M. (0400) | 8 A.M. (0800) |
| 12 noon (1200) | 4 P.M. (1600) | 8 P.M. (2000) |

GRAPHIC CHART

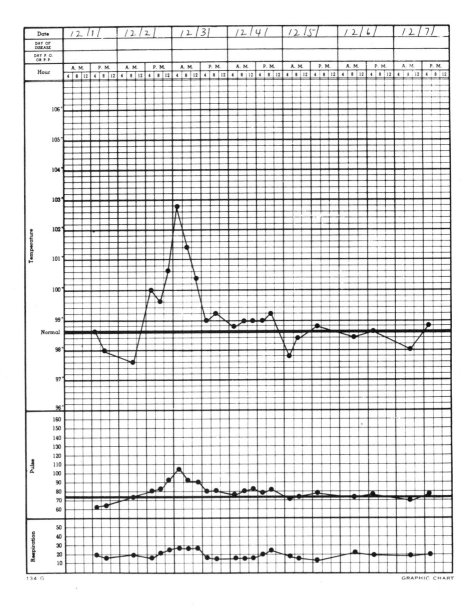

GRAPHIC CHART

Recording the Temperature

The top half of the graphic sheet is for recording the temperature. Note that the temperature range of degrees is $96°$ to $106°$ F.

1. Record in even numbers. The graphic sheet is scored so that each line equals $2/10$ of a degree. Do not use odd numbers unless you used an electric thermometer with measurements accurate to $1/10$ of a degree.

2. Place a dot on the center of the appropriate line; the dot should be at the intersection of the appropriate hour and temperature reading.

3. Using a ruler, connect the dots with a straight, accurate line.

4. If the temperature is rectal, indicate above the dot with Ⓡ.

5. If the temperature is axillary, indicate above the dot with Ⓐ.

Recording the Pulse

The pulse is charted on the same graph as the temperature, except that the pulse scale is used to locate the placement of the dot. Note that the pulse range is from 50 to 160. Each line between the bold lines represents 10 pulse beats.

Record the pulse in even numbers, such as 80, 86, 102. Using a ruler, connect the dots with a straight, accurate line.

Recording Respiration

The lower portion of the graphic sheet is used for recording the respiratory rate. Note that the respiration scale is from 10 to 50. When the respiratory rate to be recorded is one of the numbers indicated on the sheet (such as 20 or 40), then place the dot in the center of the appropriate line. Otherwise the dot is centered at the correct vertical distance between two lines.

Example: Respiration 28 is recorded as —————— 30
                                         —————— 20

Record in even numbers such as 22, 46. Using a ruler, connect the dots with a straight, accurate line.

Recording Blood Pressure

Many graphic sheets now contain a section labeled "Blood Pressure" and provide space for recording the readings. Write the systolic pressure above the slanted line and the diastolic pressure below the line.

Practice charting the following vital signs on the Graphic Chart. Be sure to enter the dates and connect the dots for one temperature reading with the dot for the next temperature reading, and do the same for the pulse and respiration values.

Day	8 A.M.	12 noon	4 P.M.	8 P.M.
1	100.2—88—20 160/88	100.8—92—22	102.4—108—24 156/86	103.2—112—24
2	99.6—96—20 148/88	100.6—200—22	100.8—102—22 134/70	98.8—80—18
3	98—76—20 130/80		98.6—72—18 144/88	
4	96.8—66—16 110/70		98.4—84—18 114/64	

Check your work for accuracy with your instructor or another student.

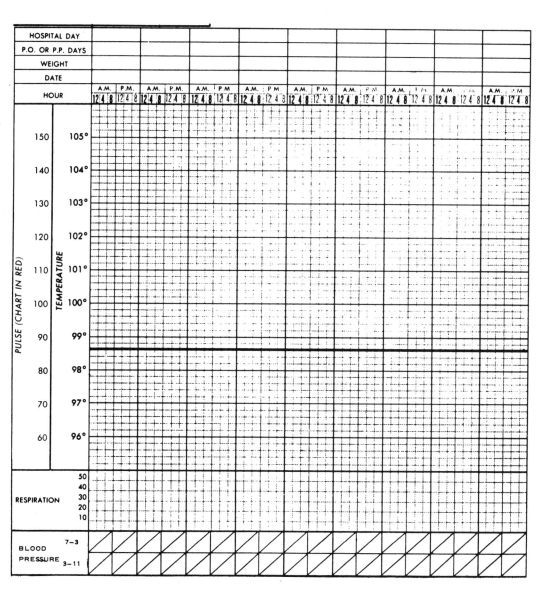

ARTISTIC PRESS, P.O. BOX 20540
LOS ANGELES, CALIF. 90006

GRAPHIC CHART

WORKBOOK ANSWERS

1. To detect early changes in the patient's condition, such as a worsening of the disease state or a return to normal.

2. 98.6°F

3. 37°C

4. 99.6°F or 37.6°C

5. to 8. Any of the following: site of measurement; weather; time of day; menstrual cycle; exercise; or patient's age, emotional state, or disease condition.

9. to 11. The following answers in any order: oral, rectal, and axillary.

12. About a 14 per cent increase.

13. 60 to 100 beats per minute.

14. The rhythm and the volume or strength of the pulse.

15. Over the apex of the heart, the pedal pulse points, or any of the following arteries: temporal, carotid, radial, femoral, popliteal.

16. Bradycardia

17. Tachycardia

18. Any six of the following: anxiety, fear, pain, fever, work, excitement, stress, hot weather, or exercise.

19. to 21. The following answers in any order: bradycardia (pulse less than 60); tachycardia (pulse over 100); or irregular pulse.

22. 14 to 20 breaths per minute.

23. Carbon dioxide

24. 1 R to 4 P

25. Regular, evenly paced, effortless, automatic, and quiet.

26. Obstructed

27. Dyspnea

28. Cheyne-Stokes breathing

29. 120/80

30. Highest

31. Diastolic

32. Pulse pressure equals systolic pressure minus diastolic pressure.

33. 140/90

34. to 38. Any five of the following responses: age, sex, pain, exercise, obesity, anxiety, fear, work, drugs, and disease.

39. Shock or circulatory collapse

40. to 41. Mercury gauge; aneroid gauge

42. On the arm at the anticubital space.

43. A faint tapping that increases in intensity.

44. A muffled change or the disappearance of the sound.

45. At eye level and from a distance of 3 feet.

46. To obtain an approximate measure of the systolic pressure.

PERFORMANCE TEST

1. In the skill laboratory, correctly and accurately take the vital signs (T, P, R, and BP) of your partner, using the procedures presented in class, e.g., oral, rectal, and axillary temperatures, and radial, femoral, temporal, carotid, and apical pulse.

2. In addition, accurately chart the vital signs you obtained on a practice nurses' notes and graphic record.

PERFORMANCE CHECKLIST

MEASURING ORAL TEMPERATURES

Demonstrate the correct method of taking an oral temperature with a glass thermometer.

1. Wash your hands.

2. Approach the patient and explain the procedure.

3. Obtain the equipment.

4. Prepare the equipment for use: clean the thermometer according to your agency regulations; rinse the thermometer in cold water if necessary.

5. Check the level of the mercury in the thermometer; if it is above $96°$ Fahrenheit, the level must be lowered by shaking the thermometer.

6. Place the thermometer in the patient's mouth:

   a. Place it under the tongue.

   b. Place it deep into the area.

   c. Ask the patient to keep the mouth closed.

7. Leave the thermometer in place for the required period of time:

   a. glass thermometers: 5 to 8 minutes

   b. electronic: until registered

   c. disposable: 45 seconds

8. Remove the thermometer, holding the top end between your thumb and index finger.

9. Wipe the thermometer with tissue, making sure to wipe from top to bottom.

10. Read the thermometer.

11. Place the thermometer in its holder.

12. Record the reading appropriately on the patient's chart.

MEASURING RECTAL TEMPERATURES

Demonstrate the correct procedure for obtaining a rectal temperature with a glass thermometer.

1. Wash your hands.

2. Identify and approach the patient.

3. Obtain the thermometer and lubricant.

4. Position the patient in Sims' position, being careful to maintain patient's privacy and warmth.

5. Insert the thermometer into the rectum: lift the upper buttocks slightly; insert the lubricated end of the thermometer about 1½ inches into the rectum.

6. Leave the thermometer in the cavity for the required period of time:

   a. glass thermometers: 3 to 5 minutes

   b. electronic: until registered

   c. disposable: 90 seconds

   Make sure to hold the thermometer during the entire time, because it could slip into the rectum.

7. Remove the thermometer and wipe it clean with gauze or tissue, wiping from top to bottom.

8. Read the temperature.

9. Record the temperature on the patient's chart.

10. Make sure to indicate that the temperature was taken rectally ®.

MEASURING AXILLARY TEMPERATURES

Demonstrate the correct method used to obtain axillary temperature.

1. Wash your hands.

2. Identify the patient and explain the procedure.

3. Obtain the thermometer.

4. Prepare the equipment for use: shake down the thermometer, if necessary; rinse and wipe it dry, if necessary.

5. Place the thermometer in the patient's axilla—make sure it is dry.

6. Leave the thermometer in for the required period of time:

   a. glass thermometers: 10 minutes

   b. electronic: until registered

   c. disposable: 90 seconds

7. Remove the thermometer, holding the top end between your thumb and index finger.

8. Wipe the thermometer with a tissue, making sure to wipe from top to bottom.

9. Read the thermometer.

10. Place the thermometer in its holder.

11. Record the reading on the patient's chart, indicating that it is an axillary temperature Ⓐ.

TAKING RADIAL PULSE AND RESPIRATORY RATE

Show the correct procedure for taking a radial, femoral, and temporal pulse and observing respiratory rate.

Taking a pulse.

1. Wash your hands.

2. Identify and approach the patient.

3. Explain the procedure to the patient.

4. Place your three middle fingertips over the appropriate artery.

5. Count the pulsations for a specific period of time — usually 30 seconds — and multiply by 2 to obtain the rate per minute. If abnormal, count for full minute.

6. Note the rate, force, and rhythm of the beats.

Observing respiration rate.

1. Count respirations for 30 seconds and multiply by 2 for the rate per minute. If breathing is abnormal, count for full minute.

2. Observe the rate, depth, and rhythm of respiration.

3. Record the procedure appropriately on the chart.

TAKING AN APICAL PULSE RATE

Demonstrate the correct procedure for determining an apical pulse rate.

1. Wash your hands.

2. Identify the patient and explain the procedure.

3. Obtain the equipment.

4. Position the patient and provide for privacy, warmth, and comfort.

5. Warm the stethoscope with your hands.

6. Insert the earpieces into your ears; the bend should be forward in the ears.

7. Place the diaphragm of the stethoscope over the apex of the patient's heart.

8. Count the beats for one full minute, noting the rate, force, and rhythm.

9. Record the information on the patient's chart.

10. Clean and replace the equipment in the proper area.

BLOOD PRESSURE

Demonstrate the correct procedure for taking a patient's blood pressure.

1. Wash your hands.

2. Identify the patient and explain the procedure.

3. Obtain the equipment.

4. Position the patient.

5. Select the cuff and apply it directly over the skin, and 1 to 2 inches above the elbow.

6. Attach the tubes from the BP cuff.

7. Close the valve of the air pump.

8. Inflate the cuff and palpate the radial or brachial artery.

9. Read the point at which the pulse fades away.

10. Deflate the cuff and wait 15 seconds.

11. Position the stethoscope over the artery.

12. Inflate the cuff 30 mm. higher than the palpated pulse point.

13. Deflate the cuff at a steady rate and note the systolic and the diastolic pressures.

14. Remeasure, if needed to determine the accuracy.

15. Return the materials and equipment to storage.

16. Record the readings on the patient's chart.

POST-TEST

Matching. For each of the measurements in Column 1, select the word that best describes it from Column 2. Consider the vital signs as those measured in a young adult.

Column 1	*Column 2*
1. P 112	a. Within the normal range.
2. T 37°C	b. Pyrexia
3. BP 164/104	c. Tachycardia
4. R 20	d. Bradycardia
5. T 98.6°F	e. Hypotension
6. P 56	f. Hypertension
7. BP/116/76	
8. T 40.1°C	
9. T 99.4°F	
10. BP 150/88	

Multiple Choice. Select the one best answer for each question.

11. Which of the following methods of taking the temperature gives the highest reading in the same person at the same time?

    a. oral

    b. rectal

    c. axillary

12. Adjustments in the body heat are made by increasing or decreasing any or all of the following factors *except* which one?

    a. hormonal action on blood vessels.

    b. external applications of heat.

    c. metabolic action on food.

    d. degree of physical activity.

13. The body temperature is lowest or in the "low-normal" range

    a. during an inflammatory process.

    b. after vigorous activity.

    c. during the late afternoon hours.

    d. upon awakening in the morning.

14. The patient is drinking a cup of coffee when you arrive to take the temperature and other vital signs. What would you do?

    a. Tell the patient you will return later when he is finished.

    b. Ask the patient not to eat, drink or smoke for 15 minutes, then take them.

    c. Take all of the vital signs then except for the temperature.

    d. Proceed to take the vital signs since hot coffee doesn't affect them.

15. Temperatures above 105.8°F or 41°C should be treated promptly to reduce the fever because of

   a. damage to the cells of the central nervous system.

   b. chemical reactions to oxygen in the blood stream.

   c. heavy perspiration reducing the amount of urine produced.

   d. the increased workload of the heart.

16. Measures to reduce excess body heat include using fans to increase the flow of air in the vicinity. This is an example of heat loss by means of

   a. conduction.

   b. radiation.

   c. convection.

   d. evaporation.

17. All of the following patients in the hospital are at risk of developing hypothermia *except* for which one?

   a. Those in a 65°F cool room.

   b. Newborn babies being exposed and bathed.

   c. Postoperative patients in the recovery room.

   d. Elderly or debilitated bed patients.

18. Accurate temperatures can be obtained most rapidly by using what kind of thermometer?

   a. disposable thermometers

   b. electronic thermometers

   c. mercury-in-glass thermometers

   d. rectal glass thermometer

19. The pulse point used most often for taking vital signs of children and adults is the

   a. apical pulse.

   b. pedal pulse.

   c. carotid pulse.

   d. radial pulse.

20. Which of these factors increase(s) the pulse rate?

   a. exercise

   b. emotional states

   c. rest

   d. all

   e. all but c

21. The normal range for the pulse in older children and adults is

    a. 115 to 130

    b. 80 to 120

    c. 60 to 100

    d. 50 to 75

22. Which of these factors increase(s) the respiratory rate?

    a. exercise

    b. emotional states

    c. fever

    d. all

    e. all but c

23. People breathe at a fairly constant rate of one respiration for every so many heart beats. The rate is one breath to how many beats?

    a. 2 beats.

    b. 4 beats.

    c. 8 beats.

    d. 10 beats.

24. The person who becomes short of breath with little exertion, such as when eating a meal, is an example of what kind of respiratory condition?

    a. dyspnea.

    b. stridor.

    c. hyperventilation.

    d. Cheyne-Stokes breathing.

25. Any kind of noisy breathing is considered to be indicative of

    a. an upper respiratory infection.

    b. an attack of asthma.

    c. an obstructed airway.

    d. an excess of secretions.

26. From the blood pressure, the nurse gains information about all of the following *except* which one?

    a. the efficiency of the heart beat

    b. adequate amount of blood volume

    c. the balance between heat production and loss

    d. the resistance of the blood vessels

27. When the heart contracts and forces blood into the arteries, the pressure is called

    a. diastolic pressure.

    b. systolic pressure.

    c. partial pressure.

    d. pulse pressure.

28. Which one of the following would be more apt to have a BP of 150/90 and still be considered to be within the normal range?

    a. a newborn infant.

    b. a young athlete.

    c. a pregnant woman.

    d. a senior citizen.

29. Prolonged hypertension causes damage to which of these tissues?

    a. brain

    b. kidneys

    c. heart

    d. all

    e. a and b

30. A fall in blood pressure, increase in pulse rate, and cold, clammy skin are symptoms of

    a. shock

    b. pyrexia

    c. infection

    d. circulatory collapse

    e. a and d

POST-TEST ANSWERS

1.	c	16.	c
2.	a	17.	a
3.	f	18.	b
4.	a	19.	d
5.	a	20.	e
6.	d	21.	c
7.	a	22.	d
8.	b	23.	b
9.	a	24.	a
10.	f	25.	c
11.	b	26.	c
12.	c	27.	b
13.	d	28.	d
14.	b	29.	d
15.	a	30.	e

Unit 22

GENERAL PERFORMANCE OBJECTIVE

When you have finished the unit, you will be able to measure accurately oral fluid intake and fluid output and maintain records as required for determination of fluid balance.

SPECIFIC PERFORMANCE OBJECTIVES

Following this lesson you will be able to:

1. Identify all food items that should be measured as fluid intake.

2. Correctly convert volumetric measurements from English and household units to metric units.

3. Measure fluid volume accurately with a graduated container.

4. Give instructions appropriate to the age and condition of the patient for keeping track of fluids taken in and the use of the bedpan or urinal for the measurement of urinary output.

5. Keep accurate records of oral fluid intake and fluid output and determine the total 24-hour I & O as required.

6. Recognize, note, and report symptoms of edema and dehydration and conditions of unusual or excessive fluid output.

VOCABULARY

anuria—failure of the kidneys to secrete urine; total lack of urination.
ascites—collection of fluid in the peritoneal or abdominal cavity.
dehydration—process that occurs when output of water from the tissues exceeds water intake.
diaphoresis—profuse sweating.
diuretic—an agent or medication that increases the secretion of urine.
edema—a condition in which the body tissues contain an excessive amount of fluid, causing swelling of the tissue; may be localized or generalized in the body.
electrolytes—chemicals that in solution separate into charged particles called ions, which can conduct an electrical current; sodium chloride (ordinary table salt) separates into sodium and chloride ions in the body fluids.
fluid compartments—the main fluid spaces: (1) *intracellular space* (filled with the liquid cytoplasm of cells) contains about two-thirds of the body water; and (2) *extracellular space* (outside cells) includes the space around cells, filled with interstitial fluid, and the space within blood vessels, containing the liquid blood plasma.
hypodermoclysis—the injection of fluids into the tissues just below the skin (subcutaneous) to supply the body with liquids when fluids cannot be taken by mouth or IV; commonly called clysis.

nourishments—extra foods, usually liquids, given between meals to supplement the diet (e.g., milk, fruit juices, crackers, ice cream, cookies).

oliguria—diminished amount and frequency of urination.

polyuria—excessive secretion and discharge of urine.

turgor—the tension or fullness of the skin; swollen or congested.

urine—the liquid wastes filtered from the blood by the kidneys, stored in the bladder, and discharged through the urethra.

INTRODUCTION

The human body is composed mainly of water, in which are dissolved many of the substances necessary for life. The digestive process involves various fluids, including saliva, gastric juices, and others, which help break down the foods we eat into simpler substances. Blood is a fluid that transports nutrients to the cells and waste products away from cells.

The fluids of the body provide the internal environment wherein many of the chemical and physical reactions take place. For this reason, the body must have a relatively stable amount of fluid at all times. Some fluid is lost continually in the form of urine and sweat, in the air that is exhaled, and in the stool, and this amount must be replaced to maintain a balance.

Many factors influence the amount of fluid that the body loses: the weather, many types of diseases, fever, surgery, stress, degree of activity, drugs, and the metabolic rate. Patients who are sick may be affected by several of these factors and therefore may not be able to maintain a fluid balance. In order to avoid serious or even fatal consequences, a record is kept of their intake and output. When the fluid intake is decreased or a loss of fluid occurs, some patients are more at risk, especially older patients who have smaller fluid reserves and infants who have a high metabolic rate and lose water about three times faster than do adults. Special attention must be given to their fluid needs.

As you can see, an important task that you will perform is keeping a record of the patient's intake and output, commonly called the I & O Record. This unit focuses on a brief discussion of the fluid compartments of the body, the role of electrolytes, and the problems of dehydration and, fluid overload. The types of fluids and foods to be measured are listed, and some equivalent amounts are listed for measuring the contents of cups, soup bowls, and other dishes. A sample intake and output form is used to illustrate the method of recording the I & O.

THE BODY'S NEED FOR WATER

ITEM 1. ᵗTHE IMPORTANCE OF BODY FLUIDS

Water is vital to health and to survival. Body water serves as the environment for the chemical changes that occur in the cells and as the means for keeping body temperatures stable, while giving form and structure to body tissues.

Fluid Compartments

The body has been described as a volume of fluid that is capable of conducting an electrical charge. The fluids consist of water, electrolytes, and nonelectrolytes that vary according to the particular fluid. Electrolytes are chemicals that break down in water into positively or negatively charged particles, or ions. They help keep the chemical balance in the body and are important in maintaining water distribution in the body and nerve and muscle function. The major electrolytes (and their symbols) are potassium (K), sodium (Na), calcium (Ca), and chlorine (Cl). You will frequently find these in reports of laboratory tests or as part of the medical treatment, such as a low sodium diet.

The quantity of body water varies according to age: It is proportionately greater in the infant and decreases as the person grows older. From 75 to 80 per cent of the infant's body weight consists of fluid. Infants use their body water three times faster than do adults. This rapid turnover of water is due to the high metabolic rate that produces the rapid growth characteristic of the first three months of life. Infants lose large amounts of water through frequent voidings and stools and through perspiration during eating and sleeping. In the adult, fluid consists of about 60 per cent of total body weight; in the aged adult, the proportion of body water is even less. Fat cells contain no water, so the proportion of body water in the obese person could be less than 50 per cent, with few reserves for use in case of sudden or severe loss.

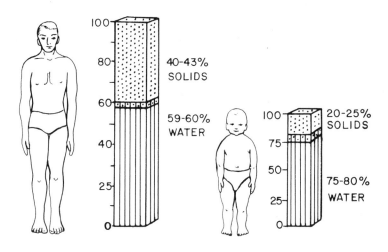

FLUID = 60-80% OF BODY WEIGHT

Fluids are located in different compartments of the body. The largest quantity of body water is contained within the cells of the tissues themselves. This constitutes 40 per cent of the total body weight and is called the *intracellular compartment.*

Fluid in the extracellular compartment averages about 20 per cent of body weight in adults, and more in infants. The extracellular compartment consists of the water that surrounds the tissues; the blood and plasma; and the various secretions, such as the digestive juices, bile, and spinal fluid, to name a few.

Fluid Balance

The body maintains fluid balance when the amount of water taken in approximately equals the amount of water eliminated. The fluids and foods of the diet provide most of the water needed each day. A small amount of water is produced during cellular metabolism as energy is released. Water is eliminated from the body in the urine, perspiration, feces, and exhaled air. Some typical volumes of water intake and output for an adult in a 24-hour period are included here:

INTAKE		OUTPUT	
Liquid	1500 ml	Urine	1400 ml
Food	800 ml	Sweat	500 ml
Metabolism	200 ml	Feces	200 ml
		Respiration	400 ml
Totals	2500 ml		2500 ml

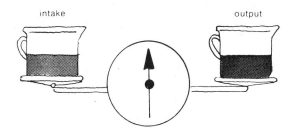

This would indicate fluid balance for this person. The amount of fluid taken in and eliminated varies in health with the temperature, activity, and habits of the person, and other factors. So vital is water to survival that if fluid intake is decreased, the body will conserve fluid by decreasing the amount of urine secreted. This is an important fact for health workers to know.

1. By now you should know at least three important roles of body fluids:

a. _____

b. _____

c. _____ .

2. What would a typical daily urinary output be for a healthy adult?

ITEM 2. PROBLEMS IN FLUID BALANCE

Even if a person has no fluid intake, the fluid loss will amount to 1500 ml per day. This is called the obligatory loss. It is something over which you have no control. We normally lose from 900 to 1000 ml daily from the evaporation of water from the skin and moisture contained in the exhaled air during respiration. In hot weather, visible perspiration on the skin increases the loss another 1000 to 2000 ml. The minimum amount of urine that is required to excrete waste products from the body is 600 ml with normal kidney function and much higher if the kidney is diseased. Even patients who are not eating or who are ordered NPO (nothing by mouth) for surgery, laboratory tests, or x-rays continue to need a minimum of 1500 ml of fluids or they will become dehydrated as fluids leave the tissues and cells.

Illness can markedly disturb the delicate balance of body fluids and electrolytes. Large amounts of fluids may be lost from the body by diaphoresis (profuse sweating), vomiting, or diarrhea. Drainage from wounds and nasogastric suction remove body fluids and electrolytes. Of course, hemorrhage or loss of interstitial fluid from a large burned surface disturbs fluid balance. These losses are especially serious for infants or young children, because more of their body tissues are liquid than are those of adults.

The daily requirement of liquids should be sufficient to replace the obligatory water loss from skin, lungs, and kidneys, which may amount to 1500 ml plus any losses from abnormal routes. The amount of water produced by the metabolism of food is about 10 ml for every 100 calories consumed, so that a 2000-calorie diet yields 200 ml. When patients are unable to drink an adequate amount of fluids, other methods must be used to supply them. Fluids are generally given intravenously or occasionally by hypodermoclysis (under the skin).

The difficulties resulting from a disturbance in the fluid balance are (1) fluid losses and (2) fluid overload. The fluid losses are the most frequently seen problems and present many challenges in nursing care.

Fluid Losses

A depletion of fluid volume results when the person has an inadequate intake of fluids or when fluids are lost through abnormal routes. Abnormal routes include gastric or intestinal suctioning, ileostomy, colostomy, draining wounds or fistulas, and weeping burns. These are actual losses of body water, but the fluid loss includes shifts of fluid from the circulating blood volume into the extracellular compartment. Fluids trapped or accumulated in the interstitial spaces or body cavities are abnormal and produce the same symptoms of dehydration.

Dehydration. Body water can be depleted rapidly, as occurs with hemorrhaging or serious oozing from extensive burns, or it can take place slowly, over a period of days. When fluid is lost rapidly, the symptoms are those of shock. The skin is cold and clammy, the pulse is rapid, the blood pressure falls, and the patient is apprehensive and restless. Unless the fluid level is restored, the patient goes into shcok, the cells are damaged, then unconsciousness and death follow. Oliguria accompanies attempts of the body to reduce further loss.

When dehydration takes place more slowly, there is a smaller blood volume circulating in the vessels and less cooling of the body, so that the face becomes flushed and the temperature rises above normal. The kidneys reabsorb more of the water by concentrating the urine, so urinary output is reduced. The patient also has weight loss, thirst, and poor skin turgor. Unless the condition is corrected, the dehydration in later stages is the same as the shock seen with rapid water loss and also leads to death.

Edema and Ascites. Do you recall the fact that body fluids must be distributed properly in the fluid compartments in order to maintain fluid balance? Sometimes excess fluid accumulates in the spaces around the cells, a condition that is called edema. Symptoms of edema include weight gain, and swelling of the subcutaneous spaces, particularly of the feet and ankles or of the face and hands.

Fluids can accumulate in the peritoneal (abdominal) cavity, and this condition is called ascites. Symptoms of ascites include weight gain, abdominal distention, and dyspnea resulting from the increased abdominal pressure.

Fluid Overload

An increased amount of fluids is corrected by the normal kidney through increasing the dilution of urine until the excess amount of water has been removed. When you drink three to four large glasses of milk or juice in a few minutes' time, the liquid expands the fluid volume as it is absorbed and the excess is transported to the kidney for excretion. Special care must be taken to prevent IV fluids from infusing too fast and causing "speed shock," or fluid overload. If the kidneys are diseased or if the increase of fluids is too rapid to be handled by the normal kidney, the following symptoms would occur: edema of the eyelids and extremities, dyspnea, and gurgling rales, which signal the beginning of pulmonary edema.

‖‖

Match the term with the correct definition.

3. _____ ascites   a. profuse sweating

4. _____ dehydration   b. scanty urine output

5. _____ diaphoresis   c. fluid in peritoneal cavity

6. _____ edema   d. parenteral fluid

7. _____ hypodermoclysis   e. swollen ankles

8. _____ oliguria   f. Na^+ (sodium particles with an electrical charge)

9. _____ ion   g. Fluid intake exceeds fluid output

     h. Fluid output exceeds fluid intake

‖‖

ITEM 3.   NURSE'S ROLE IN MAINTAINING FLUID BALANCE

An important responsibility of the nurse is to assist with the maintenance of body fluid and electrolyte balance. This involves providing and encouraging oral fluids according to individual needs, measuring and accurately reporting fluid intake and fluid loss, and then informing the doctor if the patient is not maintaining an adequate fluid balance so that parenteral fluids can be given if necessary.

In addition, the nurse observes the patient very closely and pays particular attention to complaints the patient may voice. Changes in any of the following areas may be an early sign that the patient is having a problem associated with fluid or electrolyte balance.

1. *Sensory state:* irritability, disorientation, confusion or forgetfulness.

2. *Vital signs:* elevation of temperature may signal dehydration, further depleting the fluid balance, and causing blood pressure to fall because of the loss of circulating blood volume.

3. *Physical appearance:* changes in the color, temperature, turgor, or moisture of the skin.

4. *Urinary output:* of paramount importance, as the amount indicates the adequacy of kidney function and of extracellular water circulating in the body.

5. *Body weight:* daily weight is valuable in determining fluid and metabolic changes.

6. *Muscle strength:* may signify changes in electrolyte balance. Muscle weakness and softness indicate loss of potassium; loss of sodium leads to weakness and confusion, while calcium depletion leads to twitching and convulsions.

ITEM 4.   MEASURING THE FLUID INTAKE

The Oral Fluid Intake

The average active adult requires from 2000 to 3000 ml (cc) of fluid per day, which is 2 to 3 quarts. Some agencies use cc's, or cubic centimeters, synonymously with ml's (milliliters).

Generally, the physician orders the recording of I & O for the patient.

To check the oral intake at mealtimes, you should look at the tray before it is removed from the patient's room. *Don't* count on the patient or the dietary personnel to tell you. This is *your* responsibility. The fluids you must measure on the tray include: water, coffee, tea, Jello (gelatin), ice cream and sherbet, carbonated drinks, wine, consommé, juices, milk, cream, milk shakes, infant cereals, and broth or soup.

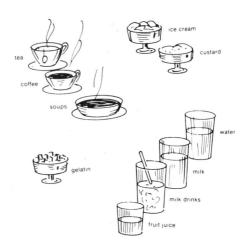

Metric and Household Measurements. Before you can record the oral intake, most agencies require that fractions and household measures be converted to ml or cc of the metric system. Because the patient's food is served in cups, bowls, and glasses, you may need to be able to convert these into metric measurements. Many agencies provide a list of the equivalent amounts contained in the type or size of dish used by the dietary department. If this information is not available for you, take a one-ounce medicine cup and measure the amount of water contained in a soup bowl, cup, or other container. A graduated container could also be used to measure the capacity.

Avoid using fractions when recording I & O, but convert these to the metric system. The following table lists some values for common household measures.

CONVERSION TABLE

Household or Apothecary Measurement	Metric Equivalent
15 drops; 15 minims	1 ml (or cc)
1 teaspoon	4 ml
1 tablespoon	15 ml
1 ounce	30 ml
1 cup (8 ounces)	240 ml
1 pint	500 ml
1 quart	1000 ml
5 ice chips to 1 ice cube (1 average ice cube = 10 teaspoons)	40 ml

COMMON EQUIVALENTS

Coffee cup	240 ml	Cream pkg.	15 ml
Iced tea glass	320 ml	Sherbert	90 ml
Juice glass	120 ml	Soup, clear	120 ml
Wax cup	180 ml	Soup, thick	180 ml
Styrofoam cup	210 ml	Jello	80 ml
Large glass	230 ml	Milk carton	240 ml

Limited or Restricted Fluid Intake. The fluid intake of patients with certain diseases of the kidney or circulatory system or with head injury may need to be limited to only the minimal amount required to prevent dehydration. You should check with your team leader or RN for the amount you must give during your 8 hours of duty. Many hospitals designate that 50 per cent of limited fluids be given during the day shift, 30 per cent during the afternoon shift, and 20 per cent during the night hours.

Recording Oral Intake

The Intake and Output Record is a work sheet used by nurses to keep track of the patient's fluid status. All of the fluids the patient drinks should be recorded at the time when they were taken. Some agencies also want you to list the type of fluid, e.g., orange juice 180 ml. Write this in the column headed *Intake* on the I & O record.

One of the following methods of measuring the amount the patient drinks from the water pitcher may be used.

1. Record each amount of liquid the patient drinks.

2. Measure the amount left in the water pitcher and subtract it from the amount in a full pitcher.

3. If the patient can take only ice chips by mouth, you may estimate that there are approximately 5 ice chips to an average ice cube and about 40 ml of water per cube.

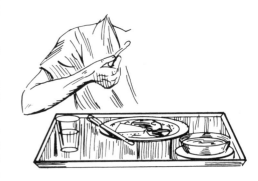

At the end of your 8-hour tour of duty, add the total intake and write the amount on the I & O record. Some patients are on I & O at more frequent intervals; if so, add intake when specified and enter it on the record. I & O may be recorded every hour for some seriously ill patients.

Follow your agency's policy for recording IV's. IV fluids are infused at a slow rate and over a longer period of time. Many Intake and Output records now specify the amount remaining in the infusion at both the beginning and the end of the recording period. The amount of fluid infused during the period can then be determined. (TBI means "to be infused.")

G-206

24 HOUR INTAKE AND OUTPUT RECORD

DATE: _5/22/XX_____

BALANCE: INTAKE MINUS OUTPUT = _____

	INTAKE							OUTPUT		
	ORAL			PARENTERAL				URINE	OTHER DRAINAGE	
TIME	TYPE	AMT.	TYPE & BOTTLE #	AMT.	TIME	AMT.	TIME	AMT.	TYPE	AMT.
8:00	Coffee	60			Start Dc'd					
	O.J.	120	#3 5% D/W	210	6 P.M. 7:50	210				
9:30	Water	60	#4 5% D/S	1000	7:50	575				
12:00	Milk	120								
	Tea	90					2 P.M.	850	Foley	
1:00	Water	30								
					8 Hr. Total =	785			8 Hr. Total =	
6-2	8 Hr. Total = 480		──────────►		──────────►	480	8 Hr. Total =			
					8 Hr. Grand Total =	1265	8 Hr. Grand Total =			
4 P.M.	H₂0	60	#4 5% D/S TBI	425	2 P.M.					
					8 Hr. Total —				8 Hr. Total =	
2-10	8 Hr. Total =		──────────►		──────────►		8 Hr. Total			
					8 Hr. Grand Total =		8 Hr. Grand Total =			
					8 Hr. Total =				8 Hr. Total =	
10-6	8 Hr. Total =		──────────►		──────────►		8 Hr. Total			
					8 Hr. Grand Total =		8 Hr. Grand Total =			

NURSES SIGNATURE	8 HOUR GRAND TOTAL =	8 HOUR GRAND TOTAL =
	24 Hr. Total Blood =	24 Hr. Total Urine —
7-3	24 Hr. Total I.V. —	24 Hr. Total Drng. =
3-11	24 Hr. Total Oral =	24 Hr. Total Other =
11-7	24 HOUR INTAKE TOTAL =	24 HR. OUTPUT TOTAL =

ITEM 5. MEASURING FLUID OUTPUT

Urinary Output

Generally, the hourly urinary output ranges between 30 ml (cc) to as much as several hundred ml, depending on the amount of intake. The average urinary output in a 24-hour period is 1000 to 1500 ml; you should report an output of less than 600 ml in a 24-hour period.

To measure urinary output, pour the urine from the bedpan or urinal into a measuring cup, commonly called a "graduate." Place the cup on a flat surface for accurate measurement. Note the level reached by the top of the fluid. Record under the column marked *Output.* Designate the time and the amount in ml. If you notice when pouring the urine in the toilet that it is a different color from the usual yellow or amber or that it smells sweet or sour, note this on the patient's chart. Describe the color, amount, and odor, and report them to your team leader immediately.

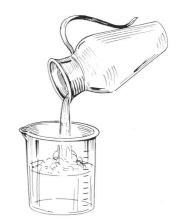

Be sure to instruct ambulatory patients and those with bathroom privileges that they are on intake and output. Ask them to urinate into a bedpan, the collecting pan placed under the toilet seat, or the urinal and to save the urine for you to measure and record. Some patients are able to keep their own intake and output record, if provided with instructions, the record, and a pencil. The RN will indicate which ones can do this.

Other Fluid Losses

Besides recording the urinary output, you should measure and record the amounts of other fluid losses if at all possible. If the patient has diarrhea, the liquid stool can be measured in the same manner as urine. Profuse perspiration that requires a change of the damp linen can be estimated as 1000 ml, and the contents of drainage or suction bottles should be accurately measured and recorded. The amount of vomitus is also recorded as output.

ITEM 6. INTAKE AND OUTPUT PROCEDURE

Instruct the patient who has been placed on I & O in the agency procedure and practice measuring and recording the intake and output.

Important Steps	Key Points
1. Explain the procedure and give instructions about I & O.	Place an I & O Record in the patient's room. Write the patient's name and room number and the date on the form. Explain that all the fluids taken in (by mouth, IV, clysis) and all fluid output are to be measured. Ask the patient to urinate or void in a collection pan, bedpan, or urinal, and not to flush it down the toilet.

Important Steps	Key Points
2. Check the water pitcher when beginning your tour of duty.	Remember to check to see if the patient is NPO (nothing by mouth) for surgery or tests. If the patient is not on restricted fluids, fill the pitcher with fresh water. Some agencies have the off-going personnel fill water pitchers — if so, check to see if it is full and how many milliliters it holds.
3. Measure and record fluid intake at frequent intervals.	Check the patient's tray *before* removing it from the room. Check the amount of fluids taken in, convert household measures to metric units and record on the Intake Record. If your agency prefers, record the amount, type of fluid, and time taken. Items considered as fluids are water (H_2O), Jello (gelatin), ice cream, carbonated drinks, consommé, milk, milk shakes, broth or soup, coffee, tea, sherbet, wine, juices, cream, and infant cereals.
4. Measure and record all fluid output.	Pour the urine into the graduate. Place the graduate on a flat surface. Read the number at the top of the fluid level. Make a note on the I & O Record each time the patient urinates so you don't forget. Be sure to indicate if the output is urine, diarrhea, or vomitus. In the nurses' notes, make a comment if the patient sweats profusely (diaphoresis), for this too is output.
5. Dispose of the output.	If a specimen is not needed for analysis, pour it into the toilet. Rinse the graduate, and empty it into the toilet — not the sink. Flush the toilet. Return the container to the bedside stand.
6. Total the I & O at the end of the shift and record in the chart.	Intake may be totaled and recorded every 1, 2, 4, or 8 hours on the special I & O sheet or the nurses' notes in the patient's chart (check your agency procedure). The fluid in the water pitcher may be recorded by the number of glasses of water taken *or* by subtracting the amount left in the pitcher from the total amount it holds. Follow your agency policy. Empty the urine from the collection bag of patients who have Foley catheters and, at the end of the 24-hour period, measure and record the intake and output on the intake and output record and empty other drainage or suction bags as directed.

WORKBOOK ANSWERS

1. Body fluids (any three of the following responses)

    —help to regulate body temperature.

    —provide water for body components such as blood and digestive juices.

    —help to eliminate waste products.

    —serve as a major constituent of cells.

    —provide an environment for the movement of solutes between cells and blood.

2. 1000 to 1500 ml

3. c

4. h

5. a

6. e

7. d

8. b

9. f

PERFORMANCE TEST

1. Determine the volume of household utensils by measuring the contents.

IIIIIIIIIIIIIIIIIIIIIIIIIIIIIIIIIIIIIIIIIIIIIIIIIIIIIIIIIIIIIIIIIIIIIIIIIIIIIIIIIIIIIIIIIIIIIIIIIIIIIIIIIIIIIIIIIIIIIIIIIIIIIIIIIIII

Supplies Needed

Intake and output bedside record	cup
water glass	soup bowl
emesis basin	water pitcher
measuring graduate	water

IIIIIIIIIIIIIIIIIIIIIIIIIIIIIIIIIIIIIIIIIIIIIIIIIIIIIIIIIIIIIIIIIIIIIIIIIIIIIIIIIIIIIIIIIIIIIIIIIIIIIIIIIIIIIIIIIIIIIIIIIIIIIIIIIIIII

A. Identify the *cup.* Fill it to the top. Using a graduate pitcher to measure, answer the following:

   1. How many ml does it hold? _____

   2. How many ml would be needed to fill the paper cup half-full? _____

   3. Fill it half-full and note the level. Repeat the procedure for one-third full _____

     and two-thirds full. _____

B. Identify the *water glass.* Fill it to the top. Answer the following:

   1. How many ml does it hold? _____

   2. Number of ml when one-third full? _____

   3. Number of ml when half-full? _____

   4. Number of ml when two-thirds full? _____

Fill the glass to each of the above levels and note the water level.

C. List four types of fluids that you would be recording on the *I & O* sheet.

   1. _____ .

   2. _____ .

   3. _____ .

   4. _____ .

D. 1. Refer to the bedside I & O sheet and record how many ml the soup bowl can hold.

     _____

   2. Fill the soup bowl with this amount to check your answer. If the patient drank all but *four* tablespoons of his soup, how many ml would he have consumed?

     (1 tbs = 15 ml) _____

   3. How many ml would be left in the soup bowl? _____

E. Refer to the bedside I & O sheet and fill the water pitcher *half-full.*

   1. How many ml would this take? _____

   2. How many ml would be needed to fill the water pitcher two-thirds full? _____

   3. How many ml would be needed to fill the water pitcher one-third full? _____

   4. How many ml would be needed to fill the water pitcher one-fourth full? _____

F. Refer to the Bedside I & O sheet and note the ml contained in a small emesis basin and in the standard emesis basin.

1. Record in ml the difference in amounts between a small emesis basin and a standard emesis basin. _____

2. If a patient vomited 250 ml, how full would a standard emesis basin be? _____ Fill the basin with this amount of water to check your answer.

2. Record oral intake and output.

‖‖‖

Supplies Needed

I & O record form   Graduated container
Toilet and sink available for use in test
A set of bottles or any containers arranged in random order, each containing a specific quantity of water (previously measured and recorded by the instructor) and labeled as follows:
  a. Urine specimen 2:30 P.M.
  b. Urine specimen 3:45 P.M.
  c. Urine specimen 4:30 P.M.
  d. Vomitus 3:00 P.M.
  e. Water pitcher: Contents as of 4:00 P.M.
                     Filled to 2000 ml capacity at 2:00 P.M.
  f. One pint of orange juice

‖‖‖

Instructions to the student: You have a patient on 2-hour I & O. The record is complete through 2:00 P.M., which is the end of the last I & O period. You are to measure and record the I & O in the order in which they normally would have been recorded according to the times shown on the labels on the bottles. Carry out all operations just as you would if these were actual specimens. You have 20 minutes to complete this assignment.

PERFORMANCE CHECKLIST

Volume measurements will vary according to the size of the cups, glasses, soup bowls, water pitchers, and emesis basins used.

ORAL INTAKE AND OUTPUT

1. Measure and record intake and output in correct sequence (as indicated by time tables).

2. Measure each output specimen correctly and enter results in ml or cc in correct column. Clean and store equipment appropriately.

3. Convert pint measurement correctly to ml or cc.

4. Measure contents of water pitcher correctly and calculate water intake correctly; refill as required.

5. Calculate and enter correct totals for 2:00 to 4:00 P.M. intake (e and f) and output (a, b, and c).

6. Measure and record 4:30 P.M. urine specimen after calculation and entry of 2:00 and 4:00 P.M. totals.

7. Make complete record on I & O form for 2:00 to 4:00 P.M.

8. Complete assignment within a time limit of 20 minutes.

POST-TEST

Matching.   For each of the measures given in Column 1, select the equivalent value for it from Column 2.

Column 1

1. quart   *1000 m*
2. teaspoon *4 ml*
3. 8-ounce glass *240 ml*
4. pint   *500 ml*
5. tablespoon *15 ml*

Column 2

a. 15 ml

b. 500 ml

c. 4 ml

d. 240 ml

e. 30 ml

f. 1000 ml

Multiple Choice.   For each of the following items, select the one answer that most correctly completes the statement or answers the question.

6. Which of the following persons would be at greater risk of having an imbalance of fluids if the fluid intake is reduced?

   a. a 40-year-old male laborer.

   b. a 30-year-old woman who is 10 lbs. overweight.

   c. a 15-year-old teenager.

   d. a one-month-old infant.

7. The reason the person in question 6 is at greater risk than the other is

   a. fat cells contain no fluids.

   b. fluids make up 60 per cent of body weight.

   c. the high metabolic rate.

   d. sex and amount of activity.

8. In the average adult, body fluids account for how much of the total body weight?

   a. 45 per cent

   b. 60 per cent

   c. 75 per cent

   d. 90 per cent

9. Fluids are continually being lost from the body. How much is lost in the form of evaporation from the skin and from the lungs each day by the normal adult?

   a. 600 ml

   b. 1000 ml

   c. 1600 ml

   d. 2000 ml

10. If the patient has diaphoresis, or visible perspiration on the skin on a warm day, what amount of fluid lost does this indicate?

    a. 2000 ml

    b. 1600 ml

    c. 1000 ml

    d. 600 ml

11. Mrs. Jane B. has been ordered to be NPO today for tests and treatments. Even if she receives no fluids whatsoever, what amount of fluids would be lost, if any?

    a. The 200 ml normally supplied by metabolizing food.

    b. None.

    c. Only the minimum amount of urine needed to excrete wastes.

    d. Urine and obligatory losses, totaling 1500 ml.

12. Mrs. B. becomes apprehensive, and you note her skin is cold and clammy. The pulse is rapid and her blood pressure is lower when you take the vital signs. These symptoms are indications of

    a. slow dehydration.

    b. electrolyte imbalance.

    c. rapid dehydration.

    d. fluid overload.

13. The most frequent cause of fluid imbalance in patients is

    a. fluid overload.

    b. colostomy.

    c. polyuria.

    d. dehydration.

14. Early changes observed by the nurse indicating a problem with the fluid and electrolyte balance would include which of the following?

    a. Changes in the vital signs and weight.

    b. Changes in the diet and sleep patterns.

    c. Changes in muscle strength and sensory state.

    d. A and C.

    e. All of the above.

15. The compartment that contains the largest amount of body fluids by body weight is

    a. the intracellular compartment.

    b. the blood vessels.

    c. the extracellular compartment.

    d. the urinary bladder.

Situation: Your patient is an adult male. His intake and output are to be recorded every four hours. Total intake and output were last recorded at 12 noon. At 12:30 P.M. the patient had lunch. He was served a bowl of soup (10 ounces), a cup of Jello (gelatin) (8 ounces), and one-half pint of milk. When you removed the tray, the milk and Jello (gelatin) had been consumed. Six tablespoons of soup remained in the bowl. His water pitcher at noon contained 900 ml. At 2:00 P.M. he urinated; you measured his output as 250 ml. At 3:00 P.M. he urinated again; you measured his output as 350 ml. At 3:15 P.M. he vomited (into a container); you measured the amount as 80 ml. At 4:00 P.M. you checked his water pitcher, it contained 600 ml of water.

The patient's fluid intake at lunch should be recorded as:

16. _____ ml of soup

17. _____ ml of milk

18. _____ ml of Jello (gelatin)

19. His total fluid intake for this period from 12 to 4 P.M. is _____ ml.

20. His total fluid output for this period from 12 to 4 P.M. is _____ ml.

POST-TEST ANSWERS

1.	f	11.	d
2.	c	12.	c
3.	d	13.	d
4.	b	14.	d
5.	a	15.	a
6.	d	16.	210
7.	c	17.	250
8.	b	18.	240
9.	b	19.	1000
10.	a	20.	680

ASSISTING WITH NUTRITION

GENERAL PERFORMANCE OBJECTIVE

You will demonstrate the knowledge and skills related to basic foods and general nutrition for adults and children and you will be able to assist the adult and the child with nutrition, after which you will make a record of oral intake.

SPECIFIC PERFORMANCE OBJECTIVES

When this lesson has been completed you will be able to:

1. Determine if patients are meeting their nutritional needs by figuring the total calories needed each day.

2. Calculate the caloric value of some foods commonly served on the diet.

3. Describe the well-balanced diet based on servings from the four basic food groups.

4. State the names of several special diets used in the treatment of patients, some foods that are allowed or restricted, and the general purpose of the diet.

5. Assist or feed an adult patient and a pediatric patient with a diet of solids and liquids.

6. Serve and collect meal trays and nourishments.

VOCABULARY

calorie—the unit of heat required to raise the temperature of one gram of water one degree Centigrade.

carbohydrates—foodstuffs with high starch and sugar content, consisting of carbon, hydrogen, and oxygen molecules. A source of heat and quick energy, they are burned up rapidly by body action.

fats (lipids)—food substances that provide heat and long-lasting energy. Some common fats are lard, olive oil, and butter. They give flavor to foods and act as a regulator for emptying the contents of the stomach.

kilocalorie—the large calorie of food calories; 1000 times as big as a small calorie; often abbreviated as kcal.

malnutrition—poor nourishment resulting from a diet deficient in essential nutrients, or the body's inability to use the food properly.

metabolism—chemical transformation (change) of food by which energy is provided for the growth of cells and substances not needed by the body are excreted as waste products (urine, feces, sweat).

minerals—chemical substances that build and repair tissues; they are important for proper cell function. Some common minerals are calcium, phosphorus, sodium, potassium, iodine, and iron.

nutrition—a branch of science dealing with the scientific laws that govern the food requirements of the human body for growth, reproduction, and energy.

proteins—food substances that build and repair tissues; they are also important in regulating the body processes. Proteins are composed of carbon, hydrogen, oxygen, and nitrogen.

vitamins—chemical substances that aid in body metabolism. When lacking in the diet, they manifest their absence by certain disease conditions. They are used to treat or prevent vitamin deficiency diseases. Some common vitamins are vitamins A, B, C, D, E, and niacin.

INTRODUCTION

As everyone knows, food is a basic need of the body and it must be supplied at frequent intervals to maintain life and the functioning of the body. The nutrients supplied by food are essential to (1) promote growth, (2) provide energy for all of the body functions and activities, and (3) replace or repair tissue through the healing process.

Hospital patients suffering from an acute injury or illness are at great risk of being malnourished. There are many reasons why they have difficulty meeting their nutritional needs and are at risk; among them are the effect of the disease itself on the digestive system, the anxiety and stress of being ill, and the effects of taking medications, of withholding the diet for various tests or procedures, and of putting the patient on NPO as part of the treatment of the disease.

When sick people have a decreased appetite and fail to meet their nutritional needs, energy needed for the body functioning is obtained from the body itself. The extra glucose stored in the liver and the muscles is the first source that is used; this supply is used up in 12 to 48 hours, depending on the body requirements. If the supply of nutrients is inadequate for more than one or two days and the stored glucose has been used, the body begins to break down deposits of fatty tissue and the proteins in muscle tissue. This leads to weight loss, higher acetone or ketone levels in the urine, delayed healing of wounds, and a greater susceptibility to infections.

Malnutrition is not difficult to see in the estimated 5 to 10 per cent of patients in acute medical-surgical units who are emaciated and appear to be only skin and bones after losing much of their body weight. Malnutrition begins long before the extreme weight loss of starvation, however. Even the patient who appears to be well nourished may not be meeting nutritional needs, and this condition is frequently not recognized by members of the health team for a variety of reasons:

— the doctors have written an order specifying the diet the patient is to receive.

— the charge nurse or team leader is attending to patient complaints of other problems or needs that are deemed to be more pressing or more serious.

— the nurse or nursing assistant taking care of the patient knows that sick patients commonly lose their appetite and send their trays back without eating the food, stating "I'm not hungry."

— the evening nurse, who may notice that the dinner tray was hardly touched, merely charts that the patient had a "poor appetite."

— other nurses who relieve for days off may comment about the condition. Everyone is aware that the patient is not eating well, but the information is often disregarded.

Helping patients meet their nutritional needs is often a challenging task for nurses. It is not enough just to order a tray and deliver it to the patient's bedside. Nurses must see that patients actually eat the food needed to meet the body requirements and provide assistance as needed to fill out the menu, to meet their food likes as much as possible, and to feed them as is necessary.

This unit focuses on how people meet their food requirements. The recommended weight ranges for men and women are listed, along with caloric requirements for a number of activities. The four basic food groups used in selecting foods to provide a balanced diet and the cultural aspects of nutrition are also discussed. Information is supplied for assisting and feeding patients, since one of your vital nursing tasks is to keep track of how well they meet their nutritional needs and, for those who do not, to report the amount and type of food that is eaten.

CARING FOR NUTRITIONAL NEEDS OF PATIENTS

ITEM 1. MAINTAINING BODY WEIGHT

Each person needs to eat enough food daily to provide for growth, healing, or the maintenance of the present body weight. During periods of rapid growth, infants and children require nearly four times as many calories for each kilogram of weight as do adults. If there is an inadequate supply of calories, those calories that are available are used, first for maintaining the body weight and second for healing. The first priority is to maintain the current weight; if sufficient food is not available, then healing is delayed and growth is stunted.

Height is a good indicator of what weight should be; a certain height usually corresponds to a certain weight. In order to make sure patients do maintain their body weight while sick or hospitalized, it is necessary to obtain their height and weight and to record this information on the hospital record. Ambulatory patients are weighed on the scale; when the patients' conditions do not permit this, a bed scale can be used, or they can be asked about their height or weight. As a last resort, the height can be measured and the weight estimated and recorded as such.

Desirable Weight Ranges

The recommended weight ranges for adults are given in the following table:

	Height (without shoes) in inches	Weight (without clothes) in pounds
Men	64	122–144
	66	130–154
	68	137–165
	70	145–173
	72	152–182
	74	160–190
Women	60	100–118
	62	106–124
	64	112–132
	66	119–139
	68	126–146
	70	133–155

Source: U.S. Department of Agriculture. Calories and Weight, the USDA Pocket Guide. (Agricultural Informational Bulletin No. 364) Washington, D.C.: U.S. Government Printing Office, 1974, p. 5.

When do you not have a table available for use, it is possible to make a rough estimate of whether the patient's weight falls within the desired range or is over or under the recommended weight. Allow 100 pounds for the first 5 feet of height, and then add 5 pounds for each additional inch of height. This figure can then be adjusted to compensate for the size of the body frame, the age, and the condition of health.

Daily Caloric Needs

Similar to the balance of fluid intake and output, the amount of calories consumed should replace those used to keep the basic life process going, plus the losses from exercise and other activities. The energy contained in foods is measured in terms of calories, that is, the amount of heat produced when they are metabolized. The amount of calories needed daily varies depending on age, sex, the amount of muscular work performed, disease, fever, and other factors. Several examples are given here to illustrate typical requirements for different groups of people:

	Age	Weight (lbs)	Calories
Infant	0 to 2 months	9 (4 kg)	480 (120 cal per kg)
Children	6 to 8 years	51	2000
Boys	15 to 18 years	130	3000
Girls	14 to 16 years	115	2400
Female	adult		1800 to 2400
Male	adult		2400 to 2800

The basic life processes of respiration, circulation, urine formation, and the regulation of body temperature require one calorie per hour for each kilogram of weight. This is referred to as the basal caloric need, and amounts to 1600 calories for a man weighing 150 lbs and 1300 calories for a woman weighing 120 lbs. The total intake of food should supply the calories needed for the basal caloric need plus the amount for other metabolic needs.

Complete bed rest	add 10 per cent of basal rate
Sitting, sedentary work	30 per cent
Moderate work	50 per cent
Heavy physical work	100 per cent

Other factors influence the caloric needs of patients. The stresses associated with surgery can increase the need to 2500 to 4000 calories in the immediate postoperative period. Patients who have had severe injuries, infections, or extensive burns may require up to 10,000 calories per day to maintain body weight. Every degree of fever above normal increases the basal metabolic rate by 7 per cent, so that a patient with a fever of 103°F (39.4°C) would need 28 per cent more calories over the basal amount.

It takes 3500 calories to equal one pound of body fat. For people who want to lose weight, it is necessary to reduce the number of calories taken in or to increase the amount of activity to use them up; however, patients in the hospital who do not eat sufficient amounts of food could lose as much as one to three pounds per day. After fatty deposits have been depleted, muscle and protein tissues are used to supply energy needed. These only provide only about half as many calories as fats, however, so thin people lose weight more rapidly.

Meeting the Caloric Needs

Many adults in this country tend to be a few pounds or more overweight and would not be in serious trouble if they lost some weight during a short illness. Patients experience a return of their appetites and a renewed interest in food as they begin to convalesce and increase their activities. The nursing staff must be aware of their nutritional status daily, however, in order to prevent problems related to malnutrition.

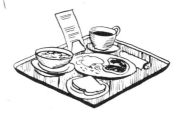

A well-balanced diet supplies the calories needed by most patients. Their nutritional needs can be met by eating the following foods daily:

- two or more glasses of milk

- two or more servings of meat, cheese, fish, or poultry

- four or more servings of vegetables and fruit

- four or more servings of bread or cereals

Additional calories are provided by fats such as butter, margarine, and salad dressings, and by carbohydrates as needed. If your patient does not eat the amount of food listed for the well-balanced diet, he or she may become malnourished. When the nutritional needs are not met, you should record the amount of food eaten as part of your observations about the patient's condition.

Daily caloric needs are generally supplied by the diet which is served in three meals during the day. You can estimate that approximately 40 to 50 per cent of the caloric intake is supplied through the largest meal, or the dinner, and that breakfast and lunch each supply about 25 to 30 per cent of the total calories. Extra nourishments or snacks may be provided during the day or evening to patients who have greater caloric needs, such as those who have undergone surgery, those who have had burns, anyone with a fever, new mothers who are nursing, and growing children.

1. Compare your weight with the recommended weight for your sex and height. Is it within the weight range, above it, or below it?

2. Compute the daily number of calories you need in order to maintain your present weight.

   a. Convert your weight from pounds to kilograms by dividing by 2.2 lbs per kg.

   b. Multiply your weight in kilograms by 24 (24 = 1 calorie per hour times the number of hours in the day).

   c. Your basic caloric need for life processes is _____ .

3. Now figure your total daily caloric need by multiplying the basic caloric amount by the percentage for your activity level and add the two figures. Total caloric need is _____ calories.

4. How many calories are needed to gain one pound of body weight?

5. The metabolic rate increases with a fever. If you have a temperature of $101°F$ ($38.33°C$), by what percentage should your total calories increase in order to maintain your current weight?

ITEM 2.   THE FOUR BASIC FOOD GROUPS

The well-balanced diet consists of foods from the four basic food groups: milk and milk products; meat and fish; breads and cereals; and the fruits and vegetables. These foods supply the nutrients that are necessary for the growth and repair of tissues; they provide the energy for the body to do the work and maintain the vital internal functions of life.

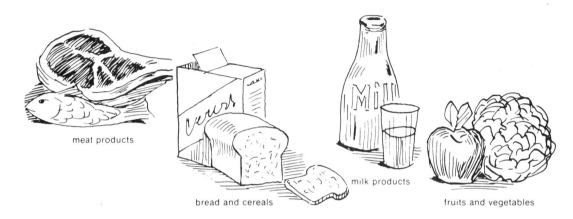

meat products

bread and cereals

milk products

fruits and vegetables

Four basic food groups.

The Milk Group

This group of foods provides a good source of calcium, proteins, and fats. Milk products such as ice cream, cheese, custards, and milk soups are used to supply some of the milk needs and add variety to the diet. The powdered nonfat and low fat forms of milk contain fewer calories and saturated fats than does whole milk, and they generally cost less too.

The recommended intake of milk is 2 to 3 cups daily for children, depending on their age and size. Teenagers should have 4 cups of milk daily, and adults should have 2 cups of milk or the equivalent in other milk products. The pregnant woman needs 3 cups a day, and when nursing the baby, the mother needs to increase her milk consumption to a quart a day.

The caloric content for several foods in this group follows:

	Quantity	Calories
Milk (whole)	240 ml	160
Cheese (cheddar)	1 ounce	105
Cheese (cottage)	1 ounce	25
Cocoa	240 ml	235
Ice Cream	½ cup	145

The Meat Group

Proteins in the diet are required for the growth and repair of body tissues and as the building blocks for enzymes, hormones, and antibodies, which regulate the body processes. The best sources of proteins are red meats, fish, and poultry. Alternative protein sources are eggs and the legumes, which include beans, peas, and lentils. Whole grains, nuts, and deep green leafy vegetables also supply lesser amounts of protein. Two servings of protein group foods are recommended daily. Although proteins are among the most expensive foods, skill and imagination can help you to prepare nutritious and appetizing dishes economically. The caloric content for some foods in the protein group follows:

	Quantity	Calories
Egg (boiled)	1 egg	80
Roast beef, hamburger	3 ounces	245
Chicken breast (fried)	3 ounces	155
Roast leg of lamb	3 ounces	285
Tuna	3 ounces	170

The Cereal and Bread Group

Cereals (the seeds of grasses such as wheat, rye, rice, oats, and so forth) are rich in starch, a carbohydrate used by the body for fuel. The cereal foods are among the most economical of the food groups, and they can be prepared in many ways. The whole grains and enriched grains provide many of the vitamins needed by the body. Four or more servings of bread, dry or cooked cereal, noodles, macaroni products, or rice should be included in the daily diet. The caloric content for some foods in this group follows:

	Quantity	Calories
Bread (white or wheat)	1 slice	60
Corn flakes (plain)	1 ounce	110
Macaroni (plain)	1 cup	190
Pancakes (4 inch)	1 cake	60
Oatmeal	1 cup	130

The Vegetable and Fruit Group

The foods in this group are high in vitamins, minerals, and fiber. Vegetables are used in soups, salads, and stews and as separate servings. Fruits contain natural sugars and make wholesome desserts. Both fruits and vegetables are good choices of foods for people who are watching their weight because both are filling and have fewer calories than other compact or concentrated foods like proteins, pastries, and nuts. Four or more servings daily are recommended from this group, including at least one citrus fruit or other source of vitamin C, such as tomatoes, and one deep green or deep yellow vegetable that is high in vitamin A. The caloric content for fruits and vegetables follows:

	Quantity	Calories
Carrots (cooked)	1 cup	45
Green beans	1 cup	30
Corn	1 cup	170
Potatoes (baked)	1 each	90
Apple	1 each	70
Banana	1 each	85
Orange juice	1 cup	110

High Caloric Foods

While the four basic food groups provide a wholesome and well balanced diet, most people add calories to the diet by eating fats and prepared foods with a high sugar content. Carbohydrates consist of sugars and the starches found in the bread and cereal group. They provide 4 calories per gram, as do proteins, so 100 grams of sugar supplies 400 calories. Fats are especially high in caloric content and supply 9 calories for each gram, more than twice as much as proteins and carbohydrates. Many of the popular foods that people like. to eat are also high in calories. A few of them are listed here:

	Quantity	Calories
Apple pie	4-inch section	345
Butter/margarine	1 pat	90
Cola drinks	12 ounces	140
Hot dog in bun	1	270
Chocolate cake (layer)	2 inches	445
Peanut butter	1 tbsp.	95
Cheese pizza	½ of 13-inch	340
Potato Chips	10 × 2-inch	115

6. Assume that your lunch consisted of the following foods and that you ate it all. How many calories did you consume?

   Cheese sandwich:

      Bread (2 slices):   _____

      Margarine (1 pat):   _____

      Cheese (1 ounce):   _____

   Coke (12 ounces):   _____

   Apple: _____

           Total   _____

7. Your patient, Mrs. Weakly, has a poor appetite. With much encouragement, she ate the following for breakfast. Approximately how many calories did she get?

   Toast with butter, 2 bites
   (about ⅛ of a slice):   _____

   Orange juice, half of
   4-ounce glass: _____

   Egg, hard-boiled, 2 bites
   (about ¼ of egg):   _____

           Total   _____

ITEM 3.   CULTURAL FOOD PREFERENCES

People eat food not only to satisfy the needs of the body for energy but also for the feelings of pleasure and satisfaction that accompany eating. Mealtime is a social event for most people, and many joyful occasions in life are celebrated with a feast.

Although food likes and dislikes are an individual matter, many attitudes and habits concerning food are the result of culture and society. National origin influences the types of foods eaten most frequently. Bread is the most important item in the Greek diet, and it is the main course of the meal in many countries. People of German descent like pork, noodles, and sauerkraut. Those of Italian heritage enjoy pastas, greens, and use generous amounts of olive oil in their cooking. People with an Oriental background use rice and fish as staple foods in their diet, and some use strong, spicy herbs for seasoning.

What is considered a food varies from one culture to another. In some places, raw fish, grasshoppers, and fried bat wings are regarded as food delicacies. A French cook prepares gourmet dishes using snails, tripe, and truffles. In the arctic regions, willow greens, salmon, and fish oils are important items in the diet. People in various parts of the United States have strong preferences for some foods. Grits and hominy are popular in many Southern states. Lobster is featured in Maine, and baked beans in Boston, and Westerners regard breakfast incomplete unless fried potatoes are served with the ham and eggs.

Food preferences are influenced by religious beliefs. Seventh Day Adventists and the strict Hindus and Buddhists eat no meat. Those of the Jewish faith avoid pork; the orthodox believers do not mix dishes containing meat with those containing milk and follow other dietary laws.

ITEM 4.   SPECIAL OR THERAPEUTIC DIETS

When people become sick and are hospitalized, they often must make some adjustments in their food preferences and food habits. Patients on a special diet may discover that it doesn't include the foods they usually eat and that spices or seasonings are not permitted; these changes may be very disturbing to them.

The patient's diet is an important part of medical treatment. When the patient is not eating the food in the diet, you should notify your team leader. Other ways may be found to encourage the patient to eat, or the dietician could be called to visit the patient. Often the diet can be adjusted to be more appealing to the patient without altering the therapeutic effect.

Patients who have been NPO as part of the treatment for their illness or injury or following surgery may be started on a special diet that progresses from clear liquids to a general or full diet as they increase their tolerance to the foods. It is most often prescribed following major surgery or in acute inflammations of the digestive tract, difficulties in chewing or swallowing, or cases of acute infections.

Clear liquid diet. Ordered when there is decreased tolerance for foods or impaired function of the digestive tract. The diet allows water, tea, coffee, clear broths, ginger ale, apple juice, and plain gelatins.

Full liquid diet. May be given to those able to tolerate more than the liquids allowed on the clear liquid diet. The diet allows additional liquids such as milk, milk shakes, cream soups, all fruit juices, and semiliquid foods such as custards, sherberts, puddings, and ice cream.

Soft diet. Consists of foods that are mild in taste, that are easily chewed and digested, and that contain almost no fiber. The diet allows white bread or toast, cooked cereals, rice, potatoes, meats, cooked fruits and vegetables, plain or sponge cakes, butter, and salt and pepper. Meats and vegetables may be chopped or strained for ease in eating, but no fried foods are allowed.

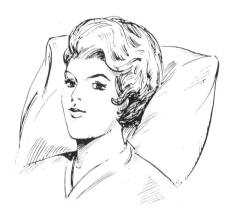

Intestinal disorder — soft diet.

Regular or general diet. All foods are allowed, but highly seasoned foods are generally not included.

Diabetic diet. Ordered for diabetic patients and may be stated as "1200-calorie ADA diet," "1500-cal soft diabetic diet," or some other similar combination. A more flexible food plan is possible with the use of the food exchange groups. The basic four food groups are expanded to six food exchange groups by adding a group for milk and one for fats. Foods within each group have approximately the same food value, so they can be substituted freely for one another. The use of refined sugars should be avoided, however, although artificial sweeteners may be used.

Bland diet. Consists of foods that are non-irritating, mild-flavored, and easily digested. It is used in the treatment of gastric ulcers, colitis, and gallbladder disease, and it excludes fried foods, onions, radishes, cabbage, coffee, tea, and very hot, very cold, or highly seasoned foods.

Low fat diet. Consists of a diet that restricts the amount of fats in the form of butter, margarine, oils, and fried foods. It is ordered as part of the treatment in diseases of the gallbladder and liver.

Low sodium diet. Restricts the amount of sodium intake in order to control the water balance in the body. Ordinary table salt is sodium chloride, the greatest source of the sodium ion. Foods are prepared without added salt; a salt substitute is used for seasoning, and foods containing high amounts of sodium are restricted from the diet. Foods with high sodium content include baked pork and beans, bacon, corned beef, baking powder biscuits, bran flakes, most breads, butter, cakes, cheeses, cookies, soda crackers, herring, margarine, mustard, olives, dill pickles, and so on.

Low sodium diets are prescribed for congestive heart disease, other cardiovascular diseases, kidney failure and renal diseases, and complications of pregnancy.

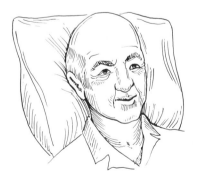

Heart disease — low sodium diet.

ITEM 5. SERVING AND COLLECTING DIET TRAYS

Part of your nursing duties may include serving the diet trays to the patients at meal times. Preparing patients for their meals before the trays arrive pays big dividends, as patients are more apt to have a better appetite, eat more, and enjoy their food more. For many of them, mealtime is a high point of the day and a time they look forward to.

Before serving a meal, provide for elimination by offering the bedpan or urinal or assisting the patient to the bathroom without waiting to be asked and perhaps interrupting the meal service. Assist the patient to wash hands and face as needed. Create an attractive and pleasant environment for eating. Remove distracting articles such as an emesis basin or a urinal, and use a spray or deodorizer to remove unpleasant odors in the room. Have the room at a comfortable temperature and see that it is well lighted. Position the patient comfortably for the meal, with the head of the bed elevated (if allowed), or assist the patient to sit up in a chair, clearing the overbed table so there is room for the diet tray.

Serving Diet Trays

Dietary personnel prepare the patient trays either in a central kitchen or in the nursing unit kitchen. In some hospitals, they are also responsible for delivering the tray to the patient's bedside. However, if you are responsible for delivering trays, serve those patients first who are able to feed themselves. In some hospitals, you may be required to check the trays with the diet order list before they are passed out in order to make sure that each patient received a tray and that it was the correct type of diet. Then deliver the trays as quickly as possible. The most common patient complaint about meals is that the food gets cold before the patient receives it.

|||||||||||||||||||||||||||||||||||||||||||||||||||||||||||||||||||||||||||||||||||||||||||||||||||||||||

Supplies Needed:

Diet tray

|||||||||||||||||||||||||||||||||||||||||||||||||||||||||||||||||||||||||||||||||||||||||||||||||||||||||

Important Steps	Key Points
1. Wash your hands.	Universal Steps A, B, and C. See Appendix.
2. Obtain the diet tray.	
3. Approach and identify the patient.	Each tray is usually labeled with the patient's name, room number, and the type of diet. The name of the tray should match your patient's wristband. Serve the right tray to each patient.
4. Place the tray on the overbed table.	Put the main dish closest to the patient. Assist if needed to remove the food covers, cut or chop the meat and vegetables, pour the beverage, or butter the bread. This takes only a minute or two and eliminates the need for the patient to ask for assistance. The likelihood of the patient rejecting the food is also minimized.

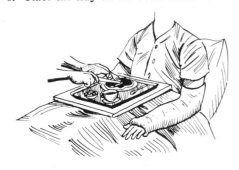

Put main dish closest to patient.

Important Steps	Key Points
5. Observe what the patient has eaten.	Allow the patient to eat without feeling rushed. During this time you can talk with patients to find out about the foods they like, the adequacy of the servings, and other information about the meals.

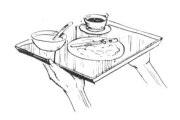

6. Remove the tray.	Universal Steps X, Y, and Z. See Appendix I. Place the food covers back on the tray and make sure that all soiled dishes are returned to the Dietary Department on a tray cart or via a dumbwaiter.
7. Return to the patient and provide for comfort.	
8. Record as appropriate.	Fluids should be recorded on the Intake and Output Record as required, and any problem in meeting nutritional needs should be documented on the chart. Charting sample: 0800. Poor appetite. With much encouragement, ate 1/3 of egg, 1/2 slice of toast, and 2 tsp. of Farina. Coffee: 60 ml.

M. Victory, PN

ITEM 6. FEEDING ADULT PATIENTS

||||||||||||||||||||||||||||||||||||||||||||||||||||||||||||||||||||||||||||||||||||||||||||||||||||||||||||||||||||||||||||

Supplies Needed:

Diet tray   Towel

||||||||||||||||||||||||||||||||||||||||||||||||||||||||||||||||||||||||||||||||||||||||||||||||||||||||||||||||||||||||||||

Important Steps	Key Points
Carry out Universal steps A, B, and C. See Appendix.	
1. Protect patient's clothing and bed linens with towel or napkin.	Spilling food or fluids is often embarrassing to patients. It only makes them more aware of their inability to do for themselves. Be patient, kind, and reassuring. Explain that you will help until the patient is well enough to eat alone.

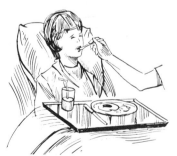

Protect clothing with small towel.

Important Steps	Key Points
2. Feed food with fork or spoon.	There are no set rules regarding the amount of each mouthful or the rate at which anyone eats. Estimate the amount of food to be placed on the fork or spoon by the patient's size and age. Older adults, as well as children, take smaller portions at a time and generally require longer periods to chew and swallow. Ask which food they prefer to start with; some people start with their meat, some with their salad, others with their liquid.
3. Offer fluids frequently. 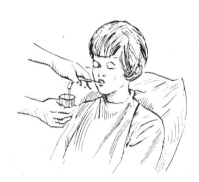	If patients do not indicate when they want fluids during the meal, offer fluids after every three or four mouthfuls of solid food. This helps the patient "wash down" food particles. If a straw (preferably flexible) is used, grasp it at the point near its middle, not at the end that goes in the patient's mouth.
4. Encourage patients to help feed themselves.	Allow (or assist) the patient to wipe the mouth with a napkin at appropriate intervals or as needed. Do not hurry the patient; give small bites, varying the foods. Alternate with liquid. Friendly, interested conversation also helps put the patient at ease and assists digestion.

Carry out Universal Steps X, Y, and Z. See Appendix.

Feeding Blind Patients

When feeding patients who have one or both eyes patched or covered with bandages, follow the same procedure as used for patients who are unable to feed themselves.

Blind people who happen to be sick may be able to feed themselves as they customarily do. You may need to place utensils in conventional positions or assist in other ways.

Describe what foods are being served and give their locations by imagining that the plate is a clock. For example, state that the bread is at 12:00, the potatoes at 3:00, the beef at 6:00, and the carrots at 9:00.

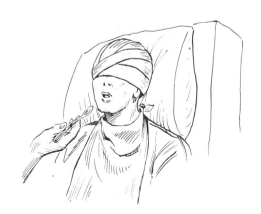

Tell what food is being offered.

ITEM 7. FEEDING CHILDREN

Newborn Infants

1. **Procedure for Feeding Formula.** A baby should usually be held while fed. Be sure to cradle the head, neck, and back. (See the accompanying picture.) Holding the infant provides a sense of security and love, both essential for sound psychological development. Without these, infants can become unresponsive, lose weight, and die.

Never prop the bottle and leave the baby with it. The infant may suck in air or too much fluid too quickly. The fluid may be vomited or sucked into the lungs (aspirated), which causes a pneumonia. This type of pneumonia could cause death very quickly.

Formulas are usually kept refrigerated on the Pediatric and Nursing Units or are ordered from a Central Supply area. The new types of prepared formula need no refrigeration; they are usually stored in an accessible work area near the patients' rooms. The amount, type, and feeding time schedule are ordered by the doctor.

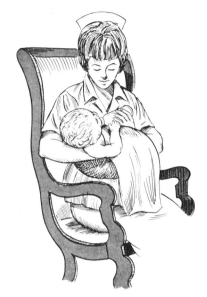

Bottle-feeding.

Supplies Needed:

Bottle of formula   Extra diaper or pad

Important Steps	Key Points
Carry out Universal Steps A, B, and C. See Appendix.	
1. Test the size of the nipple holes.	Verify the label on the bottle to see that it is the correct formula. Check the size of the nipple holes; they should be large enough to permit the baby to get the formula without undue sucking and yet not so large that the milk runs freely. The baby may have difficulty swallowing fast enough and could choke.
2. Test the temperature of the formula.	Some formulas must be warmed to take the chill off; for others, this is not necessary. If the formula is warmed in a bottle sterilizer, invert the bottle of formula and then let a few drops fall on the inner aspect of your wrist. If it feels hot, it is too warm for the infant. Allow the formula to cool awhile, then test it again before feeding the baby.

Important Steps	Key Points
3. Pick up the infant.	Carry the baby like a football, with the head resting in the palm of your hand and the back lying on your arm for support. Hold close to your body; the feet will fit between your upper arm and your chest.

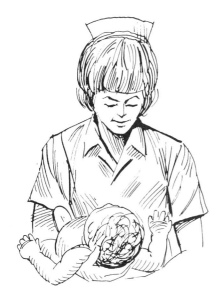
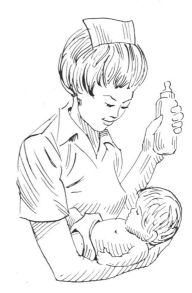

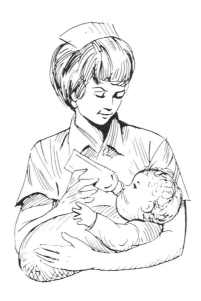

4. Seat yourself in a chair (a rocking chair is preferable).	Place the baby's bottom in your lap and support the neck and head in the bend of your elbow.
5. Insert the nipple into the baby's mouth.	Rub the nipple gently on the baby's cheek near the mouth. The infant will usually turn the mouth toward the nipple with the mouth open. This is called the rooting reflex and is normal for infants.

Important Steps	Key Points
6. Hold the bottle to avoid air bubbles.	The bottle should be held at a 45-degree angle. Be sure that the milk fills the nipple end of the bottle at all times. If you allow the angle to be too great, so that only half of the nipple is covered with milk, the baby will suck air into the stomach, causing it to become distended and painful.
7. Burp or bubble the baby periodically. 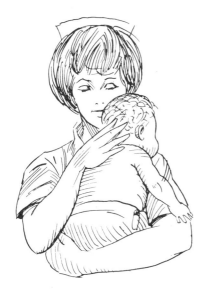	This is usually done after each ounce of formula that is consumed. Protect your uniform with a diaper or pad in case there is any spitting up. Hold the baby against your shoulder and gently rub or pat its back. This will make it easier to expel any air that might have been sucked in. In the newer collapsible feeding bottles, the danger of the baby sucking air into the stomach is almost eliminated. Therefore, you will probably need to burp only at the end of the feeding.
8. Continue feeding.	Continue until the formula is gone, or until the baby seems unwilling to take more. Burp the baby if necessary.
9. Return the infant to the crib.	Be sure that the baby's diaper is dry; if not, change it. Position infant comfortably on side or abdomen. Be sure that the siderails are up.
10. Rinse and drain the bottle.	Return it to the service area. Tidy the work area.
11. Record the feeding.	Make a notation on the appropriate chart forms. Charting example: 11:00 A.M. Similac 4 oz taken very eagerly and retained. Placed on abd. Sleeping. J. Jones, LVN

Feeding Solid Foods. Cereals, vegetables, and fruits are usually the first foods introduced to the infant. A small amount of food (usually baby food that comes already prepared in cans or jars) is given with an infant feeding spoon. The spoon should be placed well into the baby's mouth, then pulled outward and upward. If food is not placed well into the mouth, it will be pushed out again. This is a reflex action.

Children between 6 and 12 months old become fascinated with food. They want to touch it, play with it, stick it in their hair. Do not leave a child for an instant with food in front of her. If you do, guess where you are likely to find it?

Feeding the Toddler

The toddler (18 to 36 months of age) eats the same food as the older child, except that the toddler's meats and vegetables are usually diced or chopped. Young toddlers (18 to 24 months) like to feed themselves, and therefore "finger foods" are introduced. These are items such as diced cooked carrots and chopped beef that children can feed to themselves. During this time, they generally drink out of a cup. *Do not* serve liquids in glass containers; at this age, they like to chew and may bite down on a glass. If the child refuses a cup, try offering a bottle; it may provide more security during the illness.

The older toddler (24 to 36 months) may try to use a utensil to eat with; start with a spoon, not a fork. The fork tines may injure the mouth or gums and prove painful and frustrating for the child.

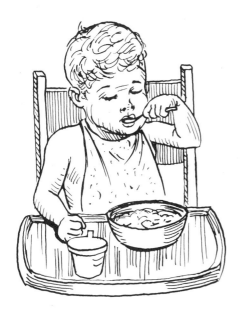

Most three-year-olds self-feed.

Feeding the Preschool Child (three to six years)

Children from three to six years old eat the same foods as toddlers, only in greater quantity. They generally eat with a "junior" fork and spoon, which are smaller than regular utensils. They enjoy eating with other children their age. It is well to have several children eat their meals together at small tables and chairs. Socializing (talking) at mealtimes helps them learn how to act and handle their utensils.

After Meals

1. Record the child's intake. Before the tray is removed, write down the amount of fluids taken in on the Intake and Output form. Also check to see if the patient ate well, moderately well, or poorly. Record this on the nurses' notes.

2. Remove the tray to the kitchen or dietary cart. Try not to leave a tray in the patient's room for an extended period of time. Also, the dietary workers have a cleaning schedule for trays; they must be washed and ready for serving the next meal.

3. Return to the patient and offer a bedpan or urinal or assist to the bathroom following a meal.

4. Provide mouth and hand care. Some children brush their teeth and wash their hands following a meal. Give them this opportunity; it is good health practice.

ITEM 8. HINTS FOR FEEDING CHILDREN

Do	Praise at intervals and at the end of the meal.
	Provide opportunities for socializing if possible.
	Promote and encourage good eating habits.
Do Not	Hurry the child.
	Punish for spilling.
	Allow to drink all of the milk first.
	Leave unattended by an adult.
	Place dessert on the tray until other foods are eaten.
	Prop the baby's bottle and leave.

WORKBOOK ANSWERS

1 to 3.   Individual answers vary.

4.   3500 calories

5.   14 per cent

6.   Cheese sandwich:

Bread (2 slices):	120
Margarine (1 pat):	90
Cheese (1 ounce):	105
Coke (12 ounces):	140
Apple:	70
Total:	525 calories

7.

Toast ($\frac{1}{8}$ slice):	19
Orange juice (2 ounces):	27.5
Egg ($\frac{1}{4}$)	20
Total:	66.5 calories

PERFORMANCE TEST

In the skill laboratory, feed your student partner, keeping in mind patient and tray identification procedures. Do not impose your eating habits on the patient; rather, provide a pleasant environment for enjoying the meal.

At the completion of the meal, record pertinent information on the sample nurses' notes.

PERFORMANCE CHECKLIST

ASSIST WITH NUTRITION

1. Provide for elimination before the meal.

2. Wash patient's hands before the meal.

3. Position the patient and the overbed tray before the meal tray is served.

4. Prepare the environment (tidy the room, remove emesis basins, bedpans, or urinals from the area).

5. Wash your hands before serving the tray.

6. Serve the tray. Match the tray label with the patient's identification band.

7. Protect the patient's gown and bed linens and arrange the food on the tray.

8. Give moderate-sized bites of food. Alternate liquids with solids (1:3 or 1:4). Ask the patient which food he prefers to eat first, i.e., salad, meat, and so forth.

9. Feed slowly, giving patient ample time to eat. Carry on a pleasant conversation.

10. Return all dietary items to the appropriate area immediately after the completion of the meal.

11. Leave the patient neat, tidy, and comfortable. Attach the call signal.

12. Chart your observations on your practice nurses' notes.

POST-TEST

Multiple Choice.   For each of the items that follow, select the one best answer.

1. When adequate amounts of food are not available for use, the body first uses the extra glucose that is stored

    a. in the pelvis of the kidney.

    b. in the liver and muscles.

    c. in the nervous system and brain.

    d. in the marrow of the bones.

2. When malnutrition leads to weight loss, one of the major results is

    a. a loss of appetite.

    b. increased thirst.

    c. higher body temperature.

    d. delayed tissue healing.

3. The patient who has been NPO for several days obtains energy needed to meet the body demands by

    a. absorbing vitamins and minerals.

    b. using the glucose in IV solutions.

    c. metabolizing fatty tissues.

    d. decreased output of growth hormone.

4. Which of the following people requires the most calories per kilogram of body weight?

    a. Working man, age 40.

    b. A teenage boy of 16.

    c. A woman nursing her new baby.

    d. The new baby.

5. The amount of food required to meet the body's nutritional need provides for all of the following *except*

    a. appeasement of the appetite.

    b. maintaining body weight.

    c. healing of tissues.

    d. body growth.

6. The number of calories required to gain or lose a pound of body weight as fat is

    a. 3500.

    b. 2500.

    c. 1500.

    d. 1000.

7. The basic caloric need refers to the calories required

   a. from the four basic food groups.

   b. to keep basic life processes going.

   c. to provide for work and activity needs.

   d. from the protein intake alone.

8. How many pounds would you allow for each inch over five feet when estimating the recommended weight range for the patient when only the height is known?

   a. two

   b. four

   c. five

   d. nine

9. Joe M. had a serious heart attack two days ago and is to remain on strict bed rest. What should his daily caloric intake be while in bed?

   a. The basal rate plus 10 per cent.

   b. The basal rate plus 30 per cent.

   c. The basal rate plus 50 per cent.

   d. The basal rate only.

10. Which of the following foods contains the greatest number of calories per gram of weight?

   a. sugar.

   b. cereal.

   c. lean meat.

   d. butter.

11. Steven, a teenage patient, is on a clear liquid diet. He can have all of the following liquids *except*

   a. coffee.

   b. milk.

   c. apple juice.

   d. ginger ale.

12. The foods that are restricted on a diabetic diet are

   a. refined sugar.

   b. carbohydrates.

   c. breads and cereals.

   d. proteins.

   e. all of the above.

13. Many patients with a heart disease are placed on a low sodium diet. The most common source of sodium is

    a. fried foods.

    b. fruits.

    c. table salt.

    d. cereal flours.

14. The purpose for restricting sodium in the diet is

    a. to promote the metabolism of fats.

    b. to balance the caloric needs with the energy used.

    c. to remove waste products from the blood.

    d. to control the fluid balance in the body.

15. The nurse carries out each of these steps when feeding a newborn infant, *except*

    a. placing the baby on the side and props the bottle.

    b. burping the baby after each ounce or so of formula.

    c. testing the size of the nipple holes.

    d. testing the temperature of warmed formulas.

POST-TEST ANSWERS

1.	b	9.	a
2.	d	10.	d
3.	c	11.	b
4.	d	12.	a
5.	a	13.	c
6.	a	14.	d
7.	b	15.	a
8.	c		

URINE ELIMINATION

GENERAL PERFORMANCE OBJECTIVE

You will achieve the capability to assist the patient (or another person) in using the designated equipment to void in a safe and effective manner, to collect specific urine specimens, and to test urine for sugar and acetone content by following the prescribed procedure.

SPECIFIC PERFORMANCE OBJECTIVES

Upon completion of this lesson you will be able to:

1. Position the patient correctly on the bedpan and remove it without spilling the contents.

2. Measure the urinary output and record it on the Intake and Output Record.

3. Record significant observations about the urinary output, such as the amount, color, odor, and time.

4. Observe the principles related to gravity drainage when caring for a patient with an indwelling catheter.

5. Obtain a routine, clean-catch, or timed urine specimen, label it correctly, send it to the laboratory, and record appropriate information on the patient's chart.

6. Obtain and test a urine specimen for sugar and acetone, using Clinitest tablets or various reagent tapes, strips, or sticks.

VOCABULARY

bladder—a hollow muscular organ for the collection of urine.
catamenia—the periodic menstrual discharge of blood from the uterus; the menses.
catheter—a hollow tube used as a passageway for fluid.
cystitis—infection of the bladder.
fracture pan—a specific type of shallow bedpan used by bed patients who have difficulty raising their hips in order to use the regular bedpan.
frequency—the condition of having to urinate often.
incontinence—the inability to retain feces or urine; lack of voluntary control over the sphincters.
kidney—glandular organ that secretes urine.
penis—the external male organ for urination and sexual intercourse.
renal—refers to the kidney.
retention—failure to expel urine from the bladder.
ureter—a tube connecting the kidney to the urinary bladder.
urethra—tube connecting the urinary bladder with the outside surface of the body.

urgency—the immediate need to urinate.

vagina—the mucomembranous tube that forms the passageway between the uterus and the external opening.

void—the process of expelling urine and emptying the bladder.

vulva—the external female genitalia.

INTRODUCTION

Another basic need of individuals is the elimination of wastes, both liquids and solids. Liquid wastes are excreted mainly through the urinary system, which regulates the amount of fluid in the body and filters out waste products that circulate in the bloodstream. The resulting urine is collected in the urinary bladder and later is eliminated. The act of voiding or emptying the bladder is under voluntary control; this control is generally achieved by age three and continues throughout life. Voluntary control is affected by illness, drugs, decreased mental awareness, and anxiety, so that patients frequently need your help to meet their elimination needs.

Although urination and the elimination of solid wastes are natural functions, people do not generally discuss these needs with strangers. When in the hospital, many patients are ill at ease and embarrassed and hesitate to ask for help when they need assistance to void or have a bowel movement. Nurses who offer the bedpan at intervals during the day help the patients to overcome feelings of embarrassment by showing that this is a normal part of the nursing care and necessary for their well-being.

As you study this unit, you will recognize that elimination of urine is a basic need, and you will learn skills that can be used efficiently and effectively to help the patient meet this need. One of the first skills is that of placing the patient on the bedpan, or assisting to use the urinal. Since the urinary output gives an indication of internal conditions of the body, it generally is measured when the patient is acutely ill, and the characteristics are described. Specimens of urine are frequently ordered to check on the patient's progress and must be collected according to instructions. Other skills you will use frequently include testing the urine of diabetic patients and taking care of patients with indwelling catheters attached to gravity drainage.

ASSISTING THE PATIENT IN URINE ELIMINATION

ITEM 1.   THE URINARY SYSTEM

The urinary system consists of two kidneys, two ureters, a urinary bladder, and the urethra. Urine is formed in the kidneys, collected in the bladder, and then excreted from the body. The urinary system is normally free of microorganisms (germs), and urine itself is sterile but does contain various chemical waste products that give it a characteristic odor and appearance.

Organs of the Urinary Tract

The kidney is a glandular, bean-shaped organ that secretes urine. It serves two purposes, as it regulates the fluid balance in the body and then removes the excess fluids and waste materials in the form of urine. Blood, which consists of water and various chemical compounds, is carried to the kidney, where it is filtered through an elaborate system of coiled tubes called nephrons. The essential chemicals are reabsorbed back into the bloodstream, and the excess amounts or waste materials are diluted with water and form urine.

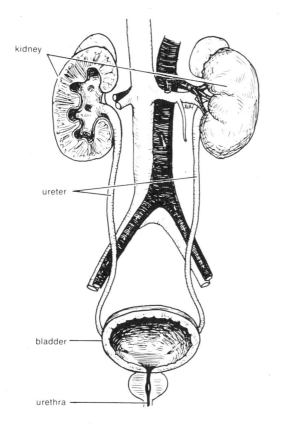

Urinary system.

The two ureters are tubes that carry the urine from the kidneys down to the urinary bladder.

The urinary bladder is a hollow, muscular organ that serves as a temporary reservoir for urine. By contraction of the muscular wall of the bladder, urine is expelled from the body through a tube called the urethra. When the amount of urine in the bladder reaches a certain level, it exerts pressure on certain nerve endings in the bladder wall and causes the urge to empty the bladder. Expelling the urine from the bladder is called urination or voiding.

The urethra is approximately ¼ inch in diameter, 1½ inches long in the female, and 8 to 9 inches long in the male. The urethra extends from the bottom end of the bladder to the exterior of the body. The external opening of the urethra is concealed between the folds of the labia in the female and at the distal end of the penis in the male.

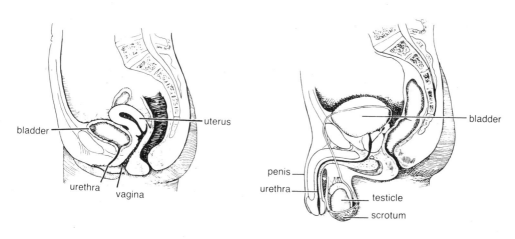

Female urinary system.   Male urinary system.

The Capacity of the Urinary Bladder

The muscle layers of the bladder wall enable it to expand and hold the accumulating urine. The capacity for urine accumulation varies in relation to the patient's health, disease state, and fluid intake; the action of food and drugs on the kidneys; and the weather. The amount of urine excreted by the body is directly related to the fluid intake. The person who drank 3000 ml of fluids will produce a larger volume of urine than will the person who had a fluid intake of only 1200 ml. The adult must put out at least 600 ml of urine in order to remove the waste products of the body; most people have a urinary output that averages 1000 to 1500 ml per day.

The number of times an individual voids during the day varies widely. Infants void from 5 to 40 times a day, the preschool child as often as every two hours, and the adult from 5 to 10 times a day. The urge to empty the bladder occurs when a certain amount of urine has accumulated and stimulates the nerve endings in the stretched bladder wall. The amount varies according to age, health, and bladder capacity; for normal adults, however, you can use these figures as a guide: males: 300 to 500 ml; females: 250 ml.

Most people have the urge to void upon awaking in the morning, after each meal, at bedtime, and after drinking additional fluids. Ordinarily, urine production is decreased during sleep, and most people sleep through the night without voiding, although others may need to empty their bladders.

Urinary retention is frequently seen in patients following surgery, the delivery of a baby, or the removal of an indwelling catheter, and in older men with enlargement of the prostate gland. In some cases of retention, as much as 3000 to 4000 ml. of urine can accumulate in the bladder because the individual is unable to void. Like an inflated balloon, the muscles become thin and there is some tearing, so that bleeding occurs. Retention is treated by inserting a catheter to drain the urine and correcting the cause of the condition medically. When the bladder is severely distended, extreme caution must be taken to prevent any blow or heavy weight on the bladder region that could rupture (break) the bladder wall. In case of bladder rupture, the patient can die within 8 hours if surgical repair is not done.

Characteristics and Components of Urine

The *normal components* are: 95 per cent water, 3.7 per cent organic wastes, and 1.3 per cent combined inorganic wastes, mineral salts, toxins, pigments, and sex hormones.

The *color* of normal urine is described in terms of varying shades of yellow. The color is due to the presence of pigments in the urine. Normal urine is a straw yellow or amber color. The lighter the shade of yellow, the more it is diluted with water.

Abnormal pigments are often found in the urine, and they too are designated or indicated by color of the urine. Smoky red or dark brown urine denotes the presence of hemoglobin or many red blood cells from bleeding in some part of the urinary tract. Blue or blue-green urine may be due to a dye or medication the doctor has ordered for the patient.

The *odor* of freshly voided urine is faintly aromatic but not unpleasant. Variations appear as the result of the ingestion of certain foods and drugs, or a decomposition of bacteria that changes the urea to ammonium carbonate and then to ammonia. An unpleasant (putrid) odor is abnormal and indicates disease.

Since sediments alter the composition of urine when it stands at room temperatures for short periods of time (as brief as 20 to 30 minutes), it is urgent that urine specimens be sent to the laboratory immediately upon collection.

The *specific gravity* is the weight of a given volume of urine as compared with the weight of an equal volume of pure water. In simple terms, it is the thinness or thickness of the liquid urine. The specific gravity is measured by an instrument called the *urinometer*. The normal numerical range is 1.010 to 1.030. Variations of the numerical values are due to the amounts of solids dissolved in the urine. The specific gravity of a healthy individual changes during a 24-hour period within the above normal limits.

The acidity or alkalinity of the urine is measured in units called *pH*. The pH of normal urine is slightly acid, ranging from 5.5 to 7.0.

The abnormal matter in the urine is composed of many pus cells, red blood cells, hemoglobin, occasional kidney stones, casts, acetone bodies, albumin, sugar, bacteria, and some parasites. Other chemicals and drugs may be present.

The urine output can be affected by two kinds of drugs: *diuretics*, which increase the flow of urine, and *antidiuretics*, which decrease the flow of urine.

Common Urinary Infections

Because the urinary tract is dark, moist, and warm, it is an excellent breeding place for germs or pathogenic bacteria.

Cystitis (inflammation of the urinary bladder) is a very common bladder infection caused by any of the following: highly concentrated urine, pathogenic bacteria, injury, irritation, or instillation of an irritating substance. Symptoms of cystitis include frequency, burning, urgency, and often a slight elevation of temperature. Patients with cystitis are very uncomfortable.

Recording the Output

During the acute stage of an illness, you and the doctor will want to know how well the patient is able to meet the elimination need. Usually the doctor orders that an Intake and Output record be kept, but nurses can keep track of the patient's fluid balance without an order. After the patient voids, measure the amount before discarding. Metal or plastic pitchers with calibrations are used for measuring and kept in the bathroom. The drainage bags used with indwelling catheters are calibrated, and the urine can be measured before the bag is emptied. Be sure to record the amount on the Intake and Output Record. See Unit 22 for additional information.

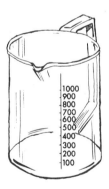

A graduate used to measure fluids.

ITEM 2. ASSISTING THE PATIENT TO USE THE BEDPAN

The *bedpan* is made of metal or plastic. Each patient has an individual bedpan stored in the bedside stand during the hospital stay. The female patient usually uses the bedpan for both urine and bowel elimination, whereas the male patient uses the bedpan for bowel elimination only.

A *bedpan cover* is made of cloth or paper, depending upon the agency in which you work. It is used to cover the pan's contents after it has been used.

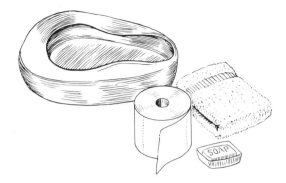

The fracture pan is used when patients are unable to sit on a regular-size bedpan. The fracture pan is made of metal or plastic. It is smaller in surface area and height than the regular bedpan. The back part of the pan is approximately 2½ inches high with a wide strip of metal across the top so that the patient is able to sit comfortably. The front, pouring side is high enough to prevent urine from being splashed or spilled in the bed.

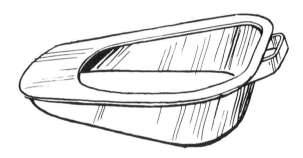

Place the patient on the fracture pan by separating the patient's legs, and slipping the pan under the buttocks. A little powder on the flat ledge helps when the patient is unable to raise the hips to assist you. The roll-to-the-side method may also be used to position the patient on the pan. This is explained in the next items.

Given a female patient who wants to void, you are to assist her to use the bedpan.

Supplies Needed

Bedpan   Washcloth
Bedpan cover   Towel
Toilet tissue   Soap and water

Important Steps	Key Points
1. Wash your hands.	Universal Steps A, B, C, and D. See Appendix.
2. Approach and identify the patient. Explain what you are going to do and gain her cooperation and confidence.	
3. Obtain the items needed.	

Important Steps	Key Points
4. Provide privacy for the patient.	
5. Ask the patient to flex her knees and raise her hips.	Slide your hand under the lower back and direct the patient to lift her hips.
6. Place bedpan under the hips.	Slide the pan into place and adjust it for the patient's comfort. The edge of the pan is placed at the end of the sacrum so that the buttocks form a seal along the rim of pan. Raise the head of the bed if allowed. Place the toilet tissue and signal cord within reach of the patient and step away.
7. Ask the patient to signal when finished.	Return after a reasonable time or when the patient signals.
8. Remove the bedpan.	Have the patient flex her knees and raise her hips. Cover the bedpan immediately and place it on a chair. Assist the patient if she is unable to clean herself.
9. Measure the amount of urine voided and record.	Pour it into a graduated container to measure the amount voided if patient is on I & O (refer to Unit 22). Empty the urine into the toilet.
10. Clean the items used and store in proper place.	Universal Steps X, Y, and Z. See Appendix.
11. Make the patient comfortable.	Allow the patient to wash her hands.
12. Record as appropriate.	Charting example: 0845. Voided 210 ml straw-colored urine. K. Cardinale, SN

U
N
I
T
24

ITEM 3. BEDPANNING THE HELPLESS PATIENT

||||||||||||||||||||||||||||||||||||||||||||||||||||||||||||||||||||||||||||||||||||||||||||||||||||||||||||||||||||||||||||||||||||||||||||||||||||||||||||||||

Supplies Needed

Bedpan	Washcloth
Bedpan cover	Towel
Toilet paper	Soap and water

||||||||||||||||||||||||||||||||||||||||||||||||||||||||||||||||||||||||||||||||||||||||||||||||||||||||||||||||||||||||||||||||||||||||||||||||||||||||||||||||

Important Steps	Key Points
Carry out Universal Steps A, B, C, and D. See Appendix.	
1. Assist the patient onto the side; position the bedpan.	Stand facing the patient's back. Place the bedpan firmly against the patient's back region at the level of the sacrum, or the top of the fold of the buttocks. Support the hip with one hand and the bedpan with the other hand. Roll the patient onto the bedpan and check its position for comfort.

Important Steps	Key Points

2. Place the call signal within easy reach, raise the siderails, and leave the room to insure privacy.

3. Remove the bedpan.

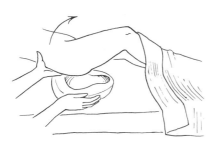

Before removing the bedpan, lower the head of the bed. Ask the patient to turn to the distal side of the bed. Hold the bedpan to avoid spilling its contents while she rolls to her side. Place the bedpan cover on the bedpan, and set it at the foot of the bed or on a chair out of the way.

4. Wipe the perineal area dry with toilet tissue.

Use a continuous stroke from the vulva across the vaginal opening to the rectum (anterior to posterior). This method of cleansing will help prevent rectal bacteria from contaminating or entering the vaginal opening or urinary tract.

Carry out Universal Steps X, Y, and Z. See Appendix.

ITEM 4.   THE USE OF URINALS

The urinal is used by male patients who are limited in physical activity by their illness or injury.

The male urinal is a plastic or metal bottle with a long, round neck, a handle, a rectangular base along one side, and a flat base at the bottom. It is not customary for the male patient to use toilet tissue when he urinates, since the urine is expelled in a straight single stream and the skin surface of the penis does not get wet.

The urinal can be used when patient is in any one of four positions: lying supine (on his back), lying on either the right or the left side or in a Fowler's position, or standing at the bedside.

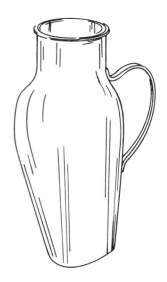

Given a male patient who is on bed rest, you are to provide a urinal for his use.

―――

Supplies Needed

Urinal
Urinal cover

Washcloth
Soap and water
Towel

―――

Carry out Universal Steps A, B, C, and D. See Appendix.

Important Steps	Key Points
1. Hand the urinal to the patient to use. 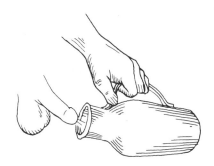	Leave the room to allow privacy while voiding, or provide assistance if needed. Turn back the top bedding, separate the patient's legs, and place the urinal between them. Place the penis far enough into the urinal so that it doesn't slip out when the patient begins to urinate. The most important aspect of this task is to remember that this is an embarrassing situation for the patient. The task is to be performed in a skillful, matter-of-fact manner.
2. Return to the room after a reasonable time or when the patient signals.	
3. Remove the urinal and cover it.	Note any unusual color or odor. Take a urine specimen if required. Allow the patient to wash his hands.
4. Empty the urinal.	Measure its contents if the patient is on "Intake and Output."
Carry out Universal Steps X, Y, and Z. See Appendix.	Charting example: Voided 500 cc pale yellow urine. <div align="right">J. Jones, NA</div>

Urinals for Female Patients

On occasion, you may have a female patient who uses the urinal for voiding when she is unable to use the bedpan or a commode. It can also be used by patients with severe limitations of movement, extreme pain, extensive sacral ulcers, or as a matter of personal preference to using the bedpan.

The female urinal is a plastic bottle with a long, wide, spoutlike top; it has a handle, a rectangular base along the side, and a flat, round base at the bottom.

The patient's position will depend on the amount of physical movement and activity that she is permitted. The opening of the urinal should be in direct contact with the perineal area. The extent of body contact with the urinal opening should reach from the rectum to the vagina. The handle should be toward the front of the patient.

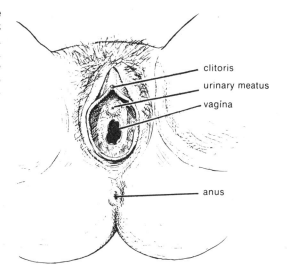

clitoris
urinary meatus
vagina
anus

External female genito-urinary organs.

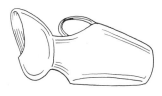

Female urinal.

ITEM 5. THE CARE OF FOLEY CATHETERS

Some of the patients you take care of will have an altered means of voiding and will have an indwelling catheter that provides continual drainage of urine from the bladder. The most commonly used indwelling catheter is the Foley catheter. It is used for a variety of purposes:

1. To help meet the patient's need for voiding. A Foley is often inserted when the patient is acutely ill, has an operation, has severe pain or limitation of movement, or is less aware of his or her surroundings or needs because of the illness or medication.

2. To keep the bladder empty and promote healing. The treatment of some infections and diseases and operations on organs of the urinary system require that the bladder not be distended because this would put strain on other structures.

3. To keep the incontinent patient dry. It helps keep the skin from breaking down and becoming infected and provides many other temporary benefits.

4. To provide a means for measuring the amount of urine produced by the kidney and keeping an accurate record of the output.

5. To assist in retraining in or restoring normal bladder control.

The Foley catheter consists of a rubber or plastic tube with two or three channels and a balloon that can be inflated with water or air to secure the end of the catheter in the bladder. The balloon serves as an anchor to keep the catheter from slipping out of the bladder. The main channel provides for the drainage of urine out of the bladder, and it is connected to tubing and a closed drainage bag. With the three-way Foley catheter, the third channel is attached to an irrigating line so that sterile irrigating solution runs into the bladder, mixes with the urine, and drains out into the drainage bag.

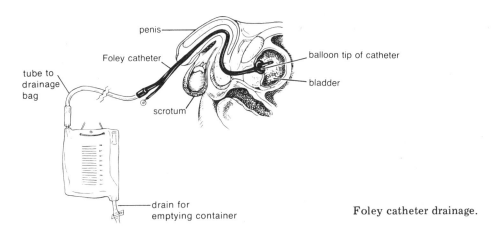

Foley catheter drainage.

Principles in the Care of Foley Catheters

Although the nurse at the beginning level has limited information about aseptic technique and normally does not insert Foley catheters, certain guidelines must be followed when caring for patients who have them.

1. Record the patient's intake and output. Patients with Foley catheters are generally quite sick, and the I & O record provides information about kidney function and fluid balance of the body.

2. Observe the tubing and the level of urine in the drainage bag each time you enter the patient's room. Report any decrease or unusual appearance of the urine to your nurse immediately.

3. Avoid contaminating the catheter or drainage system by disconnecting the catheter and tubing. Empty the drainage bag through the tube at the bottom of the container and drain into a graduate or pitcher.

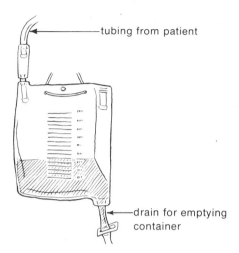

—tubing from patient

—drain for emptying
container

4. Keep the tubing free of kinking, twisting, or falling in loops below the level of the urine in the drainage bag. Pin the tubing to the bed linen or place it on top of the bed so the patient can move about easily. Loops of tubing that are below the urine level of the collecting bag interfere with the free flow by gravity.

5. Keep the drainage bag below the level of the bladder. Clamp the tubing any time the bag is raised higher than the level of the patient's bladder. This prevents the urine from running back into the bladder, causing possible infection or damage from the increased pressure.

6. Nursing care should include perineal care at least twice a day to reduce the number of organisms near the urethral opening and prevent an ascending infection along the route of the catheter. Wash the genital area thoroughly with soap and water. Many hospitals now use sterile catheter care and antiseptic solutions to reduce urinary infections. See Volume 3 for sterile catheter care procedure.

7. Measure the urine output, empty the drainage bag, and record the amount at least once every shift, or more often as needed.

8. Force fluids to more than 2000 ml per day unless contraindicated by the patient's condition or doctor's orders. Adequate fluid intake is essential to flush sediment from the urinary system.

9. The nurse uses sterile technique to obtain urine specimens from the Foley catheter for Clinitest or laboratory analysis. See Unit 4, Volume 3. A sterile syringe is used to withdraw a few milliliters of urine from the aspiration port near the catheter and tubing junction to test the urine for sugar and acetone, or a sterile cap is used to protect the ends of the catheter and the tubing if the two are disconnected briefly to obtain a specimen. Ordinarily, urine that has been accumulating in the drainage bag over a period of hours is not used for specimens.

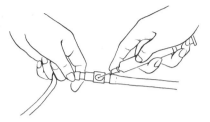

Aseptically aspirate the urine specimen using a syringe.

As a rule, patients do not have the Foley catheter disconnected when they sit up in a chair, walk around the unit, or go to other departments for therapy or treatment. The drainage bag is carried along and is either pinned to the robe or gown or put in a cardboard carton, which is then carried below the level of the bladder. When it is necessary to disconnect the catheter, follow these steps:

||||||||||||||||||||||||||||||||||||||||||||||||||||||||||||||||||||||||||||||||||||||||||||||||||||||||||||||||||||||||||||||||||||||||||||||

Supplies Needed

Alcohol sponges (2)   Sterile plug or cap
Sterile 4 X 4 dressing (2, optional)

||||||||||||||||||||||||||||||||||||||||||||||||||||||||||||||||||||||||||||||||||||||||||||||||||||||||||||||||||||||||||||||||||||||||||||||

Important Steps	Key Points
Carry out Universal Steps A, B, C, and D. See Appendix.	
1. Disinfect the connection of the catheter and tubing.	This serves to reduce the number of organisms on the surface. Use the alcohol sponge or similar disinfectant.
2. Disconnect the catheter from the tubing.	Continue to hold both tubes in your hand and avoid letting the sterile ends come in contact with anything that is not sterile.
3. Cover the end of the tubing with a sterile cap or plug.	The tubing can then be laid down, once the end has been protected from contamination.
4. Obtain urine specimen, or protect end of catheter with a sterile cap or plug.	Avoid contamination of the catheter, as germs that enter readily cause a urinary tract infection. If the sterile caps and plugs are not available in your agency, clamp the catheter and clean the catheter and drain tube with a germicidal solution as you disconnect them. Then place a thick, sterile 4 X 4 dressing around the end of each tube.
5. Remove the sterile caps or plugs from the catheter and tubing and reconnect.	

Carry out Universal Steps X, Y, and Z. See Appendix.

At times patients will say that they have the urge to urinate. You are to check the catheter and drainage through the tubing. The catheter openings in the bladder may be clogged with solid matter, and the catheter may need to be irrigated with sterile saline to remove it. This, of course, will depend on the doctor's order and your agency procedure. Another source of discomfort may be the position of the catheter in the bladder. The opening may be lying against the bladder wall, or it may be above the urine level so that it is impossible to remove the urine. Gently rotate or move the catheter so the flow will be continuous. The size of the catheter may affect the urine flow, particularly if the catheter tube is too small for adequate drainage. This can cause the bladder to become distended, and internal pressure will be exerted on the sphincter so the patient feels the urge to void.

Remember, the reproductive organs are in the perineal area of the body. Do not be surprised if the male patient expresses concern about sexual stimulation that may occur while he has the Foley catheter in place. Reassure him that is a natural phenomenon because these organs are extremely sensitive to external and internal stimulation. Maintain a matter-of-fact, gentle, and comforting manner while you care for the patient.

ITEM 6. VOIDED SPECIMEN FOR URINALYSIS

You will frequently be requested to obtain a urine specimen from the patient. Laboratory analysis of urine provides a lot of information about internal conditions of the body. There are many different types of tests performed on urine, and some of them require special steps to be taken in the method of collecting it, such as extra cleansing to reduce contamination by organisms normally found on the skin, discarding the first part of the voiding, having the person drink additional fluids at specified times, and collecting specimens at stated times. You will need to follow the instructions in the laboratory manual for these tests or follow directions given by the doctor.

No special requirements are needed for the routine urinalysis. A voided specimen is obtained as outlined in this item. The clean-catch or mid-stream urine specimen is requested of ambulatory patients and is cultured for the presence of microorganisms. It is described in the next item. The 24-hour urine specimen is in the following item, and then tests of urine for sugar and acetone are outlined.

Prompt Handling of Specimens

Urine specimens should be sent to the laboratory soon after they have been collected, unless the specimen container contains a chemical preservative. Urine specimens deteriorate quickly while standing at room temperature. The chemical composition of the urine changes rapidly if it is kept at room temperature for more than 15 minutes. If the urine specimen is left on the nursing unit for a longer period of time, the laboratory will obtain incorrect readings that could cause incorrect diagnosis and medication for your patient.

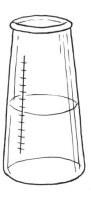

Strain All Urine

Occasionally all the urine voided by a patient is strained to catch stones from the kidney or bladder, which may be discharged through the urine. The most common method for straining the urine is to place a fine gauze 4 × 4 dressing over the spout of the graduate (some agencies may use a special sieve). Pour the urine carefully into the graduate; all stones will be caught in the fine mesh gauze. (Discard the gauze after use — take clean gauze for each straining.)

Supplies Needed

Specimen bottle and cap   Laboratory requisition slip
Bedpan or urinal

Important Steps	Key Points
Carry out Universal Steps A, B, C, and D. See Appendix.	
1. Have the patient void. 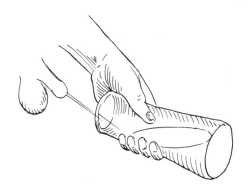	Ask the patients on bed rest and those requiring assistance to void into a bedpan or urinal. Refer to the steps in Items 1, 2, 3, and 4. For the ambulatory patient: Give the patient the specimen container and ask him to go to the bathroom, and void either in the container or in a collecting basin. The male patient can easily hold the specimen container in front of him and, as he voids, catch the urine in the container. The female patient will be able to void directly into the urine specimen container if she is able to stand in a squatting position over the toilet bowl. While she is in the process of voiding, she can hold the urine specimen container underneath the perineal area to catch the urine.
2. Collect the urine specimen.	If the patient voids into the bedpan or urinal, pour the urine into a measuring pitcher (commonly called a graduate) and note the amount. Pour at least one ounce into the specimen container. Put the lid on the container tightly. Clean and dry the outside of the container. Rinse any urine off the outside of the container under running water. Dry it with a paper towel and then discard the towel into the wastebasket.
3. Have the patient wash his hands at the sink in the bathroom.	
4. Provide for the patient's comfort and safety.	Universal Steps X and Y. See Appendix.
5. Clean and dispose of used items.	
6. Remove the container of urine from the patient's room.	
7. Label the container with the patient's name and room number.	Use the Addressograph (similar to a charge plate in a department store) to print the patient's name, and the hospital number of the laboratory requisition and charge voucher. Enter the type of test that is ordered so that the laboratory technician will know what test to perform.

Important Steps   Key Points

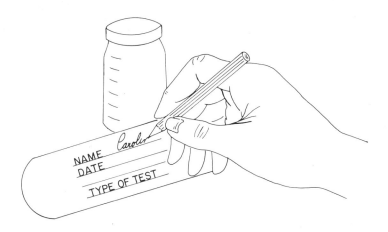

8. Take the specimen to the laboratory immediately.

9. Record on the patient's chart.

6:15 P.M. Urine specimen with requisition and voucher sent to laboratory. Specimen appeared cloudy and slightly pink. No complaints of pain on the voiding. Catamenia present.

M. Green, SN

ITEM 7.   CLEAN–CATCH OR MID–STREAM URINE SPECIMEN

This procedure is used to obtain a urine specimen for culture and sensitivity. The method provides a specimen that is free from external contamination. Two principles are involved: one is that the first portion of the urinary stream is discarded and not used for the specimen, and the other is that the external skin surfaces are cleansed to reduce contamination of the urine specimen.

Given a female patient who is able to go to the bathroom, you are to give her instructions and items needed to collect a clean-catch urine specimen for culture.

Supplies Needed

A clean-catch
   or
Specimen container and cap (sterile)
Sponges or cotton balls

Cleansing agent or soap
Unsterile glove (optional)

Important Steps   Key Points

Carry out Universal Steps A, B, C, and D. See Appendix.

1. Open the clean-catch kit or prepare the items used.

Moisten the sponges or cotton balls with water and soap. Place them within reach near the toilet, along with the specimen container. Do not touch the inside of the container at any time.

Important Steps	Key Points
2. Spread the labia apart with index finger and thumb.	Continue to hold the labia open until the cleaning is completed and the specimen is obtained.
3. Clean the middle surface with moistened sponge or cotton ball.	Wipe from the front to the back one time, and then discard the used cotton ball. Do not throw it in the toilet, because it may plug up the plumbing.
4. Repeat by cleaning the right and left sides of the vulva.	Wipe from the pubic area to the anus; discard the used cotton ball.
5. Void and discard the first portion of urine.	The first partial voiding flushes away bacteria that normally grow around and in the urethral opening.
6. Collect a specimen of the middle portion of the voiding.	Still holding the labia apart, place the sterile urine bottle in line with the urine stream and collect 30 ml or more for the test. Do not let the rim of the bottle touch the body. Place the sterile lid or cap on the specimen bottle. Rinse and dry the outer surface of the bottle.
7. Label the specimen and send to the laboratory with the request slip.	The label should include the patient's name, room number, and other information required by the agency. The requisition slip should note that it is a clean-catch specimen, the date it was obtained, and the tests that are required.
8. Record on the patient's chart.	Charting example: 2:30 P.M. Clean-catch urine specimen obtained. Sent to laboratory for culture and sensitivity. M. Green, SN

Follow the steps of the procedure, but instruct the male patients to follow these steps to cleanse the penis and collect the specimen:

1. Clean around the urethral opening of the penis with soap and water.

2. Void a small amount to clear the urethra, and discard it.

3. Collect the middle portion of the voided urine in a sterile specimen container.

ITEM 8.   THE 24-HOUR URINE SPECIMEN

A number of urine tests require a collection of urine over a period of 24 hours. The most important aspect of this task is that all of the urine voided must be kept. The laboratory analysis is done to determine the amount of a specified chemical that is excreted through the urine in a 24-hour period.

The patient's bladder should be empty at the beginning and the conclusion of the test, and all urine voided during the 24-hour period is collected. If some urine is accidentally thrown out, the test is not valid and would have to be repeated, so it is important that the patient and all of the nurses know that a 24-hour specimen is being collected.

Some tests require that the urine be kept cold over the 24-hour collection period. If so, place the labeled jug(s) in the refrigerator used for specimen collections. If there is no refrigerator on the unit for this purpose, put the jug(s) into a pan of ice in the patient's bathroom.

Supplies Needed

Gallon container, with preservative   Bedpan or urinal
   added, in cardboard box or holder   Bed sign for test

Important Steps	Key Points

Carry out Universal Steps A, B, C, and D. See Appendix.

1. Label the specimen container.

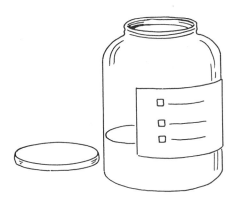

Label the container with the patient's name and room number. Write the time and date that the collection is to be started and the time and date it is to be finished. Put the jug in the patient's bathroom.

2. Place sign about test at bedside.

Make a sign (a 6 × 8 card will do) stating that a 24-hour urine collection is in progress, and tape it at the head of the patient's bed. Labels may also be inserted in the Hollister Bed Signs where these are used.

3. Have patient void at start of the test and discard the urine.

Approximately 5 minutes before the starting time of the collection, ask the patient to void into the designated equipment. Discard this urine specimen into the toilet.

4. Collect all urine voided during next 24 hours.

The test is invalid if any of the urine specimens is discarded. If this should occur, notify the charge nurse, who will notify the physician. The physician will have to decide if the collection is to be restarted. An incomplete collection could add another day to the patient's hospital stay and this is costly to the patient.

5. Have the patient void at end of the test and add to specimen.

6. Send the specimen to the laboratory.

Send the marked gallon jug(s) with the correctly marked requisition slip and charge vouchers immediately to the laboratory.

Important Steps	Key Points
Carry out Universal Steps X, Y, and Z. See Appendix.	Charting example: 3/4/xx. 0700. Instructed to save all urine for 24-hour specimen. Voided 200 ml and urine discarded. 24/hour specimen started. M. Green, SN 3/5/xx. 0700. Voided 210 ml and added to specimen. 24-hour specimen completed and sent to lab for VMA. M. Green, SN

ITEM 9. TESTS FOR SUGAR AND ACETONE IN THE URINE

Nurses frequently care for patients who have diabetes and must have their urine tested for the presence of sugar or glucose and acetone. These are not normally found in urine but may be secreted by the kidneys when the amount in the blood reaches an excessive level.

Sugar is used by the body for energy and is carried to the tissues as glucose in the blood. The amount of glucose in the blood varies between 60 and 110 mg in 100 ml and depends on the amount of food that is eaten, the amount of exercise or activity performed, and the amount of insulin available. In diabetes, the body is unable to produce or utilize enough insulin to keep the blood sugar in this range. Instead, the amount in the blood increases, and at about the level of 180 mg, the kidney begins to filter it out into the urine in the attempt to rid the body of the excess. As the amount in the blood increases, the amount in the urine also rises. Testing the urine for the presence and the amount of sugar provides the doctor with information about the amount of insulin needed by the patient.

A number of tests are used to determine the presence of sugar in the urine. The Clinitest is one of the best known; other widely used tests now available consist of tapes and strips that are dipped into a urine specimen and change color in the presence of glucose and acetone.

Testing the urine for glucose and acetone is generally done four times a day, before meals and before bedtime. The most accurate method is to obtain a double-voided specimen, in which the first voiding is set aside and the patient asked to void a short time later. This second voiding consists of the most recently produced urine from the kidney and is the best indicator of the amount of sugar being excreted at that moment, not of urine that may have been in the bladder for hours. If the patient has a Foley catheter, the specimen should be taken from the tubing, which contains the latest formed urine, not from the drainage bag.

ITEM 10. THE CLINITEST

A Clinitest kit is ordered from the pharmacy for each diabetic patient. The kit is usually stored in a safe area in the patient's bathroom. Two strengths of Clinitest tablets are commonly used. One requires 5 drops of urine mixed with 10 drops of water; the other requires 2 drops of urine mixed with 10 drops of water. Be certain that you have read the instructions on the bottle so that you are following the correct procedure.

Supplies Needed

Clinitest tablets in a bottle Test tube Eyedropper	Reaction color chart Urine specimen

Important Steps	Key Points

1. Obtain a urine specimen at the designated time.

The specimen used may be regular voiding, double-voiding, or from a Foley catheter. Take to the bathroom or the utility room for testing.

2. Add 5 drops of urine to the test tube.

Fill the eyedropper with urine. Hold it in a straight position when you place the 5 drops of urine into the center of the test tube. For accurate measurements, do not let the drops run along the sides of the test tube.

Rinse the inside and outside of the eyedropper with cold water.

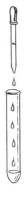

3. Add 10 drops of water to the urine.

The water and urine must be mixed for this test to be accurate.

4. Shake one Clinitest tablet from the bottle into the lid of the bottle, then pour the tablet into the test tube.

Do not use tablets that are moist or have changed color; these changes cause inaccurate testing. Good tablets are lightly spotted and bluish-white in color. Avoid putting the tablets into the test tube with your fingers, because the tablets contain a caustic soda and could irritate or burn your skin.

The dissolving tablet causes a boiling reaction and the test tube becomes hot. To avoid burning your fingers, hold the tube near the top. DO NOT ROTATE the test tube during this step.

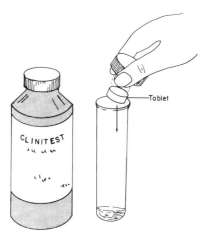

5. Compare the color changes of the specimen in the test tube with the color chart.

After 15 seconds (or after the boiling stops), shake the tube gently and compare it with the Clinitest color chart.

Note the color reaction. Usual color designations are:

Negative—the fluid will be blue, indicating that no sugar is present.

Positive— the fluid changes in color from dark green to orange; check the color change in the test tube with the block on the color chart indicating the degree of sugar content: trace, 1+, 2+, 3+, and 4+.

Important Steps	Key Points
6. Wash, rinse, and dry the equipment.	Return the bedpan or urinal to its storage space. Close the Clinitest bottle tightly, wipe up spills, and tidy the work area.
7. Record the readings on the patient's chart.	The dosage of insulin is based on the amount of sugar in the urine. The higher the sugar content, the more insulin will be given. Therefore, report the results of the test immediately to your team leader so she can give the insulin. Diabetic patients are usually taught to carry out this procedure themselves.

ITEM 11. TEST FOR ACETONE

When testing the urine of the diabetic patient for sugar, it is often necessary to test for acetone or ketone bodies as well. Acetone is an abnormal finding that indicates that the body has begun to break down stored fats to use for energy, since it is not able to use the sugar. Acetone is also found in the urine of people losing weight on a diet or in starvation. When using the Acetest tablet, follow these steps.

Supplies Needed

Eyedropper   Reaction color chart
Acetest tablet   Urine specimen
Paper towel

Important Steps	Key Points
1. Place an Acetest tablet on a clean paper towel.	
2. Put one drop of urine on the Acetest tablet.	
3. Wait 30 seconds.	
4. Compare the reaction with the color chart.	Reactions can be negative or positive. If the color of the tablet remains unchanged or becomes a cream color, it is considered to be a negative reaction. If the tablet turns from a lavender to a deep purple, it is considered a positive reaction. It is recorded as slightly, moderately, or strongly positive.

Important Steps	Key Points

5. Record and report.

Report the results to your team leader and record this information on the patient's chart.

6. Wash, rinse, and dry the equipment.

Return it to the storage area. Check to be sure that the cap is secured tightly on the Acetest bottle. Be sure to wipe up spills. Leave the work area neat and tidy.

ITEM 12. URINE TESTING BY DIP METHOD

A convenient way to test urine for sugar and acetone is to use the various strips, sticks, or tapes that react rapidly after being dipped into urine. To use these, follow these simple steps:

1. Dip the strip, stick, or tape into the urine.

2. Wait the specified amount of time.

3. Compare the reaction with the color chart.

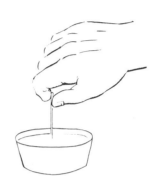

Tes-Tape Test for Glucose

Tes-tape is supplied in a dispenser similar to those used for Scotch tape. On the outside of the dispenser there is a printed color code with percentages of glucose indicated for each color. After dipping a piece of tape, wait one minute, then read the results. The color reactions are coded as follows:

Yellow — zero per cent (or sugar-free). Varying shades of green from light to dark: 1+ ($1/10$ per cent); 2+ ($1/4$ per cent); 3+ ($1/2$ per cent). and 4+ (2 per cent or more).

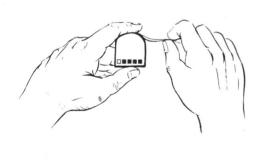

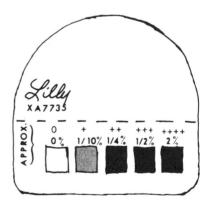

Keto-Diastix Test for Glucose and Acetone

This reagent strip combines the tests for sugar and acetone. The tip of the strip changes color when dipped into urine containing glucose or acetone. Color codes for ketone and for glucose are provided on the package. Wait 30 seconds, then compare and record the reaction for the closest matching color.

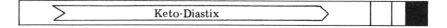

Ketostix Test for Acetone

The Ketostix is a specially treated strip that reacts when moistened with urine or blood. It is used to determine the amount of ketones present, which is indicated by variations in the color. After dipping or moistening the strip, wait 15 seconds and then compare the Ketostix with the color chart printed on the package. The color changes indicate the presence and amounts as follows:

Negative: buff color
Positive: slightly — lavender
         moderately — dark lavender
         strongly — purple

Report the results to your team leader.

PERFORMANCE TEST

In the skill laboratory, you will be asked to perform the following activities for your instructor without reference to any source material. You will need another person to take the part of the patient.

1. Given a patient who is unable to move her legs and assist herself on the bedpan, assist her to roll safely to the far side of the bed, place the bedpan under her buttocks, and position her for comfort.

2. Given a patient who is to have a 24-hour urine collection, explain the task, stressing the importance of obtaining all the urine voided in the 24-hour period. Obtain the equipment from the laboratory, mark the labels correctly on the bottle, and then indicate by signs placed on the bed and in the bathroom that the 24-hour urine collection is in progress.

3. Given a patient who is to have a clean-catch urine specimen collected, explain the task to the patient.

4. Given a diabetic patient who has voided a urine specimen, test the urine for sugar and acetone (using your agency procedure) and practice recording the results on the chart forms.

PERFORMANCE CHECKLIST

POSITIONING THE BEDPAN

1. Wash your hands.

2. Identify the patient; explain the procedure to the patient.

3. Obtain the necessary materials.

4. Provide privacy.

5. Assist the patient to the lateral position.

6. Place the bedpan appropriately, return the patient to the supine position, and elevate the patient to the sitting position.

7. Provide the patient with privacy and return when called. Lower the head of the bed, help the patient return to the lateral position, and hold the bedpan during the move to avoid spilling its contents.

8. Remove the bedpan.

9. Assist the patient with personal cleansing if necessary.

10. Provide for the patient's comfort and safety.

11. Empty the contents of the bedpan, rinse, and put away.

12. Record all significant observations of the urine.

24-HOUR URINE COLLECTION

1. Obtain the equipment with the preservative and take it to the patient's room.

2. Identify the patient.

3. Post warning signs.

4. Approximately 5 minutes before collection begins, tell the patient to void and discard that urine.

5. Transfer the urine to an appropriate jug after each voiding; make sure to measure and record the quantity.

6. Tell the patient to void approxiamtely 5 minutes before the end of the 24-hour collection and add voiding to the specimen.

7. Mark the container and the laboratory slip appropriately.

8. Arrange for immediate transfer of the specimen to the laboratory.

9. Remove the written warnings and equipment from the room.

10. Obtain the patient's chart and record all information pertaining to the collection.

COLLECTION OF A CLEAN-CATCH SPECIMEN

1. Obtain the supplies and equipment.

2. Wash your hands.

3. Identify the patient and explain the procedure.

4. Provide for the patient's privacy.

5. Cleanse the perineal area.

6. Tell the patient to void.

7. Ask the patient to interrupt voiding.

8. Collect the specimen after interruption.

9. Label the specimen with all appropriate information.

10. Arrange to have the specimen taken to the laboratory with all pertinent information.

11. Record the activity on the patient's chart.

DIABETIC TESTING

Demonstrate the procedure for the diabetic testing of a urine specimen.

1. Wash your hands.

2. Identify the patient.

3. Explain the procedure.

4. Obtain the urine specimen.

5. Transport the urine specimen to the work area.

6. Perform the indicated diabetic test.

7. Compare the reading of the test to the color chart.

8. Record the reading on the patient's chart.

POST-TEST

Matching. For each of the phrases in Column 1, select the word that it best defines from those listed in Column 2.

Column 1	Column 2
1. tube connecting the bladder with the exterior of the body	a. cystocele
	b. cystitis
2. a hollow tube that serves as a passageway for gas or liquid	c. incontinence
3. a tube that connects the kidney and the bladder	d. urethra
4. lack of voluntary control of the bladder	e. catheter
5. a urinary infection of the bladder	f. ureter
	g. retention

Multiple Choice. For each of the following items, select the one best answer to complete the sentence or answer the question.

6. Two major functions of the kidneys are (1) to remove excess or waste materials from the body and (2) to

  a. regulate the fluid balance.

  b. absorb nutrients for cellular growth.

  c. reduce the body temperature.

  d. secrete hormones needed for growth.

7. What is the average urinary output for an adult in a 24-hour period?

  a. 500 to 600 ml

  b. 500 to 1000 ml

  c. 1000 to 1500 ml

  d. 1500 to 2000 ml

8. The adult female has the urge to void when the bladder contains approximately what amount of urine?

  a. 500 ml

  b. 250 ml

  c. 125 ml

  d. 60 ml

9. The amount of urinary output depends on all of the following factors *except* for which one?

  a. age

  b. fluid intake

  c. health

  d. sex

10. In order to remove waste materials from the blood, the kidney must produce a minimum of how much urine per day?

   a. 600 ml

   b. 1000 ml

   c. 1200 ml

   d. 1600 ml

11. Which of the following characteristics of urine is abnormal and should be reported to your nurse or the physician?

   a. reddish pink color.

   b. aromatic odor.

   c. clear yellow appearance.

   d. slightly acid reaction or pH.

12. The urine test that measures the density of the urine, or its weight compared to an equal volume of water, is called

   a. Clinitest.

   b. diuretic.

   c. urinalysis.

   d. specific gravity.

13. When helping the male patient to use the urinal, the nurse carries out all of these activities *except*

   a. leaving the room to provide privacy.

   b. placing the urinal if necessary.

   c. putting toilet paper within reach.

   d. measuring and emptying the contents.

14. When using the female-type urinal, it is important for the female patient to

   a. stand at the bedside.

   b. press the urinal close to the vulva.

   c. avoid contaminating the edges of the urinal.

   d. keep the urinal in the bed at all times.

15. The Foley catheter is kept securely in the bladder by

   a. the taping of the tubing to the leg.

   b. a clamp placed near the urethra.

   c. an inflated balloon near the tip.

   d. the pull of gravity.

16. Voided urine decomposes in a short time at room temperature, so the specimen should be sent to the laboratory within what period of time?

   a. 30 minutes

   b. 60 minutes

   c. 90 minutes

   d. 120 minutes

17. Patients are catheterized for all of the following reasons *except* to

  a. keep incontinent patients dry.

  b. provide means for an accurate record of output.

  c. reduce the patient's pain, discomfort, or movement.

  d. reduce the risks of infection.

18. The nurse obtains a urine specimen from a Foley catheter and maintains the closed drainage system by

  a. using a sterile needle and syringe to withdraw urine from the tubing.

  b. removing urine from the amount in the collection bag.

  c. disconnecting the tubing from the catheter and draining urine from it.

  d. none of these.

19. The drainage bag of the Foley catheter should not be held above the level of the patient's bladder unless the tubing is clamped because this action leads to

  a. flow of urine back into the bladder.

  b. distention of the kidney with drainage.

  c. breakage of the balloon on the catheter.

  d. inaccuracy in measuring the urine output.

20. When caring for patients with a Foley catheter, the nurse should keep the tubing free of kinks and loops falling below the level of urine in the drainage bag because

  a. the tubing is part of a sterile system.

  b. this is specified in every hospital and agency policy book.

  c. it disturbs the urine flow by gravity.

  d. pressure builds up in the drainage bag.

21. Nurses should avoid disconnecting the indwelling catheter from the tubing of the closed drainage system because

  a. some urine is lost and may wet the bed linen.

  b. there is risk of contamination and infection.

  c. urine flows back into the bladder.

  d. it causes pain and discomfort for the patient.

22. When collecting the 24-hour urine specimen, it is important for the nurse to

  a. limit fluids to less than 1000 ml per day.

  b. start and end the test with the patient's bladder empty.

  c. discard the final voiding before the end of the test.

  d. force fluids to at least 3000 ml per day.

23. Urine voided by the patient was accidentally thrown out instead of being added to the 24-hour specimen that was being collected. What action should be taken by the nurse now?

    a. Tell yourself it doesn't matter, since it was only a small amount.

    b. Report to the laboratory and follow their instructions.

    c. Report to the physician and follow instructions.

    d. Report to the charge nurse and follow instructions.

24. You should transfer the Clinitest tablet to the test tube containing urine by using

    a. a 2 X 2 gauze sponge.

    b. a hemostat or forcep.

    c. the bottle lid.

    d. your thumb and forefinger.

25. The reason for obtaining a "double-voided" specimen when testing the urine of a diabetic patient is to

    a. obtain urine that is most recently produced.

    b. stop the stream and catch the middle portion.

    c. determine the amount of insulin the patient should receive.

    d. reduce the amount of urine retained in the bladder.

26. Sugar is normally present in the blood but is excreted by the kidney when the level reaches more than

    a. 20 mg.

    b. 60 mg.

    c. 110 mg.

    d. 180 mg.

27. The Clinitest is generally ordered to be done how often for the hospitalized diabetic patient?

    a. TID, after meals

    b. before meals and at bedtime

    c. every two hours when awake

    d. q4h around the clock

28. The reason for testing the urine for sugar and acetone is to

    a. determine the amount of insulin needed.

    b. adjust the amount of sugar in the diet.

    c. calculate the amount of fluids required to dilute the urine.

    d. modify the patient's level of activity.

29. When the Clinitest tablet is added to the urine and water solution, the nurse should be careful to

    a. shake the test tube to dissolve the tablet.

    b. avert the head to avoid contact with toxic fumes.

    c. place a cap over the top of the test tube.

    d. avoid burning fingers on the hot tube.

30. One of the principles involved in the collection of a clean-cloth urine specimen is

    a. it can be done only with patients on bed rest.

    b. use the bedpan and pour the urine into the specimen bottle.

    c. avoid contamination of the sterile specimen container.

    d. clean the perineal area with sterile gloves, equipment, and antiseptics.

POST-TEST ANSWERS

1.	d	16.	a
2.	e	17.	d
3.	f	18.	a
4.	c	19.	a
5.	b	20.	c
6.	a	21.	b
7.	c	22.	b
8.	b	23.	d
9.	d	24.	c
10.	a	25.	a
11.	a	26.	d
12.	d	27.	b
13.	c	28.	a
14.	b	29.	d
15.	c	30.	c

Unit 25

GENERAL PERFORMANCE OBJECTIVE

You will be able to demonstrate your ability to assist the patient in establishing and maintaining regular elimination of waste products from the large intestines, using methods appropriate to the patient's age, physical condition, and disease.

SPECIFIC PERFORMANCE OBJECTIVES

Upon completion of this lesson you will be able to:

1. Identify some of the abnormal conditions manifested in the appearance of the patient's stool, such as the presence of blood, mucus, iron, and worms or other parasites.

2. Collect a stool specimen and prepare it correctly for examination in the laboratory.

3. Promote the patient's regular elimination of waste products from the large bowel through nursing measures related to the patient's prescribed diet, fluid intake, exercise, and rest.

4. Assist evacuation of feces and flatus in the hypoactive bowel through the use of the enema, rectal tube, or Harris flush.

5. Examine for the impaction of stool in the rectum and remove it by the use of suppositories and cleansing or retention enemas.

6. Assist and teach the patient with a colostomy or ileostomy to irrigate the bowel in order to cleanse it of fecal material, to prevent obstruction, and to establish a habit of regular evacuation.

VOCABULARY

Many new words are introduced in this lesson. These words are frequently used by doctors and nurses, and you will need to learn their meanings. Because there are so many new words, those that are related are grouped together.

1. **The Small Bowel (total length 22 to 23 feet in the adult)**
   duodenum—an 8- to 10-inch portion of the small intestine connected to the lower end of the stomach and to the jejunum.
   ileum—the twisting intestine between the jejunum and the large intestine, about 13 feet long in the adult.
   ilium—part of the pelvic bone.
   jejunum—the section of the intestine between the duodenum and the ileum, about 9 feet long in the adult.
2. **The Large Bowel (total length 4 to 6 feet in the adult)**
   anus (anal)—the outer opening of the rectum between the buttocks and beyond the lower tip of the sacrum.
   appendix—a small wormlike pouch about 7.5 cm long at the end of the cecum.

cecum—the pouch at the junction of the small intestine and the ascending colon, with the appendix at the lower end.

colon—the large intestine from the cecum to the rectum, which is divided into the ascending colon, the transverse colon, the descending colon, and the sigmoid.

rectum—the lower part of the large intestine between the sigmoid and the anus, about 5 inches long.

sigmoid—the lower part of the descending colon, which is shaped like the letter "S."

3. Some Diseases and Surgical Conditions

appendicitis—inflammation of the appendix.

colitis—inflammation of the colon.

colostomy—an incision into the colon to form an artificial opening (stoma).

diverticulitis—inflammation and distention of little pouches throughout the colon.

hemorrhoids—dilated blood vessels in the anal area.

ileostomy—an incision into the ileum of the small intestine to form an artificial opening (stoma).

polyps—growths attached to mucous membranes of the nose, bladder, colon, or uterus.

ulcerative colitis—a severe inflammation of the colon with open sores of the membrane lining.

4. Contents of the Bowels

bile—an important digestive juice secreted by the liver, stored in the gallbladder; substances in bile give the brown color to feces.

chyme—the partially digested food and digestive juices; the liquid mass found in the intestines.

electrolytes—substances of a solution capable of conducting an electrical impulse or charge; important electrolytes in the body are sodium, chloride, calcium, potassium, and others.

feces—the waste material following digestion; the stool.

flatus—gas in the digestive tract (flatulence is the distention of the abdomen due to gas in the intestines).

mucus—a slippery, slimy fluid secreted by mucous membranes and glands.

parasites—organisms that live upon or in another organism or body called the host; common parasites in the intestinal tract are amoebas, flukes, pinworms, round-worms, hookworms, and tapeworms.

stool—feces; the waste matter discharged from the bowel.

5. Words Pertaining to Movement of the Intestines

constipation—sluggish action of the bowels; compacting of the feces into a hard, dense mass.

defecation—the evacuation of the bowel.

diarrhea—frequent movement of the bowels, increased number of stools per day, often liquid or semiliquid.

hyperactive—excessive movement; irritable.

hypoactive—decreased movement; less than normal.

incontinence—inability to retain feces or urine; lack of voluntary control over sphincters.

peristalsis—contraction of successive portions of the intestines followed by relaxation, which propels food content, fluids, and flatus onward.

sphincter—a circular muscle that opens and closes an opening, such as the sphincter of the anus.

6. Other Words Used in the Lesson

hemorrhage—excessive flow of blood out of the blood vessels; an abnormal amount of bleeding.

proctoscopy—examination of the rectum by instrument.

sigmoidoscopy—examination of the sigmoid colon by instrument.

stoma—mouth or opening, or an artificially created opening.

suppository—a cone-shaped, medicated substance that is inserted in the rectum, vagina, or urethra where it dissolves and is absorbed.

‖‖

That makes quite a vocabulary list. Now let's see what progress you have made in learning what the words mean. In the following list, all but one of the words on each line are related to the others. Place a check mark before the word that does not belong.

1. _____ sigmoid _____ rectum _____ mucus _____ anus

2. _____ cecum _____ ileum _____ duodenum _____ jejunum

3. _____ intestine _____ tract _____ bowel _____ colon

4. _____ appendicitis _____ diverticulitis _____ colitis _____ flatus

5. _____ chyme _____ electrolytes _____ suppository _____ bile

6. _____ polyp _____ feces _____ waste products _____ stool

Three of the words in your vocabulary are spelled in an unusual way, with the letters "r-r-h" in sequence. Match the word with its meaning and spell the word correctly.

7. _____ an excessive amount of bleeding.

8. _____ increased number of bowel movements.

9. _____ dilated blood vessels around the anus.

‖‖

INTRODUCTION

Why do you need to learn about the elimination of wastes from the bowel? Emptying a bedpan filled with stool, or feces, seems to be one of the more unpleasant tasks that nursing workers do. The sight and odor are often very unpleasant. To some of you, it might seem that we should rush through this part and get on to some more important lesson. Nevertheless, bowel elimination happens to be one of the most important subjects we study.

The appearance and the composition of the stool are important indicators of conditions in other parts of the digestive system. Obstruction or disease of the bowel may be detected by observing the stool for changes in color, the absence of color, and the presence of unusual matter such as blood. Changes in bowel habits may indicate a growth, obstruction, or disease.

In this lesson, you will learn more about the functions of the intestinal tract; conditions that change the normal composition and appearance of the stool; ways to assist the patient to achieve and maintain regular elimination of waste matter from the bowel; and procedures for problems related to elimination such as distention, constipation, incontinence, and diarrhea.

ASSISTING IN BOWEL ELIMINATION

ITEM 1. THE IMPORTANCE OF BOWEL ELIMINATION

What are the functions of the bowel that make it so important to health? They can be stated simply as those related to the absorption of nutrients and those related to the elimination of waste products.

Absorption

Absorption of vital nutrients, electrolytes, and water takes place in the small intestine and in a portion of the large intestine as the liquefied food mass moves out of the stomach and down the bowel. Elimination of the waste products at regular intervals indicates free passage of the food mass through the bowel in the time allowed for the absorption process. Absorption is reduced when the bowel moves the food mass along too quickly, or when the bowel moves so slowly that waste products collect in the absorbing parts, or when the bowel becomes obstructed or blocked. The causes of these conditions in the bowel *may* be serious enough to endanger the life of the patient.

Removal of Wastes

The body must get rid of the waste materials that are produced in the process of converting food into nutrients, which are delivered to the cells. These waste products of the body are eliminated through the skin, lungs, kidneys, and the bowel, which is the most important excretor of solid wastes. These consist of by-products of the digestive process, indigestible stuffs, water, and matter from the intestinal tract itself, such as secretions, dead bacteria, and sloughed cells.

‖‖

10. The two main functions of the intestines are

   a. _____   b. _____ .

11. Select the best answer(s) to complete the following statement. The patient's life may be endangered when absorption in the bowel is reduced by

   a. blockage of the bowel by twisting itself closed.

   b. change in the color of the stool.

   c. slow movement with no stool passed in five days.

   d. quick movement with ten stools in one day.

   e. all of the above.

12. State four of the problems related to the function of elimination.

   a. _____ ,   b. _____ ,

   c. _____ ,   d. _____ .

‖‖

ITEM 2. THE INTESTINAL TRACT

The intestinal tract is a muscular tube that extends from the stomach to the anal opening at the skin surface. The intestines are approximately six times the length of the body. In the adult, this would average about 8.5 meters, or 33½ feet.

The inner surface of the intestine has innumerable circular folds that greatly increase the area for absorption. Nutrients, water, vitamins, and electrolytes are absorbed through this surface into the blood stream. A rich supply of blood vessels around the intestines transports the absorbed materials to the cells of the entire body. The walls of the intestines also have circular muscle fibers that contract or enlarge the size of the tube, as well as longitudinal and oblique muscle fibers that allow stretching and turning of the tube.

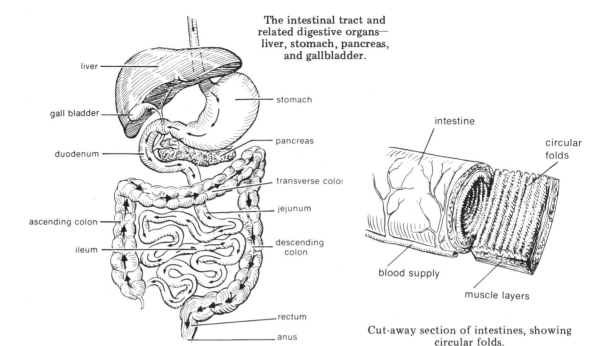

The intestinal tract and related digestive organs— liver, stomach, pancreas, and gallbladder.

Cut-away section of intestines, showing circular folds.

Small Intestine

The small intestine consists of the duodenum, the jejunum, and the ileum. The duodenum is connected to the lower end of the stomach. The jejunum forms the middle section of the small intestine, and the ileum, or twisted intestine, is the lower section that is joined to the cecum of the large bowel.

As the liquefied food mass (chyme) enters and passes through the small intestine, it is mixed with intestinal digestive juices. Absorption of nutrients and some electrolytes takes place in the small intestine. Some water is absorbed in the ileum, but greater amounts are absorbed in the large intestine.

Large Intestine

The large intestine provides a frame for the small intestines in the abdominal cavity. The cecum with the appendix is at the lower right corner of the frame and is attached to the ascending colon. The transverse colon crosses the abdomen at about the level of the navel, and the descending colon goes down the left side where it joins the sigmoid. The sigmoid colon, which gets its name from its "S" shape, crosses the abdominal cavity toward the back.

The lower segment of the large intestine is the rectum, and the anus is the outer opening of the bowel to the skin.

The main functions of the large intestines are (1) to absorb water and electrolytes, and (2) to temporarily store the residual waste products as feces. As an example of the water-absorbing capacity of the large intestine, about 500 ml of liquid chyme enters the bowel daily and all but 50 to 100 ml of water is absorbed.

Numerous bacteria are present in the normal bowel. They are found in the absorbing portion of the large intestines where they digest small amounts of food roughage, form vitamins K, B_{12}, and thiamine, and produce gas, or flatus, as a result of this bacterial activity.

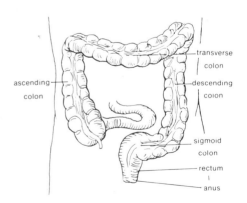

The large intestine forms a frame of the abdomen.

‖‖

13. A child's intestinal tract is approximately_____times as long as his body.

14. The long length of the intestinal tract and the circular folds provide greater surface for

_____ to take place.

15. The various parts of the intestinal tract have been described. In the following list, indicate the parts of the large intestine.

a._____ ileum   b. _____ rectum   c. _____colon

d._____jejunum   e. _____cecum   f._____duodenum

g._____anus

16. The two functions of the large intestines are   a. _____

and   b. _____ .

‖‖

ITEM 3. CHARACTERISTICS OF FECES

The digestion of food is similar to the refining of oil. Food enters the body as raw fuel and is changed by the digestive juices. The usable parts are converted to nutrients, and these are absorbed in the small and large intestines. The waste or unusable part is passed into the colon where most of the water and electrolytes are absorbed. It is then passed into the sigmoid and rectum for storage as feces until it is evacuated from the body.

Normally, the feces are composed of three-quarters water by weight and one-quarter solid material. The solid material consists of about 30 per cent dead bacteria and 70 per cent undigested roughage from food, fat, protein, and inorganic material. The brown color of the normal stool is caused by bile (one of the digestive juices) and the odor is the result of bacterial action on the foods that have been eaten.

In the newborn infant, the stool is characteristically dark greenish-black (meconium) for the first two to three days of life. After that time, the breast-fed baby has an orange-yellow colored stool and a strong smell; the stool of a bottle-fed baby has a brownish-yellow color if the formula contains malt sugars.

The color of the feces may be changed by certain drugs that the person may be taking. Vitamins and other drug preparations containing iron give the stool a black color throughout. Chlorophyll gives the stool a green color.

ITEM 4. BLOOD IN THE STOOL

Before you empty feces from any patient's bedpan or flush the toilet, you should observe the stool for any noticeable changes from the normal-appearing stool. The most serious change is the presence of blood in the stool. When you observe blood in the stool, you should report it promptly, record it on the patient's chart, and save the stool so it can be inspected by the doctor for amount of blood and clues as to when the bleeding occurred.

Blood in the stool should always be regarded as a serious matter until it has been determined otherwise. A small amount of bleeding from hemorrhoids or an irritation caused by straining at stool may clear up without any treatment. The serious causes of blood in the stool include hemorrhage from ulcer in the stomach or duodenum, severe inflammation or irritation as in ulcerative colitis or diverticulitis, cancer, and diseases that cause hemorrhage.

Bleeding that occurs in the upper gastrointestinal tract shows up in the feces as dark, almost black, in color and tarlike in consistency. During the hours that it takes the blood to move through the stomach or small intestines, it undergoes partial digestion, which changes blood to the dark, tarry substance. The partially digested blood is found thoroughly mixed in the entire contents of the stool.

Bright red blood in the stool is a sign of a recent hemorrhage or one that occurred in the large bowel. The blood is found on the surfaces of the stool and in pools but not mixed throughout the stool. The color indicates that the blood has not undergone digestion in the upper part of the bowel, nor has it been in the intestinal tract for hours.

ITEM 5. OTHER ABNORMALITIES OF THE FECES

One of the most easily observed changes in the stool is a difference in color. Color varies according to the foods eaten, but the normal stool is brown, except in infants or patients receiving formula in tube feedings, whose stools are a dark yellow. The color of the stool is important in the care of patients with disease of the digestive system because it may indicate a need to change the diet. This is especially important for the patient with an ileostomy, since the stool is evacuated through an opening in the ileum of the small bowel before maximum absorption of nutrients, electrolytes, and water has occurred. Clay color, or pale white, indicates the absence of bile or an obstruction that prevents its passage into the intestines. Chalky white color is due to chalky substances swallowed by the patient or instilled into the lower intestinal tract for X-ray purposes. Light tan color indicates undigested fat in the stool. Green, watery stools, mainly seen in infants, indicate too much sugar.

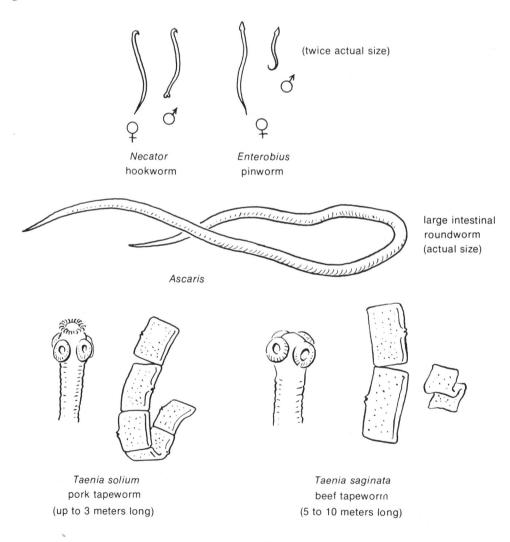

(twice actual size)

Necator
hookworm

Enterobius
pinworm

large intestinal
roundworm
(actual size)

Ascaris

Taenia solium
pork tapeworm
(up to 3 meters long)

Taenia saginata
beef tapeworm
(5 to 10 meters long)

Types of parasites.

Other abnormal characteristics of feces are the presence of large amounts of mucus, pus, or parasites, such as worms. Unusual amounts of mucus in the stool indicate an irritation or inflammation of the inner surface of the intestines. The mucus coats the stool and gives it a slimy appearance. The presence of pus indicates drainage of an ulcer that is inflamed or infected. The most common parasitic worms found in the intestines are the tapeworm, the pinworm, and the roundworm.

17. Feces consist of one-fourth_____and three-fourths_____ .

18. The color of the normal stool in an adult is_____and in the bottle-

    fed baby it is_____ .

19. One of your patients, Mr. Long, has just had a bowel movement that is black in appear-

    ance and tarry in consistency. This means that the stool contains _____ ,
    which probably came from the (duodenum) (cecum) (sigmoid colon). (Circle one.)

20. Mr. Long's hemorrhage probably occurred (10 minutes) (10 hours) (10 days) ago.

21. Hemorrhage in the large intestine produces a _____
    appearance of the stool.

22. Too much sugar in a baby's diet irritates the bowel and produces stools that are

    a. _____ b. _____ .

23. Pale, clay-colored stools are due to the absence of _____ .

24. A slick, slimy appearance of the stool is caused by _____ .

ITEM 6. BOWEL CONTROL TRAINING

In almost every culture, the child is expected to learn early in life to control the elimination of stool from the bowels. Control is usually accomplished between the ages of two and three; the child can then curb the urge to defecate to allow time to get to the bathroom or toilet. The child's success in bowel control becomes a sign of progress toward personal independence, a step toward growing up. It also gives the child a feeling of being more socially acceptable to the family and others.

To establish bowel control in the child, or bowel retraining at any age, it is essential to observe the patient's diet, fluid intake, exercise, and rest, inasmuch as these factors influence regular bowel movements.

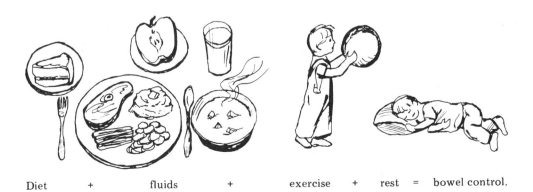

Diet   +   fluids   +   exercise   +   rest   =   bowel control.

The diet should contain roughage adequate to give bulk to the stool. The young child should take 800 to 1000 ml of fluids per day, including water, milk, juices, soups, Jello, and others. Healthy adults should drink between 2000 and 3000 ml of fluids each day. Adequate sleep and exercise are necessary for good health and the proper functioning of the intestinal tract.

The frequency of bowel movements depends on many factors and varies among individuals. It is normal for some people to have a movement every day, for others to have one every other day, and for a few to have a movement every three days. The important thing is that bowel movements occur on a regular basis. The time of the bowel movement also differs. Many adults have elimination following breakfast, but it can occur at other times of the day. Infants usually have two or three movements per day following feeding, and the young child often has a bowel movement shortly after breakfast or lunch.

Habit training for bowel control depends on recognizing the urge to defecate, establishing a regular time for elimination, providing a comfortable position, and allowing sufficient time.

Signs of the urge to defecate are a rumbling noise in the abdomen, expelling of flatus, and restlessness caused by the feeling of fullness in the rectum. The child should be toileted at a regular time each day, usually after breakfast or after lunch. Place the child in a comfortable position on a potty chair, a small commode, or toilet with a child-sized seat on it. The child should be reminded frequently and encouraged to move the bowels but should not be kept on the "potty" longer than 20 minutes. Playing with toys distracts the child from the task to be done.

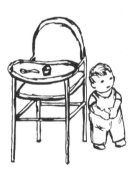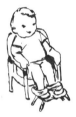

Bowel training.

ITEM 7. INCONTINENCE OF FECES

Some patients lose the ability to control their bowels during a serious illness or hospitalization. This condition is called incontinence. The patient may become incontinent of feces when the bowel is hypoactive, hyperactive, or normal. Incontinence generally occurs in patients who are not fully aware of where they are or what is going on. This lack of awareness may be due to physical disease or illness or to mental condition. Even patients who are not fully aware of what is going on about them often realize that they have had a bowel movement that soiled themselves or the bedding. Such patients often have feelings of being less of a person, lose some self-respect, become embarrassed, or suffer from anxiety and fear that they have lost all control over what is happening to them. When you take care of incontinent patients, it is important not to judge, scold, or fuss at them.

The treatment for incontinence is retraining in bowel control habits. In the beginning, it will take more time to try to establish bowel control habits than to clean up the soiled patient and change the bed. In the long run, however, you will help the patient to regain self-respect as well as control of the bowels. Special effort should be made to help the very elderly patient overcome incontinence. It should be pointed out that incontinence of urine or feces is one of the major reasons for admitting elderly patients to the extended-care facility or nursing home.

Bowel Retraining Program

The method of retraining the incontinent patient is the same as that used for training a child to control the bowels. You must see that these patients eat an adequate diet, that their daily fluid intake is at least 2500 ml, that they get the proper amount of sleep and rest, and that they get exercise within the limits imposed by their illness. Set a regular time for evacuation based on prior bowel habits and your observation of when the incontinent movements tend to occur. The patient should use the bedpan or commode or be taken to the toilet. Privacy should be provided, and 20 minutes should be allowed for the bowel movement. Many doctors order rectal suppositories to stimulate defecation on a regular schedule in the retraining period. One way of using suppositories in habit training is to give one every day for the first week, then every other day for the second and third weeks, and thereafter only as needed to maintain a regular movement every two to three days.

25. Bowel control in children is usually accomplished by age _____ .

26. To help establish bowel control, attention should be given to the child's

   a. _____ , b. _____ c. _____ , and

   d. _____ .

27. It is essential for your good health to have a bowel movement every day.

   True _____ False _____

28. Incontinence of feces means _____ .

29. The treatment for incontinence is _____ .

30. Two benefits to the patient that result from retraining bowel control habits are

   a. _____ and b. _____ .

ITEM 8. MOVEMENT IN THE INTESTINES

The liquefied food mass, or chyme, is passed along the intestines by means of movement of the muscular tube. This movement is called peristalsis. In peristalsis, the circular muscle

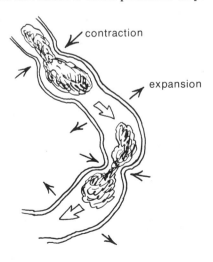

contraction

expansion

Peristalsis.

layer of the intestine contracts to squeeze and propel the portion of chyme and gas ahead of it. The circular, longitudinal, and oblique muscle layers in the segment ahead of the contracted part will expand and lengthen to accommodate the entering mass. The rumbling noise that can occasionally be heard coming from the abdomen is caused by the peristaltic movement of liquid mass and gas along the intestinal tract.

The feces are propelled along the lower intestines by peristalsis until they reach the storage portion in the lower sigmoid colon and the rectum. As more feces collect here, the rectum is filled, and the pressure on the sphincter of the anus causes the urge to open and defecate. The abdominal muscles contract to help force the evacuation of the rectum, and pass the feces through the anus.

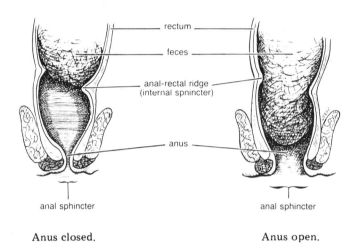

Anus closed.   Anus open.

ITEM 9. THE HYPOACTIVE BOWEL AND CONSTIPATION

A reduction or absence of peristaltic movement of the bowel results in the hypoactive bowel. Conditions that cause the hypoactive bowel are surgery, injury, disease, and bed rest. In the normal person, lack of sufficient roughage in the diet and decreased exercise may produce a sluggish or hypoactive bowel. Certain drugs such as narcotics and tranquilizers also reduce the activity of the bowel.

Constipation, one of the most common problems of the hypoactive bowel, is the irregular evacuation of feces from the bowel, causing them to become more compacted and hard while in the rectum. As additional feces are formed, they fill greater portions of the colon as well as the rectum. Constipation tends to occur when muscle tone is lacking because of inadequate exercise, irregularity of bowel movements, a sedentary life, or worry, anxiety, or fear.

The treatment includes plenty of exercise, lots of liquids, a good diet with sufficient roughage, setting a regular time for defecation, and avoiding emotional stress. When ordered by the doctor, enemas are used to empty the rectum, laxatives to stimulate bowel activity, and suppositories to stimulate the urge to defecate.

ITEM 9. THE ENEMA

An enema is the introduction of fluid into the rectum and colon by means of a tube. Rectal enemas are given to stimulate peristalsis and the urge to defecate. The cleansing enema is used to wash out the waste products or feces when the bowel is to be examined by X-ray or proctoscopy or when the bowel is distended by flatus. The commercially disposable enema, such as the FLEET's enema, is convenient and easy to use when only a small amount of fluid is needed to stimulate a bowel movement.

II Pract. 2

Types of Enemas

The type of enema to be given is prescribed by the doctor and will vary depending on the age and condition of the patient, the purpose of the enema, and the preference of the physician. The type of solution is specified, and the nurse is expected to know how to prepare it unless the commercial enema has been ordered. The most common solutions are the tap water enema (TWE), using water obtained from the faucet; the saline enema, using a saline (salt) solution; and the soapsuds enema (or SSE), using a small amount of liquefied soap in water. When other types of enemas are ordered, you may need to consult the nursing procedure book of the hospital for the ingredients and the proportions to use.

U
N
I
T
25

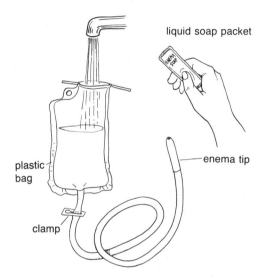

liquid soap packet

plastic bag

enema tip

clamp

Preparing soapsuds enema.

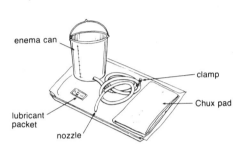

enema can

clamp

Chux pad

lubricant packet

nozzle

Enema tray.

Amount and Temperature of Solution

Disposable enema units contain about 240 ml of solution that is given at room temperature. No special preparation is needed — it is ready for use when taken from the package. The prelubricated nozzle is inserted into the rectum, and the solution is instilled by squeezing the flexible plastic bottle.

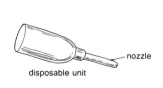

nozzle

disposable unit

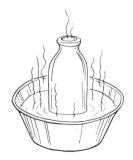

Warming saline solution.

For cleansing enemas prepared by the nurse, the amount of solution used for adults is usually between 500 and 1000 ml, and smaller amounts are used for children. The solution should run in slowly to avoid discomfort and pain as the rectum is distended by the fluid. Hold the container approximately 12 to 18 inches above the patient's anus; a greater height creates too much pressure so that the fluid runs in too rapidly and causes painful distention of the rectum and colon. It also stimulates the urge to defecate immediately so that the patient cannot retain the fluid.

The temperature of the solution should be about 105°F (40.5°C). If a bath thermometer is not available, you can test the temperature of the fluid by pouring a small amount over your inner wrist. It should be warm to touch, but not hot. Solution that is too cool usually can't be retained; hot solutions may damage the tissues of the rectum.

Recommended Position

The position of choice when giving an enema to a bed patient is the left lateral position with the hips slightly elevated. This allows the fluid, aided by the force of gravity, to flow downward along the natural curve of the rectum and descending colon. Although the right lateral position can be used if necessary, the patient may only be able to absorb a smaller quantity, since that solution has to overcome gravity to enter the sigmoid colon. If the patient is unable to turn to the other side, the supine position can be used. Enemas should not be given to a patient seated on the toilet unless it is intended only to stimulate the urge to defecate. In a sitting position, the fluid cannot flow to other parts of the colon; it merely dilates the rectum and is rapidly expelled.

‖‖

For a cleansing enema given to an adult, indicate the specific information in connection with the following:

31. Kind of solution used _____ .

32. Amount of solution _____ .

33. Temperature of the solution _____ .

34. Height of the solution container above the anus_____ .

35. State at least two possible reasons for the patient to have difficulty retaining the solution.

     a. _____ .

     b. _____ .

‖‖

ITEM 11. PROCEDURE FOR GIVING A CLEANSING ENEMA

In the skill laboratory, practice the procedure for giving an enema using the Chase doll or other model with an anal opening. Review the steps of the procedure until you are familiar with them before you give an enema to a patient in the clinical setting.

‖‖

Supplies Needed

Enema can or bag   Rectal tube or enema tip, if needed
Chux pad   Lubricant
Tubing with clamp   Solution

‖‖

Important Steps	Key Points

1. Wash hands.

Universal Steps A, B, C, and D. See Appendix.

2. Collect items and materials needed.

3. Approach and identify the patient, explain the procedure, and gain cooperation.

4. Provide privacy and drape the patient as needed.

5. Prepare the patient.

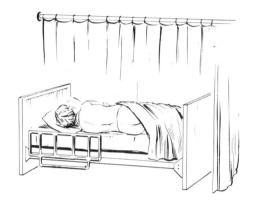

Avoid giving enemas at mealtimes, when other patients are eating in the same room, or during visiting hours, unless visitors are asked to leave the room. It is embarrassing both to the patient and to others.

If at all possible, work from the right side of the bed so that the patient can turn on the left side. Raise the bed to a comfortable working height. Lower the siderail, if one is used, and adjust the bed to a flat position. Place the Chux or pad under the buttocks.

6. Prepare the solution.

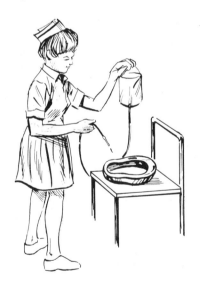

Fill the enema can or bag with the correct solution:

Amount for adult: 500 to 1000 ml
Temperature: less than $105°F$ $(40.5°C)$

Expel air from tubing by opening the clamp and allowing the solution to run through. Use the bedpan to collect this solution, then re-clamp the tubing.

7. Insert the rectal tube.

Open the packed of lubricant and lubricate the end of the rectal tube. Insert the lubricated tube gently about 4 inches.

Important Steps	Key Points
8. Instill the solution into the bowel.	Open the clamp on the tube and allow the solution to flow slowly into the bowel. Hold the solution container 12 to 18 inches above the anus. Regulate the flow according to the patient's ability to retain it. When the patient has discomfort, stop the flow by kinking the tubing or clamping it and instruct the patient to take deep breaths by mouth until the cramping and urge pass. Then continue until the patient can retain no more or the can is empty.
9. Remove the rectal tube.	Clamp the tubing and withdraw the rectal tube. Place the soiled end in the paper towel.
10. Assist the patient to the bathroom or onto the bedpan.	If the patient goes to the bathroom, ask to see the results before the toilet is flushed. Roll up the bed so that the patient is in a sitting position unless contraindicated. Place the toilet tissue and call light within reach.
11. Observe the results of the enema.	When the enema and stool have been expelled, remove the bedpan and assist the patient to clean the anal area if needed. Note the color, amount, and consistency of the stool. Empty and clean the bedpan and return it to the patient's unit.
12. Provide for the patient's comfort.	Universal Steps X, Y, and Z. See Appendix.
13. Remove all enema equipment.	
14. Report and record as appropriate.	Charting example: 1045. SS enema given. Expelled moderate amount of dark brown stool and some flatus. K. Cardinale, SN

ITEM 12.   THE RETENTION ENEMA

Often an oil-retention enema is ordered for a patient who is constipated. The oil must be retained in the rectum to soften and coat the hardened feces. Between 120 ml and 180 ml of warm oil is instilled rectally in the same manner as the cleansing enema, except that the oil should be retained at least 30 minutes. An Asepto syringe, a rectal tube or small catheter, and a small pitcher or funnel to hold the oil may be used instead of the usual equipment. Mineral oil or olive oil is most commonly used. There are several prepackaged retention enemas on the market. Follow the same procedure as when giving a cleansing enema.

ITEM 13.   DISTENTION OF THE HYPOACTIVE BOWEL

A second problem related to the hypoactive bowel is that of distention. Abdominal distention is caused by flatus (gas) when peristalsis is reduced or absent. Distention and "gas pains" occur frequently following abdominal surgery. The discomfort and pain are due to the stretching of the intestines, and to the spasms of the muscle layers. The goal of treatment is to reduce the amount of flatus into the bowel.

Procedures that you will use include the enema, irrigations such as the Harris flush, and administration of the rectal tube.

ITEM 14.   THE HARRIS FLUSH

The Harris flush is one of the most effective methods to reduce the abdominal distention caused by flatus. In some parts of the country it is called a colonic irrigation. The procedure consists of running a smaller amount of solution into the bowel, as you do in giving the enema; then, with the rectal tube still in place, the can or bag is lowered to syphon out the liquid, along with the flatus and fecal matter. The alternate filling and draining of the bowel continues at least 4 to 5 times, or until no more gas is expelled. If the solution becomes thick with fecal particles, it may be emptied into the bedpan and more clear solution can be poured into the enema can. Unless ordered otherwise, use 1000 ml of tap water at 105°F (40.5°C).

Given a patient with moderate abdominal distention following surgery of the abdomen three days ago, you are to give a Harris flush to reduce the flatus.

|||||||||||||||||||||||||||||||||||||||||||||||||||||||||||||||||||||||||||||||||||||||||||||||||||||||||||||

Supplies Needed

Enema can or bag   Rectal tube or enema tip, if needed
Chux pad   Lubricant
Tubing with clamp   Solution
Bedpan

|||||||||||||||||||||||||||||||||||||||||||||||||||||||||||||||||||||||||||||||||||||||||||||||||||||||||||||

Important Steps	Key Points
Follow steps 1 through 7 for the cleansing enema, Item 11.	
8. Instill 200 to 300 ml of the solution.	Hold the irrigating can 12 to 18 inches above the anus. Regulate the flow according to the patient's ability to retain it. When the patient has discomfort, stop the flow by kinking the tubing or clamping it, and instruct to take deep or panting breaths through the mouth until the cramping and urge pass.
9. Drain the solution.	Lower the irrigating can to a point 12 to 18 inches below the anus and allow the solution and flatus to flow back into the can.
10. Repeat steps 8 and 9.	You should continue the flushing of the bowel at least four to five times to remove as much flatus as possible.
Steps 11 through 14 are the same as for the cleansing enema, Item 11.	Charting example: 2045. Harris flush given. Solution returned clear with a large amount of flatus expelled. Abdomen soft. States feeling very relieved. K. Cardinale, SN

ITEM 15.   USE OF RECTAL TUBE FOR RELEASE OF FLATUS

When a patient is uncomfortable because of flatus in the lower bowel, a rectal tube can be inserted in the anus. This allows the gas to be expelled without the patient's straining to open the anal sphincter. The procedure is simple and effective. Obtain a rectal tube, lubricate the end, and take it to the patient's bedside in a hand towel or paper towel. Turn the patient to his or her side and gently insert the rectal tube about 4 inches. The free end of the rectal tube should be placed in the folded hand towel in case there is some expulsion of fecal material.

The rectal tube should not remain in the anus more than one-half hour. It should be removed and reinserted after several hours if the patient again has discomfort. Severe irritation of the lining of the rectum can occur from prolonged insertion. When treatment is completed, rinse the rectal tube and return it to the central processing department. If disposable rectal tubes are used by your agency, discard the tube into the designated waste container. Charting example:

1115. Rectal tube inserted. Expelling much flatus.   J. Jones, NA
1145. Rectal tube removed. States he is greatly relieved.   J. Jones, NA

ITEM 16. THE IRRITABLE OR HYPERACTIVE BOWEL

Hyperactivity of the bowel means that there is excessive movement in that area. Any condition that causes irritation of the intestines can cause hyperactivity of the bowel. The hyperactive, irritable bowel is seen in cases of diarrhea of all kinds, ulcerative colitis, diverticulitis, and certain other diseases.

Excessively strong and frequent peristaltic action moves the chyme rapidly through the intestines because the food mass may also serve as an irritant to an already irritated bowel. This rapid movement of the chyme in the bowel reduces the amount of time available for the intestines to absorb the nutrients, electrolytes, and water. It causes numerous bowel movements per day that generally are liquid or semiliquid in consistency.

The problems related to the hyperactive bowel are lack of enough food to nourish and repair the cells of the body; loss of electrolytes, which disturbs the chemical composition of the body fluids; and dehydration, which reduces the amount of water available for the body fluids. These conditions pose a serious threat to the patient's life. For example, infants and small children may die in a matter of 24 hours or less as a result of severe diarrhea.

The objectives of treating the hyperactive bowel are to reduce the irritability and to maintain adequate levels of nutrition, electrolytes, and water in the body. This requires vigorous treatment by the doctors and nurses. It is very important for the nurse worker to record the number and character of the stools per day, and the amount of food and fluid taken by the patient. It is also essential to provide an emotionally calm atmosphere for the patient.

||||||||||||||||||||||||||||||||||||||||||||||||||||||||||||||||||||||||||||||||||||||||||||||||||||||||||||||||||||||||||||||||||||||

36. The rapid movement of chyme in the hyperactive bowel interferes with _____

_____.

37. An increase in the number of bowel movements per day is called _____

_____ .

38. Disturbance of the chemical composition of body fluids is caused by loss of _____

_____.

||||||||||||||||||||||||||||||||||||||||||||||||||||||||||||||||||||||||||||||||||||||||||||||||||||||||||||||||||||||||||||||||||||||||||

ITEM 17. COLLECTION OF A STOOL SPECIMEN

Review the following procedure several times to become familiar with it before you collect a stool specimen from a patient in the clinical area.

Given a doctor's order to obtain a stool specimen for specific laboratory tests, inform the patient about the procedure. When the bowel movement is finished, collect a portion of the stool, place it in a specimen container, complete the laboratory request for examination, and then promptly send the specimen and request slip to the laboratory.

||||||||||||||||||||||||||||||||||||||||||||||||||||||||||||||||||||||||||||||||||||||||||||||||||||||||||||||||||||||||||||||||||||||||||||||||||||||||||

Supplies Needed

Specimen box with lid	Laboratory request
Tongue blades (2)	Bedpan
Paper towel	

||||||||||||||||||||||||||||||||||||||||||||||||||||||||||||||||||||||||||||||||||||||||||||||||||||||||||||||||||||||||||||||||||||||||||||||||||||||||||

Important Steps	Key Points

Carry out Universal Steps A, B, C, and D. See Appendix.

1. Tell the patient how to assist in the collection of the specimen.

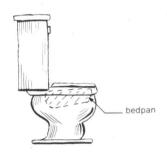

The patient should be asked to

   a. use the bedpan or bedside commode for the next bowel movement,

   b. save the stool, and

   c. notify the nurse.

The bedpan may be placed on a chair for use by the patient who has bathroom privileges, or the bedside commode may be used. In some cases, a bedpan will fit in the toilet bowl under the toilet seat as shown.

2. Collect a specimen of the stool after the patient has defecated.

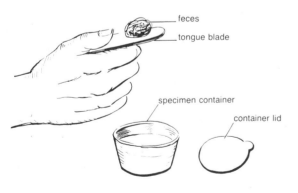

Take the bedpan and your supplies to the bathroom where you will empty the pan after obtaining the specimen. Use the tongue blades to transfer approximately one tablespoon of stool to the container. Put the lid on the container, wrap the soiled tongue blades in the paper towel, and drop them into the wastebasket. Empty and clean the bedpan or commode pan and return it to its proper place.

3. Complete the laboratory request and label for the specimen.

Check the name of the patient and the name on the lab slip to see that they are identical. This is vitally important. An incorrect label will cause the laboratory to give the wrong information on the patient. Write the patient's name, room or ward number, and the date on the lid of the container.

Important Steps	Key Points
4. Send the specimen and the request slip to the laboratory.	Make sure the specimen is taken to the lab immediately. Some laboratories accept stool specimens only during specified hours. Check your agency procedure. Stool specimens should be examined while still warm and fresh. Time and changes in temperature alter the stool. As an example, bright red blood begins to clot, dry out, and turn dark, and certain disease-causing organisms may die and thus fail to be detected.
5. Record and report as appropriate.	1110. Moderate amount of brown soft-formed stool. Specimen to lab. J. Jones, NA

ITEM 18.   FECAL IMPACTION

Fecal impaction means that the rectum and sigmoid colon become filled with fecal material. As the fecal material remains in the bowel for several days, it becomes more compacted, contains less water, and consequently becomes quite hard and difficult or painful to pass through the anus.

The most obvious sign of fecal impaction is the absence of (or only a small amount of) bowel movement for more than three days. Another important sign of a possible fecal impaction is the passage of small amounts of semi-soft or liquid stool so that there is staining and soiling of the bed linens. This occurs as bacterial action of the fecal material continues to work on the outer surfaces of the hardened impacted mass, liquefying small portions of it. It is the result of the body's effort to remove the obstructing mass.

Fecal impaction should be suspected when a patient has a hypoactive bowel with constipation, or lack of bowel movement for three days or more. As in the case of bowel incontinence, this condition usually occurs in patients who may not be fully aware of their surroundings owing to their physical condition, illness, or mental state of confusion. The very young and the very old patients are especially prone to develop fecal impaction.

The nursing treatment of a fecal impaction is to examine for the presence of an impaction, manually break it up, and remove portions of the fecal mass. This should be followed by the use of suppositories, enemas, or laxatives as ordered by the physician. Again, emphasis should be on the prevention of fecal impactions by taking measures to ensure regular evacuation of the waste products from the bowel of each patient.

ITEM 19.   REMOVAL OF FECAL IMPACTION

In the skill laboratory, go through the steps of the procedure several times until you are familiar with it. If a lifelike model of the anus and rectum is available, it can be used to help you get the feel of examining the rectum for impacted stool before you perform the procedure in the clinical area.

In this procedure, you are to examine the rectum for the presence of hardened stool, manually break it up, and remove such portions as you can in an older patient who is able to turn on his side.

Supplies Needed

Examining glove (nonsterile)   Bedpan
Lubricant   Toilet paper
Chux pad   Paper towel

Important Steps	Key Points

Carry out Universal Steps A, B, C, and D.

1. Put on examining glove.

Place the bedpan and toilet tissue on a chair that is close to the bed and within your convenient reach in order to avoid strain or injury to yourself. Put on the gloves and use lubricant on your index finger.

2. Insert gloved index finger into rectum.

The index finger should follow the wall of the rectum in a slightly curving motion. As the finger comes in contact with feces in the rectum, note the consistency; then move the finger into the lower portion of the fecal mass, again noting the consistency.

3. Break up and remove the fecal impaction.

With the examining index finger, dislodge or break off a small amount of fecal material and gently remove it, placing it in the bedpan. Continue removing as much fecal material as you can reach with your finger, or until the patient's discomfort warrants discontinuing the procedure. Remove the soiled gloves and place them in a paper towel.

4. Remove the remaining fecal material.

Often, the stimulation of removing the impaction manually will create the urge in the patient to defecate. Help the patient to the bathroom, or place the patient on a clean bedpan and provide toilet paper. If patient is still unable to defecate, follow up by carrying out the doctor's order for a suppository, enema, or laxative.

Carry out Universal Steps X, Y, and Z. See Appendix.

Charting example:
1045. Rectal examination for fecal impaction. Moderate amount of brown hard feces removed manually.

B. Rose, SN

U
N
I
T
25

ITEM 20. THE USE OF RECTAL SUPPOSITORIES

In some settings, the beginning worker in nursing may not be allowed to insert rectal suppositories. Check with your instructor, who may ask you to omit the next two items.

Rectal suppositories consist of a semisolid material that melts readily; they are somewhat cone-shaped and approximately 1½ inches long. They are made for many different purposes: some relieve pain or irritation, some contain drugs that the patient cannot take by mouth, and others promote bowel movements. The latter may do so (1) by stimulating the inner surface of the rectum and increasing the urge to defecate, (2) by forming gas that expands the rectum, or (3) by melting into a lubricating material to coat the stool for easier passage through the anal sphincter.

A nonsterile glove is worn when inserting the suppository into the rectum. After it has been inserted through the anal sphincter, the suppository should be guided by the index finger along the wall of the rectum to a point beyond the anal-rectal ridge that is about 2 to 3 inches from the outer sphincter. The suppository will be ineffective if it is pushed into the fecal mass. Correct and incorrect placement of the suppository are shown in the following sketches.

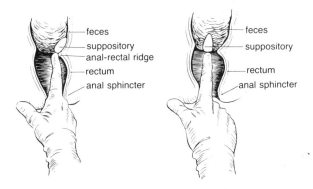

Correct placement.   Incorrect placement.

39. Purposes for using rectal suppositories are   a. _____ ,

    b. _____ ,   or c. _____ .

40. When placed correctly, the rectal suppository

    a. stimulates the outer surface of the rectum.

    b. is in contact with the inner surface of the rectum.

    c. melts inside the fecal mass in the rectum.

    d. lies between the anal sphincter and the anal rectal ridges.

ITEM 21. INSERTING RECTAL SUPPOSITORIES

You should go through the steps of this procedure several times in the skill laboratory in order to become familiar with it. Most schools do not have lifelike models of the anus and rectum, and you will not be able to insert the suppository and get the "feel" of it in the rectum until you reach the clinical area.

For your practice situation, you are to insert a rectal suppository to stimulate a bowel movement in a bed patient who can turn to the side.

Supplies Needed

Nonsterile examining glove	Suppository
Lubricant	Paper towel

Important Steps	Key Points
Carry out Universal Steps A, B, C, and D. See Appendix.	
1. Position the patient.	Adjust the bed to a nearly flat position, and lower the side rail if it is used. Place the patient in a Sims' position and fold the top bedding obliquely back over the hips to expose the buttocks. Lower the pajama pants or fold the hospital gown out of the way.

Importent Steps	Key Points
2. Put on the examining glove.	Unwrap the foil or plastic covering of the suppository, leaving it on the wrapper. Put the glove on your dominant, or working, hand.
3. Insert the suppository rectally.	Take the suppository between thumb and index finger and lubricate it. With your other hand, draw the top gluteal fold upward and toward the head to expose the anus. Ask the patient to take a deep breath at the time you insert the suppository; this helps to relax the anal sphincter. Slip the suppository into the anus, and with your gloved index finger guide it along the wall of the anus and rectum for 3 inches or the length of your finger. Withdraw your finger, and hold both buttocks tightly together for a few seconds while the patient breathes deeply until the urge to expel it has passed.

U
N
I
T
25

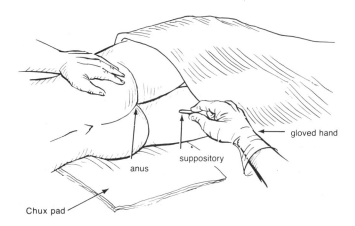

gloved hand

suppository

anus

Chux pad

| 4. Remove the glove. | Take the cuff of the glove, and pull it down over the hands so that the glove turns inside out. Place the soiled glove on the paper towel, and fold it closed. |
| Carry out Universal Steps X, Y, and Z. See Appendix. | Charting example:
0930. Glycerin suppository inserted.
<div style="text-align:right">J. Jones, NA</div>1005. Large amount of soft brown formed stool expelled with large amount of flatus. States she is feeling much relieved.
<div style="text-align:right">J. Jones, NA</div> |

ITEM 22. COLOSTOMIES AND ILEOSTOMIES

The first successful colostomy was performed in 1793. Today, thousands of people have colostomies, and a smaller number have ileostomies. Most of them have learned to manage their ostomy and to lead a normal life again. Part of their adjustment and rehabilitation depends on how well nurses and others help them adjust to having a stoma.

Colostomy refers to an opening, or stoma, made through the abdominal wall into the colon. Waste materials drain through the stoma and bypass the lower portion of the diseased or injured colon. Colostomies are performed to allow an injured or inflamed bowel time to head, or they are performed after removal of a tumor, such as cancer.

The management of the ostomy depends on the location of the stoma and the portion of colon that remains. Since the main functions of the large intestine are to absorb water, solidify waste material, and store feces until it is eliminated, the further down the colon the colostomy is located, the more the discharge will resemble a normal bowel movement. In fact, one can live with the entire colon removed or inactive, as in the case of an ileostomy. Various types of ostomy are shown in the following illustrations.

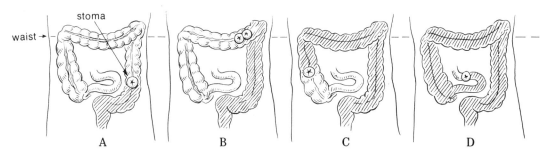

Stoma sites: A, descending colon; B, transverse colon; C, ascending colon; and D, ileostomy stoma.

Colostomies of the sigmoid, or descending, colon are the easiest to manage and to control because they are closer to the end of the large intestines. People who have colostomies in this area are able to regulate themselves so well by using irrigations that they generally can get along without a colostomy bag much of the time and need not worry about an accidental discharge. A colostomy of the ascending or transverse colon is sometimes referred to as a "wet" colostomy because the discharge is semiliquid and tends to flow at intervals during the day and night. The discharge of a "wet" colostomy may contain digestive enzymes that are irritating to unprotected skin surfaces. Refer to Unit 18, Special Skin Care, for information on how to protect the skin around the colostomy.

Care of the Patient with a Colostomy

A patient who has a new colostomy must make many adjustments following surgery. It is understandable that such patients are worried and fearful about being different now from other people, about their friends acceptance of them, and about their own feelings regarding the colostomy and loss of control over bowel actions. Perhaps most of all, they are concerned about the possibility of recovering from a disease that has required this extreme type of surgery.

As a skillful and understanding health worker, you can do a great deal to help the patient through this difficult time. First, you need to develop skills in using the colostomy appliances, in giving skin and stoma care, and in assisting the patient to gain control, if possible, through irrigations. Give frequent reassurances to the patient and family that many people in all walks of life live with an ostomy and conduct normal daily activities. If there is an ostomy club in your community, the patient can derive considerable benefit from sharing experiences with others who also have colostomies or ileostomies. You may be able to assist further by advising about the proper diet for helping to control the type of drainage and odors. Some foods, such as those of the cabbage family, beans, onions, and often, asparagus, cause increased flatus and odors. Finally, you can provide a calm, matter-of-fact atmosphere and encourage resumption of normal patterns of living. We know that emotions affect the bowel, and patients who are tense or upset will reflect this physically by developing an upset colon and increased drainage.

Ostomy Appliances

Generally, surgeons now attach an appliance on the patient's colostomy at the time of the operation, or soon thereafter. This appliance is a device for collecting the drainage from the stoma. A patient with a colostomy usually wears a lightweight plastic bag over the stoma that can be discarded after each use. The plastic is made to resist odors, but occasionally the bag may inflate with gas and look like a balloon if the patient has a lot of flatus. You can make a small hole in the top of the bag and allow the gas to escape.

Although there are many kinds of appliances on the market, most are variations of these three basic types:

1. Cloth belt supporting a two-piece combination of a disposable bag and reusable mounting ring, which may have an inner sealing ring of karaya gum, a substance that protects the skin from irritation.

2. One-piece bag with an attached square of adhesive around the stoma opening that can be worn without a belt.

3. One-piece bag with a gasket that uses no adhesive but is worn with a belt.

Those who have an ileostomy usually wear a two-piece appliance. Because the drainage from a stoma contains digestive enzymes, the skin around the stoma must be protected from contact with the drainage and the resulting irritation. Ileostomy patients need to wear a bag that can be emptied frequently without necessitating the removal of the entire appliance. Some patients with colostomies also wear this type of stoma bag, which can be emptied, rinsed with clear water, and then reclamped.

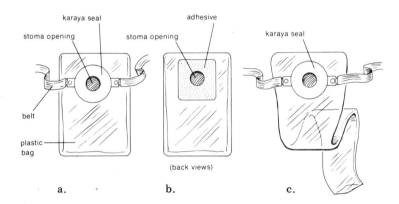

a. A karaya seal stoma bag helps promote postoperative healing. It is secured with belt.

b. Simple "stick-on" type of stoma bag, using adhesive on skin.

c. Ileostomy stoma bag, 12 to 16 inches long. Can be drained through end, then reclosed or clamped.

Stoma bags come in a variety of sizes and it is important to have one that fits closely around the stoma. Because stomas tend to shrink as healing occurs, it may be necessary to remeasure the stoma to ensure the correct size opening. Manufacturers also produce irrigations sets that contain all the equipment the patient needs for self-care. Refer to Unit 18 for instructions on stoma care and changing bags.

Preparing the Patient for Self-care

As soon as the postoperative condition allows, the patient should become involved in the care of the stoma and the surrounding skin and should learn how to control the drainage from the stoma. As the first step, have the patient watch a few times as you change the bag and clean the skin around the stoma. Then have the patient demonstrate changing the bag and cleaning the skin. Finally, patients learn to do their own irrigations. Normal activities can be resumed much sooner when patients do not have to depend on others to perform this care.

ITEM 23. COLOSTOMY IRRIGATIONS

A colostomy irrigation is simply an enema given through the stoma. Irrigations are done to (1) cleanse the intestinal tract of wastes, (2) establish control or regular evacuation of the colostomy, and (3) prevent obstruction of the bowel. For patients with a new colostomy, irrigations are carried out only with a doctor's order. Commercial irrigating sets that contain an irrigator bag with tubing, a clamp, a cone, and a plastic irrigating drain bag are available.

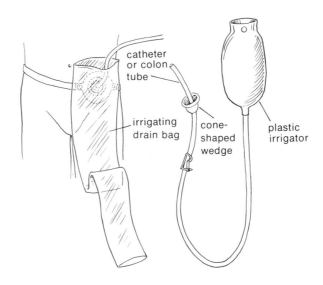

Irrigations may begin as soon as two to four days after surgery, when fecal drainage begins to come through the stoma. Remember the following rules when using colostomy irrigations to establish control of the drainage.

1. Irrigations should be done at the same time each day. Plan with the patient and select a time that will be convenient after the patient goes home as well. The time should permit undisturbed use of the bathroom for about one hour.

2. One hour should be allowed for the irrigation. The patient may be able to clamp the end of an irrigator drain and carry out other activities, but he or she should not feel rushed or pressured for time.

3. Irrigations should continue daily until control is established. Control means that there is no spillage of fecal material from the colostomy during a 24-hour period. Control can be established within a three- to ten-day period, and then maintained by irrigations every other day, or as needed.

Procedure for Irrigating a Colostomy

Given a patient who underwent a colostomy of the descending colon five days ago and is making a good recovery, you are to irrigate the colostomy with the patient sitting on the toilet or commode. You must be skillful and your manner should be accepting of the patient as a person.

||||||||||||||||||||||||||||||||||||||||||||||||||||||||||||||||||||||||||||||||||||||||||||||||||||||||||||||||||||||||||||||||||

Supplies Needed

Irrigator bag and tubing   Solution
Irrigator drain   Lubricant
Ostomy belt

||||||||||||||||||||||||||||||||||||||||||||||||||||||||||||||||||||||||||||||||||||||||||||||||||||||||||||||||||||||||||||||||||

Important Steps	Key Points

Carry out Universal Steps A, B, C, and D. See Appendix.

1. Prepare the patient.

Assist to the bathroom and provide privacy so that others cannot intrude during the procedure. Have patient sit on the toilet and help remove and dispose of the soiled colostomy bag. Have a disposable irrigating drain ready to attach to the belt, or place it over the stoma if the drain has a valve to insert the catheter through. Pull patient's gown or pajamas out of the way to keep them from soiling.

2. Prepare the solution.

Regular tap water is used, unless saline or some other solution has been ordered by the doctor. Water should be warm — about body temperature. Clamp the tubing of the irrigator, add 1000 ml of lukewarm tap water, and expel the air from the tubing.

3. Insert the catheter into the colostomy stoma.

Lubricate about 2 inches of the catheter. Insert it into the stoma about 4 inches. A cone-shaped plug placed at that distance prevents the catheter from being inserted too far and keeps the water from leaking out. If the catheter is hard to insert, *do not force it*. You could injure the colon by forcing the catheter. Open the clamp on the tubing and allow the water to flow gently, or rotate the catheter as you insert it.

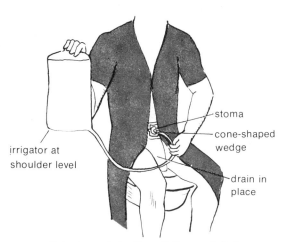

irrigator at
shoulder level

stoma

cone-shaped
wedge

drain in
place

Colostomy irrigation sitting on toilet.

4. Instill the solution into the colon.

Hold the irrigator no higher than the patient's shoulder level. Holding it higher would cause too much pressure, and water would come out as fast as it goes in. Cramps are caused by water that is too cold or being run in too fast. Run the solution in. Do not use more than 1000 ml.

Important Steps	Key Points
5. Have the patient expel the fluid.	Make sure that the irrigator drain bag is in place over the stoma opening. The first gushing return of water and fecal drainage goes directly down into the toilet. It may take up to one hour for all the fluid to return. Later, with more experience in irrigating, the patient may fold up the end of the drain, clamp it, and engage in other activities while waiting for the rest of the water and stool. If no water returns, it may be due to the fact that the catheter is inserted too far, that insufficient water was used, or that not enough time has been allowed to expel it.
Carry out Universal Steps X, Y, and Z. See Appendix.	Charting example: 1000. Tap water, 800 ml as colostomy irrigation. Solution and moderate amount of soft brown stool expelled. Did own stoma care and applied new colostomy bag. <div align="right">J. Jones, LPN</div>

Irrigation Procedure for a Bed Patient

An alternative method involves giving a colostomy irrigation to the bed patient. Use the same equipment and procedure as you would with the patient who can get up to go to the bathroom. However, after instilling the water into the stoma, place the irrigating drain securely around the opening to make sure that it doesn't leak. Either clamp the end of the drain or let the contents of the drain flow into a bedpan at the side of the bed.

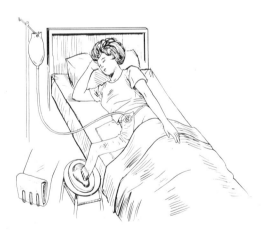

ITEM 24. CONCLUSION OF THE LESSON

You have now completed the lesson on bowel elimination. When you feel sure that you know the vocabulary, the abnormal characteristics of the feces, the problems related to the hypoactive and hyperactive bowel, and the methods of control of the bowel, and when you have practiced the procedures used, arrange with your instructor to take the Post-test.

WORKBOOK ANSWERS

1. mucus

2. cecum

3. tract

4. flatus

5. suppository

6. polyp

7. hemorrhage

8. diarrhea

9. hemorrhoids

10. a. absorption

    b. elimination of waste products

11. a., c., and d.

12. a. distention

    b. diarrhea

    c. constipation

    d. incontinence

13. six

14. absorption

15. b., c., e., g.

16. a. absorption of water and electrolytes

    b. storage of waste products

17. solid material; water

18. brown; brownish-yellow

19. blood; duodenum

20. 10 hours

21. bright red blood

22. a. green

    b. watery

23. bile

24. mucus

25. three

26. a. diet

    b. fluids

    c. exercise

    d. rest

27. false

28. inability to control elimination of feces

29. retraining for bowel control

30. a. control or continence of bowels

    b. regain self-respect

31. tap water, saline, or soap solution, or as ordered by physician

32. 1000 ml

33. 105°F (40.5°C)

34. 12 to 18 inches

35. Any two of the following:

    a. rectum overdistended with fluid

    b. solution is too cool

    c. solution is too hot

    d. solution is running in too fast

    e. solution container is held too high

36. absorption of water, nutrients, and electrolytes

37. diarrhea

38. electrolytes

39. a. to relieve pain

    b. to give medications

    c. to promote bowel movement

40. b.

PERFORMANCE TEST

In the skill laboratory, your instructor will ask you to demonstrate your knowledge and skill in performing four of the following six activities without use of reference material:

1. Describe five unusual or abnormal conditions of the stool that you could observe visually.

2. Given a recent postoperative patient with constipation due to a hypoactive bowel, you are to demonstrate the preparation and the procedure for giving a cleansing enema.

3. Given a recent postoperative patient with abdominal distention, you are to demonstrate the preparation and the procedure for giving a Harris flush.

4. Given a patient who has called you to empty feces from his bedpan, describe the steps you would take to collect a specimen of the stool and prepare it for the laboratory.

5. Given a patient who is incontinent of feces, you are to describe the measures that you would use in retraining the patient to control his bowels.

6. Given a patient with a recent colostomy of the sigmoid colon, you are to demonstrate the preparation and the procedure for irrigating the colostomy as the patient sits on the toilet. (This is an optional performance test, used at the discretion of your instructor.)

PERFORMANCE CHECKLIST

IDENTIFICATION OF ABNORMAL FECES

1. Observe the color of the feces to detect abnormalities

   a. Brown — normal.

   b. Green — too much sugar in the infant's diet.

   c. Greenish-black (meconium) — newborn infant.

   d. Orange-yellow — breast-fed infant.

   e. Green — from chlorophyll.

   g. Color of the stool is affected by some drugs.

   g. Clay — lack of bile secretion.

   h. Chalky white — ingestion of X-ray preparation solutions.

   i. Light tan — undigested fat.

2. Observe the stool for the presence of blood.

   a. Bright red blood — hemorrhage in lower bowel, or hemorrhoids.

   b. Dark brown to black blood — bleeding high in the GI tract.

3. Check the stool for mucus; mucus indicates irritation or inflammation of the intestinal lining.

4. Look for parasitic worms: tapeworms, roundworms, and pinworms.

5. Observe for pus, which indicates an infection in a portion of the intestinal tract.

6. Check for constipation.

7. Check for diarrhea.

ENEMA

1. Wash your hands.

2. Collect the materials needed.

3. Identify the patient, explain the procedure, and enlist the patient's cooperation.

4. Screen for privacy, drape, and position the patient; then adjust the bed height and lower the siderails.

5. Prepare a solution as ordered at 105°F (40.5°C) temperature.

6. Prepare to give the enema:

   a. Lubricate the tube about one inch.

   b. Expel the air from the tubing.

   c. Clamp the tubing.

7. Insert the rectal tube about 4 inches into the patient's rectum.

8. Instill the solution:

   a. Unclamp the tubing and run the solution slowly.

   b. Hold the can 12 to 18 inches above the anus.

   c. Instruct the patient to breathe deeply through the mouth. Stop the flow and wait if patient complains of cramping.

9. Remove the rectal tube and place in a paper towel.

10. Assist the patient to the bathroom or place on the bedpan.

11. Observe the results of the enema after it has been expelled.

12. Provide for the patient's comfort.

13. Remove and dispose of the used items.

14. Record the information on the patient's chart.

HARRIS FLUSH

1. Wash your hands.

2. Collect the equipment.

3. Identify the patient and inform him about the procedure.

4. Screen for privacy, drape, and position patient.

5. Prepare the solution:

   a. Lubricate the tube.

   b. Expel the air from the tube.

6. Insert the tube 4 inches into the patient's rectum.

7. Raise the can 12 to 18 inches above the patient's anus.

8. Unclamp the tube and insert 250 to 300 cc of solution.

9. Regulate the flow with the patient's ability to retain the solution.

10. Drain the solution from the colon by lowering the can to 12 to 18 inches below the anus.

11. Repeat steps 8, 9, and 10 until there is no more flatus.

12. Remove the rectal tube and place it in a paper towel.

13. Provide for the patient's comfort.

14. Remove the equipment; clean it and return it to storage.

15. Record the treatment on the patient's chart.

COLLECTION OF STOOL SPECIMENS

1. Wash your hands.

2. Gather the necessary equipment: two tongue blades, a specimen container and lid, and a paper towel.

3. Remove the bedpan and take it to the appropriate work area.

4. With a tongue blade, transfer at least one tablespoon of stool from the bedpan to the specimen container.

5. Put the lid on the container; wrap and discard the tongue blade.

6. Empty, clean, and return the bedpan to storage.

7. Write the patient's name and room number and the date in the proper place on the container.

8. Complete the laboratory requisition. Check the patient's name on the requisition and on the specimen container to be sure they are the same. Be sure to use the correct lab slip, indicating the type of test ordered, the date, and the time the stool was passed.

9. Take to the lab at once (stat). Explain why a delay in taking the specimen to the lab would alter the stool and give a false reading.

10. Record on the patient's chart.

BOWEL TRAINING

1. Describe measures used in retraining the incontinent patient.

   a. Adequate diet.

   b. Adequate liquids, at least 2500 cc of liquid daily.

   c. Sleep and exercise within the patient's physical limits.

   d. Regular time for bowel evacuation based on prior habits.

   e. Allowance of at least 20 minutes for bowels to move.

   f. Suppository, used on the doctor's order. Given daily at the same time for the first week, then every other day the second and third weeks, and then p.r.n.

COLOSTOMY IRRIGATION

1. Wash your hands.

2. Assemble the equipment.

3. Identify the patient and explain the procedure.

4. Provide privacy and prepare the patient for the procedure.

    a. Assist to the toilet.

    b. Remove the soiled colostomy bag.

    c. Prepare the irrigating drain and attach it to the belt.

5. Prepare the solution — 1000 ml water at body temperature.

    a. Pour 1000 ml of solution into the irrigator bag.

    b. Expel the air from the tubing, then clamp it shut.

6. Lubricate the tip of the catheter.

    a. Insert it into the stoma about 3 to 4 inches.

    b. Unclamp the tubing and allow the solution to run for easier insertion of the catheter.

7. Instill the solution, holding it no higher than the level of the patient's shoulder.

8. After instilling 500 to 1000 ml of solution, remove the catheter.

9. Place an irrigating drain over the stoma.

10. When all the solution and stool have been expelled, remove the irrigating drain.

11. Cleanse and dry the skin.

12. Attach a clean colostomy bag; allow the patient to do this as soon as he or she is able.

13. Provide for patient's comfort.

14. Clean and return the equipment to storage.

15. Record the treatment on the patient's chart.

U
N
I
T
25

POST-TEST

Matching.   Match each of the items in Column I with the item in Column II that best describes it. Items in Column II may be used more than once.

Column I	Column II
_____ 1. colitis	a. part of the small intestine
_____ 2. rectum	b. part of the large intestine
_____ 3. duodenum	c. part of the contents of the intestines
_____ 4. chyme	d. disease of the intestines
_____ 5. ileum	e. none of the above
_____ 6. appendicitis	
_____ 7. sigmoid	
_____ 8. flatus	
_____ 9. hemorrhoids	
_____ 10. bile	

Multiple Choice.   Select the correct or best answer for the following questions. There is only one best answer for each one.

11. In the adult, the length of the intestinal tract is approximately

    a.   20 feet long.

    b.   three times the body length.

    c.   16 feet long.

    d.   six times the body length.

12. The important function of the small intestine is to

    a.   connect the stomach to the colon.

    b.   absorb nutrients and electrolytes.

    c.   provide storage for waste products.

    d.   absorb water and gases.

13. One important function of the large intestine is to

    a.   absorb nutrients.

    b.   aid in the digestion of foods.

    c.   absorb water.

    d.   aid in transporting chyme.

14. Movement in the intestines by alternate contractions that squeeze the contents forward is called

    a.   constipation.

    b.   peristalsis.

    c.   distention.

    d.   incontinence.

15. Frequent, rapid movement of intestinal contents that results in many watery stools per day is called

  a. diarrhea.

  b. diverticulitis.

  c. peristalsis.

  d. hemorrhoids.

16. If an obstruction or twisting of the small intestine prevents the chyme from moving past the obstacle, the result is

  (1) some discomfort, but not serious.

  (2) loss of nutrients and electrolytes.

  (3) a serious threat to person's life.

  (4) decreased bowel movements.

  a. All of the above   b. (2), (3), and (4)   c. (1), (2), and (4)   d. (3)

17. Mrs. Shortly was admitted to the hospital two days ago after vomiting some blood. She passed a small stool that was black and tarry in appearance. The reason for the color of the stool is

  a. mucus.

  b. parasites.

  c. blood.

  d. medications.

18. Today Mrs. Shortly has barium while in X-ray for a GI series. The barium causes the color of the stool to appear

  a. white.

  b. green.

  c. brown.

  d. red.

19. In most cultures of the world, children are taught to control their bowel movements by the age of

  a. one year.

  b. 18 months.

  c. three years.

  d. three and one-half years.

20. When training the young child to gain voluntary control of his bowel movements, the mother or nurse should do all of the following *except*

  a. give frequent encouragement while the child is sitting on the toilet.

  b. provide roughage in the diet to give bulk to the stool.

  c. establish a regular time for bowel elimination.

  d. take the child off the "potty" after 5 minutes even if there has been no movement.

21. An older person in the hospital has not had a bowel movement for several days. In the last few hours, the patient has passed two very small, semiliquid bowel movements. The nurse suspects that the patient has

    a. an inadequate diet.

    b. an impaction.

    c. diarrhea.

    d. a hyperactive bowel.

22. The most common problem that people with a hypoactive bowel have is

    a. constipation.

    b. impaction.

    c. obstructions.

    d. infections.

23. The treatment of constipation includes all of the following *except*

    a. avoidance of emotional stress.

    b. medication for pain or discomfort.

    c. laxatives and enemas.

    d. a moderate amount of exercise.

24. When giving an enema to a patient in bed, the best position for instilling the solution is

    a. a prone position.

    b. a right lateral Sims' position.

    c. a supine position.

    d. a left lateral position.

25. The lubricated rectal tube is inserted into the anus a distance of about

    a. 2 inches.

    b. 4 inches.

    c. 6 inches.

    d. 8 inches.

26. How high above the patient's buttocks does the nurse hold the solution container when giving an enema?

    a. 4 to 6 inches

    b. 6 to 10 inches

    c. 10 to 12 inches

    d. 12 to 18 inches

27. The reason for holding the container at the correct height is to

    a. make the solution run in more quickly.

    b. have the water go up higher in the colon.

    c. avoid increasing the pressure of the water.

    d. keep the nurse's arm from getting too tired.

28. All of the following may be reasons for a patient to have difficulty taking and retaining the enema solution *except*

    a. he takes panting breaths through the mouth.

    b. the solution is too cool.

    c. the solution is too hot.

    d. the solution is running in too fast.

29. The correct position of the rectal suppository is

    a. lying in the sphincter of the anus.

    b. pushed into the fecal mass.

    c. at the flexure of the sigmoid.

    d. in contact with the lining of the rectum.

30. The most common purpose for giving a Harris flush for colonic irrigation is to

    a. relieve distention caused by flatus.

    b. cleanse the bowel of fecal material.

    c. promote the absorption of fluids.

    d. remove bacteria from the intestinal tract.

31. A rectal tube that is left in the patient's rectum for more than 30 minutes can cause

    a. total removal of all gases from the abdomen.

    b. irritation of the rectum and anus.

    c. increased absorption of water from the bowel.

    d. hyperactivity of the large intestines.

32. Patients who have a colostomy can more easily control the drainage from a stoma located in the

    a. ileum.

    b. ascending colon.

    c. sigmoid colon.

    d. transverse colon.

33. Important things the nurse can do for the patient with a new colostomy would include all of the following *except*

    a. be skillful in using the colostomy appliance.

    b. provide an accepting and matter-of-fact atmosphere for care.

    c. tell the patient not to worry and that he'll be okay.

    d. inform him about some of the gas-forming foods.

34. The colostomy appliance often used for the patient following surgery contains a karaya seal because the karaya

    a. controls the amount of drainage from the stoma.

    b. cushions and reduces the pressure of the drainage bag.

    c. keeps the odors from escaping into the drainage bag.

    d. protects the skin against the irritation of the drainage.

35. When the patient takes (or is given) a colostomy irrigation, care should be taken to

    a. hold the solution no higher than the patient's shoulders.

    b. alternate irrigation time from morning to evening.

    c. make sure the procedure is completed within 30 minutes.

    d. keep the irrigating water hot, or over $140°F$

POST-TEST ANSWERS

1.	d	19.	c
2.	b	20.	d
3.	a	21.	b
4.	c	22.	a
5.	a	23.	b
6.	d	24.	d
7.	b	25.	b
8.	c	26.	d
9.	d	27.	c
10.	c	28.	a
11.	d	29.	d
12.	b	30.	a
13.	c	31.	b
14.	b	32.	c
15.	a	33.	c
16.	b	34.	d
17.	c	35.	a
18.	a		

CARDIOPULMONARY RESUSCITATION

GENERAL PERFORMANCE OBJECTIVE

On completion of this lesson, you will be able to recognize the signs of cardiac arrest and to carry out the emergency cardiopulmonary resuscitation procedures.

SPECIFIC PERFORMANCE OBJECTIVES

When you have completed this unit you will be able to

1. Recognize and describe the signs of cardiac arrest.

2. Provide a patent airway for the victim.

3. Ventilate the victim through mouth-to-mouth resuscitation.

4. Palpate the carotid artery for signs of a pulse.

5. Maintain artificial circulation through closed-chest massage.

6. Rescue the victim with an obstructed airway by removing the foreign body with back blows, manual thrusts, and finger probes.

VOCABULARY

basic cardiac life support—the phase of emergency cardiac care that either (1) externally supports the circulation and respiration of the victim through CPR or (2) prevents circulatory or respiratory arrest or insufficiency through prompt intervention.

cardiac arrest—sudden and unexpected loss of cardiac and pulmonary function.

cardiac board—a flat board, usually kept on the cardiac arrest cart, that is placed under the patient's back to provide a firm surface for giving external heart massage if patient is in bed.

CPR—an abbreviation for cardiopulmonary resuscitation.

monitored cardiac arrest—the victim experiences a cardiac arrest while the heart is being monitored by electrocardiogram (ECG).

myocardial infarction—a heart attack, or blockage of the blood supply to the heart.

pupil—the opening in the center of the iris (the colored portion of the eye).

contracted pupils—pupils become smaller when exposed to light.

dilated pupils—pupils enlarge in darkness.

resuscitation—the act of bringing back to life.

sternum—the breastbone; a flat, narrow bone in the midline of the thorax between the ribs.

trachea—the windpipe.

xiphoid process—the lowest portion of the sternum (breastbone).

INTRODUCTION

Cardiac arrest is a sudden and dramatic event, regardless of where it occurs. People may become victims of cardiac arrest at any time and at any place. They have been struck down while playing tennis, taking a nap, driving a car, cooking a meal, or being treated in a hospital. The victims appear to be doing fine and have no particular problems until they suddenly collapse and lose consciousness. They die unless the cardiac arrest is recognized and treated in time by someone trained in cardiopulmonary resuscitation (CPR) techniques. The American Heart Association recommends that the general public, including children in grade school, be taught cardiopulmonary resuscitation as an emergency life support technique so that countless lives can be saved.*

BASIC CARDIOPULMONARY RESUSCITATION

ITEM 1. WHAT IS CARDIAC ARREST?

The term "cardiac arrest" means that the heart has stopped beating and the blood no longer circulates through the body. The victim stops breathing and loses consciousness because the brain lacks the oxygen it needs in order to function. Within 20 to 40 seconds after cardiac arrest, the person is clinically dead. After 4 to 6 minutes, the lack of oxygen has caused permanent and extensive damage to the brain and the heart. "Cardiac arrest" is the term used to refer only to those situations in which the loss of heart action and breathing occurs without warning; it is immediate — not gradual — and it is unexpected. You would not refer to deaths resulting from other causes or from a lingering, fatal disease as cardiac arrest, even though the heart action does stop.

Causes of Cardiac Arrest

There are a number of conditions that can cause cardiac arrest by interfering with the normal function of the heart or lungs. The underlying reason for cardiac arrest is believed to be a lack of sufficient oxygen to the heart muscle. The heart attack, or myocardial infarction, is a common cause of cardiac arrest. In the heart attack, a segment of the heart muscle is deprived of its blood and oxygen supply. Without oxygen, the heart muscle cells begin to die. As more cells are affected, the heart beats erratically and loses its ability to keep blood circulating adequately in the body. Each year more than one million persons in the United States suffer heart attacks, and more than half of them die. Most of the deaths occur within two hours after the initial attack. Many of these victims of cardiac arrest are adults in the most productive years of their lives.

Other conditions that may lead to sudden death are associated with hypoventilation. An obstruction of the air passages, infections such as pneumonia, or injury to the chest and lungs all involve some degree of hypoventilation. The reduction in the amount of oxygen available for the body's use exposes the person to a greater risk of cardiac arrest. Extensive burns and hemorrhage that reduce the blood volume, drug intoxication, and metabolic or electrolyte imbalances also increase the risk of cardiac arrest. Electric shock, head injury, and damage to the central nervous system are other causes.

Signs of Cardiac Arrest

When cardiac arrest occurs, the signs of death appear almost immediately, just as if someone had pushed an "off" button. Circulation stops. The heartbeat and pulse are absent. Blood pressure falls to zero. The pupils of the eyes gradually dilate. Respirations cease, and the skin looks pale and greyish in color and feels cool. If respiratory arrest occurs first and

---

*American Heart Association and National Academy of Sciences. Standards for Cardiopulmonary Resuscitation (CPR) and Emergency Cardiac Care (ECC). *Journal of American Medical Association*, 277:850, February 18, 1974, p. 838.

the heart continues to beat, the skin color will be bluish or cyanotic. Respiratory arrest rapidly leads to cardiac arrest as a result of the lack of oxygen.

Monitored cardiac arrest generally occurs in hospital settings such as the coronary care or intensive care unit, where the heart action is monitored by ECG and the nurse or rescuer responds to the alarm or actually observes the arrest on the monitor screen. As in any emergency cardiac arrest, immediate resuscitation and other advanced life support measures must be initiated.

ITEM 2. THE PURPOSE OF CARDIOPULMONARY RESUSCITATION

The purpose of CPR is to provide basic life support. This means that it is aimed at maintaining the viability, or life, of the victim's central nervous system until the body recovers sufficiently to resume these functions. In other words, you must restore the circulation and breathing. This is done by ventilating the victim's lungs and keeping the circulation going via closed-chest compression until the person revives.

The success or failure of the CPR effort depends on the speed with which the victim's breathing and circulation are restored. The need for CPR is immediate when the person suffers a cardiac arrest. There is no time to waste looking for equipment or drugs, or trying to transport the victim to a doctor or a hospital. What is needed at that moment is someone who is trained and skilled in basic cardiac life support.

ITEM 3. BASIC CARDIAC LIFE SUPPORT

You are shopping in a department store, waiting for an elevator. The door of the elevator opens and you see passengers gathered around a man who had just collapsed to the floor. They say he is dead. What might you do? Could you carry out cardiopulmonary resuscitation? With prompt CPR, the man may revive and live for years longer.

Basic life support is an emergency measure that consists of recognizing respiratory and cardiac arrest and beginning CPR to maintain the victim's life. After the heart and respiratory functions have been restored, the victim is transported to the hospital for further treatment. When coming upon a victim who has collapsed and seems to be unconscious, the A-B-C steps of cardiopulmonary resuscitation should be carried out quickly and in the order given.

A (Airway)
    +   artificial ventilation
B (Breathing)

C (Circulation)   artificial circulation

Seconds count, and CPR should be started without delay: a delay of more than 4 minutes from the onset of cardiac arrest may result in permanent brain damage, if indeed the CPR is successful in reviving the patient at all. However, there are wide variations among people with respect to tolerating lack of oxygen, so it is essential to attempt basic CPR even when more than 4 minutes have elapsed.

Cardiopulmonary Resuscitation

It is important that you practice the steps of the CPR procedure and learn to perform them competently. In an emergency, your ability to carry out CPR may mean the difference between life and death. Follow these steps:

1. Establish the victim's unresponsiveness.

2. Call for help.

3. Turn victim on back.

4. Open the airway.

5. Check for breathing.

6. Give rescue breathing.

7. Establish the presence or absence of a pulse.

8. Correct placement of the hands.

9. Closed chest cardiac compression.

It is important to determine the victim's responsiveness immediately. If there is no response to shaking of the shoulder and a loud and urgent question, "Are you all right?" the unconscious person may be in need of CPR. Even though you don't see other people around, call for help anyway. Someone may hear you and be able to assist. When collapse occurs, most people fall face down, so it is necessary to turn them before you can begin CPR. This can best be done by kneeling beside the victim, supporting the neck, and rolling the head and upper torso as in log-rolling, so there is no twisting. With the victim lying flat on the back, you are ready to begin the A-B-C of CPR.

ITEM 4. A — OPEN THE AIRWAY

In the skill laboratory, practice the skills required to begin the cardiopulmonary resuscitation procedure. Some portions of the procedure covered in later items will require the use of the Resusci-Annie mannequin. Do not practice CPR on a live, healthy person; the compressions interefere with the normal function and rate of the heart and may produce harmful effects.

Given a person who has collapsed and lost consciousness and who has no breathing activity or pulse, carry out basic cardiopulmonary resuscitation.

⸻

Supplies Needed

Resusci-Annie type of mannequin   Alcohol sponges

⸻

Important Steps	Key Points
1. Remain with the victim and tell others to summon more help.	It is essential to begin CPR without delay. Skilled medical treatment will be needed when the patient revives.
2. Turn the patient onto his or her back.	Avoid twisting by supporting the neck and log-rolling the upper part of the body.
3. Open the airway. Tilt the patient's head back by a. placing one hand under the neck and lifting it;	Often, positioning to open the airway causes the person to resume breathing on his own.

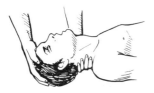

Opening airway in adult victim of cardiac arrest.

Important Steps	Key Points
b. pressing the forehead backward with your other hand.	*For infants and small children:* Avoid tilting the head back in extreme hyper-extension because this may collapse and obstruct the breathing passages. *For accident victims:* Tilting the neck back in hyperextension should be avoided when dealing with victims of diving or auto accidents in which a fracture of the neck is suspected. Avoid any movement of the neck. Immobilize the head in a neutral position with your hands at each side of the head. Place your fingers on the boney part of the jaw, not on the soft tissue. Lift the chin so that the teeth are brought close together, but don't completely close the mouth.

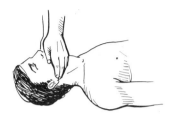

Immobilizing head and bringing chin forward when fracture of neck is suspected.

U
N
I
T
26

ITEM 5. B – BREATHING BY ARTIFICIAL VENTILATION

If the victim does not begin to breathe after the airway is open, artificial ventilation should be done at once. Practice doing mouth-to-mouth resuscitation using the Resusci-Annie or a similar type of mannequin.

Important Steps	Key Points
The first three steps were covered in Item 4.	
4. If the victim is not breathing, give mouth-to-mouth resuscitation.	Use the hand that had been pressing the forehead back. This helps prevent the escape of air during ventilation.
a. Pinch the nostrils shut.	Pinch the nostrils gently but firmly, or use your cheek to close off the nostrils.
b. Open your mouth wide and take a deep breath.	
c. Place your mouth tightly over the patient's mouth.	Make an airtight seal.
d. Blow your breath into the patient's mouth.	See the patient's chest rise as air fills the lungs; feel and hear the air as it is exhaled.
e. Remove your mouth and quickly take a breath of fresh air.	
f. Initially, repeat four times.	Do not wait for the lungs to deflate fully. This provides a supply of oxygen while you carry out the next steps of CPR.
g. Maintain a rate of 16 to 20 respirations per minute if external chest massage is not used.	The respiratory rate will be less when CPR is carried out by one person.

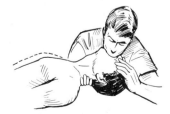

Mouth-to-mouth ventilation requires good airseal of nose and patient's mouth in order to inflate lungs.

OTHER METHODS OF VENTILATION

Artificial ventilation can also be accomplished by methods other than mouth-to-mouth. Mouth-to-nose ventilation is used when the mouth has been injured, when it is not possible to open the mouth, and when a tight seal around the mouth is difficult to achieve. With infants and children, the rescuer can cover both the mouth and nose of the victim with his own mouth. Smaller amounts of air are blown into the child's lungs and small puffs of air are used for infants — enough to raise the chest. Mouth-to-stoma ventilation is used for victims who have a permanent tracheostomy. In this case, it is not necessary to tilt the head and hyperextend the neck.

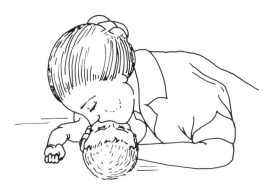

ITEM 6. C – ARTIFICIAL CIRCULATION

When you observe or are called to help an unconscious person who has probably had a cardiac arrest, first open the airway and feel for a pulse. Palpating the carotid artery for a pulse is recommended rather than trying to find a radial pulse at the wrist or a temporal pulse. The carotid arteries carry blood to the brain and the head, and a pulse can usually be felt here when other pulses have disappeared. The arteries are located on each side of the neck. The pulse can be most easily felt next to the larynx, or voice box. You should practice locating and palpating the carotid pulse on yourself and others.

Palpating the Carotid Artery

Important Steps	Key Points
5. Palpate the pulse.	Avoid compressing the artery and blocking out a weak pulse.

a. Locate the larynx. It is also called the "Adam's apple" or voice box. It is located in the front center of the neck.

b. Use the tips of your index and middle fingers.

c. Slide fingers alongside the larynx in the grooves formed by the muscles at the neck nearest you.

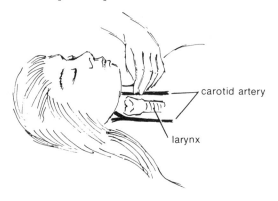

Palpating for carotid pulse.

External Chest Compressions

External chest compression is used to maintain the circulation of a cardiac arrest victim. By this method, a rhythmic pressure is applied over the lower portion of the sternum by using regular, smooth, and uninterrupted motions. This form of artificial circulation produces pulses in the body that can be felt and peaks in the systolic blood pressure over 100 mm Hg, even though diastolic pressure is zero and the carotid arteries carry about one-fourth the normal blood flow to the brain.

In the skill laboratory, practice the steps of external chest compression on the mannequin as you would perform it for a victim with no palpable carotid pulse. Do not practice chest compressions on healthy persons or non-victims, as it would interfere with the regular heart rate.

U
N
I
T
26

Important Steps	Key Points
For the first steps of the CPR procedure, refer to Item 4 and 5.	
6. If there is no carotid pulse, begin artificial circulation, using external chest compression.	If victim is in bed, insert a board under his back, full-length if possible.
a. Position yourself at the left side of the patient's chest.	You may need to get on the bed in order to compress the chest.
b. Locate the lower half of patient's sternum.	Hands are positioned two finger widths from tip of the sternum. Place a finger at the notch where the ribs meet the sternum; the other finger is placed next to the first one.
c. Place the heel of your hand over the lower half of the sternum, lengthwise next to the fingers.	Proper positioning of the hands prevents broken ribs and other injuries from excessive force.

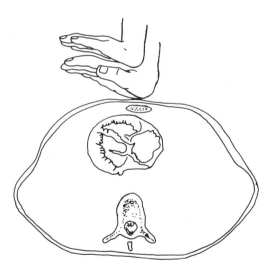

d. Put the heel of your second hand on top of the first, and move so that your shoulders are lengthwise over the patient's sternum.	Keep your arms straight and elbows locked and your fingers off the chest wall.

Important Steps	Key Points

e. Exert a firm, heavy force downward on the chest.

Adults: 80 to 120 pounds of pressure are required to depress the sternum 1½ to 2 inches. By using your entire weight, you should be able to compress the chest; this compresses the heart and forces blood into the arteries.

Children: apply pressure to the middle of the sternum and depress the chest ¾ to 1½ inch.

Infants: use the tips of your index and middle fingers to depress the sternum ½ to ¾ inch. Compress 80 to 100 times per minute.

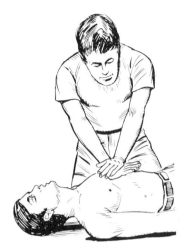

CPR by one rescuer.

f. Release the pressure, but do not remove your hands.

Develop a rhythm by pressing down with your body weight and then raising your shoulders up to allow the chest to expand and the blood to flow and fill the heart.

g. Continue compression at the rate of 80 per minute.

Continue until the patient revives or until you are relieved. Make the change without interrupting the rhythm. You will need to give two lung inflations after every 15 compressions.

h. After each minute, quickly check for the return of the carotid pulse and spontaneous breathing.

Never interrupt CPR for more than 5 seconds.

ITEM 7. BASIC CPR BY ONE PERSON

Basic cardiopulmonary resuscitation carried out by one person until additional help arrives on the scene is life-supporting and essential for the possible survival of the victim of cardiac arrest. The outline of entire basic CPR procedure follows.

1. Remain with the victim and have others summon more help.

2. Turn the patient on back.

3. Open the airway.

4. If the victim is not breathing, give four quick ventilations by using mouth-to-mouth resuscitation.

5. Palpate the carotid pulse. If it is absent, begin artificial circulation using external chest compression.

6. After every series of 15 compressions, give two quick lung inflations.

The ratio of compressions to ventilations is 15 to 2, with 80 compressions per minute.

If you are still alone, continue CPR for at least four to five minutes, then quickly phone for help from the emergency system. If a phone is not readily available, continue CPR until the victim revives or as long as you are able.

ITEM 8.   BASIC CPR BY TWO PERSONS

Basic resuscitation is easier to carry out with two rescuers. When help arrives, one rescuer continues with chest compression and the other gives artificial ventilation. Two people can continue CPR for several hours if necessary; they can change positions when the one who is doing the chest compressions becomes fatigued. The unusual position required for the hands causes strain when artificial circulation must be maintained over a period of time.

Two rescuers carry out the basic CPR procedure. The first rescuer delivers one ventilation between the fifth compression and the one following it. The compression rate is 60 per minute and the ratio of compressions to ventilations is 5 to 1.

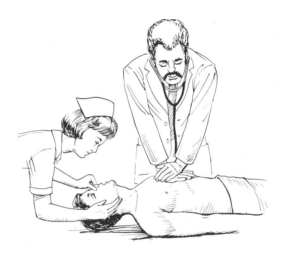

CPR by two rescuers.

ITEM 9.   CPR IN THE HOSPITAL SETTING

Cardiac arrest can occur in patients who are already in the hospital for the treatment of some other illness or injury. Patients with conditions known to have a greater risk of cardiac arrest are generally treated in special areas such as the coronary care unit and the intensive care unit. Here the patients are under the close observation of skilled nurses and doctors. Monitors are used to keep continuous track of the patient's vital signs — heart action, rate, and blood pressures such as the central venous pressure or the pulmonary arterial pressures. The detection of early changes in heart and lung functions and prompt treatment of the causes can prevent the disaster of cardiac arrest.

When arrest does occur in the hospital, basic CPR is started immediately by a trained person while the CPR team is summoned. Many hospitals use the loudspeaker or paging system, and the call "Code Blue — CCU" or "Doctor Blue — CCU" to alert members of the CPR team that a cardiac arrest has occurred and to tell them where.

The CPR tream consists of doctors and nurses who have had special training in basic and advanced methods of cardiopulmonary resuscitation. They make use of specialized equipment and various drugs to resuscitate and begin treatment of the underlying cause. An emergency cart containing all the supplies and equipment required in advanced resuscitation is rushed to the scene of the cardiac arrest. The CPR team takes over and relieves the person who has been carrying out the basic CPR.

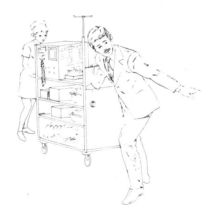

Hospital CPR team springing into action.

As a beginning worker, find out the policy of your hospital or agency regarding what is expected of you in situations where a cardiac arrest has occurred. If there is no policy, these three principles can serve as your guidelines:

1. Act to save a life.

2. Perform what you have been taught or know how to do.

3. Call for help and let the more highly trained and skilled persons take over.

ITEM 10. FOREIGN BODY OBSTRUCTION OF THE AIRWAY

An obstruction of the air passages will prevent the air from reaching the victim's lungs. When there is an obstruction, the chest neither rises with a ventilation breath nor falls when air escapes. The rescuer feels increased resistance while forcing air into the patient's mouth. There is no sound or feeling of air escaping during the exhaling phase.

The vast majority of upper airway obstructions are easily corrected, but they can cause unconsciousness and cardiopulmonary arrest. However, about 3000 people die annually as a result of foreign body obstruction, so it is important that you learn the technique for rescuing these victims.

Foreign body obstructions generally are caused by food; meat is often the culprit, although other foods are also involved. The symptoms resemble those of a heart attack and, since it often occurs when the victim is eating out in restaurants, it has been dubbed the "cafe coronary."

With complete obstruction of the air passages, the victim is unable to talk, breathe, or cough. The universal distress signal is clutching at the throat. With partial obstruction, the victim is able to breathe and is said to have "good air exchange," which permits a forceful cough that may expel the object. The person with "poor air exchange" is unable to cough effectively, has a crowing type of wheezing, and may exhibit increased respiratory distress and cyanosis. This condition should be treated as if it were a complete airway obstruction.

Maneuvers to Remove Obstructions

Airway obstructions caused by foreign bodies may be removed manually by (1) back blows, (2) manual thrusts, and (3) finger probes. Although the back blows and manual thrusts may not relieve the obstruction initially, they should be repeated. As the muscles become more deprived of oxygen, they relax, so the maneuvers may become more effective or the airway may partially open.

Back Blows. For the victim in a standing, sitting, or lying position, deliver four sharp blows in rapid succession, using the heel of your hand. Do not hold a child upside down when delivering back blows unless he is completely obstructed.

Manual Thrusts. To perform manual thrusts, make a fist and press it into the upper abdomen or lower chest in a series of four rapid thrusts to force air out of the lungs. The rush of air helps expel the obstructing body. To perform the abdominal thrust on a standing or sitting victim, stand behind and wrap your arms around the victim's waist. Place the thumb side of your fist above the navel, grasp the fist with the other hand and press it quickly with an upward thrust into the abdomen four times. If the victim is lying down on his or her back, the rescuer straddles the hips or thighs and presses a quick upward thrust into the abdomen.

Lower chest thrust may be used instead of the abdominal thrusts. In this maneuver, stand behind the victim, put your arms under the arms and encircle the chest. Place the thumb side of your fist against the sternum, grasp with the other hand, and make four quick backward thrusts. If the victim is lying down, compress the chest cavity with four external cardiac compressions as used in the CPR procedure.

The Finger Probe. Open the mouth by grasping the lower jaw and tongue and lifting the jaw forward. This removes the tongue from the back of the throat. If this action does not remove the obstruction, run your finger around the inside of the cheek and the base of the tongue and use a hooking action to dislodge the foreign body for removal.

Important Steps	Key Points

Procedure for the Conscious Victim

1. Ask the victim to speak. If unable, proceed with the maneuvers.

2. Give four back blows.

3. Give four manual thrusts.

4. Repeat steps 2 and 3 until the foreign body is removed or the victim is unconscious.

Procedure for the Unconscious Victim

1. Call for help and establish an airway.

2. Position the head and attempt to ventilate.

3. Deliver four back blows.

4. Give four manual thrusts.

5. Do the finger probe.

6. Attempt to ventilate. If unable to do so, repeat steps 3, 4, and 5 until they are effective.

Key Points:

(step 1) If the victim can speak, do not interfere with his or her efforts to clear the airway.

(step 4) Use either abdominal or chest thrusts.

(step 6) Remove any foreign object or stomach contents that may have been regurgitated. Perform mouth-to-mouth ventilation, unless the victim begins breathing spontaneously.

PERFORMANCE TEST

In the classroom or your skill laboratory, your instructor will ask that cardiopulmonary resuscitation be performed in pairs. Using the mannequin, you and your partner will demonstrate the procedure and then change positions. Each of you will demonstrate skill in performing artificial ventilation and artificial circulation.

Given a person who has suffered a cardiac arrest, is unconscious, has no pulse, and is not breathing, you and another rescuer are to give basic cardiopulmonary resuscitation.

PERFORMANCE CHECKLIST

BASIC CARDIOPULMONARY RESUSCITATION

1. Check for responses by shaking the victim's shoulder and asking, "Are you O.K.?" If not, continue with CPR.

2. Remain with the victim and have others summon more help.

3. Turn the patient on his back.

4. Open the airway.

   a. Tilt his head back.

   b. Place your hand under his neck and lift it.

   c. Press his forehead backward with your other hand.

5. If breathing is absent, give mouth-to-mouth resuscitation.

   a. Pinch his nostrils shut.

   b. Open your mouth and take a deep breath.

   c. Make an airtight seal over the patient's mouth with your own.

   d. Forcefully exhale into the patient's mouth.

   e. Remove your mouth and allow the patient to exhale.

   f. Repeat four times initially and then between every fifth compression and the one following it.

6. If carotid pulse is absent, maintain artificial circulation using external chest compression.

   a. Position yourself on the left side of the patient's chest.

   b. Locate the lower half of sternum.

   c. Place the heel of your hand over the lower half of sternum.

   d. Keep your fingers elevated from chest wall.

   e. Put the heel of your other hand on top of the first hand and lean forward so that your shoulders are parallel to and above the patient's sternum.

   f. Exert firm force downward to depress the sternum 1½ to 2 inches.

   g. Release the pressure, but keep your hands in place.

   h. Repeat steps f and g for a compression rate of 80 times per minute with one rescuer, or 60 compressions with two rescuers.

POST-TEST

Multiple Choice. For each of the test questions, there is one correct or best answer. Indicate the answer you have selected.

1. All but one of the following events happen when a person suffers a cardiac arrest. Which one does not apply?

   a. The person's circulation stops.

   b. The pulses in the body are absent.

   c. Systolic pressure is 100 and diastolic is zero.

   d. All respirations cease.

2. "Cardiac arrest" is a term that means all but which one of the following?

   a. Any death when the heart stops.

   b. Death due to a heart attack.

   c. An immediate and unexpected death.

   d. Sudden death.

3. Brain tissue is less able to tolerate a lack of oxygen than some other body tissues. Permanent damage results when the brain is deprived of oxygen for more than

   a. 20 to 40 seconds.

   b. 1 to 2 minutes.

   c. 2 to 4 minutes.

   d. 4 to 6 minutes.

4. If you are called to assist a person who has collapsed and lost consciousness, the first thing you should do is to

   a. look for injuries from the fall.

   b. establish an open airway.

   c. determine if the victim is unresponsive.

   d. provide warmth and treat for shock.

5. In many cases, the simplest method for opening the airway is

   a. tilting the victim's head back.

   b. wiping out the mouth and throat.

   c. striking the victim on the back.

   d. turning the head to one side.

6. When opening the airway of an infant, do not hyperextend the neck by tilting the head back because it

   a. causes the tongue to block the back of the throat.

   b. may obstruct or collapse the trachea.

   c. prevents making an effective seal around the mouth.

   d. leads to the accumulation of salivary secretions.

7. In giving mouth-to-mouth resuscitation to an adult, the recommended position for the patient is

    a. with the head tilted backward and the lower jaw raised.

    b. lying prone on a hard surface.

    c. lying supine on a soft surface.

    d. in Sims' position with the head turned to the side.

8. The basic underlying cause of cardiac arrest is believed to be

    a. infection of the lungs.

    b. lack of oxygen.

    c. blood clot in the brain.

    d. any disease of the heart.

9. Following a cardiac arrest, the clinical signs of death are seen within

    a. 20 to 40 seconds.

    b. 1 to 2 minutes.

    c. 2 to 4 minutes.

    d. 4 to 6 minutes.

10. The purpose of cardiopulmonary resuscitation is to

    a. give artificial ventilation.

    b. give artificial circulation.

    c. provide basic life support.

    d. stimulate the central nervous system.

11. When giving artificial ventilation, signs that the air passages are open include all of the following *except*

    a. air can be felt rushing out of the victim.

    b. you can hear the air escape when the lungs deflate.

    c. the sternum is depressed 1½ to 2 inches.

    d. the chest rises with each ventilation.

12. The number of ventilations used to inflate the lungs at the beginning of CPR is

    a. one breath.

    b. two breaths.

    c. three breaths.

    d. four breaths.

13. The indication for starting artificial circulation is

    a. contracted pupils.

    b. blood pressure of 100/0.

    c. absence of respirations.

    d. absence of carotid pulse.

14. As a result of external chest compression, the blood flow to the brain is

    a. fully restored.

    b. one-half of normal.

    c. one-fourth of normal.

    d. diverted to the heart.

15. While performing artificial circulation, the CPR rescuer applies pressure to what portion of the chest?

    a. the xiphoid process of the sternum

    b. the lower half of the sternum

    c. the left side of the chest

    d. the right side of the chest

16. When giving CPR to an infant, the rescuer would compress the chest using

    a. the index and middle fingers.

    b. the heel of one hand.

    c. the fleshy, bottom part of the fist.

    d. both hands as with an adult.

17. A force of 80 to 120 pounds is required during artificial circulation in order to compress the adult's chest how much?

    a. ½ to ¾ inches

    b. ¾ to 1½ inches

    c. 1½ to 2 inches

    d. 2 to 4 inches

18. When CPR is performed by one rescuer, after the initial ventilation the ratio of breaths to compression is

    a. 1 breath, 5 compressions.

    b. 2 breaths, 5 compressions.

    c. 1 breath, 15 compressions.

    d. 2 breaths, 15 compressions.

19. The ratio of compressions to ventilations when CPR is given by two people is

    a. 1 breath, 5 compressions.

    b. 1 breath, 15 compressions.

    c. 2 breaths, 5 compressions.

    d. 4 breaths, 15 compressions.

20. The hospital CPR team is highly skilled and trained in the use of

    a. basic CPR methods.

    b. advanced CPR methods.

    c. cardiac drugs and equipment.

    d. all of the above.

    e. all but a.

UNIT 26

POST-TEST ANSWERS

1. c	11. c
2. a	12. d
3. d	13. d
4. c	14. c
5. a	15. b
6. b	16. a
7. a	17. c
8. b	18. d
9. a	19. a
10. c	20. d

ASSISTING WITH SPIRITUAL CARE

GENERAL PERFORMANCE OBJECTIVES

Upon completing this lesson, you will be able to obtain the services of the clergyman for the patient's spiritual needs, provide for the observance of certain religious practices, and help the clergyman as may be needed. You will be expected to show respect for the patient's religious beliefs even though these may differ from your own.

SPECIFIC PERFORMANCE OBJECTIVES

When you have finished this unit you will be able to:

1. Call the religious representative requested or designated by the patient.

2. Assist patients to observe certain religious practices during their stay in the hospital if they wish.

3. Show your concern for the religious articles belonging to the patient by handling them respectfully and providing for their safekeeping.

4. Demonstrate respect for the patient's religious beliefs in all aspects of your conduct.

VOCABULARY

anointing of the sick—a Roman Catholic sacrament performed by the priest with prayers for recovery and salvation for a critically ill person or one in danger of dying; formerly called the last rites or extreme unction.

agnostic—one who believes that the existence of God or any supreme being is unknown and probably unknowable.

atheist—one who denies the existence of God and rejects all religious faith and practice.

baptism—a sacrament signifying spiritual rebirth and admission into the Christian community through the ritual use of water; many Christian faiths require one to be baptized before death in order to attain grace or to be saved.

chaplain—a clergyman serving the spititual needs of members of an organization or institution such as a hospital, college, or military unit, regardless of denomination.

clergy—ordained Christian ministers, those ordained to perform ministrations in the church.

communion—

(a) Catholic (Roman and Greek): the sacrament of the eucharist; partaking of a small wafer or piece of unleavened bread that symbolizes the body of Christ.

(b) Protestant: the sacrament of receiving both the unleavened wafer of bread and a drink of wine that symbolize the body and the blood of Christ.

pastor, priest, rabbi—a clergyman; a religious leader of a congregation who guides the spiritual lives of its members.

sacrament—a formal religious ceremony that is sacred; it is performed as a symbol of a spiritual reality, especially those instituted by Christ as a means of grace.

(a) Protestant: two sacraments are generally recognized — baptism and communion.

(b) Catholic: seven sacraments — baptism, confirmation, communion, penance, marriage, anointing the sick, and holy orders.

INTRODUCTION

The meaning of religion and God varies among the people of the world. We know that among many religions, and even among followers of the same religion, observance and interpretation of the religious doctrine differ widely. One person may be an active member of an organized religious institution, such as a church or synagogue; another may simply hold a general belief in God or a Supreme Being. Some people may claim to be agnostic or atheistic. The point to remember is that the individual's religious belief or lack of it is a matter of personal choice.

Patients bring with them their religious beliefs and needs as well as health needs when ill. Because an illness, an operation, or an injury often represents a possible threat to life, they may turn to religion for comfort and reassurance. Their mental and emotional reactions are related to and have a profound effect on their physical health. Therefore, we must be concerned with helping them to obtain support and peace of mind through their religious beliefs.

As a nurse, you should respect the patient's beliefs even though these may differ from your own. Avoid arguing points of religion or trying to convert the patient to your own views. It is very important for many patients to talk about their faith and fears when they are facing the stress of illness or surgery. Their fears may have many aspects; fear of pain, of disfigurement, of never being the same again, or of death. The chaplain or minister is a valuable member of the health team because of his or her skill in providing spiritual support for patients who want it. The nurse can also help by listening and helping patients express their feelings. Most health workers find it difficult in the beginning to listen and discuss topics like death because this subject is generally avoided in our society. It becomes easier to handle when you are able to accept the patient's right to have certain feelings; then you can proceed from there to talk about possible causes for these feelings. Usually, talking about such fears with someone who does not reject or judge them makes the fears less threatening. As you talk with patients about their feelings, it might be appropriate to ask if they would like to have a chaplain or clergyman visit them. The decision should rest with the patient.

SPIRITUAL CARE AND HEALTH CARE

ITEM 1. CARE OF RELIGIOUS ARTICLES

Many patients bring some religious articles with them when they come to the hospital. Although these articles may not seem important to you, they hold great significance for the person who owns them. Be sure to treat these possessions with respect and be careful not to drop or misplace them.

Patients who are members of the Catholic faith usually bring crucifixes, religious medals, and rosaries with them. Often the Catholic patient wishes to wear a medal, but if it is pinned to the hospital gown, it may be lost when the gown is changed. It would be better to tape or tie the medal to the patient's wrist in order to keep it from being lost.

Protestant patients may bring a Bible, prayer book or other religious reading materials to the hospital with them. Orthodox and Conservative Jewish men may wear a skull cap (yarmulke) during their daily prayers while they are in the hospital.

ITEM 2. DIETARY REGULATIONS

Certain religious denominations follow special dietary customs. Some of the most common customs you will encounter are described below:

Catholic: Although the Catholic Church has relaxed its dietary regulations, many Roman Catholics still do not eat meat on Fridays and on other specified days.

Protestant: Dietary restrictions vary among denominations, and many have no restrictions that would affect the hospitalized patient. Some, such as the Seventh Day Adventists, are vegetarians (eat no meat) and do not drink stimulants such as coffee, tea, or liquor. Other denominations prohibit smoking, or drinking of alcoholic beverages.

Jewish: Jewish doctrine (law) forbids eating pork and shellfish. Orthodox Jews (strict in observance of law and tradition) eat only kosher foods that are prepared in a manner prescribed by Judaic law. Foods containing milk are not eaten at the same meal with meat. Conservative Jews observe slightly modified dietary regulations and are somewhat less strict in their observances. Reform Jews have no dietary restrictions; their practice of Judaism can be described as a simplified and liberal approach and belief.

U
N
I
T
27

ITEM 3. REQUESTS FOR A VISIT BY A CLERGYMAN

The chaplain on the staff of a health agency provides spiritual service for patients on a nondenominational basis. If your agency does not have a resident chaplain, the patient may ask you to have a Protestant minister, a priest, or rabbi, or another religious representative come to visit. After the patient makes his request, call a local church or temple as indicated by the request and ask that one of its clergymen visit the patient. Many patients will request a visit from a specific priest, minister, or rabbi. In that case, you would obtain the necessary information about the name, the church or temple represented and its location.

When making a call to ask a clergyman to visit a patient, you should have the following information:

a. The clergyman — specified by denomination, church or temple, or name.

b. The patient — name and room number, the name of the hospital or agency, and a general statement about his or her condition, for example, whether critically ill or scheduled to undergo surgery.

c. The service to be performed — a general visit or an administration of the sacraments of communion, baptism, or anointing of the sick (extreme unction).

After you have called, tell the patient that you have contacted the clergyman and give the name and approximate time of the visit if this is known. By reporting back to the patients you are letting them know that they can depend on you and that you are concerned about their needs.

ITEM 4. HOW TO ADDRESS A MEMBER OF THE CLERGY

Most clergymen introduce themselves when they arrive at a hospital or agency to see a patient, and they give their title as well as their name so you will know how they are addressed. However, if you are in doubt as to what to call a Protestant minister, the title of Pastor or Mister is customarily used with the surname. Those with a doctor of philosophy degree would be called "Doctor." The title "Reverend" is often used incorrectly to address Protestant clergymen.

The Catholic priest is addressed as "Father" and some Episcopal ministers may also use this title. Jewish clergymen are called "Rabbi," which means master or teacher. Rabbis who have a doctoral degree would be addressed with the title of "Doctor." Any clergyman appointed to serve members of an organization such as a hospital or military unit may be called "Chaplain."

ITEM 5. THE SACRAMENT OF COMMUNION

As stated earlier, communion is an important sacrament of the Christian faith. It is a spiritual reconfirmation or rededication of faith that provides great consolation for the patient.

In most Catholic hospitals, communion is given daily to those Catholic patients who desire it. Each hospital has a procedure for notifying the priest about patients requesting communion, such as a list that gives the name of the patient and the room number. Catholic patients usually take communion before surgery and during any serious illness. In other hospitals communion is given on a PRN (as needed) basis or as requested by the patient. The priest or minister will generally bring whatever is needed for the celebration of communion.

The following procedure is generally used in Catholic hospitals and other agencies to prepare the patient for communion, especially when the priest will be administering the sacrament to a number of patients.

Supplies Needed

Face towel	Glass of water
Teaspoon	

Important Steps	Key Points
1. Obtain the items needed.	Universal Steps A, B, C, and D. See Appendix.
2. Wash your hands.	
3. Approach and identify the patient.	
4. Provide for privacy.	
5. Prepare the patient.	Offer the bedpan or urinal or assist to the bathroom, if permitted. Provide washcloth for washing hands and face. Place in supine or semi-Fowler position for comfort.
6. Prepare a work space for the clergyman to conduct communion.	Provide a clear area on the bedside stand or overbed table for the articles used in the sacrament. Cover the table with a clean towel. Place a teaspoon and another folded towel neatly on the towel. (The teaspoon and extra towel may be optional; check your agency procedure.) The towel is used by either the clergyman or the patient if needed. The clergyman will place his special kit on the work area. A glass of water may be needed to assist the patient in swallowing the water or unleavened bread.

Important Steps	Key Points
7. Leave the immediate area, unless requested to stay to assist the patient.	Allow the patient and priest (or minister) privacy, since confession may precede the sacrament of communion. Following communion, the priest or minister will probably offer a short prayer. Often the patient will meditate or nap following communion.
8. After the sacrament is over and the priest has gone, tidy the room and provide for the patient's comfort.	Universal Steps X, Y, and Z. See Appendix.
9. Record on the patient's chart.	Charting example: 0730. Communion given by Father John. <div align="right">J. Jones, SN</div>

U
N
I
T
27

ITEM 6. THE SACRAMENT OF BAPTISM

Baptism is a sacrament practiced by the members of the Catholic and many Protestant faiths. In being baptized, the participant pledges to observe the precepts of his faith and thereby becomes a full member of the religion. According to most Christian beliefs, it is essential for an individual to be baptized before dying in order to attain salvation.

In the hospital, the sacrament of baptism is important when a patient, usually a newborn baby, is in the danger of dying. When a baby is born to Catholic parents, the nurse should be prepared to baptize the baby in the absence of a clergyman. Some Protestant parents may also request that the baby be baptized when his or her life is in danger. The following procedure is used for baptism.

IIIIIIIIIIIIIIIIIIIIIIIIIIIIIIIIIIIIIIIIIIIIIIIIIIIIIIIIIIIIIIIIIIIIIIIIIIIIIIIIIIIIIIIIIIIIIIIIIIIIIIIIIIIIIIIIIIIIIIIIIIIIIIIIIII

Supplies Needed

Baptism tray with shallow basin   Face towel
   and bottle of holy water.

IIIIIIIIIIIIIIIIIIIIIIIIIIIIIIIIIIIIIIIIIIIIIIIIIIIIIIIIIIIIIIIIIIIIIIIIIIIIIIIIIIIIIIIIIIIIIIIIIIIIIIIIIIIIIIIIIIIIIIIIIIIIIIIIIII

Important Steps	Key Points
Carry out Universal Steps A, B, C, and D. See Appendix.	
1. Obtain the baptism tray and place it on a table cleared for that purpose.	Some hospitals use a baptism tray, which contains a vessel or shallow basin and a bottle of holy water (water that has been blessed by a priest).
2. Pour a small amount of holy water into the vessel.	The clergyman who is baptizing the patient will do this; otherwise you would do so.
3. Sprinkle a few drops of water on the patient's head to baptize.	The clergyman, or you, would then say the words, "I baptize thee in the name of the Father, and of the Son, and of the Holy Ghost. Amen."

Important Steps	Key Points
	If the infant is Catholic, it is preferable that a Catholic nurse baptizes him or her; however, anyone can do it. The important point is that the child is baptized.
Carry out Universal Steps X, Y, and Z. See Appendix.	Charting example: 1950. Baptized by Chaplain Miller. B. Walls, SN

ITEM 7. ANOINTING OF THE SICK

This is a Catholic sacrament of utmost importance to the Catholic patient because it is intended to prepare the soul for life after death. This sacrament is administered only once during a critical illness or a period of illness when there is danger to the patient's life (e.g., the very aged person), but it can be given several times during one's life. If a Catholic patient dies without receiving this sacrament, the priest should be notified promptly to determine whether the sacrament can still be given.

The following procedure is used in preparing the patient for the sacrament of anointing of the sick.

Important Steps	Key Points
Carry out Universal Steps A, B, C, and D. See Appendix.	
1. Remain with the patient and the priest.	You may be needed for assistance. Fold back the bed covers to expose the patient's feet. Stand respectfully at the foot of the bed.
2. The priest anoints the patient.	He will use oil to anoint the patient's forehead, eyes, nose, mouth, hands, and feet.
Carry out Universal Steps X, Y, and Z. See Appendix.	Charting example: 0100. Sacrament of anointing the sick by Father John. B. Walls, SN

ITEM 8. THE JEWISH RITE OF CIRCUMCISION

The Jewish rite of circumcising the male baby is performed much less frequently in hospitals than it was previously, when mothers and babies stayed for a week or longer after the baby's birth. Some Jewish mothers do not have their baby sons circumcised before taking them home so that the religious rites can be observed later, when the baby is about eight days old.

Circumcision is a surgical procedure of cutting away a portion of the prepuce, or foreskin, of the penis for the purpose of cleanliness. In the Jewish faith, it is a method of purification and is usually done on the 8th day after the baby's birth. Frequently a Mohel (one who has specifically trained for this procedure) performs the circumcision before a prescribed number of witnesses. Following the ceremony, there is usually a celebration at which wine and cakes are served to family and friends.

ITEM 9. THE MOSLEM RITE OF CIRCUMCISION

The Moslems also circumcise (Sunnat) their infants, although it may be done any time during a lifetime.

ITEM 10.   OTHER RELIGIOUS BELIEFS AFFECTING HEALTH CARE

As part of your job, you may come into contact with patients who have beliefs (religious or personal) different from those previously mentioned. Many individuals and religions stress the "natural order" of life. The "natural order" is a philosophy that believes that our existence depends on the balance found in nature or the environment. Many of these beliefs are beneficial to the health of individuals, but a few may pose problems in the realm of health care.

One belief that you may encounter is that of the Jehovah's Witnesses, which forbids the use of blood transfusions. A patient who holds this belief will refuse to have surgery that may require blood transfusions or transfusion for medical reasons, even though it is a matter of life and death.

Christian Scientists also stress the natural order and the positive power of faith. On becoming sick or disabled, some followers of this religion put off seeking medical help until the illness or disability becomes quite far advanced.

These are two examples of religious beliefs that may pose difficulties in matters of health care. However, people have a right to their beliefs and a right to refuse treatment that is contrary to their beliefs.

UNIT 27

PERFORMANCE TEST

In the classroom or skill laboratory your instructor will ask you to demonstrate your skill in carrying out the following procedures without reference to your lesson guide, notes, or other source material.

1. Given a Protestant patient who has requested to see a Methodist minister before going to surgery in two days, you are to make a phone call and provide the minister with the necessary information.

2. Given a critically ill Catholic patient whose family has requested that the priest be called to give the sacraments, you are to prepare the patient and assist as may be necessary in the sacrament of anointing of the sick.

3. Describe for your instructor what you might say and do in the following situations:

   a. An Orthodox Jewish patient eats only kosher foods and your hospital has no way of providing kosher foods although it does have a selective menu for patients.

   b. A Catholic patient has been prepared for surgery (had all jewelry, false teeth, and so forth removed) but wants to wear a certain religious medal to surgery for spiritual protection.

PERFORMANCE CHECKLIST

CALLING A CLERGYMAN

1. Look up the name of the church of the proper denomination in the phone book or in a list provided by the agency.

2. Make the phone call and identify yourself.

3. State the purpose of the call. (The following information may be in any order.)

   a. Give the name and the room number of the patient.

   b. State the name of the hospital.

   c. State that the patient will be going to surgery in two days.

   d. State that the patient wishes to see the clergyman before surgery.

   e. Make a statement about the general condition of the patient.

4. Obtain the name of the clergyman who will visit and the approximate time of his or her arrival.

5. Report back to the patient that the call has been made, the name of the person and the time of the visit.

6. Record the activity on the nurses' notes.

THE SACRAMENT OF ANOINTING THE SICK

1. Approach the patient and explain that the priest will give the sacrament.

2. Have the patient void and wash hands and face; assist as needed.

3. Place the patient in a comfortable position — supine or semi-Fowler.

4. Pull the curtain to provide privacy.

5. Clear a space for the sacramental articles and place a towel as a cover. Provide a teaspoon and a second towel if this is part of the agency's procedure.

6. Fold back the bed covers to expose the patient's feet.

7. Stand by respectfully as the priest gives the sacrament.

8. Replace the top bed covers over the patient's feet after the sacrament.

9. Dispose of soiled linen, clean and return the teaspoon to the proper area, and tidy the room.

10. Attend to the needs and comfort of the patient. (Ask if there is anything the patient needs.)

11. Record the sacrament of anointing the sick on the patient's chart with the time and the name of priest.

DISCUSSION OF SITUATIONS

1. The Jewish patient who eats kosher foods.

   a. Show respect for the other's religious beliefs by discussing alternative ways of meeting dietary needs.

   b. Might allow the patient's family to bring in some kosher-prepared food (check with agency procedure).

   c. Help the patient to select foods from the menu that can be eaten, such as fruits and vegetables with milk dishes at one meal, and with meat dishes at the next meal.

   d. Other alternatives include having food sent in from a kosher restaurant, "meals on wheels," or a commercial source.

2. The Catholic patient wearing a medal to surgery.

   a. May be able to tape the medal to the patient's wrist unless it would be in the area where surgery is to be done.

   b. Show respect for the other's religious beliefs by discussing alternative ways of meeting the patient's needs.

   c. Can discuss with the patient other ways in which spiritual needs could be met, such as a visit with a priest, and the taking of sacraments before surgery.

   d. Other possible ways suggested by the student.

U
N
I
T
27

Section 5

SKILLS RELATED TO MEDICAL THERAPY

INTRODUCTION

Most of the physician's orders for the treatment of a patient's condition are carried out by nurses. These orders are an essential part of the total nursing care of the patient and require your skills and competence. Some of the skills are relatively simple to perform, such as filling a bag with hot water to place on the patient's sore shoulder or to warm cold feet, but all nurses are expected to avoid burning the patient and to know which patients are less able to tolerate temperatures of water in the hot range. Other procedures, such as medical isolation precautions and preoperative and postoperative care, are more complex. They are based on the principles and rationale of fundamental skills and are used to meet the special needs of patients with infectious disease and those undergoing a surgical procedure.

Units 28 and 29, on pre- and postoperative care, describe the responsibilities of the nurse for the surgical patient. They outline the methods of preparing the patient and completing the hospital records necessary for surgery, and then for providing nursing care to the patient recovering from the effects of surgery while in the recovery room or in a bed on the nursing unit. Safety belts, jackets, and wrist holders are sometimes needed for the protection of the patient; these are described in Unit 30.

Although students in nursing programs leading to licensure and nurses practicing as LPNS, LVNS, or RNS may be expected to take more responsibilities for some aspects of the procedures, all beginning nurses must know how to care for patients who are being treated with oxygen, IV infusions, or a nasogastric tube attached to suction. Units 31, 32, and 33 describe the purposes for these procedures, the problems or symptoms indicating the need for the treatment, and the precautions to be followed. Unit 34 provides rationale and procedures for the use of hot and cold applications. Step-by-step instructions in the application of bandages and binders are given in Unit 35. The differences between medical and surgical asepsis are analyzed in Unit 36, which also includes procedures for maintaining medical isolation precautions. Finally, Unit 37 talks about caring for the dying patient, understanding one's own feelings about death, and preparing the patient's body for the morgue.

DIRECTIONS FOR THE STUDENTS

Study the units as you have previously. Whenever possible, practice the procedures in the skills laboratory before trying to do them in the clinical setting. When you feel confident that you know how to perform the procedure and the rationale or reason for the various steps, notify your instructor and arrange to take the performance test. It is suggested that the first time you perform the procedure for a patient, it should be under the supervision of your instructor or another designed nurse. You may want to review the steps of the procedure in the Performance Checklist before proceeding to the patient's bedside to carry it out.

The post-tests consist of questions that seek to test your knowledge and understanding of facts, principles, rationale, and relationships regarding the patients needs and the procedures.

SELECTED REFERENCES

Unit 28: Preoperative Care

Coburn, Dorothy: Anticipating breast surgery. Am J Nurs 75:1483-1485 (September) 1975.
MacClelland, Doris C.: Are current skin preparations valid? AORN Journal 21:55-60 (January) 1975.
Preop teaching helps. Nursing 80 10:90-91 (March) 1980.
Rayder, Melinda: A new nurse asks why properative teaching isn't done. Am J Nurs 79:1992-1995 (November) 1979.

Unit 29: Postoperative Care

Bouvett, Jeane Marie: Preoperative and postoperative care of patient with cerebral aneurysms. Nurs Clin North Am 9:655-666 (December) 1974.
Croushore, T.: Postoperative assessment: The key to avoiding the most common nursing mistakes. Nursing 79 9:47-51 (April) 1979.
Johnson, Marion: Outcome criteria to evaluate postoperative respiratory status. Am J Nurs 75:1474-1475 (September) 1975.
McConnell, Edwina: After surgery, Nursing 77 7:32-39 (March) 1977.
Metheny, Norma A.: Water and electrolyte balance in the postoperative patient. Nurs Clin North Am 10:49-57 (March) 1975.
Smith, Betty J.: Safeguarding your patient after anesthesia. Nursing 78 8:53-56 (October) 1978.
Steele, Bonnie: Test your knowledge of postoperative pain management. Nursing 80 10:76-78 (March) 1980.

Unit 31: Oxygen Therapy

Dingle, Rebecca, et al.: Continuous transcutaneous O_2 monitoring in the neonate. Am J Nurs 80:890-893 (May) 1980.
Felton, Cynthia: Hypoxemia and oral temperatures. Am J Nurs 78:56-57 (January) 1978.
Luckmann, Joan, and Sorenson, Karen: Medical Surgical Nursing: A Psychophysiologic Approach. Philadelphia: W.B. Saunders Company, 1974, pp. 884-936.
Nursing Grand Rounds: Adult respiratory distress syndrome: A true test of nursing skills. Nursing 80 10:51-57 (May) 1980.
Rifas, Ellene: How you and your patient . . . can manage dyspnea. Nursing 80 10:34-41 (June) 1980.
Segal, Sydney: Oxygen: too much, too little. Nurs Clin North Am 6:39-54 (March) 1971.

Unit 32: Assisting with Intravenous Therapy

Beaumont, Estelle: The new IV infusion pumps. Nursing 77 7:31-35 (July) 1977.
Buickus, Barbara A.: Administering blood components. Am J Nurs 79:937-941 (May) 1979.
Cullins, Laura C.: Preventing and treating transfusion reactions. Am J Nurs 79:935-936 (May) 1979.
Fundamentals of IV maintenance. A programmed unit. Am J Nurs 79:1274-1287 (July) 1979.
Geolot, Denise H., and McKinney, Nancy P.: Administering parenteral drugs. Am J Nurs 75:788-793 (May) 1975.
Hanson, Robert: Heparin-lock or keep-open IV? Am J Nurs 76:1102-1103 (July) 1976.
IMED 992, Operating Instructions: Volumetric Infusion Pump. 1978. IMED Corp., 9925 Carroll Canyon Road, San Diego, CA 92131.

Intravenous therapy: A special feature. Am J Nurs 79:1268–1296 (July) 1979.

Kurdi, William: Refining your IV therapy techniques. Nursing 75 5:41–47 (November) 1975.

Newton, David W., and Newton, Marian: Route, site, and technique. Three key decisions in giving parenteral medication. Nursing 79 7:18–25 (July) 1979.

Snider, Malle A.: Helpful hints on IV's. Am J Nurs 74:1978–1981 (November) 1974.

Unit 33: Nasogastric Tubes, Drainage, and Specimens

Giving medication through a nasogastric tube. Nursing 80 10:71–73 (May) 1980.

Griggs, Barbara, and Hoppe, Mary C.: Update. Nasogastric tube feedings. Am J Nurs 79:481–485 (March) 1979.

Hanson, Robert: New approach to measuring adult nasogastric tubes for insertion. Am J Nurs 80:1334–1335 (July) 1980.

Hoppe, Mary C.: The new tube feeding sets, or your patients are what you feed them. Nursing 80 10:79–85 (March) 1980.

Volden, Cecilia, Grinde, Jacquelyn, and Carl, David: Taking the trauma out of nasogastric intubation. Nursing 80 10:64–67 (September) 1980.

Ziemer, Mary, and Carroll, Jane S.: Infant gavage reconsidered. Am J Nurs 78:1543–1544 (September) 1978.

Unit 34: Hot and Cold Application

Hot and cold therapy. Prepared in consultation with Marion Waterson. Nursing 78 8:44–49 (October) 1978.

Unit 35: Bandages and Binders

Love-Mignogna, Susan: Taping and splinting: Seven common problems and how to avoid them. Nursing 80 10:88–92 (April) 1980.

Rinear, Charles, and Rinear, Eileen: Emergency bandaging: A wrap-up of better techniques. Nursing 75 5:29–35 (January) 1975.

Unit 36: Medical Isolation Techniques

Castle, Mary: Isolation: Precise procedures for better protection. Nursing 75 5:50–57 (May) 1975.

Donley, Diana I.: Nursing the patient who is immunosuppressed. Am J Nurs 76:1619–1625 (October) 1976.

Francis, Byron J.: Current concepts in immunization. Am J Nurs 73:646–649 (April) 1973.

Henderson, Donald A.: The eradication of smallpox. Scientific American 235:25–33 (October) 1976.

Jenny, Jean: What you should be doing about infection control. Nursing 76 6:78 (November) 1978.

Mackey, Christine, and Hopefl, Alan: Keeping infections down when risks go up. Nursing 80 10:69–73 (June) 1980.

Murray, Malinda: Fundamentals of Nursing. 2nd ed. Englewood Cliffs, N.J.: Prentice-Hall, Inc., 1980.

Selekman, Janice: Immunization: What's it all about? Am J Nurs 80:1440–1441 (August) 1980.

Shafer, Kathleen N., et al.: Medical Surgical Nursing. 6th ed. St. Louis: C.V. Mosby Company, 1975, pp. 71–91.

U.S. Department of Health, Education, and Welfare; Isolation Techniques for Use in Hospitals. 2nd ed. Center for Disease Control, Washington, D.C.: U.S. Printing Office, 1975.

Wolff, LuVerne, Weitzel, Marlene, and Fuerst, Elinor: Fundamentals of Nursing. 6th ed. Philadelphia: J.B. Lippincott Company, 1979.

Unit 37: The Dying Patient and Postmortem Care

Bunch, Barbara, and Zahra, Donna: Dealing with death: The unlearned role. Am J Nurs 76:1486–1488 (September) 1976.

Burnside, Irene M.: You will cope, of course. Am J Nurs 71:2354–2357 (December) 1971. (Experiences of a newly widowed nurse.)

Engel, George: Grief and grieving. Am J Nurs 64:94 (September) 1964.

Marks, Mary Jo: The grieving patient and family. Am J Nurs 76:1488–1490 (September) 1976.

Pennington, Elisabeth A.: Postmortem care: More than ritual. Am J Nurs 78:846–847 (May) 1978.

Ross, Elisabeth Kubler: What is it like to be dying. Am J Nurs 71:54–56 (January) 1971.

Taylor, Phyllis, and Gideon, Marianne: Cardiac arrest: A crisis for all people. Nursing 80 10:42–45 (September) 1980.

Unit 28

PREOPERATIVE CARE

GENERAL PERFORMANCE OBJECTIVE

Upon completion of this unit, you will be able to prepare a patient for a surgical operation.

SPECIFIC PERFORMANCE OBJECTIVES

When you have finished this unit you will be able to:

1. Prepare the patient for surgery by

   a. posting NPO sign and restricting food and fluids prior to surgery.

   b. preparing the skin surfaces.

   c. assisting to obtain specimens for laboratory tests and other examinations before the operation.

   d. assisting patient in personal hygiene and preparing other basic need areas as required.

   e. ensuring the patient's safety after sedative preoperative medications have been given.

2. Prepare the patient's records for surgery by

   a. seeing that a signed surgical consent form is on the chart.

   b. completing a preoperative checklist accurately.

3. Provide preoperative teaching and instructions for the patient and the family.

VOCABULARY

anesthesia—a partial or complete loss of sensation, with or without loss of consciousness, as a result of disease, injury, or administration of a drug.

asphyxia (asphyxiation)—a lack of oxygen in the blood and the increase of carbon dioxide in the tissues and blood.

aspirate—to breathe in; to get foreign material in the lungs.

barbiturates—a group of drugs used as sedatives or relaxants.

bladder sphincter—the plain muscle around the opening of the bladder.

catheter—a tube for evacuating or injecting fluids through a natural passage, e.g., a urinary catheter.

cyanosis—a Greek word for the slightly bluish-gray or purple discoloration of the skin due to a deficiency of oxygen and an excess of carbon dioxide in the blood. (Oxygen in the blood makes it look red and gives the skin a pink tone.)

hematocrit (Hct)—a test that measures the volume percentage of red blood cells in whole blood.

hemoglobin (Hgb)—the essential oxygen carrier of the blood, found within the red blood cells and responsible for the red color of blood.

hemorrhage—abnormal discharge of blood, either external or internal.

laparotomy—the surgical opening of the abdomen; an abdominal incision.

narcotics—a group of drugs producing stupor, sleep, or complete unconsciousness; used to allay pain. (Regulated by federal laws.)

nasogastric tube—a small tube that is passed through the nose down to the stomach for nutrition or evacuation of gastric contents.

NPO—nothing by mouth (Latin, nulli per os).

prosthesis—an artificial organ or part, such as an artificial limb, eyeglasses, and dentures.

red blood cell (RBC)—the laboratory count for the number of red cells (erythrocytes) in the blood.

venipuncture—withdrawal of blood from a vein by using a needle and syringe.

white blood cell (WBC)—the laboratory count of the numbers of white cells in the blood, which are also called leukocytes.

Suffixes for Surgical Procedures

-cele: tumor, cyst; hernia (as in cystocele).

-ectomy: cutting out, cutting off (as in appendectomy).

-oma: tumor (as in fibroma).

-ostomosis, -ostomy: to furnish with a mouth or an outlet (as in colostomy).

-otomy: cutting into (as in thoracotomy).

-plasty: revision, molding, or repair of tissue.

-pexy: fixation; anchoring in place.

U
N
I
T
28

INTRODUCTION

The physical and psychological preparation for surgery begins in the physician's office when the patient is examined and the decision is made that surgery is necessary. It is then that the physician explains the surgical procedure to the patient, including the effect that it will have and the risks involved; at this time, the patient has an opportunity to express concern and feelings about the procedure. After doctor and patient have completed their discussion, the physician's office nurse schedules the surgery at the appropriate hospital and reviews the specific requirements for admission with the patient.

The psychological impact of this impending operation on the emotional well-being of the patient can be categorized in various ways: fear, shock, anger, denial, acceptance, resignation, or relief. Fear of the diagnosis is probably the greatest concern. The patient may also fear loss of part of the body, unconsciousness and the inability to know or control what is happening, pain or death, separation from family, and the effects of surgery on home and employment. The nurse should provide an opportunity for the patient to describe these reactions and feelings to a stressful situation.

For some patients, religious faith is a source of strength. Meeting with a clergyman of the patient's faith and partaking of the sacraments are especially important before surgery.

The physician writes orders for the preoperative preparation, and the anesthesiologist orders the preoperative medication. In many hospitals, the writing of these orders cancels all previous orders. Be sure to check the specific details of the orders with the registered nurse.

PREOPERATIVE CARE PROCEDURES

ITEM 1. PREPARATION OF THE PATIENT

Each year more than 10 million people undergo some type of operation in this country and the vast majority have a safe and uncomplicated recovery. When they make the decision to have surgery, they literally put their lives in the hands of the surgeon and the operating room team. In order to promote the patient's safe recovery from the operation, there are several principles to be considered when preparing the patient for surgery.

1. Surgery is an important event in any individual's life. For most people, it represents a serious decision involving their body and their health. They must understand what is proposed, including all the risks, and give their consent for it.

2. Surgery produces physical stress on the body relative to the extent of the surgery and the injury to the tissue involved. Operations classified as minor surgery ordinarily pose little or no real risk or danger to the patient, are less complex, require less anesthesia, and are of relatively short duration. Those classified as major surgery take longer, are more complex, usually require general anesthesia, and pose a potential risk or hazard to the patient's wholeness of function or to life itself. The physical stress of surgery is greatly magnified by the psychological stress of anxiety and worry, which uses up energy that is needed for healing of tissues in the postoperative period.

3. Surgery produces actual physical damage to tissues of the body. The incision is a cutting of the skin and other tissues, and the internal organs and tissues of the body are handled by the surgeon and the assistants. This causes bruising, injury, and inflammation of the tissues, and results in pain after the anesthesia wears off.

4. Incisions through the skin and mucous membranes penetrate the protective barrier of the internal organs and put the patient at risk of bacteria entering the body and causing serious infection. For the greatest protection of the patient, surgery requires strict attention to aseptic technique, the use of sterile materials, and thorough disinfecting of the skin around the operative site.

5. The effects of anesthesia and other medications tend to last well into the postoperative recovery period. These drugs have a depressant effect on the body by decreasing pain and awareness of one's surroundings. The effect on body systems, such as the gastrointestinal (GI) tract, is to slow them down and make them hypoactive, particularly the bowel.

Thus, the nursing goals in preparing the patient for surgery are

1. to assist the patient to reach the best physical and mental condition possible;

2. to reduce stress and anxiety; and

3. to reduce or eliminate sources of postoperative discomfort or possible complications through preoperative instructions or teaching.

Since surgery affects the whole person, attention must be given to each of the following areas during the preoperative period.

Vital Signs

The patient's temperature, pulse, respiration, and blood pressure are taken at designated intervals throughout the preoperative days and nights. Any deviation noted in these readings helps the physician to determine existing abnormalities that would indicate the need for a delay in surgery.

Fluids and Nutrition

Patients generally receive a regular meal the night before surgery, unless a special diet or NPO is ordered as part of the treatment of the disease or condition. Then they are to be NPO from bedtime or 12 midnight on, until orders are written in the postoperative period for food and fluids. Restricting food and fluids reduces the danger of aspirating fluid in case the patient should vomit in reaction to the anesthesia.

You should post a sign saying "NPO for Surgery" at the patient's bedside as a reminder to all persons that the patient is not to eat or drink. All food and liquids are removed from the bedside, and the water pitcher is emptied. Stress the importance of NPO restriction to the patient's family and friends in case the patient requests fluids. The temptation to quench a dry mouth with "just a few sips" of water is often difficult to resist. However, if the patient drinks or accidently eats from a tray of food, the surgery would have to be cancelled and rescheduled at a later date, thereby prolonging the hospitalization and causing greater expense for the patient.

Some patients scheduled for a local or spinal anesthesia or for surgery later in the afternoon may be allowed a liquid or light breakfast and then will be NPO until surgery.

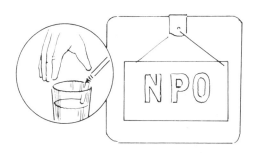

Elimination

Enemas are ordered and usually given the evening before surgery, although in some cases they are given the morning of surgery. An enema is given preoperatively so that the patient will be spared the strain and exertion of moving his bowels during the immediate postoperative period, which could cause pain or hemorrhage in the operative areas. General anesthesia and other drugs produce relaxation and hypoactivity of the intestines. Finally, some types of abdominal surgery require cleansing of the colon to remove all fecal material in order to lessen possible contamination of the wound during or following the operation.

When the patient is taken to surgery, the bladder should be empty. Patients with bathroom privileges may go to the bathroom to void until the preoperative medications are given. After the sedative medications have been given, the patient becomes sleepy and woozy and should use the bedpan or urinal rather than risk the chance of a fall or an injury.

If there is an indwelling catheter, empty the catheter drainage bag immediately before the patient goes to surgery. Record the amount of urine removed on the proper record (nurses' notes, Intake & Output record).

Personal Hygiene

Bath. The patient should bathe the evening before or the morning of surgery. If surgery is scheduled for very early in the morning, it is best to have the patient bathe the evening before.

Nails and Hair. Details of personal grooming such as trimming the nails and shaving should be completed before surgery. All metal objects such as bobby pins should be removed from the hair; during surgery they may be lost or could injure the patient's scalp.

Most patients will shampoo their hair before admission for surgery. Those who have been hospitalized for some time preoperatively may have a shampoo at the hospital if they are able and the doctor gives permission. Long hair may be braided to keep it neat and out of the way. Most hospitals provide turbans or some similar head covering for patients to wear to the operating room. These serve the double purpose of preventing the straying of loose hair in the operating room and keeping the patient's hair clean and in place during the operation and the recovery from anesthesia.

Attire. The patient is given a clean hospital gown. Some patients may request to wear their own gown or pajamas to surgery, but as a rule this is not permitted. During most operations, the patient's gown is removed and placed in the soiled linen hamper before the sterile drapes are put in place. Another hospital gown is put on the patient at the conclusion of the operation. The operating and recovery rooms do not have the facilities for taking care of the patient's private clothing, which would probably be lost in the hospital laundry.

For added warmth, some hospitals provide patients with long, white flannel stockings or boots to wear to the operating room.

Prostheses. In most hospitals, the patient is asked to remove dentures so that they will not become broken or dislodged and cause respiratory obstruction during the administration of anesthesia. This includes all bridges, partial plates, and full dentures. Other prostheses such as glasses, contact lenses, or limbs must be removed before surgery. Be sure that the small items are placed in a container labeled with the patient's name and room number. Dentures should be kept moist with water or a denture cleansing solution. All prostheses are costly and easily broken or lost; *take extra care to keep them safe.*

Mouth Care. All patients should have thorough mouth care before surgery; a clean mouth makes them more comfortable and prevents the aspiration of particles of food that may be left in the mouth. Chewing gum is not permitted, since it too may be aspirated.

Makeup. Because the color of the face, lips, and nailbeds is watched carefully for cyanosis during surgery by the anesthesiologist, patients are asked to remove their makeup and nail polish. Cyanosis may be caused by certain gases and drugs, asphyxiation, or any condition interfering with the entrance of air into the respiratory tract or lungs.

Jewelry. Jewelry should be removed for safekeeping. A valuable ring might slip off the finger of an unconscious patient and be lost, or stones may loosen and fall out. If the patient prefers to leave the wedding band on, it may be taped to the finger, or a piece of gauze may be threaded under it and tied to the wrist. Be careful not to tie it too tightly or circulation will be impaired. Although taping the ring is the most common safeguard used, some patients are allergic to tape of any kind, and gauze would then be preferred.

The policies for preoperative preparation are designed for the safety of the patient. Try not to lose sight of this, or to enforce meaningless rules as an assertion of authority or discipline. Sometimes exceptions can be made by the physician if in doing so the patient will be spared acute embarrassment.

Preoperative Medication

Usually medications are given to help the patient relax before surgery. Sedatives are often given the evening before surgery to help the patient sleep. About an hour before surgery a narcotic such as morphine or Demerol is administered to relieve apprehension. Although the patient may awaken or be awake when taken to the operating room, the medication dulls the patient's awareness of the experience and makes it easier to relax and take an anesthetic.

Atropine may be administered with the narcotic to dry up secretions if a general anesthetic is to be given. This decreases the likelihood of respiratory complications resulting from aspiration of secretions. It makes the patient's mouth feel very dry. Explain this so that the patient will not become concerned about this discomfort.

Skin Preparation of the Operative Site

The purpose of skin preparation (commonly called a prep) is to make the skin as free of microorganisms as possible, thus decreasing the possibility during surgery of bacteria entering the wound from the skin surface. The skin is shaved to remove the hair on it because microorganisms cling to hair and become a source of infection at the operative site. The wide area of skin around the site of the incision is shaved and cleansed to further reduce the possibility of infection. If surgery is planned on the wrist, the arm would be shaved beyond the elbow, and surgery involving the chest involves shaving both the anterior and posterior of the body.

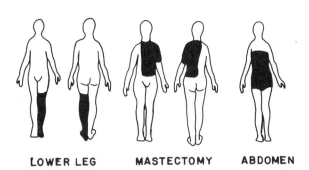

LOWER LEG   MASTECTOMY   ABDOMEN

Each agency has its own policy regarding the skin preparation of patients. The preps may be done the afternoon or evening before surgery by the nursing personnel on the nursing unit or by members of the prep team who shave all the patients scheduled for the following day. In some agencies, preps are done in the surgery department just prior to the operation.

When you are responsible for preparing the skin, check the doctor's orders for the type of operation or the area to be shaved, and then refer to a chart if necessary to determine the extent of the prep.

ITEM 2. THE SURGICAL SKIN PREPARATION

Supplies Needed

Shaving kit containing razor, blade, basin, cotton balls, and soap
Nail file or clippers if needed

Disinfectant solutions or soaps as ordered
Gooseneck light, or flashlight

Important Steps	Key Points
1. Wash your hands.	Universal Steps A, B, C, and D. See Appendix.
2. Collect the equipment needed.	
3. Approach and identify the patient and explain the procedure.	
4. Provide for privacy and drape as necessary.	

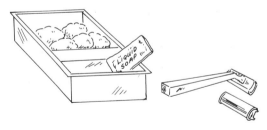

5. Apply soapy solution to the skin.	Use moistened sponges and work up a lather.
6. Hold the skin taut to shave it.	Use a new or sterilized razor and a new blade. Tautness of the skin makes the hair rise and become easier to remove.
7. Stroke in the same direction as the hair grows.	This produces a clean, smooth shave and is less irritating to the skin.
8. Begin in the center and work outward.	Avoid causing nicks, cuts, or scratches that could become infected.
9. Scrub the entire area, rinse, and dry.	Cleanse skin folds, umbilicus, and nails thoroughly when these are in the area shaved.

Important Steps	Key Points
10. Inspect for removal of all hair.	Use the light or flashlight and closely inspect all skin surfaces to see that all of the hair has been removed.
11. Provide for the patient's comfort.	Universal Steps X, Y, and Z. See Appendix.
12. Remove and dispose of used supplies.	
13. Record the procedure.	Charting example: 2000. Surgical prep of the abdomen from nipples to midthigh. <div align="right">M. Victory, PSN</div>

ITEM 3. PREPARATION OF THE PATIENT'S RECORDS

In addition to preparing the patient for surgery, the hospital record must be complete and contain all of the information that may be needed by the doctors and nurses in the operating room or later in the recovery room. It should contain the patient's history and physical reports of laboratory tests and x-ray examinations, recorded vital signs, the medication record, and the nurses' observations charted completely on the nurses' notes. Usually the patient's identification card or addressograph plate is sent to surgery along with the chart.

Consents

The patient is asked to sign a statement giving consent to have the surgery performed. If the patient is a minor or is confused or comatose, the next of kin with legal responsibility will be asked to sign the consent for the patient. This consent implies understanding of the nature of the surgery to be undertaken. A signed consent is required for each surgical procedure regardless of the length of time the patient stays in the hospital. In this way, the patient is protected from having surgery to which consent has not been given, and the hospital and the doctor are protected against claims that unauthorized surgery has been performed. See Unit 7 for signing and witnessing consents.

Laboratory Procedures

It is customary to collect urine and blood specimens from the patient for routine testing the day before the scheduled surgery. Emergency surgery requires collection of specimens immediately in the emergency room, or as soon as the patient arrives on the nursing unit and is put to bed. A designated amount of blood is removed by venipuncture in order to determine the patient's complete blood count (CBC), hemoglobin (Hgb), and hematocrit (Hct). The results of these studies help to detect the presence of infection and the general ability of the body to provide oxygen to tissue and to withstand blood loss and the added stress of surgical injury to tissues. The physician may order a blood typing and crossmatch for a specific number of pints of blood if it is known or suspected that the blood lost during surgery will need to be replaced.

A clean specimen of urine is obtained and tested. The results of the test determine the presence of infection or abnormalities in the patient's urinary system that may alter the schedule of the surgery.

X-ray Procedures

A chest X-ray is taken preoperatively to determine the condition of the patient's lungs. The result may influence the type of preoperative medication ordered as well as the kind of anesthesia used during surgery.

Checklist for Preoperative Care

Some hospitals put a checklist or reminder sheet on the front of the chart of each preoperative patient. You are required to initial and note the date and time of the activities you are responsible for performing in the preoperative period.

The items in this checklist may include:

1. Operative consent signed and on the chart.

2. Blood report on the chart.

3. Urine report on the chart.

4. X-ray report on the chart.

5. Identification wristband on the patient.

6. Operating area prepared.

7. Enema(s) given.

8. Douche given.

9. NPO at_____.

10. Tube inserted: Nasogastric _____ Catheter _____ Other _____

11. Jewelry removed: _____

12. Prosthesis: What was removed _____

    What remained on _____

13. Hair prepared or covered.

14. Bathed and gowned for surgery.

15. Voided or catheterized.

16. Morning TPR, BP charted.

17. Preoperative medication given.

18. Bed lowered and siderails up.

19. To surgery: Time_____ Date _____

    Wristband checked by _____
    (O.R. Personnel)

    _____
    (Floor Personnel)

ITEM 4. PREOPERATIVE TEACHING AND INSTRUCTIONS

Nursing research has shown that preoperative teaching is effective in reducing patients' anxiety and discomfort in the postoperative period. The teaching may be in short formal sessions or informally at the bedside while other tasks are being performed. Teaching and demonstrations should be recorded on the nurses' notes, as should observations and other procedures that are done. Usually teaching is done by licensed nurses and should focus on helping patients understand what to expect in the way of restrictions in their activities, the type of pain they may have, things they might do to promote their recovery, and aspects of their care they might plan with the nurses.

Types of information provided in preoperative teaching include instructions regarding turning, coughing, and deep breathing every hour when awake, especially for those who have had general anesthesia. Restrictions of their activities, diet, and fluids are also discussed, as is

U
N
I
T
28

possible use of an IV to provide fluids postoperatively and a Foley catheter to drain urine from the bladder. All patients experience some degree of pain after an operation, so the teaching should include a discussion concerning what type of pain might occur, how to notify the nurses when medications are needed, and what other things have helped to reduce pain in the past. You may also need to explain the special aspects of the care that follows particular types of surgery, such as the use of the nasogastric tube, log-rolling, the use of splints or appliances, and the need for various types of respiratory therapy. Informed patients who know what to expect in terms of restrictions, discomfort, treatment, and nursing care can better cope with their fears and often experience less pain and discomfort.

Following the operation, most patients go to the recovery room, where they stay until they are awake and responding from the effects of the anesthesia. During this period the nurses take the vital signs every 15 minutes or so, check dressings and tubes, give medications, and monitor the IV fluids. After patients are awake and in stable condition, they are transferred back to their rooms for further care. The usual rule is that no visitors are allowed in the operating rooms or the recovery room, so you should direct the families of patients to the waiting room. Others may wish to know the location of the cafeteria or the restrooms.

ITEM 5. PREPARATION THE DAY BEFORE SURGERY

Explain the preoperative routine to the patient. Wash your hands and identify the patient.

Supplies Needed

Urine specimen container   Stethoscope
Consent form   Enema tray (if needed)
NPO sign   Shaving kit (if needed)
Thermometer   Blood pressure cuff

Important Steps	Key Points
Universal Steps A, B, C, and D. See Appendix.	
1. Take and record patient's vital signs.	Record them on the graphic sheet and on the preoperative list.
2. Collect a urine sample.	Explain to the patient that a urine test is routinely done before any operation. (Refer to Unit 24, Urine Elimination.)

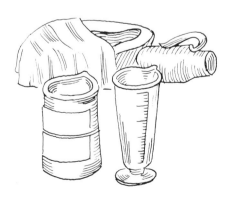

Important Steps	Key Points
3. Explain the laboratory and X-ray procedures.	Tell the patient that a lab technician will be taking some blood for tests. In some agencies, the preop laboratory and X-ray work is done at the time of admission to the hospital *before* the patient is sent to his room. In this case, step 3 would be omitted.
4. Prepare a consent form.	This is usually done by an RN or unit clerk. Consent forms are generally kept at the nursing station. In the area designated write or stamp the patient's name, age, sex, and room number, the hospital number, the doctor's name, and the date. Ask the RN to check for accuracy when you are completing the surgeon's name and kind of surgery. Follow your agency's policy to obtain the patient's signature on the consent form.
5. Post an NPO sign and explain the restriction of food and fluids.	Tell the patient not to eat or drink anything, not even a sip of water, after the specified hour. Most patients go to surgery in the A.M. and are NPO until after bedtime or midnight at the latest. Different times may be specified for patients who go to surgery later in the day.
6. Give an enema, if ordered.	Explain that an enema is given to clean out the lower bowel for surgery and to reduce the need to have a bowel movement in the first days after surgery, when straining causes discomfort or pain.
7. Explain the need for skin preparation.	Tell the patient that some time during the evening before surgery, an OR technician or other designated person will come in to clean and shave the area surrounding the site of the incision.
8. Provide personal hygiene.	If the patient wishes a shampoo and an order is obtained, give the shampoo. Remove nail polish if worn. Use acetone or nail polish remover. Explain that the anesthesiologist checks the color of the nails as an indication of the amount of oxygen the patient is getting. If surgery is scheduled for very early in the morning, the patient may wish to take a bath the night before; see that this is made possible.

Universal Steps X, Y, and Z. See Appendix.

U
N
I
T
28

ITEM 6. PREPARATION THE DAY OF SURGERY

||||||||||||||||||||||||||||||||||||||||||||||||||||||||||||||||||||||||||||||||||||||||||||||||||||||||||||||||||||||||||||||||||||||||

Supplies Needed

Thermometer	Denture cup (if needed)
Blood pressure cuff	Soap, wash cloth, towels
Stethoscope	Tooth brush and paste
Hospital gown	Surgical checklist

||||||||||||||||||||||||||||||||||||||||||||||||||||||||||||||||||||||||||||||||||||||||||||||||||||||||||||||||||||||||||||||||||||||||

Important Steps	Key Points
Carry out Universal Steps A, B, C, and D. See Appendix.	
1. Take the patient's vital signs and record them.	Take temperature, pulse, blood pressure, and respirations, and record them on the patient's chart.
2. Give A.M. care.	Assist the patient to wash face and hands, and to clean teeth.

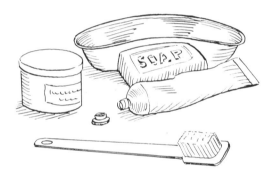

3. Give hair care.	Brush the patient's hair neatly. If it is long, you may braid it for neatness. (Refer to Unit 19, Special Care of Hair.) Cover with a surgical cap or turban, if these are used by your hospital.
4. Dress the patient in a hospital gown.	Assist patient to remove own pajamas and put on a hospital gown. Only sterile linens and drapes are used during an operation. Generally, the gown worn by the patient is removed, so personal gowns or pajamas are easily lost when discarded in the soiled linen.
5. Have the patient remove dentures, make-up, and jewelry.	Explain that makeup becomes smeared during surgery and masks the color of the skin. Have the patient give the jewelry to a member of the family for safekeeping, or put in a valuables envelope and lock it up. All dentures, bridges, or partial plates should be removed and placed in a labeled denture cup.
6. Have the patient void and empty the bladder.	Assist to the bathroom or with the bedpan or urinal immediately before the preoperative medication is given.

Important Steps	Key Points
7. After preoperative medication is given, use extra safety precautions.	Place the bed in the low position with siderails up. Caution the patient to remain in bed and not to smoke, because the medication causes decreased awareness, sleepiness, dizziness, and lack of coordination.

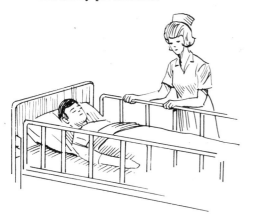

8. Complete your checklist.	Check each item for which you are responsible; write your initials and the time. Notify the RN when the list is completed. Record in the appropriate place on the nurses' notes or the surgical checklist.
9. Assist with the transfer of the patient to the OR cart.	When the OR orderly comes to take the patient to surgery, check the name of the person to be picked up; the name on the chart; and then the patient's wristband. *All of these must match.* Assist in moving the patient from bed to cart and secure the straps for safety. Sign off the chart in the nurses' notes by writing the time, the date, and "Patient to Surgery."

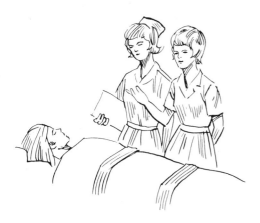

10. Direct the family to the waiting room facilities.	Show them where the waiting area for surgery and the restrooms are located. Also, tell them where coffee, tea, or food may be purchased.

PERFORMANCE TEST

1. Complete the nurses' notes and preoperative checklist for the following situation. Read through the case and record the appropriate information on the nurses' notes and on the preoperative checklist.

    A young woman, 26 years of age, was admitted by stretcher to room 223 at 0745. She was complaining of severe pain over the entire abdomen. The intern ordered an ice bag to be applied to the abdomen. The TPR were: (rectal) $101.4°F$ $- 92 - 22$. At the time of admission, the patient was unable to void; however, two hours later she voided 400 ml. A urine specimen was sent to the laboratory. The lab technician drew blood for a CBC. When Dr. Sommers called at 0930, the patient was still complaining of pain and was extremely nauseated although she had not vomited. Dr. Sommers visited shortly thereafter to examine the patient and to write the history and physical reports. He then scheduled the patient for an appendectomy for 6:30 that evening. The consent for surgery was signed by the patient.

    The OR technician performed the surgical skin prep, and a cleansing enema was given by the nurse's aide. Since her preop medication was ordered to be given by the RN at 5:00 P.M., the patient was prepared for surgery at 4:30 P.M. The TPR remained the same as it was on admission, with a BP of 124/72. The patient voided at this time. She had no dentures but she did remove her contact lenses, hair pins, and nail polish. A solid gold watch and $20.00 in four bills were placed in a valuables envelope and locked in the nurses' station.

    The preop medication was given at 5:00 P.M., and the bed was placed in the low position with the siderails up. The patient slept until 6:25 P.M., at which time she was taken to surgery via stretcher.

2. With a partner in the skills laboratory, prepare the patient for a cholecystectomy that is scheduled for tomorrow at 0900. Follow the steps outlined in your procedure. Record your activities on practice nurses' notes.

PERFORMANCE CHECKLIST

PREOPERATIVE CARE OF A PATIENT

1. Complete the preoperative entry in the nurses' notes, observing the rules for charting.

    a. Enter each preop activity with a complete description, the time, the date, and your signature.

    b. Sign specimens out to the laboratory in the stated manner (from the Unit 24, Urine Elimination) and follow other laboratory and X-ray procedures.

    c. Chart the prep, noting the time, type, and person performing the prep.

    d. Chart the disposal of valuables.

2. Complete the preoperative checklist with the required information on the form (observing the above rules).

PREPARATION THE DAY BEFORE SURGERY

1. Wash your hands, identify the patient, and explain the procedure.

2. Take the vital signs.

3. Collect the urine specimen.

   a. Correctly label the specimen and attach a label to the prepared requisition.

   b. Provide for the transmittal of the specimen to the lab.

4. Explain the laboratory and X-ray procedures that will occur.

5. Prepare a surgical consent form and obtain the patient's signature.

6. Explain the food and fluid restrictions.

7. Give an enema.

8. Explain the "prep."

9. Provide personal hygiene, for example, shampoo, shower, oral hygiene, and removal of nail polish.

10. Chart the activities on the patient's chart.

PREPARATION THE DAY OF SURGERY

1. Wash your hands, identify the patient, and explain the procedure.

2. Take the vital signs.

3. Give A.M. care, care for the hair, and dress the patient in a hospital gown.

4. Remove any dentures, makeup, and jewelry. Put valuables in a secure place (with the family or in the agency's safe).

5. Have the patient void (be able to explain why this is necessary).

6. Apply safety measures (bedrails up, bed in the low position, and smoking articles removed).

7. Complete the preoperative checklist.

8. Assist in transferring the patient to the OR stretcher.

9. Direct the family to the waiting room.

POST-TEST

Multiple Choice. Select the best answer for each of the following items.

1. The preparation of the patient for surgery begins at the time

    a. the consent for surgery is signed.

    b. the patient is admitted to the hospital.

    c. the decision is made that surgery is necessary.

    d. the operation is listed on the surgery schedule.

2. Patients are ordered to be NPO before an operation because

    a. an empty stomach prevents aspiration of material.

    b. the anesthesia stops the digestive process.

    c. there may be vomiting during the recovery period.

    d. energy from food isn't needed during surgery.

3. Patients scheduled to have surgery during the morning hours generally are NPO from what time?

    a. For six hours prior to the time scheduled.

    b. From midnight on the day of surgery.

    c. From noon of the previous day.

    d. After breakfast on the day of surgery.

4. All of the following characteristics are true for the patient scheduled for minor surgery *except* for which of the following?

    a. The operation produces little or no psychological stress.

    b. The procedure tends to be less complex in nature.

    c. The operation takes a shorter period of time.

    d. The surgery poses little or no real risk to the patient's life.

5. The surgical incision made into the skin or mucous membrane increases the patient's risks of

    a. inactivity.

    b. delayed healing.

    c. severe pain.

    d. infection.

6. The main reason that preoperative medications and anesthesia are given before an operation is to

    a. constrict the blood flow.

    b. depress the mental awareness.

    c. promote the clotting of blood.

    d. stimulate the cellular activity.

7. During the operation, the surgeon handles, cuts, and bruises tissue; this causes which of the following postoperatively?

   a. Infection.

   b. Drainage.

   c. Pain.

   d. Fever.

8. When preparing the patient for surgery, the goal of nursing actions is to

   a. reassure the patient that there is nothing to worry about.

   b. have the family participate in postoperative care.

   c. put the patient in the best condition possible.

   d. make sure the vital signs remain stable.

9. One of the major effects that surgery produces in the individual is that of

   a. an increase in body temperature.

   b. nausea and vomiting after the anesthesia.

   c. a prolonged hospital stay.

   d. physical and mental stress.

10. The reason for checking the vital signs frequently before the patient goes to surgery is to

   a. detect abnormalities or signs of infection.

   b. determine the clotting ability of the blood.

   c. reduce anxiety and fears about surgery.

   d. ensure nursing observations and contact with the patient.

11. After the preoperative medications have been given, the patient should be cautioned by the nurse to

   a. use brighter lights for reading.

   b. stay in bed and not smoke.

   c. go to the bathroom to void before surgery.

   d. drink lots of fluids to quench dry mouth.

12. Dentures and bridges are removed before sending the patient to surgery, because during the operation they could

   a. obstruct the respiratory tract.

   b. easily fall out of the mouth and get lost.

   c. cause injury to the anesthetist's fingers.

   d. become damaged from the anesthetic gases.

13. The purpose for shaving hair from the skin in preparation for surgery is

   a. for easier removal of perspiration of the skin.

   b. to reduce pulling of hair when tape is removed.

   c. to prevent accumulation of drainage from the wound.

   d. to remove as many microorganisms as possible.

U N I T 28

14. Preoperative teaching is helpful for the patient, since it is an effective means of

    a. increasing dependence on the nurse and family members for care.

    b. reducing awareness during the operation itself.

    c. reducing anxiety and discomfort during the postoperative period.

    d. restricting the amount of activities during the convalescent period.

15. One of the topics the nurse includes in preop teaching of the patient who is to have a general anesthesia is

    a. turn, cough, and take deep breaths postoperatively.

    b. the details of the surgery itself.

    c. the complications that could occur.

    d. give reassurance that everything will turn out OK.

POST-TEST ANSWERS

1. c	9. d
2. a	10. a
3. b	11. b
4. a	12. a
5. d	13. d
6. b	14. c
7. c	15. a
8. c	

POSTOPERATIVE CARE

GENERAL PERFORMANCE OBJECTIVE

You will be able to assemble the required equipment and provide postoperative care to the unconscious or helpless patient who is recovering or who has fully recovered from anesthesia. You will do this to protect the patient's safety by the early detection and prevention (when possible) of postoperative discomforts and complications. Proper care at this time will promote recovery.

SPECIFIC PERFORMANCE OBJECTIVES

Upon completing this lesson you will be able to:

1. Maintain an open airway for the unconscious or helpless patient.

2. Promote adequate ventilation of the lungs during recovery from anesthesia and during convalescence.

3. Take the vital signs every 15 minutes or as specified until stable.

4. Connect all tubes to suction or drainage as appropriate.

5. Inspect all surgical sites and keep the dressings dry and intact.

6. Keep accurate record of the intake and output from all sources and monitor the IV infusion.

7. Provide for the safety of the patient by using appropriate measures.

8. Ensure that the urinary output is adequate by having patient void within a specified period of time or through use of the indwelling catheter.

9. Provide for the patient's comfort and relief from pain.

10. Carry out nursing actions to prevent discomforts and complications during convalescence.

11. Promote the goals of early ambulation and return to independence in activities of daily living.

VOCABULARY

1. **Words Related to the Level of Consciousness**
   coma, comatose—state of being unconscious; unresponsive to stimuli.
   conscious—state of being awake; responsive, alert.
   disoriented—state of being confused; lack of response or inappropriate response to stimuli.
   semi-conscious (semi-comatose)—state of being able to respond to physiological stimuli, but capable only of reduced response to mental stimuli.
   unconscious—state of being unaware; unresponsive to all stimuli.

2. Words Related to Postoperative Complications

apnea—stopped breathing; lack of respiration.

atelectasis—a diffuse blockage of tiny air sacs in the lungs caused by bits or plugs of mucus, or by a surgical opening into the chest cavity.

embolism—obstruction of a blood vessel by a foreign substance, i.e., air bubble, fat globule, purulent matter, or blood clot.

embolus (plural is emboli)—an embolism floating in the blood stream.

evisceration—the separation of an incisional wound, with the exposure of an organ through the separation or opening.

hemorrhage—excessive flow of blood out of the blood vessels; an abnormal amount of bleeding.

hypoxia—decrease in the supply of oxygen.

hypoventilation—decreased or reduced column of air taken into the lungs.

shock—a clinical syndrome resulting from inadequate circulation, or impending circulatory collapse, due to various causes.

thrombus—a blood clot that develops within a blood vessel, either attached to the vessel wall or lodged within the vessel.

thrombophlebitis—a condition in which inflammation of the vein wall has preceded the formation of the thrombus.

3. Other Words Used in the Lesson

airway—the air passages of the body: the mouth, nose, larynx, pharynx, trachea, bronchi, and lungs; also, a plastic or metal tube inserted in the mouth and pharynx to insure clear air passage.

aseptic—a condition free of contamination or germs; sterile.

anesthesia—the absence of pain; drugs that block perception of pain, with or without loss of consciousness.

cannula—a short hollow tube or pipe.

cyanosis—bluish color of tissue resulting from lack of oxygen.

electrolyte balance—dissolved chemicals in such body fluids as blood and serum, capable of conducting an electrical charge; ionized particles in balance.

larynx—the voice box.

pharynx—the back of the throat.

pulmonary—refers to the lungs and the function of breathing.

INTRODUCTION

The operation is over. The surgeons have used their knowledge, skills, and talent to perform an operation designed to prolong the patient's life or to improve the quality of some aspect of that life. However, the very nature of the operation produces injury and stress to the patient's body. The anesthesia administered during the surgery reduces the patient's ability to respond to both internal and external stimuli. This, then, is the state of the patient entering the postoperative period; the body has undergone a deliberate injury, and response to stimuli has been reduced.

Patients literally entrust their life and welfare to the doctors and nurses during surgery and the postoperative phase of illness. If something were to go wrong, they often could not even signal for help, much less take steps to correct the problem themselves. The surgical injury combined with the reduced ability to respond to stimuli makes these patients dependent upon the help and assistance of the nurse. The less patients are able to respond, the more the nurse must be their eyes, ears, touch, judgment, and muscles, as well as their physiological watchdog.

In postoperative nursing, the *helping* and *caring* aspects of nursing become dramatically clear. Patients recovering from a spinal anesthesia are unable to turn themselves, so the nurse turns them frequently. The unconscious patient is unable to control secretions trickling down his throat, so the nurse controls them by positioning and by suctioning. In helping surgical patients, the nurse is guided by the doctor's orders for postoperative treatment and therapy, but the helping aspect of nursing is evident even as the nurse bathes perspiration from the patient's forehead or adjusts the light so that it doesn't shine directly in his eyes.

The caring aspect of nursing is the feeling that is extended to patients and experienced by them. It is the part of nursing that requires being with the patients, tending to their needs, heeding their responses, protecting them from dangers, and providing them with compassion, tenderness, concern, consideration, and respect. Through this caring aspect of nursing, we are able to nurse the patient, not just tend to the disease.

The helplessness of the postoperative patient makes it essential that the nurse have the skills and knowledge to help maintain the life processes, provide safety and comfort, and prevent complications. This lesson is designed to give you the *beginning skills* that you will need in order to provide postoperative care to patients under the direction of the doctor and the nurse.

POSTOPERATIVE CARE PROCEDURES

ITEM 1.   WHERE POSTOPERATIVE CARE IS GIVEN

Regardless of the location in which postoperative care is given, the same meticulous and skillful nursing care is required. Surgical patients receive postoperative care in (1) a recovery room, sometimes called the PAR (Post-anesthesia Room), (2) an intensive care unit (ICU), or (3) their own rooms.

Following surgery, most patients are taken to the recovery room, which is generally located near the operating rooms. It is staffed with skilled nurses and equipped with all the things needed to handle most postoperative emergencies. There, doctors and anesthetists from the operating room check on the condition of the patients frequently and can be reached quickly when needed.

Postoperative patients remain in the recovery room until they have recovered from the anesthesia or are able to respond to the stimuli around them; this generally takes from two to six hours. During this period the nurses give constant and complete care to the patients, with particular attention to the vital signs, which are taken every 15 minutes. When the patient has recovered and the vital signs are stable, the doctor writes an order to transfer the patient back to the room on the nursing unit. Recovery rooms in many smaller hospitals are not open during the night hours, when only emergency surgery is performed.

Intensive care units have been established in many hospitals to provide highly specialized and complex nursing care in one central area. Some surgical patients are taken directly to the ICU following a complex and serious operation. Such patients may remain there for several days if their condition continues to be unstable. As a beginning worker in nursing, you *should not* be assigned to work in the recovery room or an ICU until you have gained clinical experience.

Postoperative care of the patient during convalescence takes place mainly on the nursing unit. Before the availability of recovery rooms became widespread, all patients were returned from the operating room directly to their rooms. The nursing staff on the unit stayed with the patients until they recovered from anesthesia and continued care through the recovery period until the patient was discharged from the hospital. In hospitals that have recovery rooms, the patient will already have recovered from the anesthesia before being returned to the room. Nevertheless, you will need to check the patient frequently during the first 72 hours or so and to provide greater assistance for personal needs during this early postoperative period.

1. In the postoperative period, the effects of surgery and the anesthesia on the patient are characterized by

    a. _____ and b. _____ .

2. The functions of nursing consist of the a. _____

    and b. _____ aspects.

3. Orders for the postoperative care of the patient are written by

    a. the charge nurse.

    b. the doctor.

    c. the ward clerk.

    d. the anesthesiologist.

4. As a beginning worker in nursing, where would you most likely give postoperative care

    to the patient? _____ .

5. When is the patient transferred from the recovery room to his or her own room?

    _____ .

ITEM 2. PREPARING THE POSTOPERATIVE UNIT

In order to provide postoperative care to the patient, certain equipment is essential. You should prepare the unit and collect the equipment before the patient arrives from surgery or the recovery room, so that observation and care of the patient can begin immediately. The patient's bed should be made up as a postoperative bed, as described in your lesson on bedmaking (Unit 9). Even if the patient has recovered from the anesthesia, transfer onto the bed is easier if the top bedding has been folded back. Many patients will experience some nausea and vomiting or have some drainage, so the bed should be protected with a pad or towel at the head and a plastic sheet, drawsheet, pad, or Chux on the middle portion of the bed. These pads can easily be changed if they become soiled.

On the bedside stand, supply the following items: tissues, an emesis basin, a thermometer, a sphygmomanometer, a stethoscope, nursing records, paper, and a pencil.

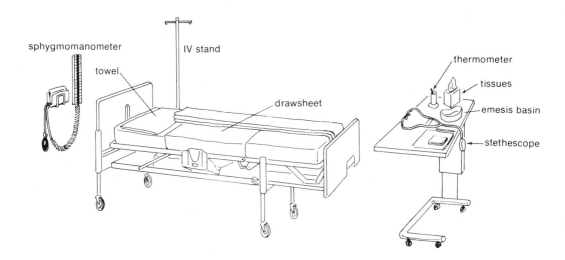

Even the reacted patient should have vital signs checked every 15 minutes at least four times. When the vital signs have been stable for some time, the doctor or the nurse may instruct that they be taken less frequently or discontinued. Most patients who have had major surgery will also have an IV running during the early postoperative period in order to supply the fluids that they are unable to take orally. An IV stand should be at the bedside to hold the bottle of fluids.

Other equipment may be needed at the bedside, depending upon the type of operation performed or the patient's condition. The team leader or the nurse in charge will be able to tell you what may be needed. For instance, some patients will have Levin tubes that will be connected to suction machines or wall suction outlets; others may have urinary catheters connected to drainage sets; still others may need special traction or weights after orthopedic surgery; and those who have had tonsils removed may require ice packs to soothe their throats.

In the skills laboratory, you should practice collecting the required equipment and preparing the patient's bed so that postoperative care can be given to the patient who is received on the nursing unit from the recovery room or directly from surgery.

Supplies Needed

Linen pack with drawsheet	Tissues
Sphygmomanometer	Emesis basin
Stethoscope	Intake & Output record
IV stand	Special equipment (as needed)

Important Steps	Key Points
1. Confer with your team leader or the charge nurse for special instructions.	Based on knowledge about the patient's condition and type of surgical procedure being performed, the nurse may ask you to have special equipment such as a throat or gastric suction machine, oxygen equipment, or orthopedic appliances.
2. Collect the equipment and supplies needed and take them to the patient unit.	A thermometer is usually in the patient unit; if not, be sure to take one with you.
3. Make a postoperative bed.	Follow the instructions given in the lesson on bedmaking. The top bedding should be folded to the side or to the bottom of the bed, and the pillow placed on the overbed table or on a chair. The bed should be equipped with side-rails for safety.
4. Arrange the other items at the bedside.	Place the IV standard at the side or the foot of the bed. On the bedside stand, place the tissues, emesis basin, thermometer, sphygmomanometer, stethoscope, and Intake & Output record. Arrange other special equipment if needed.
5. Prepare for stretcher access to the bed.	Move furniture, such as chairs, out of the way so that there is a clear path at least 4 feet wide from the entrance of the room to the side of the bed for the stretcher transporting the patient. It is often easier to transfer the patient from the stretcher to the bed if the bed is pulled out so that the head of the bed clears the front of the bedside stand.

ITEM 3. CARDINAL RULES FOR POSTOPERATIVE CARE

Following the operation, patients are sent to the recovery room for care until they recover from the anesthesia and their condition has stabilized. They are under the direct observation of the nurses at all times, and are not transferred to the nursing units until they are able to summon help as needed when the nurse is not in the room.

Regardless of the type or extent of the surgery, the postoperative care for every patient is primarily concerned with making sure that the physiological needs of the body, particularly those involving oxygenation, fluid balance, and nutrition and elimination are met while the patient is recovering from anesthesia.

1. *Maintain an open airway and adequate respiratory function.*

2. *Take vital signs until the patient's condition is stable.*

3. *Maintain fluid balance and record fluids taken.*

4. *Check the operative site for excessive drainage.*

5. *Provide for the patient's safety.*

6. *Provide for the patient's needs.*

Each of these cardinal rules will be explained in greater detail as we progress. The physiological needs of the surgical patient are of paramount importance. Once these needs have been met, the patient's psychological and social needs can be met. First things first; it does little good to help reduce the patient's anxiety about a job if the patient is hemorrhaging from a wound. Attend to the hemorrhage first, then the anxiety.

ITEM 4. MAINTAIN ADEQUATE RESPIRATORY FUNCTION

In the recovery room, one of the main concerns of the nurse is that an open airway and adequate respirations are maintained in the surgical patient. The airway can become obstructed when the patient's jaw and tongue relax, causing the tongue to fall back into the pharynx, or when secretions collect and block the passage of air.

The unconscious patient will usually arrive in the recovery room with an airway that was inserted by the anesthetist to keep the tongue in place and the air passages open, as shown in the sketch. By turning the unconscious patient's head to one side, you can help to keep the tongue from obstructing the airway. The airway is spit out or removed when the patient begins to wake up and the swallowing reflex returns. Many patients are routinely given oxygen during the time they are in the recovery room to prevent hypoxia.

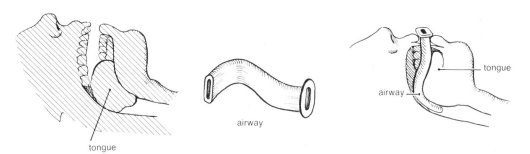

Tongue blocking pharynx.   Airway in place.

Saliva, mucus, and other secretions often collect in the back of the unconscious patient's throat and interfere with breathing. Such secretions may be drawn into the lungs, where they cause irritation to the lung tissue and further interfere with breathing. You can tell by the moist, rattling sounds of the breathing whether secretions are obstructing the passageway. These secretions should be suctioned from the mouth and throat as soon as possible. Again, the patient's head should be turned to one side so that some of the secretions can drain from the corner of the mouth.

To prevent respiratory complications in the postoperative period, you should carry out these nursing measures:

1. Turn the patient at least every two hours so that pressure of the lungs is relieved and all parts can expand with air.

2. After patients have recovered from anesthesia, they should be encouraged to take 5 deep breaths every hour, to cough and remove mucus and secretions, and to move their arms and legs. You may need to do passive exercises of the extremities if they are unable to move about.

Respiratory Complications

Postoperative complications of a respiratory nature occur more often than all the other problems combined. Respiratory function is often compromised in the surgical patient. The combination of drugs given to produce anesthesia or to reduce pain, as well as the body response to the trauma of surgery itself, affects respiratory function. The respirations become shallow, and the rate of breathing is usually slow. This reduces the amount of air moving in and out of the lungs, a condition called hypoventilation. Hypoventilation and obstruction of the air passages are common causes of a decrease in the amount of oxygen available to the body, or hypoxia.

Common early signs of decreased respiratory function are (1) shallow breathing and (2) a slow respiratory rate. Late signs of respiratory distress are rapid, gasping types of respirations, and cyanosis (dusky, bluish color of the skin and the nailbeds). The treatment of hypoventilation consists of giving oxygen and of nursing measures that increase the respiratory function: deep breathing, coughing to clear mucus from the passages, and frequent turning to relieve pressure on the lungs and to allow lung expansion. Without treatment, hypoventilation may progress to respiratory failure. This can occur several days after surgery, as the patient tries to be more active and places greater demand on a poorly functioning respiratory system.

Postoperative (or hypostatic) pneumonia is a common complication of hypoventilation. Air sacs in the lungs that are not expanded with air become filled with fluid or collapse. They become a fertile field for the growth of viruses and germs that cause pneumonia. Decreased respiratory function and the possibility of infection occur when the air sacs are plugged by mucus in a condition called atelectasis. The treatment of both pneumonia and atelectasis includes ventilating the lungs and administering antibiotics or other drugs.

U
N
I
T
29

|||||||||||||||||||||||||||||||||||||||||||||||||||||||||||||||||||||||||||||||||||||||||||||||||||||||||||||||||||||||||||||||||||||||||||||

6. Hypoventilation should be suspected when the respirations are

   a. _____ and b. _____ .

7. The unconscious patient should be turned every _____ hours.

8. The common obstructions of the airway are a. _____ and

   b. _____ .

9. Why is it advisable to turn the unconscious patient's head to one side?

   _____ .

10. The underlying cause of most respiratory complications is _____ .

11. To increase respiratory function, you should assist and encourage the postoperative patient to a. _____ b. _____ , and c. _____ .

12. Two complications that result from decreased respiratory functions are

    a. _____ and b. _____ .

||||||||||||||||||||||||||||||||||||||||||||||||||||||||||||||||||||||||||||||||||||||||||||||||||||||||||||||||||||||||||||||||||||||||||||||||||||||||||||

ITEM 5. TAKE VITAL SIGNS UNTIL STABLE

The vital signs are indicators of the physiological condition of the patient and comprise measurement of the temperature, pulse, respiration, blood pressure, and level of consciousness. Specifically, the blood pressure and the pulse rate reveal the state of the circulatory system; whereas the respiratory rate is concerned with the breathing function. The temperature and the level of consciousness indicate the functioning of the central nervous system and the brain.

The normal ranges for the T, P, R, and BP are given in Unit 21, The Vital Signs. For a particular individual, the vital signs may fall anywhere within or above or below the normal range yet be usual for that person. Thus, the normal range for the specific patient should be determined by comparing the present vital signs to those taken when the patient was well or in a stable condition. Stable vital signs refer to T, P, R, and BP readings that do not vary from the patient's other *recent* measurements.

The level of consciousness should be recorded as part of the vital signs. Various levels of consciousness are described as:

1. Unconscious — The patient does not respond to stimuli and the reflexes are absent; he is unable to swallow or to blink his eyes. General anesthesia produces unconsciousness.

2. Semiconscious — The patient responds to painful stimuli, moves about restlessly, and has reflexes (e.g., swallowing reflex) but has difficulty understanding or responding to verbal directions.

3. Disoriented — The patient may be able to respond to all stimuli but is confused about reality with respect to persons, time, place, or events. Speech is often irrelevant and behavior may be inappropriate.

4. Conscious — The patient is able to respond to all stimuli, is alert, and is in command of intellectual skills.

During the time patients are in the recovery room, the vital signs must be taken every 15 minutes and recorded. Changes in the vital signs are often the first signs of shock. The doctor may order that vital signs be taken less frequently after the patient has responded from the anesthesia and the vital signs have remained stable for one hour or more.

As patients begin to respond from the anesthesia, they need reassurance from the nurse and must be oriented in terms of time, person, and place. You may need to reassure them several times, for although patients respond and seem to talk rationally, the medications and anesthesia diminish their ability to remember. They need to be told that the operation is over, that they are doing well, that you are there to watch over them closely, and that they are in the recovery room (or their own room).

Patients should *not* be slapped, shaken, or yelled at in order to make them react or rouse more quickly. The response you would get from the patient would not be a true awakening from anesthesia but a defensive response to avoid pain or injury. The patient's body needs time to break down the chemicals in the medications and anesthesia and to begin eliminating them before emerging from their effects.

ITEM 6.   SHOCK AS A COMPLICATION

Shock is one of the complications seen in postoperative patients and can occur at any time. It is the body's response to inadequate circulation, and the first evidence of shock is changes in the vital signs. Shock leads to a persistent decrease in the blood pressure, along with an increase in the pulse rate and pale, clammy skin.

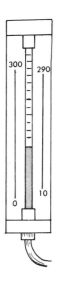 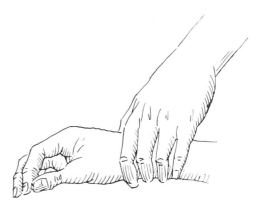

Radial pulse.

U N I T 29

The most common cause of shock in the postoperative patient is the loss of blood. The stress of surgery, the anesthesia, and the injury from the incision itself can lead to shock. Progressive and prolonged shock leads to death, so the faster the state of shock can be reversed, the better are the patient's chances for recovery. Unless circulation is restored, damage may occur to the brain, kidneys, or other organs resulting from the lack of blood and oxygen. With prompt and adequate treatment, shock is reversible and the patient will recover.

The signs of shock are related to the effects of inadequate circulation. The symptoms are:

1. **Skin** — pale in color, clammy to the touch.

2. **Blood Pressure** — progressive, consistent fall in pressure is the earliest indication of shock.

3. **Pulse** — rapid (often over 120 beats per minute), thready, or quivery.

4. **Respirations** — rapid and shallow, often grunting as if hungry for air.

5. **Cyanosis** — blueness of fingernail beds or lips due to lack of oxygen; use inner lip for detection in a dark-skinned person.

6. **Urine output** — scanty or absent because of decreased circulation through the kidneys.

The anxiety and apprehensiveness exhibited by the patient at the onset of shock turns to listlessness and finally unconsciousness as the shock progresses. The early signs of impending shock are apprehension, a rapid and thready pulse, and air hunger. Profound shock is characterized by a change in the level of consciousness, profuse sweating, and markedly low blood pressure.

Treatment of Shock

The best treatment for shock consists of prevention and early recognition. Shock can be prevented by careful physiological and psychological preparation of the patient for surgery. Postoperatively, it can be avoided by the replacement of the blood and fluid lost, careful movement of the patient, judicious use of drugs that depress circulation or respiration, and retention of body warmth through the provision of light covers and a warm room. *Do not* apply external heat directly to the body, however, because this dilates superficial blood vessels in the skin and further reduces deep circulation. Keep the patient in a flat position and give him a sense of security through skillful care performed in a calm, quiet atmosphere.

Early signals of shock are detected by carefully observing the patient and the vital signs. If your observations indicate that the patient may be going into shock, you should *immediately* summon help and report the signs so that the doctor can be notified. *Do not leave the room* unless instructed to obtain supplies or carry out other duties.

You can help in the treatment of shock. Keep the patient warm by providing additional blankets and help put in Trendelenburg's (shock) position by mechanically elevating the foot of the bed or placing it on "shock blocks." *Exceptions:* Patients who are recovering from a spinal anesthesia or who have had brain surgery *must not* be placed in shock position *but should be kept flat.* The doctor will order the replacement of blood or fluids, so that if the patient does not have an IV running, you should have the equipment ready. Oxygen and various drugs may also be ordered to treat the shock. Close observation of the patient and the vital signs is essential until recovery from shock is established.

‖‖

13. In the postoperative patient, the cause of shock is usually _____ .

14. A patient going into shock would have early signs that include a. _____ ,

     b. _____ , and c. _____ .

15. When you observe signs of shock in your patient, what is the first thing you should do?

     _____ .

16. The treatment of shock by the nurse-doctor team, in which you also participate, consists of:

     a. _____   b. _____   c. _____

     d. _____   e. _____   f. _____ .

‖‖

ITEM 7. MAINTAIN FLUID BALANCE AND RECORD FLUIDS

During surgery, the patient has lost blood and tissue fluid as a result of the surgical procedure. Moreover, fluids have undoubtedly been restricted for several hours before surgery. These lost fluids, in addition to the 2000 to 2500 ml of fluids needed by the adult to maintain normal fluid balance, need to be replaced either during surgery or in the early postoperative period.

Immediate Postoperative Period. The doctor's postop orders will state the kinds and amounts of fluids the patient is to have:

Typical orders for fluids postoperatively are:

1. NPO (nothing by mouth), followed by an order for IV fluids.

2. Clear liquids as tolerated.

3. Full liquid diet.

4. Force fluids to 2000 ml daily.

5. IV: 5 per cent D/W 1000 ml, run in 10 hours, to follow present bottle.

In order to keep track of the postoperative patient's fluid balance, a careful Intake & Output record is kept. All fluids given to the patient are recorded and all output is measured from all sources if possible.

Patients are often NPO for one or more days following major surgery under a general anesthetic. Intravenous fluids are given during this time to replace fluids lost in surgery and to maintain the fluid balance. Blood transfusions are given to replace large blood losses. IV fluids are ordered so that a certain amount runs into the vein in a specified period of time. The nurse adjusts the rate of flow so that the proper amount runs in, observes the needle site frequently to assure that it is in the vein, and supports the IV site when moving the patient.

In the recovery room, oral fluids are never given to unconscious or semiconscious patients because the swallowing reflex is diminished or absent. Surgical patients who have had a spinal or local type of anesthesia are usually allowed "fluids as tolerated" by the doctor in the postop orders. Conscious patients are given small sips of water at a time; more can be given later if they are able to keep it down.

It is important that the kidneys continue to function and produce urine after surgery. The patient should void within the 8- to 12-hour period following an operation. Be sure to report to the charge nurse if any surgical patient is unable to void within eight hours. Some postoperative patients will have a catheter in place so that the urine in the bladder drains continually and the amount of urine produced within a specified time can be quickly measured in the drainage bag. Note the amount of urine in the bag and check the drainage system at least every hour when your patient has an indwelling catheter. Hourly measurement of urine output is easier when you use a urometer instead of a soft pliable collection bag.

UNIT 29

ITEM 8. CHECK THE OPERATIVE SITE

Dressings. When the patient has come from surgery or the recovery room, you should check the operative site as soon as possible. Look to see if the dressing over the wound is dry and in place so that it protects the wound. Some dressings may have a small amount of slightly bloody drainage on them, and it is important to check them frequently to see if the bleeding continues or increases. Be sure also to check the bed linen for signs of bleeding. Cases have occurred in which the dressing appeared dry, but blood seeped under it and formed a pool beneath the body.

One word of caution: Do not change or reinforce a surgical dressing unless you are specifically instructed to do so by the doctor or the nurse in charge. Report to them about any bleeding or drainage that has soiled the dressing, because this may be a sign of complications. For more about sterile dressings, see Volume 3.

Drainage Tubes. You should find out if the patient has tubes in place and whether these are to remain clamped or connected to suction. The tubes should be secured to the bed in such a way that they do not pull on the patient. Moreover, they should not be kinked or lying under the patient's body. The usual tubes are a urinary catheter, which is attached to the urinary drainage tubing and bag; a Levin or other type of gastrointestinal tube attached to suction; a nasal tube, which carries oxygen; and various tubes or drains left in an incision to assist in the flow of drainage. Commonly used drains would be catheters, Penrose (cigarette) drains, chest tubes, and others.

||||||||||||||||||||||||||||||||||||||||||||||||||||||||||||||||||||||||||||||||||||||||||||||||||||||||||||||||||||||||||||||||||||||

17. What is meant by fluid balance? _____ .

18. An adult who is convalescing well after surgery has a total output of 2150 ml for the 24-hour period. What should the intake have been? _____ .

19. When is the patient expected to void following surgery?

_____ .

20. The most common types of tubes the patient may have following surgery are

   a. _____ , b. _____ , and c. _____ .

||||||||||||||||||||||||||||||||||||||||||||||||||||||||||||||||||||||||||||||||||||||||||||||||||||||||||||||||||||||||||||||||||

ITEM 9. PROVIDE FOR THE PATIENT'S SAFETY

Preoperative medication, anesthesia, and injury produced by surgery all combine to reduce the patient's awareness. The hospital and nurses are legally responsible for protecting these patients from harm. The nurse should be in constant attendance during the early postoperative period. This means that you must be where you can readily observe the patient and be at the bedside to help within a second or so.

Siderails. Make it a habit to use siderails on the bed for the postoperative patient. Siderails help to keep patients from falling out of bed, especially when they are not fully aware of their surroundings. If the patient is extremely restless, it may be helpful to attach a safety belt to his or her waist. The safety belt should not be attached to the immoveable frame because raising the head or foot of the bed will tighten the belt and squeeze the patient. In some recovery rooms, postoperative patients are kept on stretchers instead of being transferred into beds. These stretchers should be equipped with siderails and safety belts for the patient's security. Siderails also can be used to assist in turning; the patient can hold one siderail while turning toward it.

Positioning. Changing the patient's position is another way of providing for his safety. You should know and use the procedures to immobilize or support parts of the body and to reduce pressure areas. Other principles of the postoperative positioning follow: (1) No head pillow is used for the unconscious patient or for 8 hours following a spinal anesthesia; (2) the head is turned to one side when the patient is in the supine position so that secretions can drain from the mouth and the tongue cannot fall back into the throat to block the air passages.

Prevent Infection. One of the most important ways to provide for the patient's safety is to prevent the possibility of infection. The patient's resistance to infection is decreased by the surgery. You can reduce the chance of infection by washing your hands before and after working with each patient, by maintaining sterility around the incisional wound, by turning the patient frequently to prevent respiratory infections, and by avoiding contact with patients when you yourself have a cold, sore throat, boils, or other type of infectious disease.

||||||||||||||||||||||||||||||||||||||||||||||||||||||||||||||||||||||||||||||||||||||||||||||||||||||||||||||||||||||||||||||||||

21. To reduce the possibility of danger or harm to the patient in the first hours following surgery, you would take the following steps:

   a. _____ , b. _____ , c. _____ , d. _____ .

22. Which of the following statements refers to a nursing activity that provides for the patient's safety?

   a. The nurse closely observes the patient to help maintain his respiratory and circulatory functions.

   b. The nurse takes care to prevent dislodging the IV needle from the vein when turning a patient who is receiving IV fluid.

   c. After assisting the patient to use the bedpan for voiding, the nurse washes her hands before taking the patient's vital signs.

   d. Every two hours, the nurse assists and encourages the patient who has recovered from anesthesia to breathe deeply, cough, and turn.

||||||||||||||||||||||||||||||||||||||||||||||||||||||||||||||||||||||||||||||||||||||||||||||||||||||||||||||||||||||||||||||||||

ITEM 10. DISCOMFORTS FOLLOWING SURGERY

Although the discomforts are less serious than the complications of surgery, the patient may feel miserable unless they are promptly and effectively relieved.

Pain. A certain amount of pain is expected aftery surgery, the most severe occurring during the first 48 hours. It will normally decrease with each passing day. The doctor's orders for postoperative care prescribe the medication to be given for pain; however, there are things you can do to help relieve the pain. You should make the patient comfortable, for example, by helping him turn or change his position or by giving him a backrub. When a patient complains of pain, try to find out the kind of pain and the probable cause. If it is pain in the operative site, pain medication should be given promptly, because minutes seem like hours if the patient has to wait. Often a lesser amount of medication will be needed if given promptly. If pain persists over a period of time, a larger dose usually will be needed. Often you will find that patients have less pain if they can talk about their worries and anxieties. Patients may resist turning, doing exercises, or getting up during the first few days, when pain is severe. You should discuss with the team leader the best time for assisting patients with these activities in relation to their medication for pain.

Nausea and Vomiting. Vomiting is less a postoperative problem today than it was some years ago when ether was the main agent used in general anesthesia. Ether is still used but not to the extent it was in the past. Although vomiting is less likely, most patients will have some nausea and lack of appetite after surgery.

One of the goals for postoperative patients is to regain the normal function of the gastrointestinal tract as soon as possible. Generally, patients will begin to take food and fluids within a short time after recovering from the anesthesia. You can help them to overcome nausea and vomting by giving small sips of liquid. Tap water (not ice water), tea, and ginger ale are tolerated best, although small children may want only milk. If the patient seems nauseated, suggest taking several deep breaths through the mouth until the feeling passes. Abrupt movements and activity should be avoided. Patients should be encouraged to taste the food when it arrives on their meal trays, even if they don't have an appetite.

Care of the Vomiting Patient

Patients who are nauseated may begin to vomit at the sight of a tray full of food. To avoid this ask them if they would like to try one or two dishes and then take only those items into the room. You can provide emotional support and physical cleanliness for the patient who is or has been vomiting. The patient is distressed by the discomfort, the illness, and the dependency upon someone else to clean up the vomitus. It is important that you perform this task skillfully and effectively in a matter-of-fact, pleasant, and gentle manner.

U
N
I
T
29

Supplies Needed

Emesis basin	Tissues
Graduate for measuring	Basin of water, wash cloth, and towel
Mouthwash	Linen (as needed)

Important Steps	Key Points
1. Closely observe a patient who complains of nausea or who may vomit.	Put the emesis basin and tissues within the patient's reach. Notify the team leader, who may be able to administer medication to help control the nausea and vomiting.

Important Steps	Key Points
2. Assist the patient by explaining how to reduce the nausea and vomiting.	Have the patient rest quietly and avoid sudden movement. Remove or reduce odors that may stimulate the "gag" reflex. Instruct the patient to take short, panting breaths through the mouth when feeling the urge to vomit. Remember, sick people are highly sensitive to odors. It is important that you avoid using perfumes, lotions, cigarettes, gum, and other substances that produce odors that may be offensive to patients.
3. Help the patient who is vomiting or has vomited.	Wash your hands. Position the patient's head on one side and place an emesis basin under the cheek. Use tissues to wipe vomitus from the nose or mouth in order to avoid possible inspiration of the vomitus material into the lungs.

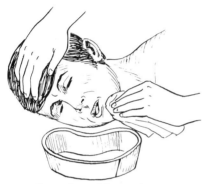

Care of vomiting patient.

Important Steps	Key Points
4. Assist to wash face and rinse mouth.	Vomiting leaves a foul taste in the mouth, as well as a disagreeable odor. Some patients may simply want to rinse out their mouths with tap water to avoid further nausea or vomiting. Others will want to use a mouthwash or brush their teeth.
5. Measure and discard the vomitus.	Measure the amount before discarding it. Record the amount as output on the Intake and Output record. Wash and dry the basin and return it to the night stand for future use. Note the color, odor, consistency, and other characteristics of the vomitus. The following terms are used when charting incidents of nausea and vomiting:

      a. hematemesis — blood in the vomitus

      b. tarry — looks black, usually from old blood

      c. partially digested food — from a recent meal

      d. odor — describe any unusual smell; sweet, fruity, sour, fecal, etc.

      e. amount — the measured amount, or an estimate (i.e., small, moderate, or large)

      f. projectile vomiting — sudden, forceful emesis

Important Steps	Key Points
Carry out Universal Steps X, Y, and Z. See Appendix.	Charting example: 1330. Emesis of partially digested food, approx. 100 ml. Linen changed. Still c/o nausea. 1345. Emesis — 120 ml of greenish-yellow fluid. <div align="right">J. Jones, NA</div>

ITEM 11. CARE DURING THE CONVALESCENT PERIOD

Patients are transferred from surgery, the recovery room, or the intensive care unit to the general nursing units when their condition has stabilized. Here they stay while recuperating from the operation until they are discharged. Most patients make rapid progress in their recovery following surgery, regaining their ability to meet their own basic needs with less assistance from the nurse each day. However, your nursing care should include the following activities, especially for patients who had a general or a spinal anesthesia:

1. Maintaining adequate ventilation of the lungs.

2. Monitoring vital signs for signs of complications.

3. Maintaining Intake and Output record for fluid balance.

4. Providing physical care and safety.

5. Encouraging early ambulation.

6. Minimizing pain and postoperative discomforts.

7. Preventing postoperative complications.

Respiratory Function

Nurses continue to monitor the respiratory function of postoperative patients long after they leave the recovery room and return to their own rooms. During the days and sometimes weeks that follow in the convalescent phase, the patients need to be reminded to turn, cough, and take at least five deep breaths every hour while awake. These actions often cause considerable discomfort to patients following certain types of surgery, so they often need encouragement to cough and deep breathe, as well as assistance to turn from side to side.

Many postoperative patients will have doctor's orders for special treatments by the respiratory therapist to improve their breathing and ventilation. The object of such treatments is to have patients breathe deeply and expand all areas of their lungs more fully. A number of simple types of breathing devices may be ordered for use with your patients, such as blow gloves, blow bottles, inspirators, and rebreathers. Some specialists have reservations about their use, since patients may merely expire or use air from the oral passages to blow, and show little or no evidence that they are taking a deeper breath with the use of the device.

Vital Signs

Vital signs must be taken and recorded for postoperative patients at least once a day during the usual hospital stay, although they are taken more frequently in most hospitals. When the temperature is elevated beyond normal, the vital signs are taken at least four times a day (q4h) until the temperature has been normal for 24 hours.

Vital signs should be taken whenever the nurse or health worker wants to check on the patient's physiological condition. Even slight changes in these signs may be the first clue that the patient is developing a postoperative complication. A rise in temperature may indicate an infection; a fall in the blood pressure with an increase in the pulse rate may be an early sign of shock or hemorrhage. A slow respiratory rate should alert the nurse to problems associated with hypoventilation. These changes should be reported to your team leader without delay. Vital signs are an important part of postoperative care.

Fluid Balance

It is still important to keep an accurate record of the patient's intake and output of fluid during the convalescent period. Patients who have had major surgery have undergone a great deal of trauma that has upset or altered the physiological status of the body. Anything can then upset this delicate balance, including inadequate fluid intake. Anesthesia, pain following surgery, medications, and inactivity all serve to decrease the appetite. Other fluids may be lost owing to drainage, bleeding, suctioning, or emesis; even more seriously a decrease in urinary output could mean that kidney function may be decreased.

All fluids taken in by the patient, whether orally or by IV, are recorded on the Intake and Output sheet. All output, including urine, vomitus, and drainage from all tubes, should be measured and recorded. The Intake and Output record provides the doctor and nurse with valuable information about the patient's fluid balance. However, you should know about each patient's fluid intake and output without a written order from the doctor to record it.

Physical Care and Ambulation

During the postoperative period, patients need your assistance for their personal hygiene. They should be encouraged to take care of many of their hygienic and personal needs as they gain strength in the days following surgery. On the first day after surgery, patients may be able to brush their teeth and wash their face and arms without becoming overfatigued or uncomfortable. You will need to provide the supplies and to finish bathing them. During the patient's bath period, you should see that the joints are put through the range-of-motion exercises. When the patient is resting in bed, the body should be in good alignment, with supportive aids to maintain good position and with protective aids to reduce and prevent formation of pressure areas.

It is common practice to get patients out of bed hours after surgery, instead of keeping them in bed for prolonged periods. The harmful effects of bed rest were discussed in the lesson on patient movement and ambulation (Unit 13). You should remain with the patient the first few times that he is out of bed. Assist him to dangle his feet at the side of the bed for a few minutes so that the circulatory system can adjust to the change of position. When no longer dizzy or light-headed, assist the patient to stand, take a few steps, and sit in a chair. In the postoperative orders, the patient's doctor will specify when the patient is to be ambulated, how often, for how long a period of time, and with what, if any, limitations.

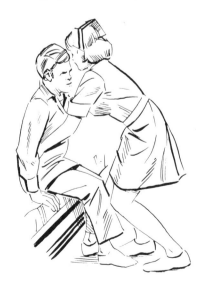

Mrs. Lily returned from the recovery room a short time ago. You have taken the vital signs and have noted the following:

Time	BP	P	R
1115	128/78	88	20
1130	112/70	100	20
1145	108/60	112	20

23. What might this indicate to you? _____ .

24. What should you do now? _____ .

25. Mr. Willis had surgery last week and his vital signs have been within the normal ranges for several days. However, this morning his temperature was 37.6C (approximately 99.8F) at 0600. How often should you take his vital signs today? _____

_____ .

Postoperative Pain and Discomforts

During the convalescent period, surgical patients often experience various discomforts as well as pain. The effects of anesthesia and drugs on the intestinal tract cause it to be hypoactive, and patients who have surgery involving the digestive tract or the abdomen itself often have no bowel sounds or peristalsis for several days postoperatively. Nausea, vomiting, lack of appetite, abdominal distention, "gas pains," and constipation may then cause discomfort for the patient.

Incisional Pain. Most patients begin to feel pain in the operative site as they react from the effects of the anesthesia. The cutting of the incision, clamping, and handling of organs during the operation causes damage to nerves and other tissues. The damage causes inflammation with its cardinal signs of swelling, pressure, and pain. The pain produced by the injury of tissues is most severe during the first and second day and then gradually subsides as healing occurs. By five to seven days postoperative, most patients are comfortable with no further need for other than mild pain medication, if even that.

The patient's pain should be controlled during the convalescent period, as continued pain increases anxiety, alters the vital signs, and may lead to hypoxia, decreased activity, and other complications associated with surgery. Most pain medications control the discomfort for four to six hours, so if you know when the patient last had something for pain, you will be able to anticipate when the pain might recur. Potent narcotics are given during the first two or three days after surgery and cause most patients to become drowsy and sleepy. They prefer to rest then rather than bathe, get up in a chair, or engage in other activities. This should be considered as you plan when to carry out these tasks.

Abdominal Distention and Flatus. The distention of the abdomen with flatus occurs as a result of a hypoactive bowel. Medications, anesthesia, handling of the bowel in some types of surgery, inactivity following surgery, and change in diet habits all contribute to the hypoactive bowel. By the second or third postoperative day, flatus accumulating in the hypoactive bowel causes the abdomen to become distended and painful. The discomfort from "gas pains" has been described by many patients as being the worst part of having an operation. Narcotics and other medications given for pain tend to slow down bowel activity and further contribute to the discomfort of distention.

The doctor usually prescribes a rectal tube, enema, Harris flush, or medication to stimulate the passage of flatus. As the patient passes gas, the distention is relieved, often within a matter of minutes. You can help relieve the discomforts of distention by helping the patient to turn frequently and to get up if allowed to ambulate. Hot liquids and solid food help to reduce distention; but iced liquids seem to aggravate the condition. When the rectal tube is used, remove it after 30 minutes. The tube can be reinserted in an hour or so if the patient becomes uncomfortable again. Positioning can help in many cases. Sims' position and the prone position make it easier to pass the flatus. Some patients may be able to use the knee-chest position for a short time to get rid of some gas, but most postoperative patients will not be able to tolerate this position during the first few days after surgery.

Constipation. When the surgical procedure has been a minor one, the patient will probably experience no change in bowel habits. Some patients, however, will not have a normal bowel movement until the third or fourth day after surgery, owing to decreased intake of foods and fluids, less movement and exercise, and the hypoactive bowel. Narcotics and other medications, anesthesia, and surgery all contribute to decreased bowel activity.

You can help the patients who are constipated by encouraging them to eat a diet with normal amounts of roughage, to drink large amounts of fluid, to get some form of exercise, and to walk about if able. Provide privacy and time when the patient is attempting to move the bowels. An enema or a suppository may be given when ordered by the doctor.

Other Discomforts. Less frequently, the patient may develop (1) *parotitis*, (2) *urinary retention*, or (3) *hiccups* (singultus) during the postoperative period, and these can be just as distressing as the problems already discussed.

Parotitis is an inflammation of one or more of the salivary glands and is seen in patients who have not eaten or taken fluids orally for a period of time, or who have not had good mouth care regularly and have thus lacked stimulation of the salivary gland. Frequent mouth care will prevent this condition.

Urinary retention is the inability to void or to empty the bladder when voiding does occur. Small, frequent voidings are often a sign of overflow from a full and distended bladder. Position, privacy, a high fluid intake, and reassurance are all important when you assist the patient to empty the bladder.

Having the patient breathe into a paper bag will often relieve the hiccups, but persistent hiccups require more vigorous treatment prescribed by the doctor.

|||||||||||||||||||||||||||||||||||||||||||||||||||||||||||||||||||||||||||||||||||||||||||||||||||||||||||||||||||||||||||||||||||

26. Almost without exception, the postoperative patient will experience the discomfort of

     of _____ .

27. The depressing action of drugs and anesthesia causes hypoactivity of the bowel and

     contributes to the discomforts of a. _____ and

     b. _____ .

28. The patient had surgery about ten hours ago and is allowed to take fluids and diet as tolerated but continues to have moderate nausea. Some actions you might take to reduce the patient's nausea are:

     a. _____   b. _____   c. _____

     d. _____   e. _____ .

|||||||||||||||||||||||||||||||||||||||||||||||||||||||||||||||||||||||||||||||||||||||||||||||||||||||||||||||||||||||||||||||||||

ITEM 12. WOUND COMPLICATIONS

Wound Infection. The two types of wound complications are infection and the breaking open of the incision. During recent years, some organisms have emerged that are resistant to the action of various antibiotics. It is still very important to prevent wound infections because the use of antibiotics may prove ineffective in treating the infection.

Prevention of infections of the wound depends on careful handwashing, scrupulous cleaning of equipment, use of sterile supplies, and practice of aseptic techniques by the nurse.

The first sign of wound infection is increased pain in the incision. In normal recovery, pain decreases each day. The incision shows signs of infection by becoming reddened, warm, and swollen, and by draining puslike material. If a patient develops a wound infection, it is important to prevent it from spreading to others. The treatment prescribed by the doctor may include antibiotics to fight the infection, drainage of the pus, and often, application of wet or dry heat.

Wound Separation. Wound separation (the breaking apart of the edges of the incision) may occur in some patients during the sixth to eighth day after surgery. The causes of wound separation are malnutrition, which interferes with the normal healing process; defective suturing; and excessive strain on the wound from retching, coughing, and so forth. When the wound separates so completely that body organs (viscera) are exposed, the condition is called evisceration. Usually the patient will feel that something "has broken loose" or "given way." You should have the patient stay at complete bed rest, inspect the dressing for pinkish drainage, look to see if the wound has separated, relieve strain on the wound, and reassure the patient by saying that you would like the doctor to check the dressing. The nurse in charge and the doctor should be notified immediately. If there is evisceration, the nurse will cover the wound with a sterile dressing moistened with sterile saline solution to protect the exposed organs.

U
N
I
T
29

ITEM 13. CIRCULATORY COMPLICATIONS

Hemorrhage. Hemorrhage can occur as a complication during the immediate postoperative period, and such loss of blood has been mentioned as one cause of shock. With external hemorrhage, the bleeding is visible. Since the volume of blood in circulation is reduced, the other symptoms of hemorrhage are the same as those for shock: pale color, anxiety or apprehension, rapid pulse, and lower blood pressure. In addition to taking the vital signs (BP, then P), the dressings, drainage, and bedding of the postoperative patient should be inspected frequently for signs of bleeding. Dark-brownish color of the blood in drainage or on dressings indicates that the bleeding occurred some time ago, while bright red blood is a sign of fresh bleeding. Report the color and the amount to the charge nurse and record it on the patient's chart.

The treatment for hemorrhage is (1) to stop the bleeding, and (2) to treat the shock. If your patient starts to hemorrhage, you should call for help immediately, notify the nurse in charge and the doctor, attempt to control the bleeding if possible, and treat the shock. Place the patient in a flat position or a shock position, provide additional blankets if necessary, and collect the supplies and equipment needed to replace the lost blood with IV's or transfusion.

Thrombophlebitis. Another complication is called thrombophlebitis (thrombo = blood clot, phleb = vein, itis = inflammation). It is an inflammation of the vein and commonly occurs in the leg, which has a sluggish blood flow that leads to the formation of a clot. The condition may be caused by the patient's prolonged inactivity or by pressure caused by a pillow under the knee or by a tight strap around the arm or leg that restricts venous circulation. The formation of a blood clot in a vessel is illustrated in the following figures.

The immobility of the surgical patient slows the rate of his blood flow. This sluggish flow of blood is further aggravated by bed rest and the former practice of putting pillows under the knees. Blood flowing slowly through the legs will begin the clotting process within a matter of a few hours. Clots (thrombi) have been known to grow in size and length until they are the length of the leg itself.

The symptoms are pain, heat, redness, and swelling around the affected area of the leg. Treatment consists of complete bed rest, elevation of the limb, application of warm wet packs to the area, and drugs as ordered by the doctor. Thrombophlebitis is not as common a complication today because postoperative patients are encouraged to move about and ambulate early.

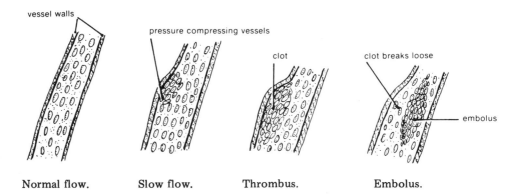

Normal flow.   Slow flow.   Thrombus.   Embolus.

Embolism. The most dreaded possible consequence of thrombophlebitis occurs when the blood clot dislodges from the vein and travels through the blood stream to the heart and the lungs. This is called a cardiac or pulmonary embolism, which at its best produces pain and an extended period of illness but at its worst causes sudden collapse and death. The symptoms are severe chest pain, cough, and difficulty in breathing. Because of the danger and possible tragedy from pulmonary embolism, all efforts should be made to prevent thrombophlebitis and embolism in the blood stream. Preventive measures include early ambulation or exercising the legs, using elastic stockings or wrapping the legs with elastic bandages, and slightly elevating the foot of the bed to improve venous return of blood. Because of the danger of dislodging possible clots, one essential rule to remember is: Avoid rubbing or massaging the legs of the postoperative patient, even as a comfort measure.

---

29. Mr. Sloan had an operation on his stomach three hours ago. Which of the following conditions would lead you to suspect that he may be hemorrhaging? More than one answer may be correct.

    a. You notice more dark reddish-brown drainage on his abdominal dressing.

    b. He has started moving restlessly from side to side, his eyes seem to roll around, and he is moaning.

    c. In the last few minutes, the Levin tube has filled with bright red drainage.

    d. His IV fluids have slowed down to a rate of 20 drops per minute.

    e. His pulse is now 116 beats per minute, but had been around 60 to 80 in surgery.

30. The day after surgery, Mr. Sloan asked you to put a pillow under his knees to ease the strain on his abdomen and also wanted you to rub his legs because they seemed sore. What would you do and why?

    _____ .

31. Name those measures you can take to prevent thrombophlebitis from becoming a complication for Mr. Sloan.

    a. _____

    b. _____

    c. _____

32. Wound infections produce inflammation; the symptoms of inflammation are:

a. _____ b. _____ c. _____

d. _____ e. _____ .

33. Evisceration means the exposure of _____ .

ITEM 14. CONCLUSION OF THE LESSON

You have now completed the lesson on postoperative care of the surgical patient. After sufficient practice in the skills laboratory, you should be able to collect the necessary equipment and prepare the patient's unit for his arrival following surgery so that there is no delay in giving him care. Your responsibility for the patient is based on the cardinal rules of postoperative care, knowledge of ways to identify and prevent complications, and methods to reduce the patient's discomforts.

Make an appointment with your instructor and arrange to take the post-test. After that, you should be able to use your beginning skills to provide safe and effective nursing care to the postop patient in the clinical area.

WORKBOOK ANSWER SHEET

1. a. a deliberate injury to the body

   b. reduced response to stimuli

2. a. helping

   b. caring

3. b

4. on the general nursing unit.

5. When patient is recovered from anesthesia and vital signs are stable.

6. a. shallow

   b. slow

7. two

8. a. the tongue

   b. secretions

9. To allow secretions to drain and to keep the tongue from falling back into the throat.

10. hypoxia

11. a. cough

    b. deep breathe

    c. turn

12. a. hypoventilation

    b. hypostatic pneumonia

13. blood loss

14. a. rapid, thready pulse

    b. fall in blood pressure

    c. pale, clammy skin

15. Summon help.

16. The following answers in any order:

    a. adding blankets for warmth.

    b. placing in shock position.

    c. replacing blood or fluid balance.

    d. providing oxygen.

    e. giving drugs.

    f. close observation of vital signs, and patient.

17. intake of fluids equals fluid output or loss.

18. the same (2150 ml) or more

19. within 8 hours

20. The following answers in any order:

    a. urinary catheter

    b. nasogastric or Levin tube

    c. oxygen

21. The following answers in any order:

    a. stay with patient until fully conscious.

    b. keep siderails up.

    c. change patient's position frequently.

    d. use aseptic techniques to prevent infection.

22. All answers are correct.

23. Falling BP and rising pulse may be signs of shock.

24. Report changes to the team leader.

25. four times a day, or q4h until the temperature returns to normal.

26. pain

27. a. abdominal distention or gas pains

    b. constipation

28. The following answers in any order:

    a. give sips of fluids if allowed.

    b. have patient rest quietly.

    c. have patient take deep panting breaths through the mouth.

    d. remove or reduce odors.

    e. give only foods patient thinks will be retained.

29. c and e

30. Would not use a pillow under the knees or rub the legs because of the danger of thrombi and emboli. Explain that it would be better to move, change his position, and exercise his legs.

31. The following answers in any order:

    a. encourage early ambulation, movement, and exercise of the legs.

    b. encourage use of elastic stockings.

    c. avoid rubbing or massaging legs.

32. The following answers in any order:

    a. pain

    b. redness

    c. heat

    d. swelling

    e. drainage of pus

33. an internal organ

PERFORMANCE TEST

Your instructor will ask you to perform the following procedure in the skills laboratory without reference to other resource material.

1. Given an adult male patient returning from surgery, collect the equipment needed and prepare the patient's unit for his arrival in such a way that you would be able to begin his postoperative care safely and without delay. For the purpose of this exercise, the patient will have an IV running and will have a urinary catheter in place.

2. To improve your skills in charting, record the observations you would make about the patient's condition and indicate some of the ways in which you would assist the postoperative patient. Chart on the nurses' notes used by your hospital. You may use the following information as a guideline, but you will need to add more details of your own.

   Mrs. Goodwill had her gallbladder removed early this morning and has been transferred from the recovery room to her own room. She is awake and has no complaints at this time except for a dry mouth. She has a nasogastric tube, an IV is running in her left arm, and she has an indwelling catheter. You have been taking care of her since she arrived back on the unit and have taken her vital signs twice:

   T — 98, P — 88, R — 16, BP — 132/82

   15 minutes later, they were: P — 84, R — 16, BP —130/82

PERFORMANCE CHECKLIST

PREPARATION OF PATIENT UNIT

1. Obtain instructions for securing special equipment (the type of equipment is dependent on patient's condition and the surgery procedure performed).

2. Collect appropriate equipment, including at least the following items:

   a. Linens

   b. Tissues

   c. Sphygmomanometer

   d. Stethoscope

   e. Intake and Output record

   f. IV standard

   g. Airway

   h. Paper and pencil

3. Prepare a postoperative bed (refer to the unit on bedmaking if necessary).

4. Arrange the equipment appropriately.

5. Ensure that the bed is accessible by stretcher.

6. Maintain an open airway.

7. Connect the drainage tubes.

8. Take the vital signs as directed.

9. Observe and record fluid intake and output.

10. Check the operative site.

11. Maintain the IV (if appropriate).

12. Provide for the patient's safety.

13. Report and record the care given, as appropriate.

CHARTING OF POSTOPERATIVE CARE

1. Follow the instructions for charting for your hospital. One example of charting is shown here:

HOURS		NURSING OBSERVATIONS
A.M.	P.M.	
	1:30	From Rec. Rm. per stretcher. To bed in Rm 410. Siderails up. IV of 5% D/W running at 30 gtts/min in L. Arm. Foley catheter draining well — straw-colored urine. NG tube attached to low suction. Mod. amount of green-colored fluid. Abd. dressing dry and intact. Awake and responding. T 98, P — 88, R — 16, BP — 132/82
	1:45	P — 84, R — 16, BP — 130/82 No complaints of discomfort.
		C. Allen, RN

U
N
I
T
29

POST-TEST

Matching. Select a word from List II that most accurately defines the phrase in List I. Not all of the words in List II will be used.

List I	List II
1. reduced amount of air inhaled into the lungs	a. unconscious
2. a device to keep the tongue from falling back into the throat	b. thrombus
	c. cannula
3. a clot circulating within the blood vessels	d. airway
4. the bluish-tinged color of the skin and nails	e. atelectasis
5. inadequate circulation of blood	f. hypoventilation
6. a blood clot formed in the inner wall of a blood vessel	g. cyanosis
7. unresponsive to all stimuli	h. antisepsis
8. state of being unaware of pain	i. shock
9. blockage of air sacs in the lungs with mucus	j. embolus
10. excessive amount of bleeding	k. apnea
	l. anesthesia
	m. hemorrhage

Multiple Choice. For each of the following situations, you are to select the one best answer to the question.

11. Your patient, Mr. Blake, has gone to surgery to have an operation for a bleeding duodenal ulcer. Your team leader has assigned you to prepare Mr. Blake's unit for his return and has mentioned that he will probably have a Levin tube in place. In setting up his unit and bed for postoperative care, you would provide

   a. an Output record to keep track of all drainage from the Levin tube.

   b. extra blankets and hot water bottle to conserve his body heat in case of shock.

   c. an extra airway you could insert to keep his tongue from blocking the air passages.

   d. a suction machine to withdraw drainage from the stomach or upper bowel.

12. After the operation, Mr. Blake is taken to the recovery room. He has had a general anesthesia and while unconscious, he

   a. needs the nurse's assistance to cough.

   b. is unaware of any stimuli.

   c. reacts to stimuli, but feels no pain.

   d. is unable to swallow salivary secretions.

13. The nurses in the recovery room have started their post-op care of Mr. Blake. The *first* observation they make is to

   a. see that he is breathing.

   b. take the blood pressure and pulse.

   c. evaluate the level of consciousness.

   d. inspect the dressings for bleeding.

14. The recovery room nurse noticed that Mr. Blake's vital signs at the end of the operation were: BP — 124/80, P — 84, and R — 16. Now, a half hour later, the vital signs are BP — 118/80, P — 92, and R — 10. From these readings, the nurse suspects that Mr. Blake may be

a. bleeding internally.

b. in the early stage of shock.

c. developing a thrombus.

d. underventilating his lungs.

15. As part of Mr. Blake's care in the recovery room, the nurse has taken his vital signs every 15 minutes, checked the dressing, which has remained dry, and noted the dark, greenish-brown drainage from the Levin tube. Now, Mr. Blake has become more restless, moving his arms and moaning. As he groggily opens his eyes several times and starts to spit out the airway in his mouth, the nurse knows that

a. she should remind him to leave the airway in place.

b. he is restless because of pain and should have medication.

c. he is beginning to recover from the anesthesia.

d. his restlessness is a symptom of impending shock.

16. Mr. Blake is now waking up, and the nurse hastens to reassure him by saying, "Your operation is over, and you are in the recovery room. I'm Miss Jensen and I'm taking care of you." In addition, Miss Jensen also asks him

a. to keep his head turned to one side so secretions will drain out of his mouth.

b. to take several deep breaths, cough, and move his legs in the exercises.

c. whether he is thirsty, and what type of fluid he would prefer to drink.

d. to lie quietly so that the Levin tube and the dressing on the incision will not be disturbed.

17. Miss Jensen helps turn Mr. Blake to his side, and he dozes off. The reason she turned him was

a. to help make him more comfortable.

b. to relieve pressure areas on his back.

c. to promote the expansion of the lungs.

d. all of the above.

18. A short time later, Mr. Blake complains of pain and is given medication for it, since he has fully recovered from the anesthesia and his vital signs are quite stable. Stable vital signs indicate that

a. there is no change from the previous reading.

b. there are no postop complications or discomforts.

c. the readings are within the patient's normal range.

d. there is rapid recovery from the general anesthesia.

19. You have been notified that Mr. Blake is being transferred from the recovery room to his own unit. When he arrives, you notice that he is very relaxed from the medication and that he has an IV still running in one arm. As you help settle him in his bed, you are careful to

    a. avoid dislodging the IV needle from the vein.

    b. elevate the knees of the bed to prevent strain on his abdominal muscles.

    c. raise the siderails before leaving the bedside.

    d. take his vital signs every 15 minutes for one hour.

    e. all except b.

    f. all except c.

20. Now that Mr. Blake is back in his room, it is important that you

    a. check his condition frequently.

    b. stay with him constantly until the IV is completed.

    c. help him to turn, cough, and breathe deeply every 4 hours.

    d. massage his back and legs as a comfort measure.

21. It is now nearly 8 hours since Mr. Blake had his surgery. You offer him a urinal and ask him to void. The reason for doing this is that

    a. you need to write down the amount as output on the Intake and Output record.

    b. distention of his bladder with urine causes him additional discomfort and pain.

    c. you want to make sure his kidneys are putting out urine following the surgery.

    d. the doctor needs to know how long to keep him on IV fluids.

22. Since Mr. Blake returned to his room, you have assisted him to turn and encouraged him to breathe deeply, to cough, and to move his legs at least every 2 hours. By coughing, Mr. Blake will be less likely to develop the postop complication of

    a. embolus.

    b. pneumonia.

    c. shock.

    d. hemorrhage.

23. By moving his legs every 2 hours, he is less likely to develop the complication of

    a. pain.

    b. shock.

    c. thrombus.

    d. hypoventilation.

24. The second day aftery surgery, the doctor removes Mr. Blake's Levin tube and leaves an order for fluids as tolerated and a liquid diet. Mr. Blake is eager to try taking fluids. What would you recommend that he do?

    a. Wait until his liquid diet arrives at the next meal time.

    b. Go ahead and drink all the water he wants.

    c. Take at least 2000 ml of fluids daily.

    d. Start with small sips at first to see if it is retained.

25. Later that day Mr. Blake complains of gas pains in his abdomen. The most probable reason for the gas pains would be that

    a. his bowel is hypoactive following surgery.

    b. the Levin tube was removed too soon.

    c. he has not had enough solid foods.

    d. his fluid intake has been too high.

26. You can help relieve Mr. Blake's gas pains by which of the following nursing measures?

    a. Providing a paper bag for him to breathe in.

    b. Assisting him to turn or to get up and walk around.

    c. Giving him only ice-cold fluids to drink.

    d. Having him breathe deeply and pant through his mouth.

27. On his third postoperative day, Mr. Blake stated that he did not feel well. He had a lot more pain in his incision. You call the team leader, and both of you inspect his incision. You notice that the area around the lower end of the incision is very red. From the symptoms, you would suspect that Mr. Blake has developed

    a. an embolus.

    b. strained muscles.

    c. an evisceration.

    d. a wound infection.

28. Suppose that Mr. Blake had been on complete bed rest for several days after surgery, that he had not moved his legs, and that he has kept a pillow under his knees. If he then complained of soreness and pain in one leg, what probably had happened?

    a. He had cramping in his leg muscles due to lack of exercise.

    b. He had become weak due to the prolonged bed rest.

    c. He had an inflammation and blood clot in a leg vein.

    d. He had developed a contracture from flexion of the knees.

29. Mr. Sloan, who is in the room next to Mr. Blake, went to surgery today and has just returned to his room from the recovery room. He had a spinal anesthesia for his operation less than 4 hours ago. If he were to develop symptoms of shock, what should you *avoid* doing when helping to treat the shock?

    a. Provide warmth to his body with extra blankets.

    b. Lower the head of his bed in the shock, or Trendelenburg's position.

    c. Remain with the patient at all times and give reassurance.

    d. Take and record the vital signs until they have stabilized.

30. One of the doctor's postop orders for Mr. Sloan was "Diet as tolerated." Mr. Sloan began taking some liquids by mouth in the recovery room but now is experiencing a great deal of nausea. You have suggested that he do all but one of the following until the nauseated feeling passes. Which one does *not* apply?

    a. Breathe deeply through his mouth several times.

    b. Cough several times and turn frequently.

    c. Take small sips of any liquid he chooses.

    d. Lie quietly in one position or on his right side.

POST-TEST ANSWERS

1.	f	16.	b
2.	d	17.	d
3.	j	18.	c
4.	g	19.	e
5.	i	20.	a
6.	b	21.	c
7.	a	22.	b
8.	l	23.	c
9.	e	24.	d
10.	m	25.	a
11.	d	26.	b
12.	b	27.	d
13.	a	28.	c
14.	d	29.	b
15.	c	30.	b

USE OF RESTRAINTS

GENERAL PERFORMANCE OBJECTIVE

Upon completing this lesson, you will be able to apply various types of restraints that will help to immobilize or support a part of the body.

SPECIFIC PERFORMANCE OBJECTIVES

When you have finished this unit you will be able to:

1. Apply a wrist restraint or limb-holder to partially immobilize a patient's arm or leg in such a way that it does not interfere with circulation or cause injury.

2. Apply a body or jacket restraint to partially immobilize a patient who is in bed or to support a patient in a chair or wheelchair in a manner that provides for safety and comfort.

3. Apply an elbow restraint safely and effectively on an infant or young child to prevent flexion of the elbow.

4. Apply a belt restraint or safety belt around a patient's waist in such a way as to provide a feeling of safety and security.

VOCABULARY

discipline—training that corrects, molds, or perfects the behavior or moral character; to correct or train.
limb-holder—a cloth tie or restraint that keeps a limb (arm or leg) in a certain position or limits its full range of motion (sometimes called a soft restraint).
Posey belt—a commercially made restraint belt or strap.
punishment—act of subjecting to penalty, pain, loss, or other affliction for some offense or transgression.
restrain—to hold back from action, to check or keep under control, to repress, to deprive of liberty.

INTRODUCTION

In the field of health, restraints are used only as a safety measure. The most common reasons for using restraints are to immobilize a part of the body wholly or partially, to assist in the support of part of the body, or to prevent possible harm to the patient him/herself or to others. There are legal restrictions concerning the use of restraints that forcibly interfere with the patient's right to liberty, and these must be observed. Restraining a person (or patient) in a locked room, for instance, is subject to certain legal requirements.

Restraints may be indicated in the care of patients based on the patient's need for safety, or on the doctor's judgment of a need to limit the patient's movements for medical reasons. You must know the principles involved in the use of restraints and the correct method of applying them. In this unit, you will learn procedures for using restraints on an extremity or on the body.

ITEM 1. PRINCIPLES RELATED TO THE USE OF RESTRAINTS

There are certain principles involved in the use of restraints for patient care in any health facility. These principles and the attitudes about restraints as described in this unit may differ from those taught or practiced by other workers in nursing. The emphasis here is on patients and their needs and on how the use of the restraint will benefit them.

Principle 1. The Use of Restraints Must Meet a Safety Need or Help the Patient

At times total and partial immobilization of a patient is required in order to provide support for a part of the body or to prevent the patient from harming himself or others. Restraints are used only, however, when the patient is unable to accomplish these activities owing to his or her physical or mental condition and when other methods have been tried without effect.

As an example, a patient may be receiving an IV in his left arm, which is supported on a board. After receiving a medication for pain that dulls awareness, the patient tries to pull out the IV. As a safety measure, a loose wrist restraint might be applied to the right wrist that would allow some movement, yet not enough to reach the IV.

Another example is the patient who has periods of mental confusion, as is often seen in the elderly. A body jacket or safety belt may be required for the patient who is in bed or sitting in a wheelchair. Without the reminder of the jacket or belt, these patients might try to get up without assistance and suffer further injury.

Principle 2. All Restraints That Limit Movement or Immobilize Must Be Ordered By a Physician

Most agencies have specific policies and regulations about the use of restraints. You should learn these. In every state, there are legal requirements and regulations about providing for the safety of patients, and limiting the patient's liberty or movements by forcible means. When the patient's movements must be limited for medical reasons, there has to be an order for the restraint, either a specific written order or an agency policy statement that stipulates when and what kind of restraints may be used.

Principle 3. Restraints Must Not Be Used as a Means of Punishing or Disciplining the Patient

The use of restraints or the threat of tying the patient down as a method of coercing, threatening, punishing, or disciplining should not be tolerated in any health agency. If a bossy, dictatorial, "Do as I say, or else" approach is taken with the patient, it often leads to anger on both the part of the patient and the worker, and the probable use of force and restraints. The "caring for" and "caring about" approach to the patient would be more effective in understanding his need for our help.

Perhaps it would be better if health workers referred to restraints as "safety belts." The very word "restraint" conveys a sense of punishment or discipline.

Principle 4. Restraints Are Applied Snugly To a Body Part, But Not Tightly Enough to Interfere With Blood Circulation

Care must be taken when applying safety belts or restraints so that the patient's restless movement or tugging does not close off the circulation. Impaired circulation to the part will cause the following symptoms: coolness of the skin, pallor or bluish color, numbness, and loss of sensation or movement. The restraint should be loosened or removed immediately, and the part gently massaged to restore the circulation.

*Principle 5.   The Patient's Position Should Be Changed Every Two Hours
When Restrained, and Active or Passive Exercise Should Be
Given: The Restrained Part is Released Unless Contraindicated*

The change of position for the patient is necessary to relieve pressure, to increase circulation, to improve body functioning, and to provide more comfort. Positioning, changing, and exercising the restrained part help to reassure the patient that the restraint is truly a safety measure and not a punishment.

ITEM 2.   TYPES OF RESTRAINTS AND SAFETY BELTS

Restraints come in many sizes and shapes. Increasingly, hospitals and health facilities are using commercially made restraints made of a strong cloth or canvas; the belts are usually webbing or tightly woven strong twill. Some agencies use folded sheets, bathrobe belts, woven strips of material or webbing, or gauze as a means of immobilizing a part of the body. A few examples of the commercial type of safety belt or restraint are described below.

Safety belt or restraint — made of webbing or twill with a buckle on one end. It is available in a variety of lengths but is often 5 or 6 feet long. Longer lengths are used to secure the patient on stretchers, when turning a patient on a Stryker frame or a Circ-O-lectric bed, and for other purposes. It is often used to provide safety for patients in wheelchairs. See the sketch below for the safety belt.

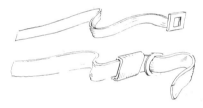

Safety belts.

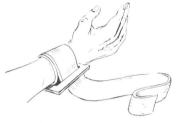

Limb-holder or
wrist restraint.

Limb-holder or wrist restraint (also called a soft restraint) — made of strong cloth about 3 inches wide with an 8- to 10-inch soft flannel padded end that is wrapped around the wrist or ankle. The padded end has a slit in it so the longer belt part can be drawn through it to encircle the wrist or leg. Some people may refer to it as a Posey, which is the name of one of the leading manufacturers of restraints.

Body restraint — made of canvas or strong material; it has a short belt that buckles around the patient's body and is attached to the middle of a much longer belt that can be tied to the bed or around a wheelchair. (See the following sketch.)

Jacket restraint — made of canvas or strong material; it has a portion that fits over the patient's chest with straps or belts that go over the shoulders and others that go around the waist. The straps or belts may be crossed or tied behind the patient's back. It is generally used as a safety measure and to support the patient's trunk in an upright position while he is in a wheelchair. (See the sketch on following page.)

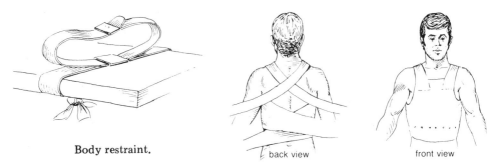

Body restraint.   back view   front view

Jacket restraint.

Elbow restraint — made of a folded, thick cotton or flannel material and used to restrain infants and small children from flexing their elbows to reach their face in cases of severe skin rashes or surgery of the face, such as the repair of a hairlip. (An example of an elbow restraint is shown below.) It is approximately 12 inches long, 10 inches wide, with six or eight slots in which are inserted tongue blades or plastic slats and three or four double ties along one edge used to secure the restraint around the elbow. One double tie at the top of the restraint is used to secure the restraint onto the child by crossing the back and tying under the opposite arm. If the ties for securing the restraint under the arm are missing, use safety pins to attach the restraint to the infant's shirt.

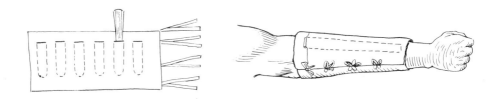

Leather restraint — made of leather with a buckle that has a locking device. A key must be used to unlock the buckle to remove the restraint. This is used only as a last resort when a patient is so disoriented that he becomes dangerous to himself, to other patients, or to the health workers. This type is being used less and less today, and always requires a doctor's written order when it is employed.

ITEM 3.   TYPES OF KNOTS USED

Velcro fasteners are now found on many limb-holders and soft restraints; they secure the restraints without causing constriction of the circulation of the involved limbs. The ties still must be secured to the bed or the chair by some form of knot; however, you should avoid tying unnecessary knots in restraints. In case of danger to the patient (such as a fire) or when emergency treatment is needed, restraints may have to be removed in a hurry. In such cases, you may have to cut the restraint if there are numerous knots or if the knots are tied so tightly that it is difficult and time-consuming to untie them. A word or two about knots is therefore important.

Clove hitch — may be used to apply a wrist-type restraint to an extremity. The advantage of this type of knot is that it permits the patient some mobility while it will not cut off the circulation to the extremity. The clove hitch is made as shown. Your observational skills are needed when you have any patient in restraints to assure that circulation in the extremity is maintained.

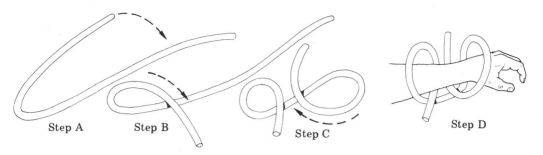

Step A   Step B   Step C   Step D

Square knot — may be used to secure the restraint to an extremity or to secure the ends to the bed frame or the wheelchair. The advantage of the square knot is that it does not slip and will not tighten if pulled on. It also will not loosen when the stress or pull on the ties is released. The square knot is made as shown in the following diagram.

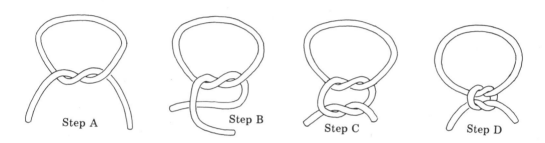

Step A   Step B   Step C   Step D

Take the left tie and pass it over, under, and across the right tie. It is now on the right side. Take the original right tie, pass it under, over, and across the other tie. Place the first crossover where you want the knot to be located and tighten the second crossover to form the square knot. Notice that the two crossovers form a partial loop at each end, and the ties on each side of the loop are in the same position; see step C.

Half-bow knot — used to secure the restraint to the bed frame or the wheelchair. It is much easier to untie than the square knot, because you merely pull the loose tie end to remove the bow portion, and then loosen the crossover tie. It also will not slip even when stress or pull is exerted on the secured portion of the tie. You already know how to make the half-bow knot because you use it when tying your shoelaces, except that for a restraint you make only one loop in the bow.

These types of knots are likely to be the ones you will use to apply and secure restraints.

One final precaution should be noted before you begin practicing the procedures. When a restraint is secured to the bed frame, *do not tie* it to the *moveable siderails* or to the *immoveable portion* of the bed. If the siderails are lowered, it may pull the restraint too tightly or cause strain on the patient's body where it is being immobilized. Raising or lowering the head of the bed may produce the same effects if the restraint is tied to the immoveable portion of the bed frame.

ITEM 4. APPLYING A LIMB-HOLDER OR WRIST RESTRAINT

Supplies Needed

Limb-holder or soft wrist restraint (2)   Padding (ABD pad or washcloth)
(If not available, use roller gauze or
   ace bandage)

Important Steps	Key Points
1. Check for a doctor's order or agency policy before restraints are applied.	This is a legal requirement when a patient's movements and freedom are to be curtailed.
2. Wash your hands.	Universal Steps A, B, C, and D. See Appendix.
3. Obtain the cloth restraint that is to be used.	
4. Approach and identify the patient.	
5. Explain to the patient what you plan to do and why.	
6. Apply the limb-holder to each wrist. a. Wrap the padded end around the wrist. b. Pull the tie end through the slit in the wrist portion. c. Attach the tie end to the spring frame of the bed with a half-bow or square knot.	If a commercially made limb-holder is not available, you can improvise: use roller gauze, preferably 2 or 3 inches wide and at least 3 to 4 feet long. Use a washcloth or ABD pad to wrap around the wrist.
7. Check the extremity distal to the restraint for adequate circulation.	Good circulation in hands and feet is indicated by warmth, normal color, and movement.
8. Change the patient's position every two hours.	Remove one restraint at a time; give active or passive exercise to the joints, then replace the restraint. If the patient's behavior is unpredictable because of confusion, mental illness, or disease of the brain, you should have an assistant to help you when you release the restraint.
9. Provide for the patient's comfort and welfare.	Place the signal cord where it can be reached, even with the restrained hand. *Do not leave your patient unable to signal for you.* Adjust the position of the bed as allowed or desired. Make sure the body is in good alignment.
10. Remove the restraints when the time specified by the doctor has elapsed, or the need to immobilize has passed.	
11. Record the pertinent information on the patient's chart.	Charting example: 0930. Speaking in confused way, keeps calling out for "George" and pulled out the IV. Some bleeding at the needle site and bandaid applied. Soft restraints applied to both wrists after IV was started by the nurse. M. Dolan, NA

ITEM 5. APPLYING A JACKET RESTRAINT

The following procedure is used to apply a jacket restraint to a patient who is in a wheelchair. It could also be used for patients in bed, although they would have to be turned from side to side.

II

Supplies Needed

Jacket restraint

IIIIIIIIIIIIIIIIIIIIIIIIIIIIIIIIIIIIIIIIIIIIIIIIIIIIIIIIIIIIIIIIIIIIIIIIIIIIIIIIIIIIIIIIIIIIIIIIIIIIIIIIIIIIIIIIIIIIIIIIIIIIIIIIIIIIIIIIIIIIIIIIIIIIIIIIIIIIII

Important Steps	Key Points
Carry out Universal Steps A, B, C, and D. See Appendix.	
1. Place the jacket over the chest.	Be sure that the wheelchair brakes are locked. Have the patient lean forward slightly while you stand behind the chair. You may need an assistant to help hold the patient.
2. Cross the lower side and shoulder straps each behind the back.	
3. Tie each set of straps in knots behind the wheelchair.	Tie them in a half-bow knot or square knot at the back of the wheelchair.
Carry out Universal Steps X, Y, and Z. See Appendix.	Charting example: 1000. Up in wheelchair. Jacket restraint applied for safety. M. Dolan, NA

U
N
I
T
30

ITEM 6.   APPLYING AN ELBOW RESTRAINT

IIIIIIIIIIIIIIIIIIIIIIIIIIIIIIIIIIIIIIIIIIIIIIIIIIIIIIIIIIIIIIIIIIIIIIIIIIIIIIIIIIIIIIIIIIIIIIIIIIIIIIIIIIIIIIIIIIIIIIIIIIIIIIIIIIIIIIIIIIIIIIIIIIIIIIIIIIIIII

Supplies Needed

Elbow restraints (2), with Velcro fastener or safety pins

IIIIIIIIIIIIIIIIIIIIIIIIIIIIIIIIIIIIIIIIIIIIIIIIIIIIIIIIIIIIIIIIIIIIIIIIIIIIIIIIIIIIIIIIIIIIIIIIIIIIIIIIIIIIIIIIIIIIIIIIIIIIIIIIIIIIIIIIIIIIIIIIIIIIIIIIIIIIII

Important Steps	Key Points
Carry out Universal Steps A, B, C, and D. See Appendix.	
1. If necessary, prepare the elbow restraint.	You may have to slip a tongue blade into each of the insert pockets unless the restraint has built-in rigid supports.
2. Wrap the restraint around the arm with ties or Velcro fasteners on the outer side.	To secure the restraint, pin it to the baby's shirt or, if it has ties, place it around the body and tie it under the other arm.
3. Remove the restraints every two hours to allow flexion of the elbows.	Remove one at a time and for passive or active range of motion exercises.
Carry out Universal Steps X, Y, and Z. See Appendix.	Charting example: 1300. Elbow restraints applied to both arms. Incision on upper lip dry and clean. M. Dolan, NA

ITEM 7. APPLYING A SAFETY BELT OR RESTRAINT STRAP

||||||||||||||||||||||||||||||||||||||||||||||||||||||||||||||||||||||||||||||||||||||||||||||||||||||||||||||||||||||||||||||||||||||||||||||||||||||||||||||||||||||||||

Supplies Needed

Safety belt, strap, or sheet

||||||||||||||||||||||||||||||||||||||||||||||||||||||||||||||||||||||||||||||||||||||||||||||||||||||||||||||||||||||||||||||||||||||||||||||||||||||||||||||||||||||||||

Important Steps

Key Points

Carry out Universal Steps A, B, C, and D. See Appendix.

1. Apply the safety belt or restraint strap around the patient's wrist.

   With the patient sitting in a chair, place the strap around his waist, bringing both ends behind the chair and tying them in a half-bow or square knot, or fasten the buckle if there is one;

   or

   place the strap or belt completely around the patient's waist, cross the ends in the back, then bring both ends behind the chair and tie them in a half-bow or square knot (or fasten the buckle);

   or

   place the strap around the patient's waist, tie it at one side in a square knot, bring the ties to the back of the chair, and fasten them with a half-bow or square knot.

This can be done for the patient who is lying in bed, sitting in a wheelchair, or lying on a stretcher. It is not commonly used for the bed patient, however, because siderails are generally adequate to protect the patient from falling out of bed.

There are several ways to apply the safety belt or strap. You may find that one method works well for one patient and another method is better for a different patient.

Carry out Universal Steps X, Y, and Z. See Appendix.

Even for the patient who is sitting up, the position must be changed or weight shifted frequently to relieve pressure. Charting example:
1015. Up in wheelchair. Safety belt applied around waist.

M. Dolan, NA

PERFORMANCE TEST

In the classroom or skill laboratory, your instructor will ask you to perform the following activities to demonstrate your skill without referring to any source material. You may use Mrs. Chase (the mannequin) or another student in the role of patient.

1. Given a patient receiving an IV in the left arm who tries to remove the needle from the vein, apply a limb-holder, or similar soft restraint, to the right wrist. Tie the restraint at the wrist with a knot so that the patient's tugging on it will not cut off circulation to the hand.

2. Given a patient with a muscular disease involving the muscles of the trunk, apply a jacket restraint to support the body while patient is sitting in a wheelchair, using the method that provides the most safety for the patient.

3. Given a 4-month-old child who has a severe rash on the face and neck, apply elbow restraints to both arms and describe the care you would give the child during the time the restraints are used. The care referred to would be in addition to bathing, diapering, feeding, or holding the child.

4. Given an elderly, slightly confused patient in a wheelchair who is not to bear any weight on the left leg, place a safety belt or restraint strap around the patient's waist and fasten the ends of it behind the wheelchair, using the method and knots of your choice from those described in the procedure.

UNIT 30

PERFORMANCE CHECKLIST

APPLYING LIMB-HOLDER

1. Check for the doctor's order.

2. Wash your hands.

3. Obtain a limb-holder or similar soft cloth restraint.

4. Approach and identify the patient.

5. Explain what you are going to do and why.

6. Apply the limb-holder or wrist restraint to the right wrist correctly.

    a. Place a padded end around the wrist, or pad it.

    b. Pull the tie through the slit, or make a clove hitch or square knot at the wrist.

    c. Tie the loose end to the spring portion of the bed.

    d. Make clove hitch, square, or half-bow knots correctly.

7. Check the wrist and hand to see if circulation is good.

8. Provide for the patient's comfort and welfare.

    a. Adjust the bed to the allowed position.

    b. Leave the signal cord within reach.

    c. Make sure that the patient is in good body alignment.

9. Change the patient's position every two hours.

10. Record pertinent information on the patient's chart.

APPLYING A JACKET RESTRAINT

1. Check for the doctor's order. (Some agencies may not require an order for support, but it would be better to have one.)

2. Wash your hands.

3. Obtain a jacket support or restraint.

4. Approach and identify the patient.

5. Explain what is to be done and why.

6. Apply the jacket restraint to the patient in a wheelchair.

   a. Lock the wheels of the wheelchair.

   b. Have an assistant support the patient while the jacket is being applied.

   c. Place a large portion of jacket correctly over patient's chest with the shoulder straps at the top.

   d. Stand behind the chair while your assistant supports the patient, cross the lower side ties behind the patient, and tie them behind the wheelchair.

   e. Take the shoulder straps, cross them behind the patient's shoulders, and tie them behind the wheelchair.

   f. Make a square or half-bow knot correctly.

7. Provide for the patient's comfort and welfare.

8. Record pertinent information on the patient's chart.

APPLYING ELBOW RESTRAINTS

1. Check for the doctor's order.

2. Wash your hands.

3. Obtain elbow restraints and tongue blades if needed.

4. Approach and identify the patient.

5. Prepare the elbow restraints by inserting tongue blades.

6. Apply the elbow restraints, one on each arm.

   a. Wrap it around the arm, leaving the tie edge outermost.

   b. Wrap the ties around the arm and tie them in half-bow knots.

   c. Pin the restraint to the baby's shirt.

7. Remove the restraints every two hours to do range of motion exercises of the elbow.

8. Provide for the child's comfort.

9. Record pertinent information on the patient's chart.

APPLYING A SAFETY BELT OR RESTRAINT STRAP

1. Check for the doctor's order.

2. Wash your hands.

3. Obtain a safety belt or restraint strap.

4. Approach and identify the patient.

5. Explain what you are going to do and why.

6. Apply the safety belt or restraint strap around the patient's waist while patient is sitting in a chair.

   a. Place a strap around the patient's waist and back of the chair, then tie or buckle it; *or*

   b. place the strap around patient's waist, cross the straps behind, and tie the ends behind the chair or buckle them; *or*

   c. encircle the strap about patient's waist, tie it to one side in a square knot, and then tie it behind the chair.

   d. Make a square or half-bow knot correctly.

7. Provide for the patient's comfort and welfare.

8. Tell the patient that he or she will be checked in two hours or sooner.

9. Record pertinent information on the patient's chart.

U
N
I
T
30

POST-TEST

Directions: Mark the answer that makes the statement complete.

1. The use of restraints must meet some need or help the patient. They are used in all of the following cases except

    a. for the elderly, confused wheelchair patient.

    b. when the patient attempts to pull an IV out of arm.

    c. to discipline the patient.

    d. when the disoriented patient becomes combative.

2. All restraints that limit movement or immobilize the patient must be ordered by a physician. All of the following statements are true except

    a. The order is written by the physician.

    b. There are legal requirements and regulations about providing for the safety of patients.

    c. The agency policy may determine restraint use.

    d. Restraints are used to coerce the patient.

3. To eliminate the patient's feeling of being threatened when he is restrained, use the following phrase

    a. These are safety belts.

    b. These are restraints.

    c. These are belts to keep you in bed.

    d. These straps are used to keep you immobilized.

4. Restraints are applied snugly to a body part, but not tightly enough to interfere with circulation. All of the following are symptoms of circulation impairment except

    a. pallor or bluish color.

    b. numbness.

    c. blanching.

    d. loss of sensation or movement.

5. The patient's position should be changed when restraints are utilized. The restrained part should be exercised unless contraindicated (choose the one correct answer)

    a. at least every 1 to 2 hours.

    b. at least every 3 to 4 hours.

    c. at least every 2 to 5 hours.

    d. at least every 3 to 6 hours.

6. The change of position for the patient is necessary for all of the following reasons except

   a. to relieve pressure.

   b. to increase circulation.

   c. to improve body functioning.

   d. to increase flexion of the part.

7. Restraints come in all sizes and shapes. The following types are examples of commercial restraints except

   a. folded sheets.

   b. a jacket restraint.

   c. a limb-holder.

   d. a leather restraint.

8. The following knots are used when applying restraints except

   a. clove hitch.

   b. half-bow knot.

   c. double knot.

   d. square knot.

9. Restraints should be tied to the following part of the bed

   a. the siderails

   b. the moveable part of the bed frame (spring attachment)

   c. the immoveable part of the bed frame

   d. the head and foot boards

10. When restraints are attached to the bed frame, the safest knot used is

    a. the half-bow knot.

    b. the double knot.

    c. the square knot.

    d. the plain knot.

U
N
I
T
30

POST-TEST ANSWERS

1. c	6. d
2. d	7. a
3. a	8. c
4. c	9. b
5. a	10. a

Unit 31

GENERAL PERFORMANCE OBJECTIVE

You will be able to demonstrate your knowledge of the various oxygen therapies as well as the nursing care indicated when caring for patients who are receiving oxygen therapy.

SPECIFIC PERFORMANCE OBJECTIVES

Upon completion of this lesson and your laboratory practice you will be able to correctly:

1. Describe and identify the methods of oxygen therapy administered to patients.

2. Show how to regulate oxygen flow and how to care for a patient with an oxygen tent, nasal cannula, nasal catheter, oxygen mask, Venturi mask, or IPPB (intermittent positive pressure breathing apparatus), and properly record your activities.

3. Demonstrate and discuss safety precautions that must be observed when patients are receiving oxygen therapies.

VOCABULARY

alveoli—clusters of grape-like air sacs in the lung.
anoxia—a reduction or lack of oxygen.
atelectasis—a lack of air in the lungs due to blockage of small bronchial tubes.
bronchioles—the terminal ends of the bronchi.
bronchus (plural, bronchi)—one of two branches of the trachea.
diaphragm—the muscle separating the abdominal and thoracic cavities.
diffusion—a chemical process whereby a liquid or gas mixes its chemical components.
dyspnea—difficult or labored respiration.
expiration—exhaling air from the lungs.
hemoglobin—oxygen-carrying substance in red blood cells.
humidifier—an apparatus used to increase the moisture content of the air.
hypoxemia—low oxygen content in the blood.
hypoxia—low oxygen content in the tissues.
inspiration—the act of breathing air into the lungs.
nasal catheter—a tube of rubber or plastic used to give oxygen through the nose.
nebulizer—an atomizer or sprayer.
pleura—the covering of the lung.
respiration—the act of breathing (inspiration and expiration).
therapeutic—pertaining to treatment given for the purpose of healing.
trachea—the windpipe, a 4½-inch-long tube extending from the larynx to the bronchial tree.

INTRODUCTION

One of the most basic needs of life is an adequate supply of oxygen. Oxygen is needed by all of the cells of the body in order to metabolize, or burn, nutrients and produce the energy needed to function. Without oxygen, cell metabolism slows down, and some cells begin to die in as little as 30 seconds. Through the act of breathing, we take in air that contains about 20 per cent oxygen. An exchange of gases takes place in the lungs as oxygen is absorbed into the blood stream and carbon dioxide, a waste product of cell metabolism, is removed in the exhaled air.

When people are healthy, and the cardiorespiratory system is functioning normally, few think at all about breathing; it is a routine and semi-automatic activity. The moment that something interferes with getting enough oxygen to meet the body's needs, however, breathing becomes a conscious effort and assumes paramount importance. Perhaps you remember having a severe cold at some time in your life, and how difficult it was to breathe through a stuffy and runny nose. It took so much more energy to breathe that you weren't as active as before. It was more difficult to read your assignments or to study your lessons. You felt tired and wanted only to take it easy and rest.

For most people, upper respiratory infections and obstructed nasal passages make it more difficult to breathe and to obtain sufficient oxygen to carry out their usual activities. So it is with patients. Those with conditions or diseases that affect their ability to breathe easily and without effort become aware of the difficulty in taking each breath and the increased work that it takes. As nurses, we need to identify as soon as possible those patients with breathing problems, to take appropriate nursing actions to help relieve obstructions of the airway, and to initiate or maintain oxygen therapy competently when it is used in the patient's treatment.

In this unit, you will learn about the signs and symptoms associated with hypoxia, or the lack of sufficient oxygen to meet the body's demands. Obstructions of the airway are the most common causes of hypoxia, and a number of nursing actions that you can use to clear the airway are described. Also discussed are various types of equipment for oxygen therapy, such as delivery of oxygen by means of nasal cannula, catheter, Venturi mask, and use of IPPB. Finally, principles are presented as guidelines for you to follow as you help your patients meet their oxygenation needs.

UNIT 31

NURSING AND OXYGEN THERAPY

ITEM 1. THE PHYSIOLOGY OF BREATHING

Breathing is the means by which oxygen is brought into the body and excess carbon dioxide is removed. Once in the lungs, oxygen is transported to the cells of the body. The transport system can be readily understood if we think of oxygen as cargo, the hemoglobin in the red blood cells as the vehicles that carry the oxygen, and the system of blood vessels as the paths by which the vehicles travel to deliver the cargo to the destinations, that is, the cells.

Take a few minutes to review the anatomy of the respiratory tract.

Air enters the body through the nose, where it is warmed, moistened, and filtered by the fine hairs in the nasal cavity. The air continues down the throat to the trachea, or windpipe. This is a 4½-inch-long tube extending from the larynx to the bronchi, which lead directly into the lungs. Here the bronchi branch into many smaller tubes called the bronchioles. Since it resembles a tree, this part of the respiratory tract is commonly called the bronchial tree.

The tiny bronchioles lead to the alveoli, or air sacs, in the lung. The alveoli are surrounded by a network of tiny blood capillaries, and it is here that O_2 and CO_2 gases are exchanged. The oxygen is picked up by the hemoglobin in the red blood cells and circulated to all the tissues of the body. Various chemicals in the venous blood then carry carbon dioxide back to the heart and to the lungs, where it is exhaled from the body.

Drawing air into the body is an active effort that requires the work of various groups of muscles. The diaphragm is a large dome-shaped muscle that separates the chest and abdominal cavities. It moves down and out during inhalation while the intercostal muscles, located between the ribs, move the rib cage up and out to enlarge the chest cavity during inhalation. This movement draws air into the lungs and it is the movement you observe when counting the patient's respiration rate. Patients with difficulty in breathing have more labored and pronounced muscular effort, which is called dyspnea. Exhalation for the normal person is a passive activity that occurs when the muscles relax and air leaves the lungs easily.

The rate at which we breathe is regulated by the respiratory centers in the brain and in the walls of large arteries that respond to the amount of oxygen and carbon dioxide in the blood. They are particularly sensitive to the CO_2 level. When it increases, respirations become more rapid and deep in order to remove the excess amounts. Normal rates of respirations are 40 per minute for newborn babies; 30 per minute for infants and small children; and 14 to 20 per minute for adults.

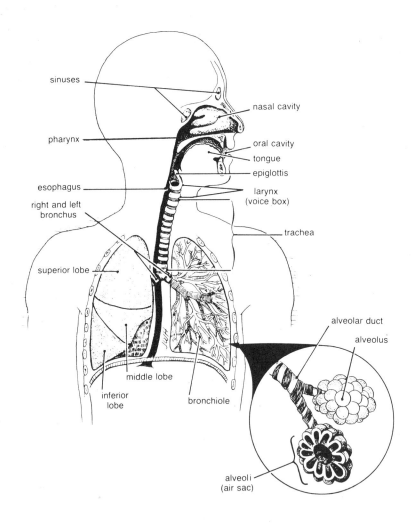

ITEM 2. RESPIRATORY PROBLEMS OF INSUFFICIENT OXYGEN

Patients with an infection or disease of the respiratory tract typically have some difficulty in breathing, and every nurse should be aware of the problem and the treatment for it. What may not always be recognized is that any patient, at any time, may develop problems when the oxygen supply is inadequate to meet the needs of the body. This condition, called hypoxia, may arise suddenly when the airway becomes obstructed; very often, however, it is a gradual and insidious condition found in patients with no complaints, who lie quietly in bed and have slow, shallow breathing.

Patients At Risk of Hypoxia

The following diseases and conditions often interfere with the patient's ability to breathe and obtain enough oxygen to supply the body needs adequately. Obstructions of the airway are the most common causes of hypoxia and often are the most easily corrected. Patients who have undergone surgery with general anesthesia, however, are especially prone to develop some degree of hypoxia, unless treatment is given. Be alert to signs of insufficient oxygen in patients with these conditions:

1. Any obstruction of the airway. The airway can be obstructed by secretions, mucus, or any type of foreign body; reduced in size by spasms or by swelling due to inflammation of areas near the tract; or cut off by near-drowning.

2. Any decreased movement of the chest. Conditions that limit the movement of the rib cage include abdominal surgery, chest injuries, obesity, arthritis and other diseases of the spine, and inflammations such as peritonitis.

3. Any impaired function of the neuromuscular system involved in breathing. This especially includes brain injuries, coma, use of general anesthesia, stroke, and other diseases that cause paralysis, for example, poliomyelitis and multiple sclerosis.

4. Interference with the diffusion of gases in the lungs. This condition may be due to tumors in the lung and diseases such as emphysema, emboli, and injury.

5. Less oxygen in the air due to environmental factors. The "thin air" of higher atmospheres is a natural example of this; some man-made examples are the smog, smoke, and heat excess in the air.

U
N
I
T
31

Symptoms of Insufficient Oxygen

Many patients are able to call for help when they experience an abrupt onset of a respiratory obstruction or dyspnea. They sit upright and change their pattern of breathing in an attempt to get additional oxygen. They state, "I can't breathe," or "I feel like I'm suffocating," and seem breathless as they pant for more air. You should notify the nurse or doctor immediately, identify the cause of the condition, and begin treatment. As patients become extremely anxious and even panicky when they have trouble breathing, it is important for nurses to remain calm and give reassurance by rapid and competent care in treating the condition.

In the more gradual onset of decreased oxygenation, the signs are less clear or dramatic as the body tries to adjust to the lower amounts of O_2 that are available. All tissues of the body need oxygen, but some cells are more sensitive to a reduction than are others. Areas affected first by hypoxia are the retina of the eye, the brain, and the heart — all organs that are important for survival. Many of the earliest signs result from changes in the patient's behavior and the function of these organs. With reduced oxygen, the most notable symptom is a reduction in activity, with an increase in fatigue; other signs may be detected before this one, however. You should suspect that patients are not meeting their oxygen needs when you observe these symptoms:

1. There is an abrupt change in the visual acuity or ability to see things.

2. The patient is increasingly restless or irritable, with dulling of the intellect and changes in judgment.

3. There is a decrease in muscle coordination and strength.

4. In the early stages, the BP, P, and R rates increase as the heart beats more rapidly to circulate the limited oxygen available to the cells.

In the later stages of inadequate O_2 supply, the symptoms include cyanosis, crowing type of respirations, retraction of the muscles used in breathing, and a decrease in the BP and P rates. At this time, patients are unable to move about or carry out other activities of daily living. From 30 to 50 per cent of their energy is diverted to the hard work of breathing.

ITEM 3. TREATMENT OF DECREASED OXYGEN INTAKE

Whenever your patient complains of breathing problems or shows symptoms that indicate a decreased intake of oxygen, promptly notify your team leader or the doctor. The treatment for insufficient oxygen is to supply more oxygen, so the doctor generally orders this for the patient. This may be on a continuous basis until the underlying cause is corrected or on a p.r.n. basis as it is needed by the patient. Oxygen therapy is supervised and managed by nurses, although more complex treatments are performed by respiratory therapists using various drugs, exercises, and respirators and other equipment.

In managing the care of patients with dyspnea and hypoxia, nurses employ the following actions or techniques:

1. Maintain an open airway. Clear obstructions of the air passages by any of these methods:

   a. Use suction to remove secretions and mucus when the patient is unable to cough them out.

   b. Use an airway to keep the tongue from falling back into the throat and obstructing the passage of air. Airways are most often used in comatose or unconscious patients.

   c. Thin out secretions by using steam inhalation treatments, nebulizers, and medications, either with or without IPPB (intermittent positive pressure breathing).

   d. Proper positioning.

2. Encourage or assist the patient to cough, to turn frequently, and to take deep breaths several times each hour. This is one of the most important nursing actions you can take to help your patients to meet their oxygen needs. The cough is nature's way of ridding ourselves of an obstruction or blockage of the respiratory tract. A sneeze is a similar action to relieve the respiratory tract of a foreign object. Yawns and sighs are two forms of deep breaths that help expand the alveoli in the lung. A yawn is a deep, long inspiration usually due to mental or physical fatigue. A sigh is a prolonged inspiration followed by a long expiration.

3. Increase the oxygen content of the inhaled air by giving oxygen via one of several ways: by nasal cannula, prongs, catheter, mask, or Venturi mask, or even with the use of a hyperbaric chamber.

4. Positioning. Additional energy and oxygen are needed when patients are anxious and have tense, rigid muscles. You can help patients with dyspnea to relax, expand the chest more fully, and use less of their limited oxygen supply by good positioning. Bed patients with dyspnea are placed in good alignment and in high Fowler position unless this is contraindicated by their condition. You can help relax the shoulder muscles and allow expansion of the chest by supporting the forearms on pillows at the sides. Patients with obstructive diseases like emphysema breathe easier when they sit at the side of the bed or in a chair and rest their arms on two or three pillows placed on a table or night stand in front of them. Turning the head to one side helps to prevent the pooling of secretions in the back of the throat of unconscious, weak, or helpless patients. Postural drainage is also used to promote the removal of secretions from the lungs.

ITEM 4. PRINCIPLES AND PRECAUTIONS FOR OXYGEN THERAPY

Oxygen is a colorless, tasteless, and odorless gas that is present in the air. Although it is essential for life, the use of oxygen is not without its disadvantages. One of the properties of the gas is that it supports combustion. High concentrations of oxygen can cause fires to burn very rapidly, and when used medically in the treatment of patients, great care must be taken to prevent fires from occurring. A second hazard in the use of oxygen is the possibility of infection occurring if contaminated articles are used in the treatment of the patient. Bacteria thrive in the presence of oxygen and more easily enter the body through the already impaired respiratory tract. The third disadvantage associated with the use of the gas is that it is very drying to the tissues of the respiratory tract. Unless moisture is added, the dried tissues become cracked and provide less resistance to infection.

When caring for patients who are receiving oxygen therapy, these principles can serve as a guide for your actions.

1. Give the proper amount of oxygen as ordered for the individual. While a little oxygen is often lifesaving, a lot of oxygen may be fatal for some patients. It is like any medication: A small amount is good, but a large amount is not necessarily better.

2. Maintain an open airway through correctly positioning and suctioning the patient or through the use of an airway. You should be alert to wet, gurgling respirations in the unconscious patient and see that suctioning is done by either you or another nurse. Assist the conscious patient who complains of any breathing difficulty.

3. Give oral hygiene every 3 to 4 hours because oxygen therapy is drying to the tissues, which often makes the mouth smell or taste bad. Inspect the skin around the nose and mouth for irritation from the equipment or the tape if used to secure the nasal catheter.

4. Prevent infections by removing, cleaning, or replacing nasal catheters every 6 to 10 hours, or according to your agency's policy. Sterile equipment should be used by the respiratory therapist when using respirators and ventilators for therapy. Change the catheter from one side to the other in order to reduce irritation of the tissues.

5. Monitor the activities of patients. The patient who requires oxygen therapy while on bedrest has a physical intolerance to additional activity if it produces shortness of breath, dizziness, or complaints of chest pain. You should provide nursing care as needed and allow frequent periods of rest.

6. For patients with O_2 p.r.n., do not discontinue the oxygen flow and then ask patients to immediately increase their activity by getting up to sit in a chair or going to the bathroom. Allow time for patients to adjust to room air before carrying out additional activities. The level of oxygen in the blood falls drastically as soon as the O_2 is turned off and may take 5 to 10 minutes or longer to return to normal.

U
N
I
T
31

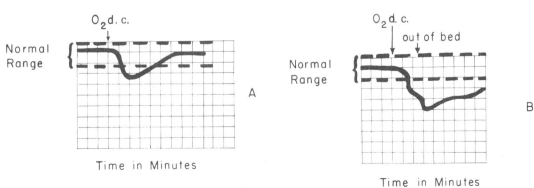

Return to normal O_2 level in blood with rest (A) and deficit with activity demand (B) after O_2 therapy is discontinued.

7. Observe safety measures to prevent explosion or fire.

    a. Place "No Smoking" signs at the door of the room and at the bedside.

    b. Instruct staff, patient, family, and visitors about the hazards caused by use of lighters, matches, candles, and other items that could cause fire.

    c. Electrical equipment used in the area must be in good working order and properly grounded, using the 3-prong outlet, to avoid electrical sparks.

    d. Avoid using wool blankets, nylon, and other materials that produce static electricity.

8. Oxygen tents are not used as extensively as in the past, but when an overbed tent is used for your patient, observe the following:

    a. Provide additional warmth if needed by using cotton blankets because the air flow inside the tent is cooling. Do not use wool or synthetics, which could cause sparks.

    b. Avoid using electrical equipment inside the tent because the oxygen concentration creates an extremely inflammable environment and could cause a fire. This includes electric razors, radios, suction machines, and call lights.

9. Take the patient's temperature rectally, so that the patient's breathing isn't impaired by an oral thermometer.

ITEM 5.   EQUIPMENT FOR OXYGEN THERAPY

The respiratory therapy department is usually given the responsibility of providing the equipment needed, setting it up, and supervising its use, but when respiratory therapists are not available, nurses may find it necessary to do this so that patients receive the needed oxygen. Nurses most often start oxygen for patients who receive it on a p.r.n. basis, monitor its use, and then discontinue it when no longer needed, so they need to know the basic function of the equipment used.

The equipment needed for the administration of oxygen therapy are the oxygen source, the flowmeter, the humidifier, the tubing, and the appropriate appliance for the method being used. In most hospitals, the equipment is assembled by the respiratory therapist, who often initiates the treatment and replaces used items when necessary. When respiratory therapists are not available, the nurse may collect the equipment, begin the treatment, and manage the therapy to meet the patient's oxygen needs.

The Flowmeter and the Humidifier

Today, most hospitals have a central oxygen supply with outlets mounted in the wall near the patient's bed. The flowmeter is attached to the piped-in O_2 and regulates the amount given. The rate of flow is prescribed by the physician in terms of liters per minute (liter/min) and may range from 2 to 12 liters/min. The flow rate is based on the patient's condition and the report of the blood gases that measure the amount of O_2 and CO_2 in the patient's blood. While rates of 4 to 6 liters/min are common, patients with emphysema and other obstructive lung diseases are given only 2 liters/min, because higher concentrations of O_2 further reduce the respiratory rate.

The rate of flow is adjusted by turning the valve to the "on" position, and continuing to turn it until the desired flow level is indicated in the gauge just above the flow adjustment valve. Different manufacturers may place the flowmeter control valve at different places on the meter, for example, at the top or the side of the gauge.

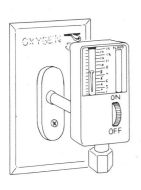

Flow meter

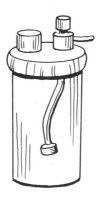

Humidifier bottles

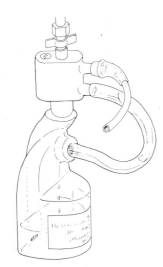

The humidifier is attached to the flowmeter and is usually situated between the flowmeter and the tubing. The oxygen bubbles through the container of water and is moisturized before entering the air passages. Check the level of fluid in the container at intervals during the day to make sure that it is working satisfactorily. When the fluid level is low, notify the respiratory care department so that the unit can be replaced or refilled with distilled water, if this is the policy in your agency.

Methods of Administering O_2

Tubing is attached to the humidifier and to the equipment used in the administration of the oxygen. Methods of administration include the use of nasal prongs (or cannula), a nasal catheter, face masks with or without a bag, a face tent, a Venturi mask, and the T-piece, which can be attached to an endotracheal tube.

Catheter. Oxygen is given by nasal catheter when high concentrations (up to 35 per cent) of oxygen are required. The nasal catheter may be rubber or plastic. It is about 16 inches long, with several small holes in the tip of the catheter so that the oxygen can come out of the tube in several places. The type and size of the catheter for an adult is usually a #14 French.

This method is frequently used because it is efficient, it is not frightening to most patients, it permits easy observation of the patient by nursing personnel, and it gives the patient freedom to move about in bed. The catheter may cause some irritation to the nasal passages if it is left in for a long period of time; therefore, a humidifier is always used with this type of administration to keep the passageways moist. Although as a beginning nurse practitioner you will not initiate the use of the various nasal oxygen techniques, you may be responsible for starting and stopping the oxygen flow per doctor's or patient's request.

Cannula. The nasal cannula consists of a rubber or plastic tube with short curved prongs that extend into the nostril about ¼ to ½ inch. The cannula is held in place with an elastic band that fits snugly around the head and attaches to the cannula and can be easily adjusted for the patient's comfort. There is no need to fasten the cannula to the patient's face with tape; therefore, with this method of oxygen therapy the skin will not become irritated. This may be useful for patients requiring oxygen during meals.

Masks. Various types of masks are available for the administration of oxygen in concentrations ranging from 24 to 55 per cent at flows of 3 to 7 liters/min. Oxygen concentrations above 60 per cent are rarely used because of the danger of oxygen toxicity. Some patients may dislike this method of oxygen administration, since the mask must be placed over their face and they feel that the mask will suffocate them.

The Venturi mask is made to provide oxygen mixed with room air in precise proportions to deliver an oxygen concentration of 24, 28, 35, and 40 per cent to the patient. Usually the respiratory therapist performs and supervises its use.

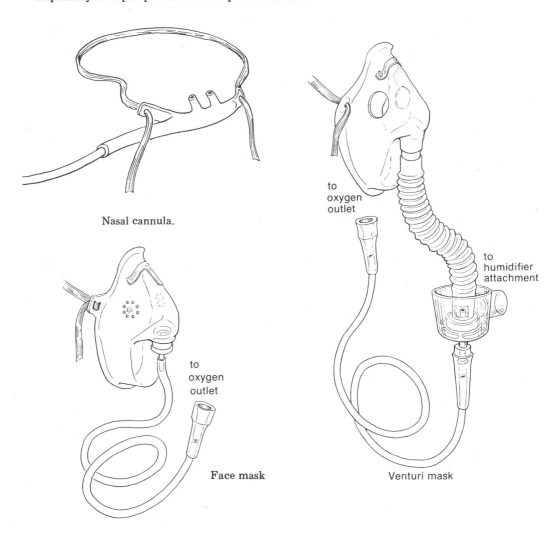

Nasal cannula.

Face mask

Venturi mask

ITEM 6.   ADMINISTERING OXYGEN THERAPY

You should be aware of the techniques for beginning administration so that you can assist the nurse or doctor and the patient. You must know how to regulate the oxygen flowmeters.

In the skill laboratory, given an emergency patient who is having severe breathing problems, assist in obtaining, assembling, and initiating oxygen by using a nasal catheter, nasal prongs or cannula, or oxygen mask.

Supplies Needed

Flowmeter	Oxygen delivery equipment:
Humidifier	Nasal catheter and lubricant
Tubing	Nasal cannula (prongs)
"No Smoking" signs	Oxygen mask

Important Steps	Key Points
1. Wash your hands, approach and identify the patient, and explain what is to be done.	Universal Steps A, B, C, and D. See Appendix.

2. Assemble the necessary equipment.

3. Connect the apparatus.

Attach the flowmeter to the piped-in oxygen outlet on the wall by pressing it firmly into the outlet. Attach connector tubing to the humidifier and the nasal catheter, cannula, or mask.

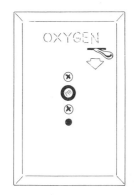

Wall-mounted oxygen outlet.

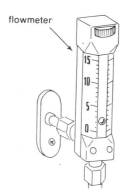

flowmeter

4. Turn on the oxygen.

Set the wall-mounted oxygen flow at 3 liters per minute. This is done by turning the flow adjustment valve toward the "on" position.

Test the oxygen flow by inserting the tip of the nasal catheter in a glass of water. The oxygen will bubble out through the holes in the catheter. If it does not, check to see if the holes are plugged.

5. Put the nasal cannula or mask in place, or insert the nasal catheter.

To insert the nasal catheter, carry out these steps:

a. Measure the length of the catheter to be inserted from the tip of the nose to the ear lobe.

b. Lubricate the tip with a water-soluble lubricant. Do not use mineral oil or vaseline, which can cause lipid pneumonia.

c. Introduce the catheter along the floor of the nasal passage straight toward the ear.

d. Check the location at the back of the throat on one side of the vulva.

e. Secure the catheter to the face with tape (1) to the side of the nose or (2) over the bridge of the nose and on the forehead.

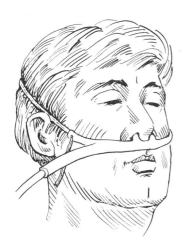

Cannula in place.

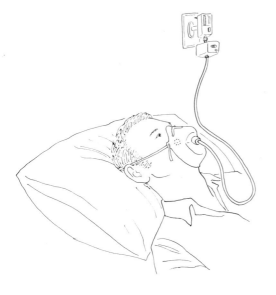

Face mask in place .

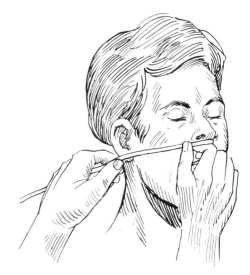

Measuring nasal catheter.

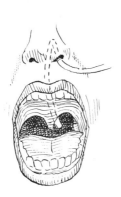

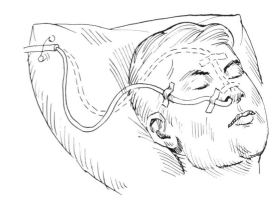

Nasal catheter in place.

Important Steps	Key Points
6. Adjust the oxygen flow.	Set it at the rate prescribed by the physician. (You may have done this under step 4.)
7. Place a "No Smoking" sign strategically.	Put signs on the head of the bed, on the oxygen equipment, and on the patient's door. Warn visitors against smoking.
8. Provide for the patient's comfort.	Universal Steps X, Y, and Z. See Appendix.
9. Record the oxygen therapy.	Remember, the *Initiation* of the oxygen treatment is usually done by the nurse. The oxygen may be ordered p.r.n., however, and you may be responsible for turning the flowmeter on or off as the patient requests. Be sure to record each administration. Charting example: 1015. Nasal oxygen started at 3 liters/min. Respirations 20 and less labored, color is pink. Seems less apprehensive. <div align="right">R. Olsen, SN</div>

ITEM 7. IPPB THERAPY

Although IPPB (intermittent positive pressure breathing) treatments are generally administered by the respiratory therapy department, you will be required to observe patients receiving these treatments as you would any patient receiving oxygen therapy. Give frequent oral hygiene and maintain the previously stated safety precautions. If you do give IPPB treatments, you will undoubtedly be given special training.

IPPB is a method of inflating the lungs with air or oxygen given under slight pressure on an intermittent basis. The best positive pressure ventilators can be adjusted to the requirements of the individual patient. IPPB treatments are given for 15 to 20 minutes three or four times a day and are utilized for:

1. Preoperatively familiarizing the patient in anticipation of postoperative use.

2. Preventing atelectasis by increasing the depth of respiration.

3. Promoting the clearing of bronchial secretions in pulmonary edema, pneumonia, asthma, bronchitis, and emphysema.

4. Delivering aerosol medications to dilate the bronchi and relieve bronchospasm.

5. Lessening the effort of breathing for patients who have certain respiratory diseases.

6. Facilitating the exchange of oxygen and carbon dioxide, and improving alveolar ventilation.

IPPB treatment can be given on a p.r.n. (as needed) basis or continuously, depending on the needs of the patient. Some types of positive pressure ventilators are used on a continuous basis for patients who have had severe head injuries or whose respirations are critically reduced by drugs, disease, or surgery. In these cases, an interruption of the regular respiratory rate for more than 2 minutes can lead to death. Most patients needing mechanical ventilation on a continuing basis are cared for in medical or surgical intensive care units during the acute period of their illness. Since an artificial airway is needed, constant supervision of these patients is required.

U
N
I
T
31

ITEM 8. ADMINISTRATION OF OXYGEN BY TENT

Oxygen tents are used less frequently than they were 25 years ago. They supply a relatively high concentration of oxygen (50 to 60 per cent) and provide a means of circulating the moist air around the patient. The temperature of the air can be somewhat controlled and it provides comfortable air-conditioning for the patient. The oxygen tent is not economically efficient because of the high volume of oxygen needed to maintain the designated concentration, as well as loss of oxygen when the tent is raised to permit working with the patient. You should plan your work so that you do not have to loosen the oxygen tent frequently; on those occasions when you do loosen the tent, carry out as many procedures as possible to reduce the number of times the tent must be raised.

While many patients like the oxygen tent because they can move about freely, they sometimes have a feeling of isolation. You must therefore talk with these patients frequently. If you speak loudly and clearly, they can hear you without your disturbing the tent.

Most oxygen tents now in use are electrically cooled models. When taking care of children in pediatrics, an apparatus is used similar to the oxygen tent. Called a mistogen tent, or Croupette, it provides both oxygen and very high humidity. The Croupettes are commonly used for children who have respiratory congestion or a disease process.

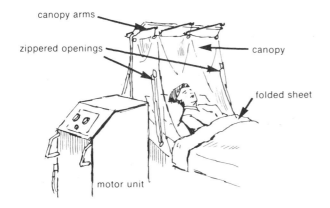

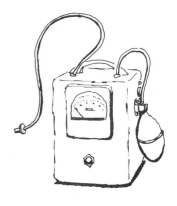

Oxygen analyzer
(records oxygen
concentration).

In the skill laboratory, given a young male patient who has pneumonia, you will assist in setting up and regulating the oxygen tent.

Supplies Needed

Console control unit with canopy
Flowmeter and tubing
Drawsheet

Oxygen analyzer
"No Smoking" or "Oxygen in Use" signs

Important Steps	Key Points
Carry out Universal Steps A, B, C, and D. See Appendix.	
1. Place the control console at the head of the bed. 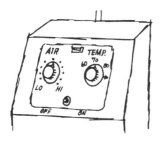	Move the tent to the head of the bed. Place it along one side of the bed with the regulating dials facing away from the patient. Extend the canopy arm to a horizontal position.
2. Plug in the unit and turn it on.	Plug the cord into the electrical outlet. Check the cord to be sure it is not frayed. Turn the motor on and set the control knobs on the control panel. Set the temperature at 70°F. Set the circulation dial halfway between low and high.

Important Steps	Key Points
3. Connect the oxygen to the control unit.	Attach the oxygen flowmeter to the wall outlet; then connect the oxygen outlet from the tent to the flowmeter.
4. Start the oxygen at 15 liters/min.	Some units use ice for cooling and have a water tray at the back of the machine. If yours does, fill it with ice, check it often, and empty the accumulated water.
5. Place the canopy over the head of the bed and secure the sides.	Arrange the canopy over the patient, but do not drag it over the patient's face. Secure the edges by folding a drawsheet in half lengthwise, laying it across the patient's abdomen, then placing the bottom edge of the tent canopy securely under the mattress at both sides of the bed and at the head of the mattress. Be sure that zippered openings in the sides of the canopy are tightly closed.
6. Check the oxygen concentration in the tent.	Utilize the oxygen analyzer routinely at 2- to 4-hour intervals to determine the concentration (per cent) of oxygen in the tent. Allow 15 minutes for oxygen concentration to increase and stabilize after the tent has been opened.
7. Adjust the oxygen flow between 10 and 15 liters/min. to maintain desired concentration.	After the initial analysis the flow rate may be reduced to maintain the desired concentration but should never be below 10 liters. Flow below 10 liters does not allow for adequate removal of CO_2.
8. Post signs for "No Smoking" or "Oxygen in Use."	
Carry out Universal Steps X, Y, and Z. See Appendix.	Charting example: 2030. Frequent spasms of tight, non-productive coughing. T — 102.8, P — 110, R — 32 with some dyspnea. BP — 134/90. Placed in oxygen tent at 15 liters/min. O_2 concentration = 50%. 2115. Resting quietly. Color good. P — 88, R — 24. No coughing at this time. M. Mann, RN

U
N
I
T
31

ITEM 9. USING THE OXYGEN CYLINDER

Obtain the oxygen cylinders (tank) and accessory equipment from central service or the respiration therapy department (as designed by your agency). Observe and maintain the following safety measures before the first step of the procedure is begun.

1. Stand the cylinder securely in its carrier in order to keep it from falling.

2. Put the cylinder beside the head of the bed, away from doors, doorways, heaters, and areas that have continuous, concentrated traffic.

3. Check the oxygen cylinder tag, which has a perforated design to indicate the following information: "Full," "In Use," "Empty." When the cylinder is turned on for the patient, remove the "Full" segment, leaving the "In Use" marker visible. When the tank is empty, remove the "In Use" segment, leaving the "Empty" marker visible. At this point notify the respiratory therapy department to remove or replace the cylinder.

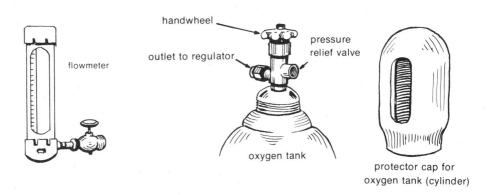

Supplies Needed

Oxygen equipment:
  Tubing
  Humidifier
  Nasal catheter, cannula, mask,
    or tent

Oxygen cylinder (on carrier)
Wrench
Flowmeter or regulator
"No Smoking" signs

Important Steps	Key Points
1. Stand at the side of the cylinder.	Direct the oxygen outlet away from people and warn the patient of the impending noise.
2. Slowly turn the handwheel clockwise to slightly open the cylinder and close immediately.	The handwheel is on the top of the cylinder. The slight opening removes dust particles and is known as "cracking the valve." The slow motion prevents the sudden uncontrolled release of gas under pressure.
3. Attach the regulator to the valve outlet connection.	Using a wrench, tighten the regulator nut onto the outlet valve until the nut is tight and holds the regulator firmly.
4. Attach the top of the humidifier to the oxygen regulator flow gauge or flowmeter.	Be sure that the flowmeter is set at "off" when you connect it with the oxygen outlet or cylinder.
5. Open the handwheel slowly and adjust the flow gauge or flowmeter to the prescribed liter flow.	This turns on the cylinder regulators.
6. Proceed to utilize the oxygen equipment prescribed for the patient (nasal catheter, mask, nasal cannula, or tent).	Refer to the application and safety steps in Item 6.

ITEM 10. HYPERBARIC OXYGEN CHAMBERS

Hyperbaric oxygen chambers are especially constructed rooms that provide for very high oxygen concentrations; they are used to treat patients who have anaerobic (without oxygen) infections, or patients whose hemoglobin is not carrying enough oxygen to the tissues. Inasmuch as these units are installed in few health agencies at this time, we will not describe their operation. If you are assigned to this type of patient, you will undoubtedly receive some training in working with a hyperbaric chamber before your assignment.

PERFORMANCE TEST

1. Regulate the oxygen flowmeter to give (1) 4 liters of oxygen per minute, and (2) 10 liters of oxygen per minute. Be sure to have your instructor check you at each point. Practice recording the activity in the nurses' notes.

2. Demonstrate the equipment used and discuss the purpose of oxygen administration by means of a nasal catheter, cannula, or mask.

PERFORMANCE CHECKLIST

REGULATION OF FLOWMETER

1. Wash your hands.

2. Approach and identify the patient, and explain the procedure.

3. Check the flowmeter to be sure that the humidifier bottle is 2/3 filled with water.

4. Adjust the flow by opening the flow valve until the gauge reads 4 liters/min (to be checked by your instructor).

5. Continue adjusting the flow valve until the gauge reads 10 liters/min.

6. Adjust the flow to read 4 liters/min.

7. Record the activity on nurses' notes.

USE OF OXYGEN THERAPY EQUIPMENT

1. Wash your hands.

2. Identify the patient, and explain the procedure.

3. Assemble the appropriate equipment and position the bed to a comfortable working height.

4. For the catheter:

   a. Measure the catheter length for insertion from the nose to the ear lobe.

   b. Lubricate the tip with water-soluble lubricant.

   c. Insert the catheter and check the length by looking into the patient's mouth.

   d. Secure the catheter with tape.

5. For the cannula and mask:

   a. Place the equipment in or over the patient's nose.

   b. Adjust the head strap for comfort.

6. Regulate O_2 flow per the physician's order.

7. Post "No Smoking" signs.

8. Leave the patient comfortable and in good body alignment.

9. Record the activity on the patient's chart.

POST-TEST

Directions.   Choose the answer that will make the statement complete.

1. Common methods of delivering oxygen to patients include all of the following except

    a. the nasal cannula.

    b. a mask.

    c. an oxygen tent.

    d. IPPB.

2. The respiratory system consists of all of the following except

    a. the nose.

    b. the larynx.

    c. the bronchi and trachea.

    d. the esophagus.

3. The equipment needed for the oxygen set-up includes all of the following except

    a. an oxygen flow meter.

    b. a nasal catheter.

    c. an oil-based lubricant.

    d. a connecting tube.

4. All tissues of the body require a continuous supply of oxygen because

    a. O_2 surrounds and bathes the cells.

    b. it is used to produce energy.

    c. O_2 fights off infectious organisms.

    d. it helps the cells to grow and multiply.

5. Normal breathing is characterized by each of the following statements except for which one?

    a. Inspiration is a passive activity.

    b. Breathing is a routine and semi-automatic activity.

    c. Muscles raise and lift the rib cage during inspiration.

    d. The diaphragm moves down and out when inhaling.

6. The exchange of the gases O_2 and CO_2 takes place in

    a. the bronchi.

    b. the nares.

    c. the alveoli.

    d. the large arteries.

7. In the normal, healthy person, the rate of breathing is regulated more by which of these factors?

   a. The O_2 level in the blood.

   b. The CO_2 level in the blood.

   c. The anxiety level of the person.

   d. The amount of hemoglobin in the blood.

8. How does an upper respiratory infection affect the person who has some swelling of membranes in the nose?

   a. The person works harder to breathe and has less oxygen.

   b. Usually has no effect because the obstruction is minor.

   c. The amount of oxygen in the blood remains unchanged.

   d. There is less oxygen in the air that is taken in.

9. The most common cause of decreased oxygen intake, or hypoxia, is

   a. impairment of nerves and respiratory muscles.

   b. difficulty in the diffusion of the gases.

   c. pollution of the environmental air.

   d. an obstruction of the air passages.

10. The first symptom of a reduction in the supply of oxygen needed to meet the body's demands is

    a. increasing restlessness, or irritability.

    b. panting type of respiration.

    c. cyanosis of the nailbeds of the fingers.

    d. retraction of muscles used in breathing.

11. In providing nursing care for patients who are having difficulty breathing, it is important to reduce the patient's anxiety because it

    a. increases the pulse and respiratory rate.

    b. causes tense muscles that need more oxygen.

    c. causes needless fear and worry.

    d. delays recovery and healing of injured tissues.

12. The type of patient who is more apt to have insufficient oxygen intake to meet the needs of the body is

    a. the hyperactive patient.

    b. the quiet, immobile patient.

    c. the patient following abdominal surgery.

    d. the patient with cancer of the lung.

    e. all except a.

    f. all except b.

13. One nursing measure you could use to help the patient relax who is having difficulty breathing is to

    a. suction the trachea.

    b. turn to the Sims position.

    c. sit with arms resting on pillows.

    d. assist to walk about the room.

14. All of the following are hazards associated with oxygen therapy. Which one is not specifically mentioned in this unit?

    a. Possibility of fires

    b. Infections from contaminated items

    c. Arrhythmias of the heart

    d. Drying of respiratory tract tissues

15. The patient with dyspnea has oxygen running at 2 liters/min. and is breathing somewhat easier. Since the O_2 seems to be helping, what would you do?

    a. Increase the oxygen to 4 or 6 liters/min.

    b. Discontinue the oxygen.

    c. Leave it at 2 liters/min as ordered.

    d. Begin patient activities, such as the bath.

16. Masks used to give oxygen may frequently cause the patient to complain of

    a. skin irritation.

    b. a feeling of smothering.

    c. face pain.

    d. a feeling that the mask is too small.

17. When you use any oxygen, important safety factors include all of the following except

    a. "No Smoking" signs.

    b. nonfrayed electric cords.

    c. use of woolen blankets.

    d. water in the humidifier.

18. The IPPB treatment is utilized for all of the following except

    a. the prevention of atelectasis.

    b. delivery of aerosol medications to constrict the bronchi.

    c. the improvement of alveolar ventilation.

    d. to relax the respiratory muscles.

UNIT
31

POST-TEST ANSWERS

1.	d	10.	a
2.	d	11.	b
3.	c	12.	e
4.	b	13.	c
5.	a	14.	c
6.	c	15.	c
7.	b	16.	b
8.	a	17.	c
9.	d	18.	d

ASSISTING WITH INTRAVENOUS THERAPY

GENERAL PERFORMANCE OBJECTIVE

When you have completed this lesson, you will be able to maintain an IV and to give daily care to the patient who is receiving IV therapy. You will apply good safety measures throughout the procedure.

SPECIFIC PERFORMANCE OBJECTIVES

Following this lesson you will be able to:

1. Describe the parts of a primary IV.

2. State four purposes for patients to receive IV therapy.

3. Explain at least four principles to follow when caring for a patient with an IV.

4. List the points to observe when checking the patient's IV to see that it is running well.

5. Calculate the rate of flow of IV fluids when the amount of fluids and period of time is known.

6. Assist the patient as needed with daily care, bathing, dressing or undressing, eating, and ambulating with an IV running.

U
N
I
T
32

VOCABULARY

amino acids—the end products of protein digestion; there are 22 known amino acids.
bore (needle)—the inside passageway of a needle through which liquid passes.
flask—a bottle or container for liquids.
glucose—a simple sugar; dextrose
gtt—an abbreviation for "drops," used in the calculation of IV flow.
heparin lock—a supplementary IV line used at intervals to give doses of medications.
hyperalimentation—the parenteral administration of solutions of nutrients to provide total or supplemental calorie needs.
hypertonic—having greater osmotic pressure than body fluids.
hypotonic—having less osmotic pressure than body fluids.
infiltrate—collection of fluid in the tissue when the needle is not properly placed in the vein.
infusion— the act of pouring into, commonly associated with the introduction of liquids into a vein
intermittent IV—the giving of doses of medications intravenously and at intervals using a needle or cannula attached to a short tubing containing heparin known as a heparin lock or heparin well.
isotonic—having the same osmotic pressure as body fluids.

lumen—a hollow passageway.

macrodrop—a large drop, usually one tenth of a milliliter (i.e., 10 drops per ml).

microdrop—a small drop, usually one sixtieth of a milliliter (60 drops per ml).

pH—a term used to indicate alkalinity (high pH) or acidity (low pH).

parenteral—referring to the introduction of materials into the body by routes other than the intestinal tract (orally).

piggy-back IV—a second flask or bottle added to a primary IV line.

saline—sodium chloride (NaCl), or salt.

TPN—total parenteral nutrition; supplying all of the patient's nutritional needs through the intravenous route.

transfusion—the act of transferring blood or its component parts (plasma, serum, packed cells) from one person to another.

viscous (viscosity)—pertaining to a substance that is sticky or gummy in consistency.

INTRODUCTION

In recent years, the intravenous route has become exceedingly popular as a method of supplying the patient with fluids and medications when the patient is unable to take them orally or rectally. Of all of the parenteral routes (that is, routes other than the intestinal tract), the intravenous route has the advantage of making the drug or solution instantly available, since it is injected directly into the bloodstream and circulated to all tissues. The disadvantage is that the material cannot be retrieved if an error has been made. Additionally, because a needle or catheter is used to provide entry into the blood vessel, all material must be sterile in order to avoid introducing bacteria into the circulation, where it could cause widespread infection.

Your responsibilities relating to IV therapy may vary according to what you are taught in your nursing program and what is specified in the hospital policies where you work. Nursing assistants generally provide nursing care, see that the IV is running, and observe the needle site for signs of infiltration. On the other hand, student nurses may be designated to adjust rates of flow, add bottles of fluids, or terminate IV's with or without supervision. Some students in RN programs are allowed to give medications via the IV route. You may carry out those tasks that have been designated by your instructors, team leader, or supervisor.

Many of your patients will be receiving fluids or medications by this route, so you will need to know some basic information about IV equipment, the type of solutions that are used, principles related to the use of this route, and the way to monitor or keep track of the rate of flow. Most of the patients who require fluids by the IV method should be on Intake and Output, and careful record should be kept of the amounts to be infused during the shift or period of time.

When you enter your patient's room, you should quickly observe the condition of the patient — whether awake or asleep, the level of consciousness if awake, and any visible sign of difficulty or discomfort. Next, you should observe the special equipment that may be in use, particularly any tubes attached to the patient, such as an IV, oxygen or nasogastric tube, or a Foley catheter. Pay special attention to where the tube enters or is attached to the body and then follow the tubing to its source or origin to see that it is working as it should.

In this Unit, we will discuss the use of IV therapy, principles related to it, and care of the patient with an IV. Items in the Unit discuss in quite basic terms such topics as reasons for using the IV method, the types of solutions that are commonly used, a brief description of IV equipment, principles involved in using the IV route, other types of IV's, ways of monitoring the rate of flow, and steps in giving care to patients who have IV's. For additional information on IV's, refer to Unit 7 in Volume 3, Medication Administration: Intravenous Medications and Infusions.

THE ADMINISTRATION OF INTRAVENOUS THERAPY

ITEM 1. WHY ARE IV'S GIVEN?

IV's are given to supply the body with needed elements that cannot be supplied as rapidly or efficiently by other means. These elements may be:

1. Blood, plasma, or other blood components.

2. Nutritional requirements in the form of glucose, amino acids, or saline.

3. Fluids and salts when the patient is unable to receive enough of these by mouth (orally).

4. Medications that the patient is unable to take by any other means.

The sites most frequently used for IV's are the veins of the forearm and hand. The veins that are so prominent on the inner surface of the elbow are not used extensively for IV infusions because movement of the elbow causes infiltration or damage to the vein. This makes it impossible to use veins distal to that point. IV's are seldom started in the veins of the legs of adults unless no other vein is available, because of the increased danger of causing phlebitis or thrombosis. Scalp veins are often used for IV purposes in infants because the veins in the arms and legs are too small or difficult to enter with the needle.

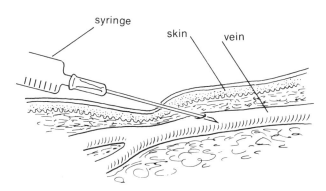

ITEM 2. TYPES OF IV SOLUTIONS

The physician orders the type of solution to be given, the amount to be infused, and the rate by either the number of hours it is to run or the volume per hour. There are many types of solutions available, and still others can be prepared to meet specific needs of the individual patient. As a nurse at the beginning level of practice, you need to be able to recognize the most commonly used types of fluids, even though you are not responsible for starting, adding fluids to, or discontinuing the IV. The solutions most frequently used are those containing glucose, saline, electrolytes, vitamins, and amino acids. In addition to these, blood and blood products are given intravenously. Some of the more common solutions follow:

- Normal Saline. This is an isotonic solution of 0.9 per cent sodium chloride, or salt. It resembles most body fluids in density and osmotic pressure, and it combines well with blood.

- One-half Normal Saline. The solution is half the strength of normal saline, or 0.45 per cent concentration. It is hypotonic, which means that it is drawn into cells such as red blood cells.

- 5 per cent Dextrose in Water. One liter of solution contains 50 gm of glucose and supplies 4 calories per gm, or a total of 200 calories per liter.

- 5 per cent Dextrose in Saline. This solution contains glucose in isotonic saline.

- Ringer's Solution. This is a solution of normal saline with potassium and calcium added to help maintain or restore electrolyte balance in the body.

- Solutions for TPN. Total parenteral nutrition (TPN) supplies all of the body's nutritional needs through a special type of IV usually placed in a large vein that empties into the heart. Hypertonic solutions of glucose, amino acids, electrolytes, and lipids (fats) are given slowly and usually by means of an infusion pump.

- Blood and blood products. Whole blood and its components — plasma, platelets, and packed red cells — are given by transfusion.

The amount of IV fluids to be given in a 24-hour period will depend on many factors. Generally, the average adult will require between 2000 and 3000 ml per day to maintain the fluid balance as described in Unit 22. More will be required if the patient is losing fluids by some abnormal route such as vomiting, diarrhea, wound drainage, or serum loss in extensive burns.

ITEM 3. MANAGING THE IV.

According to the Kardex, the doctor has ordered the following IV fluids for your patient: #1 — 5% D/S, 1000 ml to run 10 hours, and #2 — 5% D/W 1000 ml to run 10 hours. As a beginning level student, what are your responsibilities for the IV? What are you expected to know or to do about it? How will it affect the care you are to give the patient?

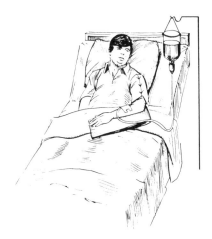

The assignment of responsibilities differs from one agency to another and varies according to the level of nursing. General procedures and principles are described here to serve as guidelines as you care for patients receiving IV's.

Who Starts IV's?

The fluid therapy through intravenous route involves placing a needle or cannula in a vein. It is necessary to puncture the skin, which causes some degree of discomfort for the patient. Unless the needle is inserted skillfully and accurately, the vein could be damaged and other tissues bruised by unsuccessful probing. Most general hospitals and health agencies have an IV policy that states who is allowed to start IV's and how they qualify for this responsibility. Most policies specify that licensed nurses, either RN's or LPN's, may start IV's if they have completed a course of instruction and are certified by the hospital. Just having a license is not sufficient; nurses must have additional training and instruction.

In many larger hospitals, there is a team of IV nurses responsible for starting all IV's, giving IV medications, trouble-shooting when there are problems in keeping the IV's running, and starting transfusions. In some hospitals, a doctor must be present to start the transfusion of blood or its components.

Keeping the IV Running

Your primary responsiblity will be to check the IV each time you see the patient and to see that it is running properly. You should check frequently, every half hour or so, and observe each of these points as your eyes travel from the bottle, down the tubing and to the needle site:

1. The level of fluid remaining in the bottle or flask. When there is 50 to 100 ml left, be sure to notify the nurse so that a new bottle can be added before the current bottle is completely empty.

2. The IV flow. The solution should drip into the chamber at regular intervals, unless a volume infusion pump is being used.

3. The rate of the infusion. Is there a time strip indicating that by a certain time this amount of fluid should have run in? Or is the IV to run at a rate of so many drops per minute? Count the rate. If it is too fast or too slow, it should be adjusted by the designated nurse so that the correct amount of fluid is infused per hour.

4. The needle site. Are there any signs of infiltration (solution leaking out of the vein into the surrounding tissue)? If infiltration is occurring, there is swelling and blanching of the skin. Redness at the site may be an indication of inflammation.

UNIT 32

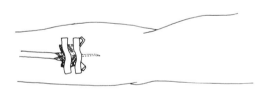

5. Complaints by the patient. After the IV has been started, it should not cause any pain or discomfort. Complaints of pain, difficulty breathing, itching, or other symptoms indicate problems that should be reported, and appropriate actions should be taken.

The IV bottle is hung from an IV standard or pole so it will not fall or tip over. The tubing should be long enough to provide enough room for the patient to move about in bed, to turn over, or to carry out necessary activities. An armboard is used to support the arm and to prevent excess movement that might cause the IV to infiltrate. Soft restraints are needed for children and confused patients who might pull out the IV or cause it to infiltrate. Infants are often placed in a "mummy" restraint. The child is "mummied" by wrapping a sheet or blanket folded in fourths around the body so the arms are bound lightly to the sides of the body and only the head, neck, and feet are free. It is important that the child not be kept restrained for a long period of time, because movement is so restricted.

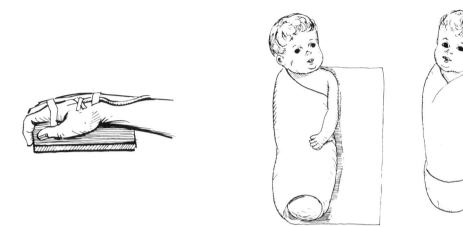

Restrain infant for IV.

When caring for the patient receiving IV therapy, be sure to keep the solution sterile. The tubing should not be disconnected at anytime, and other bottles of fluid or medications are added to the IV only by the designated nurse.

ITEM 4. TYPES OF IV EQUIPMENT

Many types of IV administration sets are manufactured and available for use. They include the standard or primary administration sets, the "Y" set, tubing for tandem or series infusions, sets with injection ports for "piggy-back" infusions, and controlled volume sets. These are illustrated and described in more detail in *Nursing Skills*, Volume 3. The primary IV consists of the bottle of sterile fluids, the IV tubing with its drip chamber, a clamp to regulate the flow, and the needle or cannula that is inserted into the vein.

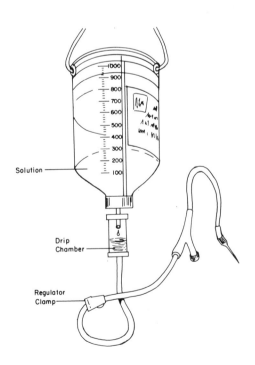

The primary IV tubing set is selected according to the size of the drop to be delivered into the drip chamber. There are three major sizes:

1. *Regular drops* (15 drops/ml of fluid, or as specified by the manufacturer): used for administering IV therapy to most adult patients.

2. *Macrodrops* (10 drops/ml): used for thick, viscous fluids, such as blood.

3. *Microdrops* (60 drops/ml): used when very small amounts of fluid are required or when extreme care must be used to measure the exact amount. Most often used when giving IV fluids to infants and children.

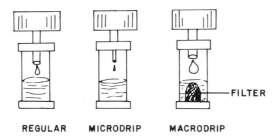

REGULAR   MICRODRIP   MACRODRIP

Piggy-Back Method. Another type of IV that is commonly used is the "piggy-back" method, which uses a tubing set with one or more injection ports so that a smaller bottle of IV medications with its tubing can be added to the primary IV. The smaller bottle of medication is hung higher than the level of fluid in the primary bottle so that it will run in first. When it is empty, the solution in the lower bottle will begin to run in at the same rate of flow, unless of course the tubing had been clamped off for some reason. The designated RN or IV nurse is responsible for adding medications "piggy-back" to the IV.

Intermittent IV Line. Some patients do not require large amounts of fluid by the IV route but may need to receive IV medications at intervals. An intermittent IV line is established by inserting a needle that is attached to a small length of tubing that is capped and contains a heparin solution to prevent the blood from clotting in the needle. This is called a heparin well, heparin lock, Jelco plug, or other similar trade name.

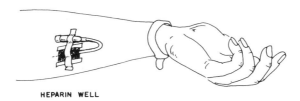

HEPARIN WELL

Infusion Pump. Infusion pumps are used in many hospitals to regulate the flow or rate of IV fluids, especially when patients receive hyperalimentation or medications for which it is essential that a certain amount be infused in a certain time period. The pumps tend to vary, so you will need to have a demonstration of how to handle the tubing and bottle when your patient needs a clean gown.

ITEM 5. THE RATE OF FLOW

When IV therapy is administered, the fluid enters the circulation immediately. The adult adapts best to fluids given at a steady rate of 20 to 60 regular drops per minute, that is,

U
N
I
T
32

between 80 and 250 ml per hour. Larger amounts of fluids increase the work of the heart, and the fluid overload could lead to congestive heart failure.

Factors that influence the rate of flow of an IV solution are the size of the needle, the height of the flask, and the viscosity of the fluid. Fluids flow less rapidly through a needle with a small bore than through a needle with a larger bore. The higher the container is held, the faster is the flow of fluid. Blood is more viscous and requires a larger needle; thus, the macrodrip administration set is used.

If your hospital policy requires you to be responsible for regulating the amount of fluids the patient is to have by IV during a given period of time, you must know how to calculate and regulate the drip rate.

The physician generally orders IV fluids, 1000 ml, to be run in during an 8-, 10-, or 12 hour period. This amount should infuse at an even rate so that equal amounts are given each hour. When the number of hours is stated, many nurses prepare a time strip to be placed on the bottle that shows the amount to be infused each hour and the level of the solution remaining in the bottle at 0900, 1000, 1100, and so forth.

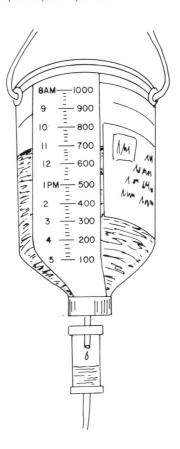

Keep the IV on time by regulating the drip rate. If the IV fluids are infusing behind schedule, recalculate or reschedule the time in consultation with your team leader or the physician.

How to Calculate. If you have questions about how to calculate the IV drop rate, check with your instructor. There are charts available that have already calculated the rates for the various drip chambers and for the period of time ordered to run in standard amounts, such as 1000 ml. If you do not have one of these charts, it is necessary to solve the problem mathematically. The basic formula for calculating the rate of flow follows:

$$\frac{\text{amount of solution} \times \text{number of drops per ml}}{\text{time in minutes}} = \text{drops per minute}$$

Calculation of Rate Using the Regular IV Drip Chamber

Problem:	How many drops per minute are required for the physician's order of "1000 ml 5% dextrose in water in 12 hours"?
Known Facts:	15 gtts are released by the drip chamber for each ml.
	60 minutes = one hour.
	IV to run for 12 hours.
	Amount is 1000 ml.
Solution:	12 hours $\times$ 60 minutes = 720 minutes to run IV.
	1000 ml $\times$ 15 gtts/ml = 15,000 gtts to be given.
	Divide 15,000 gtts by 720 minutes = 21 gtts /minute.
	Rate is 21 gtts per minute.

Calculation of Rate Using the Micro-drip Chamber

Problem:	How many drops per minute are required for an order of "500 ml 5% dextrose in normal saline in 10 hours" for a child?
Known Facts:	60 gtts are released by the drip chamber for each ml.
	60 minutes = one hour.
	Since there are 60 drops in a ml and there are 60 minutes in an hour, the micro-drip will deliver drops at a ratio of 60:60, or 1:1.
Solution:	Divide 500 ml by 10 hours = 50 ml per hour.
	The ratio of gtts per ml and minutes per hour is 1:1.
	Therefore, the rate is 50 gtts per minute.

U
N
I
T
32

Calculation of Rate Using the Blood Transfusion Drip Chamber

Problem:	How many drops per minute are required when the physician's order states: "Give 500 ml whole blood in 4 hours"?
Known Facts:	10 gtts are released by the drip chamber for each ml.
	500 ml are to be given in 4 hours.
	60 minutes = one hour.
Solution:	500 ml $\times$ 10 gtts/ml = 5000 gtts.
	4 hours $\times$ 60 minutes = 240 minutes.
	Divide 5000 gtts by 240 minutes = 21 gtts/minute.
	Rate is 21 gtts per minute.

RATE OF DROPS REQUIRED TO INFUSE A VOLUME OF FLUIDS IN A SPECIFIED PERIOD OF TIME

Time (hours)	1000 ml Volume			500 ml Volume	
	Amount per hour (ml)	Regular Drops (15 gtts/ml)	Macrodrops (10 gtts/ml)	Amount per hour (ml)	Microdrops (60 gtts/ml)
12	83	21	14	41	41
11	91	23	15	45	45
10	100	25	17	50	50
9	111	28	19	55	55
8	125	31	21	63	63
7	143	36	24	72	72
6	167	42	28	83	83
5	200	50	33	100	100
4	250	63	41	125	125
3	333	83	56		
2	500	125	83		

ITEM 6. PRINCIPLES RELATED TO IV THERAPY

A number of principles can be drawn from the previous material regarding the use of IV's and the nurse's responsibilities in caring for the patients. Consider these when you care for a patient with an IV:

1. Protect the sterility of the fluid. Make sure that everything coming in contact with the solution is sterile, including the inside surfaces of the drip chamber, tubing, and needle, as well as all connecting points between the bottle and the drip chamber and between the tubing and the needle.

2. Protect the needle site from contamination to avoid possible infection. Many hospitals now apply an antibiotic ointment and an airtight dressing over the needle site. This should not be removed unless the IV is being discontinued.

3. Remove air bubbles from the tubing and do not allow the current bottle to run dry before adding the next one.

4. Fluids flow through the tubing by the force of gravity, and with negative pressure in the IV line, blood will flow back into the tubing. This is disturbing to patients because the flow should be the other way — into the vein.

5. Keep the bottle of fluids above the level of the needle site, but avoid having it too high, as it significantly increases the pressure of gravity and the rate of flow.

6. Regulate the rate of flow to keep the infusion on time. If the IV is behind schedule, do not open up the clamp and run in a large amount of fluid at one time to "catch up"; rather, recalculate either (1) the span of time for the infusion or (2) the rate of drops per minute.

7. Keep an accurate account of the patient's intake while receiving IV fluids. Input and Output records now provide space to chart the quantity in the bottle at the beginning and end of the time period, as well as the amount absorbed.

DATE: _____

			INTAKE					OUTPUT			
ORAL or TUBE			PARENTERAL					URINE		OTHER	
TIME	TYPE	AMT	TYPE	AMT. IN BOTTLE	TIME Start	TIME ABS	AMT. ABS	TIME	AMT.	TIME	TYPE	AMT.
0645	NPO		5% D/S #3	250								
							250					
0930			1000 5% D/W #4		0930							
1500				450			550					
7-3 TOTAL				8 HR. TOTAL		I.V. BLOOD	800	8 HR. TOTAL		8 HR. TOTAL		
1500			5% D/W #4	450								
3-11 TOTAL				8 HR. TOTAL		I.V. BLOOD		8 HR. TOTAL		8 HR. TOTAL		
11-7 TOTAL				8 HR. TOTAL		I.V. BLOOD		8 HR. TOTAL		8 HR. TOTAL		

24 HOUR ORAL _____	24 HOUR I.V. _____ 24 HOUR BLOOD _____	24 HOUR URINE _____	24 HOUR OTHER _____ _____

24 HOUR INTAKE _____   24 HOUR OUTPUT _____

U N I T 32

IV fluids are recorded on the Intake and Output Record.

8. When a second bottle is attached "piggy-back" to a primary IV line, the solution in the highest bottle runs in first. It is not necessary to clamp the tubing of the lower bottle, because it will not begin to flow until all other fluid higher than its level has run in.

9. Be alert for signs of infiltration and reactions. The usual sign is pain or discomfort due to misplacement of the needle, puncture of the vein, irritation of vein or formation of blood clots. Vital signs should be taken several times a day in order to detect early signs of reactions.

10. Reactions to transfusions of whole blood usually occur shortly after the start of the transfusion; they are less apt to occur when only components such as packed red cells, plasma, or platelets are given. The reactions most commonly seen are hives, itching, facial flushing, chills, and fever. If any of these occur, notify the nurse who will stop the transfusion and contact the doctor for further orders.

ITEM 7.   CARING FOR A PATIENT RECEIVING IV THERAPY

Important Steps	Key Points
1. Remove the patient's hospital gown.	Remove the gown from the arm without disturbing the IV. Keep the patient covered with a bath blanket to avoid exposure and chilling. Remove the IV bottle from the stand or hanger. Holding the bottle with one hand, pull the gown over the patient's arm and tubing and over the bottle. Remember: to *undress* a patient, the IV arm is *last*; to *dress* a patient, the IV arm is *first*. Rehang the bottle on the IV stand.
2. Bathe the patient.	Proceed according to Unit 17, Baths and Hygiene Measures. Wash gently around the area where the needle is inserted. Be sure not to loosen the tape that holds the needle secure. When drying the patient, pat gently over the vein to avoid dislodging the needle.

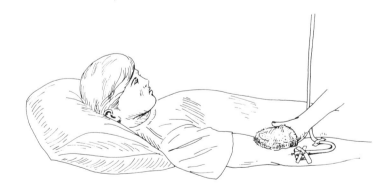

Important Steps	Key Points
3. Dress the patient.	Remove the IV bottle from the hanger. Pull the sleeve of the gown over the bottle and rehang the bottle on the IV stand. Continue carefully to thread the sleeve of the gown over the tubing and arm. Then finish dressing the patient as you would any other.
4. Assist the patient to eat.	If the IV is infusing in the hand or arm that the patient uses to eat, you will have to assist by cutting the food and preparing the liquids. You may need to feed the patient; if so, use the techniques described in Unit 23, Assisting with Nutrition. Even if the IV is attached to the arm that the patient does not use to eat, you will cut the meats and prepare the drinks. The food and utensils should be nearby for convenience. Assist as required; usually after the food is cut up, the patient can manage alone.
5. Ambulate the patient who is receiving IV therapy.	Provide a portable IV standard on wheels. Assist the patient out of bed as you were taught. Observe closely for weakness or dizziness. Support the IV arm to assure a continuous flow from the IV. A sling may be used for the patient to rest the arm in. If able, the patient may grasp the IV pole with the hand that has the IV in it. This provides support for the arm, enables the patient to move the pole at his or her own pace, and leaves the other arm free. Tell the patient to walk along one side to avoid blocking the corridor and to keep from bumping into people.

6. Observe the IV for proper functioning.	Check the patient's IV every 30 minutes. You should know the amount of fluids to be given per hour and the time at which it should be completed. Count the rate of drops and take appropriate action or report to your team leader any of the following situations:
	  a. Drops running too fast or too slow.
	  b. Low fluid level left in bottle.
	  c. Swelling around the needle site.
	  d. Patient reaction to the IV fluid, such as twitching, flushing, or blanching of skin, and increased respiration or pulse.

UNIT
32

Important Steps	Key Points
7. Apply the patient's restraints if ordered.	Follow your agency policies regarding the use of restraints, the type, and their application. Check the restraints frequently to see that circulation is not inhibited and that the fluid is running in correctly.
8. Chart on the nurses' notes and the I & O Record (if it is being used).	Charting example: 0945. Bed bath given. Ambulated in hall for 15 minutes. Returned to bed. IV running at 20 gtts/min. No redness or swelling around needle site. 200 ml solution remaining in bottle. J. Jones LVN

PERFORMANCE TEST

In the skills laboratory, bathe, feed, and ambulate a patient receiving IV therapy in the right arm. Maintain frequent checks as outlined in the unit of instruction.

When you have finished this part, complete the Intravenous Therapy Worksheet.

PERFORMANCE CHECKLIST

INTRAVENOUS THERAPY

1. Dress and undress a patient receiving IV therapy without dislodging the needle. (For additional detail, refer to the checklist in Unit 16, Dressing and Undressing.)

2. Give assistance with meals when needed. (For additional details, refer to Unit 23, Assisting With Nutrition.)

3. Bathe the IV site during the regular bath without causing pain to the patient or dislodging the needle. (Refer to Unit 17, Baths and Hygiene Measures, if required.)

4. Assist the patient with an IV to ambulate. (Refer to Unit 13, Patient Movement and Ambulation, if required.)

5. Check the functioning of the IV often:

   a. The IV fluid level.

   b. Swelling around the needle.

   c. The patient's reaction to the IV.

   d. The rate of flow.

UNIT 32

INTRAVENOUS THERAPY WORKSHEET

Directions: Proceed through the following items. After each situation, answer the questions on this worksheet and record the appropriate information on the nurses' notes. Discuss the situations and charting with your instructor.

Item I

Situation: Mrs. Rowe, the patient in Room 333, has a continuous intravenous drip going into the right forearm. A bed bath was given at 9:30 A.M. The nursing assistant then helped Mrs. Rowe to walk in the corridor for 15 minutes. When getting into bed, Mrs. Rowe slipped and moved her arm suddenly to balance herself on the bed. The IV drip slowed down but continued to drip. Later, the area around the insertion of the needle appeared slightly swollen.

Question: What action should the nursing assistant take?
What should be charted? Record the appropriate information in your nurses' notes.

Item II

Situation: Mr. Budd, in Room 624, is on continuous bed rest because of extreme weakness. He has been getting blood transfusions daily. Miss Wood, RN, started a blood transfusion (500 cc) at 11:00 A.M. in the left anticubital space. At 11:40 A.M. he rang the call light. When the nurse answered, she found Mr. Budd's face extremely flushed. He said he was chilled and needed more covers. She observed tremors around his lips. The blood transfusion was dripping rapidly and approximately 300 ml had been absorbed. Mr. Budd complained that he ached all over.

Question: What action should the nurse take?
What will the nurse chart? Record the appropriate information in your nurses' notes.

Item III

Situation: Baby Vincent had brain surgery and has an intravenous running in the left inner ankle. The left leg is securely restrained. The intravenous has been ordered to drip at a rate of 10 gtts per minute. When the student nurse had given 2 oz of Baby Vincent's formula, she noted that the IV bottle was empty and had blood coming back in the IV tubing near the needle.

Question: What action should the student nurse take?
What will the student nurse chart? Record the appropriate information in your nurses' notes.

Item IV

Situation: Mr. James, a 38-year-old healthy male was hospitalized after fracturing the right femur. An open reduction was done and Mr. James was received on the Orthopedic Ward with an IV running. The doctor ordered the present IV to be followed with 1000 ml 5% dextrose and water to be run during a period of 12 hours.

Question: At how many gtts per minute would the IV be set to complete in 12 hours?

Item V

Situation: Mr. George suffered a severe laceration on his left arm. The doctor ordered 500 ml of whole blood Type O to be infused at 200 ml per hour.

Question: How many gtts per minute would be given?

POST-TEST

Multiple Choice: Select the one best answer for each of the items.

1. Whenever you enter your patient's room, what is the first thing you should observe?

    a.   The neatness of the bed linens.

    b.   The condition of the wound dressing.

    c.   The condition of the patient.

    d.   The rate of drops in the IV.

2. The major advantage of the intravenous route over other parenteral routes is that the fluid

    a.   is immediately circulated to the tissues.

    b.   can be given over a longer period of time.

    c.   can be given in larger amounts.

    d.   is less apt to cause an adverse reaction.

3. The usual site used to insert the IV needle in adult patients receiving intravenous therapy is

    a.   the veins of the scalp.

    b.   veins in the legs.

    c.   the inner part of the elbow.

    d.   veins in the forearm.

4. The amount of IV fluids needed per day for the average adult patient who is NPO is about

    a.   500 to 1000 ml.

    b.   1000 to 1500 ml.

    c.   1500 to 2000 ml.

    d.   2000 to 3000 ml.

5. Which one of the following groups are allowed to start IV's according to the policies of most hospitals?

    a.   The nurse assigned to give medications.

    b.   The head nurse in charge of the unit.

    c.   Licensed nurses who are certified by the hospital.

    d.   Nurses who have one year's experience or more.

6. After the IV has been started, the patient continues to complain of pain at the site of the needle. Which of the following actions would you take?

    a.   Reassure the patient this is common, but it goes away.

    b.   Report it to the nurse because an IV should not cause pain.

    c.   Wrap the arm in a towel to provide soothing warmth.

    d.   Notify the nurse so that medication for pain can be given.

7. All of the following parts of the IV must remain sterile *except*

   a. the fluid being infused.

   b. the inner surfaces of the tubing.

   c. the outer surface of the bottle.

   d. the needle shaft in the vein.

8. The most common reason for an IV to stop dripping is that

   a. it has infiltrated.

   b. blood backs up in the tubing.

   c. the solution is too thick.

   d. the vein is too full.

9. A heparin well is inserted in the patient's vein and is used for giving

   a. large amounts of fluids per day.

   b. nutrients by the parenteral route.

   c. blood for laboratory specimens.

   d. doses of medications at intervals.

10. Large amounts of IV fluids, up to 700 to 1000 ml per hour, are not given to patients because of the following reason:

    a. it greatly increases the work of the heart.

    b. the fluids are lost as increased urinary output.

    c. The solution lowers the body temperature.

    d. it is impossible to run fluids fast enough for that.

11. The IV administration set that delivers 15 drops per ml is most often used with which group of patients?

    a. Critically ill patients.

    b. Infants and children.

    c. Those receiving blood transfusions.

    d. Patients receiving hyperalimentation.

    e. Adults who aren't critically ill.

12. A child is to receive 500 ml of fluids in a 10-hour period, or 50 ml per hour. What is the drop rate per minute, using a micro-drip set?

    a. 20 drops.

    b. 30 drops.

    c. 50 drops.

    d. 15 drops.

13. Adverse reactions to blood transfusions generally occur within what period of time?

    a. one hour.

    b. four hours.

    c. one day.

    d. one to two minutes.

14. The nurse has attached a small bottle of medicine in solution as a "piggy-back" to your patient's primary IV. In order for the medicine to run in first, where should the bottle be located?

    a. Closest to the patient's heart.

    b. Above the level of the first bottle.

    c. Below the level of the first bottle.

    d. Below the level of the patient's heart.

15. If your patient's IV has been running slowly and with much difficulty and is now nearly three hours behind schedule, what action should you take?

    a. Coax it along and do the best you can.

    b. Notify the nurse, who will reschedule it.

    c. Discontinue it, since the IV isn't doing as it should.

    d. Open the clamp and run it wide open until it's caught up.

POST-TEST ANSWERS

1.	c	9.	d
2.	a	10.	a
3.	d	11.	e
4.	d	12.	c
5.	c	13.	a
6.	b	14.	b
7.	c	15.	b
8.	a		

U
N
I
T
32

Unit 33

GENERAL PERFORMANCE OBJECTIVE

At the completion of this unit, you will be able to employ the correct techniques for taking care of patients with various gastrointestinal tubes—tubes with or without suction and tubes used for special feedings and for obtaining sputum or gastric specimens for special laboratory tests.

SPECIFIC PERFORMANCE OBJECTIVES

When you have finished this unit, you will be able to:

1. Identify four kinds of tubes used in the gastric analysis procedure.

2. Assemble equipment and assist with the insertion of the various GI tubes.

3. Feed a patient with a gastrostomy tube.

4. Identify and describe the action of the common types of suction apparatus: portable electric suction, wall-outlet suction, or a Gomco Thermotic Pump with intermittent or continuous action.

5. Collect a gastric content specimen and prepare it correctly for delivery to the laboratory.

6. Instruct and assist the patient to produce sputum without undue discomfort and distress, and collect the sputum specimen correctly for delivery to the laboratory.

7. Identify and care for various types of drains, such as Penrose, cigarette, and T-tube drains and portable bellows type of suction.

VOCABULARY

aspiration—the act of drawing in or out of a cavity of the body by suction; withdrawal of fluid from a body cavity by suction with an instrument called an aspirator.
Cantor tube—a single long tube used for intestinal decompression; it has a mercury-weighted balloon at its distal tip to facilitate moving the tube into the intestine.
decompression—the removal of air or drainage from a wound, cavity, or passageway.
distention—the state of being stretched out or bloated, as the abdominal cavity may be with gas or fluid.
emesis—vomiting.
enteral—occurring or situated within the intestines.
esophagus—the muscular tube that connects the oral cavity with the stomach.
Ewald tube—a specific rubber tube with a large lumen that is passed through the mouth into the stomach to withdraw stomach contents for various laboratory examinations.

expectorate—to spit out or expel mucus or phlegm from the throat or lungs.

flatus—gas that is expelled rectally; expelling gas orally is called burping or eructating.

gag reflex—an involuntary (not controlled by the will) retching or vomiting action caused by stimulation of certain nerve endings in the back of the throat that in turn stimulate the vomiting center in the brain.

gastric—refers to the stomach.

gastrostomy—a surgical operation making a temporary or permanent opening through the abdominal wall into the stomach for feeding purposes.

gavage—feeding through a tube inserted through the nose and down the esophagus into the stomach.

Gomco Thermotic Pump—a special electric suction machine commonly used with various gastrointestinal tubes.

lavage—the washing out of a cavity; gastric lavage is the washing out of the stomach contents, as in emergency cases.

Levin tube—a long plastic or rubber tube that is inserted through the nose or mouth to the stomach and used to drain off fluids and decompress the stomach.

lumen—an opening.

Miller-Abbott tube—the most common double-lumen GI rubber tube used with an inflatable rubber bag on the distal end to drain or decompress the small intestine.

nasogastric tube—a rubber or plastic tube that is inserted through the nose and down the esophagus to the stomach.

peristalsis—the involuntary, wavelike motion of the digestive tract that moves food through the alimentary canal.

sputum—a substance from the lungs that is coughed up and spit out of the mouth; it contains saliva, mucus, and sometimes pus.

suction—the act of sucking up (or drawing up) by reducing air pressure and creating a partial vacuum.

INTRODUCTION

During an acute illness, many patients will have various types of nasogastric (NG) and drainage tubes as part of the treatment of their condition. You will encounter a number of them in your nursing experience. The man with a bleeding ulcer has an NG tube so that bloody drainage from the stomach may be suctioned out. The patient going to surgery in the morning for a bowel resection has an order to have a Levin tube inserted preoperatively. The elderly woman admitted with a suspected bowel obstruction now has a tube that is being advanced into the intestines, while in the Emergency Room a small child has a tube inserted to remove the pills that were mistaken for candy. As you can see, nasogastric tubes are used for many purposes, and a number of your patients will require them in the treatment of their medical and surgical conditions.

It is not difficult to care for patients with NG tubes or wound drainage tubes. The nasogastric tube is inserted through the nose or the mouth and into the stomach or lower in the intestinal tract. It remains in place for days or even weeks, until the condition requiring its use is corrected. Baths, oral hygiene, and backrubs are given as usual, the bed is made, and the patient may even get up in a chair or walk in the halls with an NG or drainage tube.

In this unit, you will learn the purposes for which nasogastric tubes are used and the types of tubes that are available. Although nursing assistants generally do not insert short nasogastric tubes, other students in nursing programs leading to licensure as RNs or LPNs may be expected to intubate patients when this is needed. Procedures are included for passing the tube, irrigating it to keep the lumen open, feeding patients via an enteral tube, and collecting gastric and sputum specimens. Several types of wound drains are described as well.

UNIT
33

NURSING CARE FOR NASOGASTRIC AND DRAINAGE TUBES

ITEM 1. USE OF NASOGASTRIC TUBES

Each year millions of people suffer from diseases involving the gastrointestinal tract, and many of them are hospitalized for medical or sugical treatment. For many of them, part of the treatment entails a nasogastric tube.

Purposes for Use

Inserting a nasogastric tube is a relatively common procedure. It is ordered by the physician, who generally passes the long intestinal tubes and surgically places the enteral tubes, although nurses introduce short tubes and manage all of them. The tubes are used for the following reasons:

1. For suction drainage of the stomach and intestinal tract
   a. to remove accumulated gas and secretions causing distention after abdominal surgery.
   b. to empty out the digestive tract before surgery on the stomach or intestines.
   c. to remove fluids when unable to move through the tract due to paralysis or an obstruction.
   d. to relieve persistent vomiting.

2. For diagnosis in order to identify a disease or the cause of pathology, as in gastric ulcers or tumors.

3. For evacuation of the stomach contents after ingestion of poisons.

4. For establishment of a route for feeding someone unable to take food by mouth.

Patients who have an NG tube are placed on NPO, and a careful record is kept of their fluid intake and output. The drainage removed by suction is emptied and recorded each shift. As much as 3000 ml of stomach contents can be suctioned out in a day, so these patients are very susceptible to developing disturbances of their fluid and nutritional needs.

Types of Tubes

Various types of tubes, designed for specific uses, are available.

Gastric Tubes. Short tubes, which are about 3 feet long, are used to intubate the stomach and duodenum. The short tube has one lumen, or open inner space, except for the sump tubes. The most common types of short tubes are the Levin tube, Rehfuss tube, and the gastric sump tube.

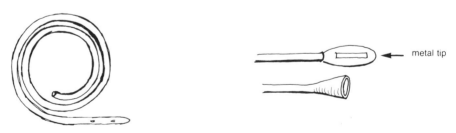

Rehfuss tube.

metal tip

Levin tube.

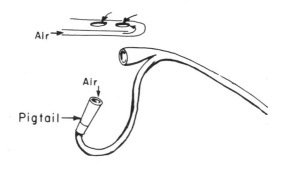

Gastric sump tube.

The Levin tube is a popular type of tube. It is about 3 feet long, comes in various diameter sizes, and is made of plastic or rubber. Popular sizes are 14, 16, and 18 French. The plastic disposable nasogastric tube is convenient to use and is tolerated quite well by patients. The rubber style of tube must be chilled in a pan of ice to make the tube stiff for easier insertion. The Rehfuss tube is similar but has a metal tip on the end that makes it easy to see in X-ray examinations. The gastric sump tube has a double lumen, with one channel open to the room air to prevent the build-up of suction within the tube. The air channel is called the pigtail. This type of tube is used more often following surgery on the stomach, as it affords protection to the suture lines.

Other types of short tubes that are seen more often in clinics and emergency rooms are the Jutte tube with a metal mesh tip, and the Ewald tube with large openings in the tip. The Ewald tube is used for gastric lavage, or to wash out the stomach, and for obtaining gastric specimens of thick stomach contents containing undigested or partially digested food.

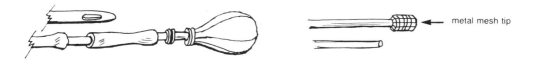

Ewald tube.   Jutte tube.

Nasogastric tubes are used to feed patients who are unable to take food orally, as in the case of patients in prolonged coma, diseases, or cancer of the mouth and throat. The Levin tube can cause severe irritation of the nose and throat when left in place for longer than a few days, so the trend is toward the use of smaller and more pliable tubes.

Among the newer feeding tubes, the Dobbhoff tube comes in a #8 French size, which is one half the diameter of the formerly used #16 French Levin tube. It has a column of mercury on the end to weight it for easier placement. The Keofeed tube is similar in size and also has the mercury-weighted tip. These smaller tubes are easily plugged, so the formula may need to be pumped in using the special infusion pumps.

Intestinal Tubes. The Cantor, Harris, and Miller-Abbott tubes are long tubes used to reach parts of the bowel beyond the stomach. They are used in bowel obstructions and other conditions in which it is necessary to remove gas and secretions to decompress the bowel. All are from 6 to 10 feet in length, and each has a bag or a balloon containing mercury on the end. The weight of the mercury helps advance the tube through the intestines.

UNIT
33

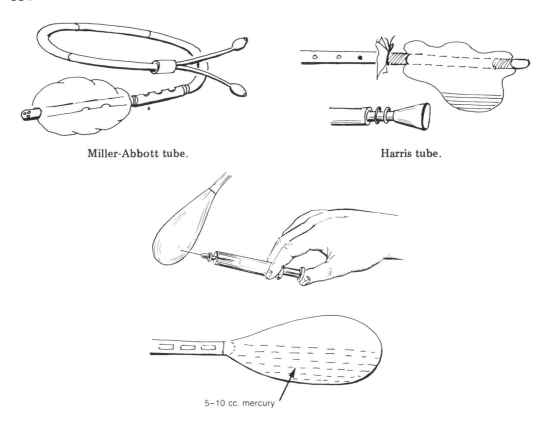

Miller-Abbott tube.   Harris tube.

5–10 cc. mercury

Cantor tube.

The Cantor and Harris tubes have a single lumen. The balloon or bag on the end is filled with a small amount of mercury before it is inserted through the nose to the stomach and advanced into the intestine. The Miller-Abbott tube has a double lumen. One is the passageway for the drainage; the other is connected to the balloon that is used to add or remove the mercury.

The long tubes move along in the bowel by peristalsis, so the doctor usually writes an order for the nurses to advance the tube one or two inches per hour until the desired length has been reached. Only then is the tube taped in place.

ITEM 2.   SUCTION MACHINES

The short nasogastric tubes and longer intestinal tubes are connected to suction as ordered by the doctor. The suction withdraws the contents from a cavity by means of decreasing the air pressure, or creating a negative pressure. Low pressures are used on a continuous or intermittent basis to avoid sucking the tissues of the stomach or intestines into the holes of the NG tube. The gastric secretions are collected into a tightly closed bottle that is connected by tubes to the machine and to the NG tube. At least once every shift, the nurses take off the cover of the bottle to measure and empty the contents. The amount of drainage is recorded as output on the I & O record.

Most health agencies now have suction outlets in the wall at the head of the patient's bed. This eliminates the necessity of cluttering the patient's room with extra equipment. Wall suction units are particularly useful in special care units (ICU, CCU, and others). Occasionally there is a problem of maintaining enough suction in the entire system which supplies all patients. Some physicians are therefore reluctant to use this system. Your responsibility will be to see that the suction is working, that the NG tube is draining, and that the drainage bottle does not overflow.

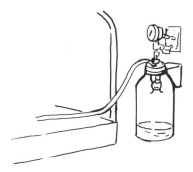

A very popular type of suction apparatus is the Gomco Thermotic Pump. It is a portable electric machine that is brought to the bedside and plugged in. It provides intermittent suction that can be regulated by a "low" or "high" control button to obtain the negative pressure ordered by the doctor. With few exceptions, "low" pressure is used for patients with nasogastric or intestinal tubes.

When your patient has a portable suction machine, be sure that it is plugged in and turned on. On some models, a green light flashes as the pressure is on to create a suction and goes out when there is no suction. Again, close observation of the drainage bottle contents is important to prevent overflow. Check the workings of the machine frequently to be sure it is pulling the drainage from the stomach or intestine.

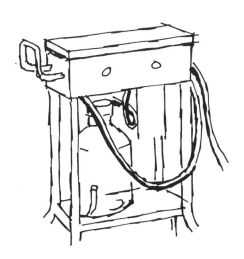

U
N
I
T
33

Emptying Drainage Bottles

▬▬

Supplies Needed

Graduate for measuring   Paper towels

▬▬

Important Steps	Key Points
1. Turn off the suction momentarily.	This will break the suction in the system, allowing easy removal of the rubber stopper on the drainage bottle.
2. Remove the rubber stopper from the bottle top.	Unclamp the holding bracket if there is one.
3. Pour the contents into a graduate.	Measure the contents and record the time, amount, color, odor, and consistency after reassembling the system.
4. Rinse the graduate and the drainage bottle.	Dry the outside of the drainage bottle with paper towels and discard them in the wastebasket.
5. Clean and replace the rubber stopper on top of the cleaned drainage bottle.	Make sure that is is airtight and held in place, with the clamps securely tightened.
6. Turn the switch back to the "on" position on the suction machine.	This will reestablish the suction system. Observe the flow of drainage for a few minutes. Tell the patient when you will return.
7. Make the patient comfortable and record the amount of drainage on the chart of the I & O sheet.	

ITEM 3. NURSING CARE

The nursing measures that must be observed include frequent special mouth care for these patients. Since they are NPO, the mouth becomes very dry and tastes bad, and the lips may become cracked. These become ideal locations for pathogens to enter the body. To keep the mouth and lips moist, swab the oral cavity with a cotton swab that has been moistened in equal parts of glycerin and lemon juice. This liquid comes prepackaged for use in most agencies; if not, you can mix the solution, which is very refreshing to the patient. Mouthwash may also be used if the patient is able to spit the liquid out; mouthwash should not be swallowed.

The nostrils often become dry and tender. When you take care of patients with the various gastrointestinal tubes, you should remember the following:

1. Demonstrate kindness, gentleness, and quiet concern for their comfort.

2. Give meticulous and frequent oral hygiene and nose care.

3. Provide for freedom of movement as much as possible by securing the suction tubing to the patient's clothing or skin to permit maximum activity.

4. See that the patient does not lie on the tubing; do not permit the tubing to be kinked, because the suction will be cut off, stopping the fluid drainage.

5. When you are checking to see if the suction machine is operating satisfactorily, first check to see that it is properly attached to the patient and the wall outlet, that the machine is turned on, and that the tubes are not kinked. If you have checked all of these points and made sure that the drainage bottle is not overflowing, but you see that the machine is *not* working, report at once to your team leader. This situation can be crucial to the well-being of your patient because there may be a plugged tube.

6. Observe, report, and record the contents of the drainage bottles accurately. Report and record any unusual contents promptly to your charge nurse.

Because patients are usually very ill and apprehensive, you must keep the environment quiet, clean, tidy, and well-ventilated. Patients are often supersensitive to odors and can become nauseated very easily.

Answer the call lights promptly and check on your patients frequently. Patients requiring this type of treatment provide a challenge to nursing care. They often relax if you give an extra backrub or change bed linens p.r.n. Your quiet solicitousness when caring for these patients can hasten their recovery.

ITEM 4. INSERTION OF THE NASOGASTRIC TUBE

Most patients do not look forward to having a nasogastric tube inserted, but it can be passed with much less difficulty when the nurse gains the patient's cooperation and then proceeds in an assured and competent manner. The procedure should take only a few minutes to do when the nurse coaches the conscious patient about what to do and gives encouragement. An explanation that swallowing the tube is like swallowing a long piece of spaghetti has been helpful for numerous patients and reduces the gag reflex. Another point you can stress is the purpose of the tube or the way in which the tube should help the patient.

At this time you will not be expected to insert the gastric tube; however, you will need to practice getting the patient and supplies ready, and you should know the steps of the procedure so you can assist as necessary.

||||||||||||||||||||||||||||||||||||||||||||||||||||||||||||||||||||||||||||||||||||||||||||||||||||||||||||||||||||||||||||||||||

Supplies Needed

NG tube
Irrigating set including the following:
  Basin
  Solution container
  Irrigating syringe
  Lubricant, water soluble
  Towel
  Protector cap, or tube plug

Tape
Tissues
Stethoscope
Glass of water and straw

U
N
I
T
33

||||||||||||||||||||||||||||||||||||||||||||||||||||||||||||||||||||||||||||||||||||||||||||||||||||||||||||||||||||||||||||||||||

Important Steps	Key Points
1. Wash your hands.	Universal Steps A, B, C, and D. See Appendix.
2. Collect the items needed.	
3. Approach the patient, explain what you are going to do, and gain cooperation.	
4. Provide for privacy.	
5. Position the patient.	Fowler's position is usually assumed because it enables the tube to move by gravity down the digestive tract. Hand the emesis basin and the tissues to the patient. Otherwise, place the emesis basin close beside patient's face with the tissues near the pillow.
6. Check the air flow through the nostril.	Close one side of the nose and check the air flow through the other. Pass the tube through the nostril with the best air flow. If changing the NG tube, insert it in the nostril other than the one previously used to avoid further irritation of the tissue.

Important Steps	Key Points

7. Measure the tube for distance to be inserted.

Find the target distance for inserting the tube by measuring from the tip of the nose to the tip of the ear, and then to the tip of the xiphoid process. Mark it with a small piece of tape.

A scale is available that measures the distance more precisely, since NEX may be too long for short patients and too short for taller adults.

Some tubes have approximate target markings on them: one black band indicating the length of tubing needed to reach the stomach, two bands for the pylorus, and three bands for duodenum.

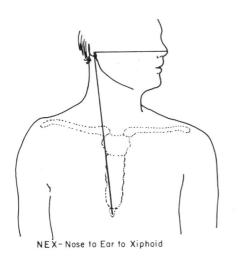

NEX– Nose to Ear to Xiphoid

8. Lubricate the tip of the tube and insert in the nose. Aim the tube down and toward the ear.

For easier insertion, use water or a waterbase lubricant to moisten the tip of the tube. *Do not use an oil-base lubricant:* the possibility of lipoid aspirational pneumonia is to be avoided.

If you encounter a severe resistance, withdraw the tube and insert it in the other nostril. Do not forcibly push it, because you could injure tissues and cause bleeding.

9. As tube reaches back of the throat, have patient drop head forward and begin to swallow.

Tell the patient to bend head forward and to swallow a mouthful of water as the tube is passed down the esophagus to the stomach. Check the position of the tube as it passes down the back of the patient's throat by having patient open mouth and hold down tongue with tongue depressor. (See diagram.)

If the tube is coiled up in the mouth, withdraw it into the nose and begin again by having the patient bend head forward and swallow. The patient can signal you to stop for a moment to rest, if necessary, but avoid waiting too long.

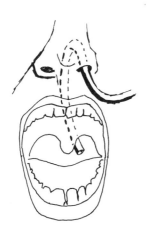

10. Advance the tube each time patient swallows or sucks air.

Continue to have the patient swallow water or ice chips as the tube is passed; the esophageal peristalsis and the fact that you work in a reassuring manner will help the patient tolerate the procedure.

Important Steps	Key Points
11. Check the placement of the tube.	When the target point on the tube has reached the nose, the tube should be in the stomach; you should verify this, however. Any or all of these methods may be used, and if still not sure, X-ray may be needed to confirm its location.

11. Check the placement of the tube.

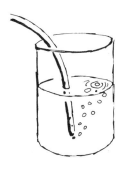

When the target point on the tube has reached the nose, the tube should be in the stomach; you should verify this, however. Any or all of these methods may be used, and if still not sure, X-ray may be needed to confirm its location.

a. The return of gastric juice in the tube is an obvious sign. Use the irrigating syringe to pull back using gentle suction and aspirate stomach contents. If none are obtained, turn patient onto left side, insert the tube another one to two inches and try again.

b. Inject 10 to 20 ml of air into the tube with the irrigating syringe and listen with the stethoscope placed to the left of the tip of the ziphoid. The air makes a "swooshing" sound as it enters the stomach, but patient may belch if the tube is in the esophagus.

c. Place the end of the tube in a glass of water and observe for the rise and fall of water in the tube with each inspiration and expiration as well as air bubbles that indicate that the tube is in the trachea. Keep the glass of water well below the insertion level of the tube to prevent aspiration of water into the lungs.

If the patient has dyspnea, coughing, or cyanosis or is unable to talk or hum, the tube is in the trachea and must be removed and reinserted.

12. Tape the tube securely to the face.

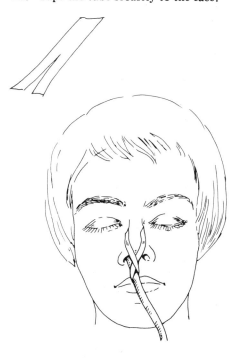

Use the chevron method of taping by placing the midportion of a piece of tape around the back of the tube, crossing one end over the other, and securing them to the bridge of the nose. Avoid pressure caused by the tube against the nasal tissues.

U
N
I
T
33

Important Steps	Key Points
13. Attach the free end of the tube to the suction machine.	Make sure the machine is plugged in and turned on "low" pressure. If suction has not been ordered, clamp, plug or cover the end of the NG tube so that it won't leak gastric contents. When the patient is allowed out of bed, loosely loop the tubing in a circle, secure it with adhesive tape, and pin it to the patient's gown. This will help prevent pulling that would be uncomfortable for the patient.
14. Provide for the patient's comfort.	Universal Steps X, Y, and Z. See Appendix.
15. Remove used articles and leave bedside unit neat and tidy.	
16. Report and record the procedure.	Charting example: 0930. Continues to complain of nausea and vomiting. Emesis of 350 ml. dark green fluid. Abdomen distended. 0945. Levin tube inserted and attached to low suction. Draining large amount of dark green fluid and some gas. <div align="right">A. Brown, RN</div>

ITEM 5. IRRIGATING THE NASOGASTRIC TUBE

The process for clearing the blocked or plugged passageway of the gastric tube is called irrigation. If the tube becomes plugged, the physician orders an irrigation to be done at stated intervals or p.r.n. This is a clean procedure, not a sterile one, and unless ordered otherwise, usually 30 to 60 ml of normal saline solution is enough to flush the tube.

Other means can be utilized to unplug the tubing:

a. Change the position of the tube by gently pushing it in and pulling it out.	Occasionally an eyelet opening of the tube adheres to the wall of the stomach, preventing drainage. Pulling the tubing from the lining of the stomach permits full drainage to occur.
b. Use a gentle "milking action" on the tube to free blockage. (Hold the tube securely in place while milking.)	Thick material may plug the passageway of the tube between the patient's nose and the drainage bottle. Gently squeeze the tubing between your palm and fingers. Move carefully along the tubing in this manner until suction is restored.

Supplies Needed

Irrigating set containing: Solution: Normal Saline or water
  Syringe, irrigating
  Solution container
  Drainage receptacle
  Antiseptic sponges
  Protective cap for tube
  Underpad, or drape

Important Steps	Key Points

Carry out Universal Steps A, B, C, and D. See Appendix.

1. Fill the syringe with the irrigating solution.

Hold the syringe between your index finger and thumb. Place the tip of the syringe in the solution and pull the plunger up to obtain at least 30 ml of solution.

2. Disconnect the gastric tube from the drain tube on the machine.

Turn off the suction power. Secure the drain tube to the holder on the machine. Hold the gastric tube in a fistlike grasp with the last three fingers of your hand.

3. Attach the filled syringe to the free end of the gastric tube and irrigate.

Inject 10 to 15 ml of solution into the tube. Pull back gently on the plunger to withdraw, if possible. Often the solution cannot be withdrawn but goes into the small bowel.

Repeat this process until the passageway is clear. Do not injure the mucous lining of the stomach. If fresh bleeding is apparent, stop the procedure and notify the physician immediately.

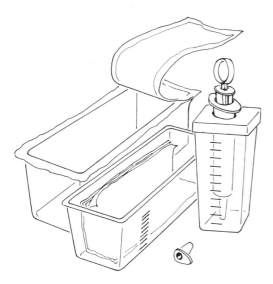

Typical disposable irrigation set

4. Observe the contents of the irrigating solution.

The color, odor, consistency, and amount (absence or excess) must be noted and accurately recorded on the patient's chart.

5. When the irrigation is completed, attach the gastric tube to the drain tube of the suction machine.

Turn the power of the machine on. Check to see whether there is an NPO sign.

Carry out Universal Steps X, Y, and Z. See Appendix.

Charting example:
1430. NG tube not draining. Irrigated with saline, and now draining moderate amount of thick, dark brown fluid.

A. Brown, RN

ITEM 6.   INSERTION OF LONG INTESTINAL TUBES

In the procedure, you will again be assisting with insertion of the tube. You need to know the procedure and be ready to help as needed. Stand opposite the person inserting the tube and talk reassuringly to the patient.

U
N
I
T
33

In larger hospitals, the patient is sent to the Gastroenterology Department, GI clinic, or laboratory where the intestinal tube is inserted. The patient is then returned to the nursing unit with orders for the tube to be advanced and connected to suction.

Important Steps	Key Points

Refer to steps 1 through 11 of Item 4.

12. After the tube reaches the stomach, inflate the balloon.

The doctor or nurse will use a sterile syringe and needle to inject 5 to 10 ml of mercury or air into the outlet connecting the air passageway to the balloon. The inflated and weighted tube then passes into the small intestine.

13. Place the patient in *right Sims'* position.

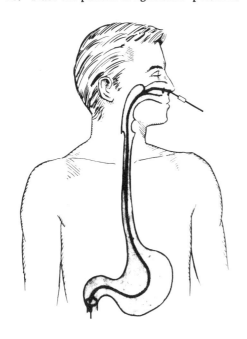

This makes the passage of the tube faster and easier by helping the peristaltic action and gravity to move the tube from the stomach to the small intestine.

The tube should not be secured until it is finally inserted into the small intestine. This can be determined by the ring markings on the outside of the tubing as well as by the appearance of the drainage. When the tube reaches the intestines, it is attached to a suction machine. The outside tip of the tube is secured to the patient's face with adhesive tape and pinned to his gown to permit freedom of movement.

The nursing care and observation of the equipment and drainage are the same as for other patients with gastrointestinal suction and drainage.

Remove the tubing as follows:
a. Deflate the balloon; use an appropriately sized syringe to remove the air or mercury.
b. Pinch and slowly pull the tubing a few inches every minute or so.
c. Avoid stimulating the gag reflex and causing the patient to vomit.

ITEM 7.   ENTERAL TUBES FOR NUTRITION

Enteral tubes are those introduced into the digestive tract and used for feeding. As stated earlier, one of the purposes of the short nasogastric tubes is to supply nutrients to patients who refuse to eat or who are unable to eat food orally. This method of feeding patients by tube is also called gastric gavage. Patients of any age may be fed in this manner, from the very small infant to the elderly geriatric patient. Other types of enteral tubes include the gastrostomy tube, which is surgically inserted through the abdominal wall into the stomach, and the needle catheter jejunum (NCJ) tube, which is surgically threaded into the jejunum of the small intestine.

Some patients who will require a tube for their nutrition for long periods of time have a gastrostomy tube inserted. A small incision is surgically made in the upper left abdominal wall and the tube is sutured in place to prevent it from slipping out of the incision. In about 10 days the wound is healed and the tube can be taken out and reinserted p.r.n.

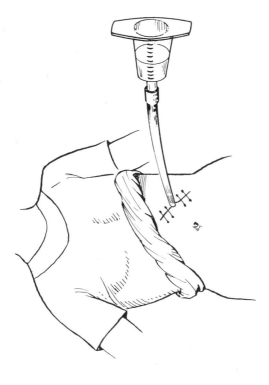

A gastrostomy or enterostomy tube in place.

Types of Tubes Used

Any short nasogastric tube can be used for tube feedings, and the Levin tube has been used extensively for this purpose. With more emphasis on providing adequate nutrition for hospitalized patients, some patients receive tube feedings for several weeks or even longer. The larger Levin tube causes extensive irritation and ulceration of tissues in the nose and esophagus, so the trend today is to use much smaller and more flexible tubes.

The newer tubes are about one half the diameter of the Levin tube or smaller. Several now on the market are the Dobbhoff and Keofeed tubes, which have a weighted column of mercury on their tips to help keep them in place, and the Med Pro, the smallest of the three. An infusion pump is usually needed to pump the formula through these small tubes.

Tube Feeding Formulas.

An increasing number of special formulas are prepared commercially, although some hospitals may still prepare tube feedings in their diet kitchens. The formulas vary in the number of calories and the amount of fats and proteins they provide and in the electrolytes, if any, that they contain.

The following are among the popular brands of commercial formulas:

Name	Calories per liter	Protein (grams per liter)
Isocal	1000 (or 1/ml)	34
Ensure Plus	1500 (or 1.5/ml)	54
Vivonex	1000 (or (1/ml)	21

These formulas are also provided in 250-ml containers that are convenient for feedings given intermittently during the day, as well as for those given continuously. An administration set similar to that used for IV administration is used to give the solution slowly and over a long period of time. If a syringe is used, the formula should flow in by gravity; it should not be pushed in as a bolus or in large amounts.

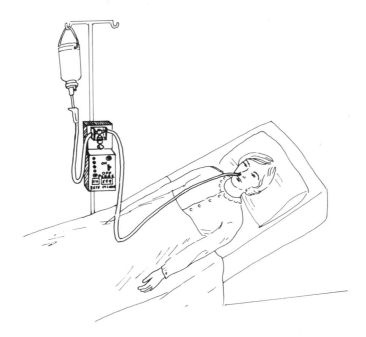

Continuous tube feeding using an infusion pump.

Principles for Tube Feedings

Because tube feedings contain a high level of glucose in order to provide the necessary calories, they should be given very slowly to prevent diarrhea and sugar in the urine. The preferred method is to give the feedings slowly over a 24-hour period. When feedings are ordered for four or more times a day, the doctor usually begins with a small amount, that is at half strength and then increases the rate as the patient shows tolerance for it.

Some of the principles to observe when giving patients tube feedings follow:

1. Elevate the head of the bed 30 degrees before and after feeding, or at all times if on continuous feedings.

2. Note the position of the tube before each feeding or at least once a shift.

3. Give the formula at room temperature by bag, syringe, or infusion pump. Hang only a 4- to 8-hour supply at one time.

4. Perform a Clinitest every 4 to 6 hours or as ordered for glucosuria.

5. If nausea occurs, stop the feeding and notify the nurse.

6. Record an accurate Intake and Output. Dehydration can occur owing to diarrhea or simply to the high glucose content of the formula.

ITEM 8. GIVING AN INTERMITTENT TUBE FEEDING

When patients are to be given nasogastric or gastrostomy tube feedings at specified times of the day, the following procedure is used.

Supplies Needed

Irrigation set (syringe, funnel,
administration set, glass of
water)

Formula (as specified)

Important Steps	Key Points
Carry out Universal Steps A, B, C, and D. See Appendix.	
1. Elevate the head of the bed 30 degrees.	The head of the bed should remain elevated during the feeding and for one half hour afterwards, as gravity helps the flow of the formula into the stomach.
2. Remove the cap or plug from the tube.	
3. Verify the placement of the tube.	Before you begin feeding, make sure the tube is in the stomach and not in the trachea or lung. Use the syringe and aspirate gastric fluid. If no fluid is obtained, check the tube placement by introducing air through the tube and listening with the stethoscope or by placing the tube end in water and watching for air bubbles, as shown in Item 4.
4. Aspirate for residual gastric fluid and reinstill it.	It is returned to the stomach because it is high in electrolyte content. When more than 150 ml is obtained, report it to the nurse, since it is an indication that the feeding is not well tolerated.
5. Pour the formula into the barrel of the syringe or a funnal.	Formula should be given slowly; gravity pull will draw it in. You can regulate flow by raising and lowering the receptacle as demonstrated in the adjacent diagram.

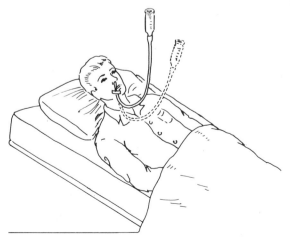

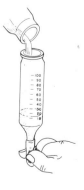

U
N
I
T
33

Important Steps	Key Points
6. Add formula to keep the neck of the receptacle filled.	If you allow the formula level to fall below the neck of the syringe, air will enter the tubing and the stomach, causing great discomfort due to distention of the stomach. Continue adding formula to the syringe until the prescribed amount is given.
7. Follow the formula with 1 to 2 ounces of water to clear the tube.	When the formula feeding is finished, pour in fresh water to clear the tube. Again, be sure to keep the liquid above the neck of the syringe to prevent air bubbles from collecting in the system or in the patient's stomach.
8. Clamp the tube.	Insert the plug in the end of the tube, cover with a cap protector, or tighten the clamp on the tube to prevent backflow of the formula.
Carry out Universal Steps X, Y, and Z. See Appendix.	Charting example: 0800. Ensure formula 250 ml given by NG tube, followed by 50 ml water. Retained. No complaints of discomfort. <div align="right">A. Brown, RN</div>

ITEM 9. WOUND DRAINAGE TUBES

Drainage Without Suction

Let us discuss common methods of draining secretions from incisions without suction.

The *Penrose drain*, a tube frequently employed, is a flat, soft rubber drain available in various widths from ¼ inch to 2 inches. The physician inserts one end of the drain into the wound at the designated site, using strict aseptic technique. The free end of the tube resting on the skin may be held securely in place with a stitch of surgical suture or a safety pin. The tube is covered with sterile dressing to catch the drainage. The dressing is changed p.r.n. Care must be taken not to dislodge the tube when changing the dressing (usually done by the doctor or nurse, using strict aseptic technique to prevent infection). Careful observation of the amount, color, odor, and consistency of the drainage is vital to the physician's treatment planning for the patient. Therefore, the observations and recordings must be accurate.

A *cigarette drain* is a Penrose drain with a gauze bandage pulled through the lumen, like tobacco in a cigarette, to act as a wick. It may be used as the doctor deems necessary. The same precautions are to be taken in placing, caring for, and removing the cigarette drain as those described for the Penrose drain.

A *T-tube rubber drain* is commonly used to drain bile from the liver into the intestine—often following a cholecystectomy (surgical removal of the gallbladder). Care must be taken not to dislodge the catheter. Since a large amount of bile may be excreted in 24 hours, the T-tube may be attached to an external tubing system that empties into a drainage bag or bottle attached to the patient's bedside. T-tubes are inserted at the time of surgery.

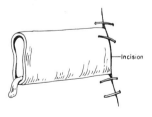
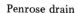

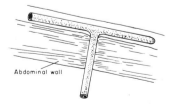

Penrose drain   T-tube placed in bile duct.

Catheters may also be used to drain surgical incisions. The size of the lumen must be large enough to accommodate the drainage; a large lumen is used if a large amount of thick fluid is to be drained. Since catheters come in varying sizes, the actual size is selected on the basis of need. The choice is made by the physician.

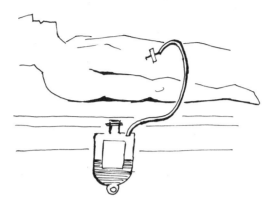

Catheter in abdominal incision.

Drainage With Suction

The portable wound suction unit is a commercially made plastic apparatus used to remove bloody drainage and pus from wounds. The unit is composed of a needle, needle protector, wound tube, connector tube, bellows (container), and belt strap.

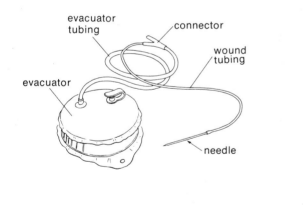

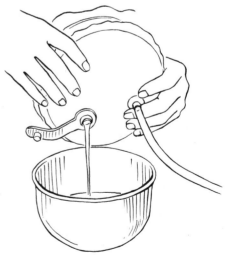

Opening outlet to remove drainage.

The wound suction tube is inserted in the wound by the physician. The implantation is usually done in surgery, but it can be accomplished elsewhere as long as a sterile field and technique are maintained.

The wound tube has an attached 5-inch needle, approximately 25 holes along the midsection, and 12 inches of closed tubing extending beyond the midsection. The end of this extension is inserted into one of the open ends of the double-ended connector tube. The connector tube is attached to the port side of the bellows. The drain plug (on top of the bellows) is opened, and pressure is applied to depress the bellows. At this step, the drain plug is reinserted and a vacuum then exists.

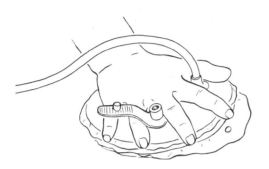

Compressing bellows unit to form vacuum.

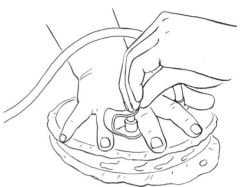

Placing plug in outlet to retain suction.

This vacuum pressure causes the drainage from the wound to flow into the bellows, where it will remain until the nurse opens the bellows, empties it, and measures and records the amount of drainage on the Intake and Output sheet of the patient's records. The discarding of the drainage is a procedure that must be repeated until drainage no longer exists and the unit is removed from the wound.

ITEM 10. COLLECTION OF THE SPUTUM SPECIMEN

In this section, we will be considering primarily the patient with a possible respiratory problem and a cough. It may be necessary to obtain specimens of sputum from the coughing patient to aid in the diagnosis of the disease and in the patient's progress toward recovery. It is important to know that in certain medical and postoperative situations the patient may be encouraged to cough in order to clear mucus from the respiratory tract and from the lungs. This promotes adequate expansion and ventilation of the lungs. In other postoperative conditions, however, such as eye surgery or hernia repair, it is advisable to inhibit coughing.

Sputum specimens are requested most often from patients who are suspected of having a respiratory disease such as pneumonia, tuberculosis, or bronchitis. Obtaining the specimen may be difficult or painful, and so you must know how to assist the patient.

There are times when it is very painful for the patient to cough. If the patient has pain in the abdominal or chest area when he coughs, obtain a drawsheet or a folded large sheet and wrap it around the painful area of the body. Hold the sheet securely with minimal pressure so that the affected area is supported. This gives the patient the external pressure necessary to equalize the internal pressure occurring during the coughing period, and it minimizes the pain and discomfort. *Do not hold the sheet too tightly* or you will defeat your purpose by causing pain and increased difficulty in breathing.

In the classroom or skills laboratory, you should practice the steps of the procedure until you are familiar with them and can carry them out skillfully.

‖‖

Supplies Needed

Specimen container with cover tissues   Laboratory requisition
Label for specimen   Small paper bag — (optional)

‖‖

Important Steps	Key Points

Carry out Universal Steps A, B, C, and D. See Appendix.

1. Tell the patient how to collect the sputum specimen.

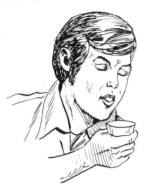

Explain that sputum is the mucus coughed up from the lungs, *not* the saliva in the mouth. Ask the patient to cover his mouth with tissues when coughing, and to spit the coughed-up sputum into the container. This will keep him from coughing germs into the air that you and others breathe.

2. Assist the patient to produce an immediate specimen if possible.

Ask the patient to breathe deeply and cough in order to bring up the sputum from the lungs, and not merely from the back of the throat.

Collect at least 1 to 2 tablespoons of sputum unless directed otherwise. Observe the patient carefully and assist when necessary; offer encouragement.

It may be easier for the patient to produce the specimen early in the morning. Mucus that has collected in the lungs during the night is more apt to be coughed up at this time. Have the patient notify the nurse who will pick up the specimen.

3. Arrange for delivery of the specimen to the laboratory.

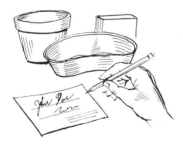

Avoid contamination. Keep the outside of the container and your hands free of the sputum when you are collecting it and transporting it to the laboratory.

After the patient coughs the sputum into the container, seal it with the lid. Put the labeled container in the paper bag for delivery to the laboratory with the lab requisition slip. (Some agencies do not require that the specimen be enclosed in a paper bag. Follow your agency procedure for transporting sputum specimens to the laboratory.)

Carry out Universal Steps X, Y, and Z. See Appendix.

Charting example:
0730. Has episodes of deep, productive coughing. Moderate amount of thick greenish grey mucus spit out. Specimen to the lab for culture.
M. Victory, PN

U
N
I
T
33

ITEM 11. COLLECTION OF A GASTRIC SPECIMEN

A sample of the gastric contents can be obtained for analysis (1) from the emesis produced by a vomiting patient and (2) from an inserted gastric tube by aspirating the necessary amount; this procedure is described in the following steps.

〓〓〓

Supplies Needed

Gastric analysis tray, including   Tissues
  Nasogastric tubes   Glass of water with straw
  Water soluble lubricant
  Towel or drape
  Aspirating syringe
  Specimen bottles with caps

〓〓〓

Important Steps	Key Points
Carry out Universal Steps A, B, C, and D. See Appendix.	
1. Insert the nasogastric tube.	Follow the procedure given in Item 4.
2. Withdraw a sample of the gastric contents.	Use an irrigating syringe to obtain at least 10 ml of fluid.
3. Place the specimen in the designated containers and put on the lids.	If test tubes are used, apply stopper lids. Avoid contaminating the outside of the container; if it has been soiled, use paper towels to wash and dry it. Label each specimen container with the patient's name and room number, the hospital number, the time, the date, and the number of the specimen. Specimens are numbered in the sequence in which they were obtained. Check the laboratory manual for the number and times for specimen collections.
4. Remove the tube.	When all of the specimens have been collected, pinch the tube near the patient's nostril or mouth and pull it out. Pinching the tube prevents gastric fluid that is left inside the tube from dripping down the patient's trachea and causing aspirational pneumonia.
5. Send or take the specimen to laboratory.	Include the laboratory requisition slip. Some hospitals require that the specimen and the lab slip be put in a paper bag for delivery to the laboratory. Some agencies use other methods; ask the nurse. Arrange to have them taken by a messenger service or take the specimens to the laboratory yourself.
Carry out Universal Steps X, Y, and Z. See Appendix.	Charting example: 0900. Levin tube inserted. Aspirated gastric fluid before and after test meal. Specimens to the lab. A. Brown, RN

PERFORMANCE TEST

In the classroom or the skills laboratory, your instructor will ask you to demonstrate the following procedures. You should be able to do so accurately, without referring to your study guide, notes, or other source material.

1. Given a patient who has abdominal distention and vomiting, you are to collect the items needed and describe the steps the nurse uses to insert a nasogastric tube and attach it to suction.

2. Given a patient with a gastric suction apparatus and a drainage bottle three-fourths full, you will empty the bottle and reattach it to the suction machine using the procedure you have just learned. Upon measuring the drainage, you will record the output on the appropriate records.

3. Given a patient with a feeding tube, you will assemble the equipment, prepare the patient (or the mannequin, Mrs. Chase), and give a feeding followed by 50 cc of water as outlined in the lesson, maintaining safety precautions. You will practice recording the activity on the nurses' notes.

4. Given a patient with a suspected respiratory disease, you are to instruct and assist the patient to produce a specimen of sputum, and prepare the specimen for delivery to the laboratory.

PERFORMANCE CHECKLIST

INSERTING A NASOGASTRIC TUBE

1. Wash your hands.

2. Collect the items needed.

3. Approach the patient, explain the procedure, and gain cooperation.

4. Provide for privacy.

5. Position the patient in high Fowler's position.

6. Check the airflow through the nostril.

7. Measure the tube for distance to be inserted.

8. Lubricate the tip of the tube.

9. Insert in the nose, aiming down and toward the ear.

10. When tube is in back of throat, have patient drop head forward and begin to swallow.

11. Advance the tube each time the patient swallows or sucks air.

12. Check the placement of the tube by aspirating gastric juices, injecting air, or testing for air bubbles in water.

13. Tape the tube securely to the face.

14. Attach the free end of the tube to the suction machine.

15. Provide for the patient's comfort.

16. Remove the used items and tidy the unit.

17. Report and record the procedure.

UNIT
33

EMPTYING THE DRAINAGE BOTTLE

1. Wash your hands.

2. Identify the patient.

3. Explain the procedure to the patient.

4. Turn off the suction.

5. Remove the stopper from the bottle.

6. Pour the contents of the jar into a graduate cylinder.

7. Attach the empty drainage jar to the apparatus.

8. Replace the rubber stopper.

9. Turn on the suction machine (put it in operation for several minutes).

10. Measure and record the volume, color, odor, and consistency of the drainage.

11. Rinse and dry the materials used.

12. Provide for the patient's comfort and safety.

ENTERAL TUBE FEEDING

1. Wash your hands and prepare the equipment.

2. Approach and identify the patient.

3. Elevate the head of the bed at least 30 degrees.

4. Remove the cap or plug from the tube.

5. Verify the placement of the tube by aspirating gastric contents, inserting air or checking for air bubbles.

6. Aspirate for residual gastric fluid, measure, and reinstill.

7. Pour formula into barrel of syringe or funnel and regulate flow by gravity.

8. Add more formula to keep neck of receptacle filled.

9. Follow the formula with 1 to 2 ounces of water to clear the tube.

10. Clamp the tube.

11. Provide for the patient's comfort and leave bed elevated for at least half an hour.

12. Clean and store equipment.

13. Report and record the procedure.

COLLECTION OF A SPUTUM SPECIMEN

1. Wash your hands.

2. Obtain the necessary items and prepare the labels correctly.

3. Identify the patient.

4. Instruct the patient on how to collect a specimen.

5. Provide for the patient's privacy.

6. Assist the patient as needed.

7. Avoid contamination of your hands, your uniform, and the container by the patient's sputum.

8. Seal the container; wash and dry the outside of the container.

9. Apply a label to the container.

10. Put the labeled container and laboratory slip in a paper bag for delivery to the laboratory.

11. Provide for the patient's safety and comfort.

12. Arrange for delivery of the specimen to the laboratory.

13. Record the pertinent information on the patient's chart.

POST-TEST

Directions: Choose the one best answer for each item.

1. Which of these tubes would be used to decompress the bowel of a patient suspected of having a bowel obstruction?

   a. Miller-Abbott tube.

   b. Gastric sump tube.

   c. Levin tube.

   d. Jutte tube.

2. The most commonly used short tube for gastric intubation and suction is called a

   a. Miller-Abbot tube.

   b. Levin tube.

   c. Cantor tube.

   d. Harris tube.

3. When the Levin tube needs added stiffness for insertion, the following is done:

   a. It is immersed in a pan of water at 105°F.

   b. It is immersed in a pan of ice for 15 to 30 minutes.

   c. Another tube is placed inside it.

   d. It is placed under cold, running tap water.

4. Patients are uncomfortable during this procedure and will probably

   a. complain of pain.

   b. have spasms of coughing.

   c. gag and retch.

   d. have a stuffy nose.

5. During the procedure, the patient is usually placed in what position?

   a. Sims' position.

   b. Trendelenburg position.

   c. prone position.

   d. Fowler's position.

6. The length of a short nasogastric tube is

   a. 12 to 18 inches.

   b. 3 feet.

   c. 4 to 6 inches.

   d. 6 feet.

7. Short nasogastric tubes are used for all of these reasons *except*

   a. to cleanse out the intestine before surgery.

   b. to feed patients unable to take food orally.

   c. to reduce postoperative distention of the abdomen.

   d. to obtain specimens of gastric contents.

8. The one feature of the gastric sump tube that distinguishes it from other short tubes is

   a. the end is weighted with mercury.

   b. it has an inflatable balloon near the tip.

   c. the extra large lumen for removing thick contents.

   d. it has two channels, one open to the room air.

9. The use of a tube and suction to decompress the stomach or abdomen means that

   a. the suction stimulates peristaltic movement.

   b. the tube inhibits the secretion of gastric juices.

   c. fluids and gas are removed from the tract.

   d. nothing by mouth reduces the internal pressures.

10. Patients who have nasogastric tubes and suctioning should be on accurate Intake and Output recording because

   a. they are NPO and don't take anything orally.

   b. they easily develop fluid or nutritional imbalances.

   c. suctioning is very irritating and drying to the throat.

   d. it is an order by the doctor and part of the treatment.

11. The target distance that you would insert the nasogastric tube is found by measuring the patients from

   a. their fingertips to the shoulder.

   b. the nose to the ear to the tip of the ziphoid.

   c. the tip of the ear to the nose to the umbilicus.

   d. the bridge of the nose to the middle of the ziphoid.

12. All except one of the following types of suction are used with tubes to decompress the stomach or the intestines. Which one is not used?

   a. Continuous pressure

   b. Intermittent pressure

   c. Low negative pressure

   d. High negative pressure

13. How often are suction drainage bottles emptied and the contents measured?

   a. Once a shift.

   b. Once an hour.

   c. Once in 24 hours.

   d. Only when the bottle is full.

14. When inserting a nasogastric tube in a conscious patient, the nurse should

   a. work quietly and gently.

   b. promise that everything will be better.

   c. coach and encourage the patient's actions.

   d. let gravity and peristalsis move the tube to the stomach.

UNIT
33

15. What is the best sign that the nasogastric tube is properly located in the stomach?

    a. Coughing, gasping, and burping.

    b. Air bubbles from end of tube placed in water.

    c. A return of gastric juice in the tube.

    d. The "swoosh" sound of injected air in the stomach.

16. The purpose for irrigating the nasogastric tube is to

    a. ensure that it is draining freely.

    b. check for any bleeding or clots.

    c. wash out the stomach.

    d. remove the build-up in pressure.

17. Enteral tube feedings refer to which of the following?

    a. Nasogastric tube for feeding.

    b. Gastrostomy tube.

    c. Enterostomy tubes like the NCJ.

    d. All of these.

18. When a tube feeding is given too rapidly, what two probelems are likely to occur?

    a. Nausea and vomiting.

    b. Rise in blood pressure and temperature.

    c. Diarrhea and glucose in the urine.

    d. Constipation and fluid overload.

19. Why is a Clinitest done several times a day for patients receiving enteral tube feedings?

    a. To see if sugar is spilling over into the urine.

    b. To test for nutritional imbalance.

    c. The patient is probably a diabetic.

    d. Because the tube interferes with gastric secretions.

20. An acceptable method of clearing the gastric tube without saline irrigation is to

    a. use a gentle "milking action."

    b. blow air through the tubing.

    c. irrigate the tubing with oxygen.

    d. pull the tube in and out approximately 3 to 4 inches.

POST-TEST ANSWERS

1.	a	11.	b
2.	b	12.	d
3.	b	13.	a
4.	c	14.	c
5.	d	15.	c
6.	b	16.	a
7.	a	17.	d
8.	d	18.	c
9.	c	19.	a
10.	b	20.	a

U
N
I
T
33

Unit 34

HOT AND COLD APPLICATIONS

GENERAL PERFORMANCE OBJECTIVE

Upon the completion of this lesson, you will be able to apply heat and cold as treatments for the patient's condition accurately, effectively, and safely.

SPECIFIC PERFORMANCE OBJECTIVES

Upon the completion of this unit you will be able to:

1. Apply heat locally to a portion of the patient's body efficiently and safely, using a hot water bottle, heating pad, heat cradle, or aquathermia pad.

2. Apply cold locally to a portion of the patient's body efficiently and safely, using an ice bag, cold pack, or hypothermia machine.

3. State the groups of patients who have a high risk of having burns of the skin following application of heat and describe the action to be taken to prevent burns.

4. Assist in setting up and operating the hypothermia/hyperthermia machine for the general application of heat or cold to the patient's body correctly, efficiently, and safely.

VOCABULARY

aquathermia—a small, electric, jarlike container that is used to hold an alcohol/distilled water solution; it has outlets to permit circulation of the fluid through tubes and a hollow vinyl pad (K-pad).

autonomic nervous system—the part of the nervous system not under voluntary control; it governs the heart, glands, and smooth muscle in the body.

Central Service (CS)—a supply area in the hospital that provides sterile and unsterile equipment and supplies used in the care of patients.

cornea—the clear and transparent tissue of the eye that covers the iris and the pupil and permits light to enter the eye.

electrolyte—a charged particle (ion) capable of conducting an electrical charge; electrolytes are essential for normal body functioning.

hyperthermia—body temperature above the normal range (hyper- = more, above).

hypothermia—body temperature below the normal range (hypo- = less, below; -thermia = temperature).

infrared lamp—a special device that has light rays beyond the red end of the visible light spectrum.

light spectrum—light is the sensation produced by electromagnetic radiation that strikes the retina of the eye; spectrum refers to the distribution of the various lengths of light rays.

metabolism—the entire process by which the body is nourished, maintained, and provided with energy.

suppuration—the formation of pus.

systemic—relating to the whole system; the whole body.

toxin—a poisonous or noxious substance.

ultraviolet lamp—a special lamp that emits light rays outside the visible spectrum at the violet end.

INTRODUCTION

The application of heat or cold to the skin surface is important in treating certain infections and traumatic conditions. Usually a physician's order is necessary before one uses any of these treatments because of the related and opposing effects produced elsewhere in the body.

In this Unit, you will learn the effects of heat and cold on the body. Principles are given to guide your performance of procedures using applications of heat and cold. You need to know the precautions to take with groups of patients who are at greater risk of suffering burns to the skin when heat is applied. Procedures are included for the use of disposable hot and cold packs, aquathermia pads, hot water bottles, heating pads, heat cradles, ice bags, and the hypothermia machine.

PATIENT CARE AND THE APPLICATION OF HEAT AND COLD

ITEM 1. PRINCIPLES RELATED TO HEAT AND COLD

In order to understand the use of heat and cold applications and their effect on the body, you need to know about some of the principles involved:

1. Heat causes dilation of blood vessels and increases the supply of blood to the area.

2. Heat stimulates metabolism and the growth of new cells and tissues.

3. Cold causes contraction of blood vessels and decreases the supply of blood to the area to which it is applied.

4. Cold retards metabolism and decreases cell activity or growth.

5. Applications of heat and cold to portions of the body cause autonomic nervous system responses throughout the body.

6. Because the blood volume of the body is constant within a closed system, an increase in the blood supply to the skin causes a decrease in the blood supply to other portions of the body; conversely, a decrease in the blood supply to the skin increases the blood supply elsewhere in the body.

7. As a conductor of heat and cold, water is more effective than air.

Effects of Heat

These principles explain the effects of heat and cold on the body. Let us consider heat first. Heat is applied to the skin surfaces to provide general comfort and to speed up the healing process. The elevated temperature or fever that so often accompanies an illness or infection is the body's way of combating the illness and promoting the healing process.

Heat dilates the blood vessels in the area of application. This increases the blood supply, adds nutrients and oxygen to the tissue, removes toxins and excess tissue fluid, and reduces pain caused by pressure on the nerve endings. The dilated blood vessels and the increased blood supply in the area of heat application cause the skin to appear pinkish or reddened, although this color is more difficult to detect in dark-skinned or black patients. Heat is used to decrease inflammation and to promote the formation of pus (suppuration).

U
N
I
T
34

The dilation of blood vessels caused by heat application and the constriction of vessels resulting from application of cold are shown in the figures that follow.

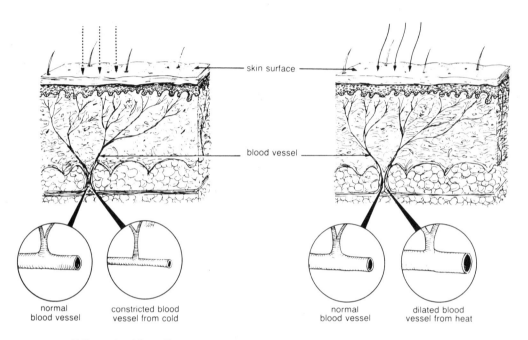

| skin surface |
| blood vessel |

| normal blood vessel | constricted blood vessel from cold | | normal blood vessel | dilated blood vessel from heat |

Effect of cold application.   Effect of heat application.

Effects of Cold

Cold applications are used to prevent or reduce swelling, to stop bleeding, and to decrease suppuration. When cold is applied to the skin surface, it contracts the muscles, which in turn squeeze the blood vessels to reduce the blood supply further. The blood vessels themselves contract, the diminished blood supply reduces the nutrients and oxygen to the cells, and cell activity is cut down. Since cold applications slow the metabolism of the body, the body can be cooled for prolonged surgery to decrease the stress of trauma and blood loss.

Prolonged cold reduces sensation and therefore lessens pain. If cold continues to interrupt the circulation, however, it can lead to necrosis (death of tissue), as is seen in severe frostbite. When a cold application is removed from the skin, there occurs a secondary reaction as the circulation returns to normal. The blood vessels dilate and give the skin a warm, glowing pink color.

Effects on the Autonomic Nervous System

Applications of heat and cold to the skin activate the autonomic nervous system. For example, the nerve endings in the skin send a message to the control center in the brain that heat has been applied. In an effort to maintain the body temperature at an even level, the control center acts to dilate the blood vessels and increase the circulation to the area. Other blood vessels to the internal organs are constricted so that the temperature of those organs is maintained to prevent disturbance of other delicately balanced body functions. Although the procedure of applying heat or cold to the body is relatively simple, the effect on the body is much more complex.

ITEM 2. IMPORTANT CONSIDERATIONS

Physician's Orders

When electric or nonelectric appliances are used for heat or cold in patient care, an order must be written by the physician on the patient's chart. The order must state the kind of appliance and the frequency and length of its application for the designated treatment.

Heat and cold treatments can be either dry—such as hot water bottles, heating pads, and ice caps—or moist, such as baths, soaks, and compresses. Moist applications have a more effective action because water is better than air as a conductor of heat and cold. Dry heat is tolerated better than a moist heat application of the same temperature, which may cause pain or burning.

Heat and cold can be applied to large or small body areas. A general application is one that is applied to the entire body; a local application is one that is used on a specific part of the body. The following figures show some examples of general and local applications.

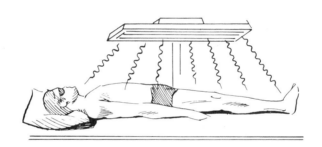

Example of general temperature application.

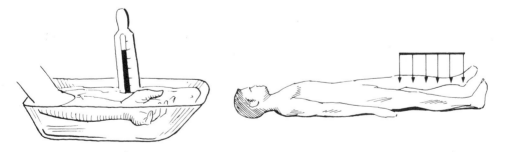

Examples of local temperature applications.

Safety for the Patient

As in all procedures, the nurse is concerned with the patient's safety. When using heat or cold applications, it is important to follow a number of principles that will reduce the danger of burns to the skin or electrical shock when electrical appliances are used.

Protection from Burns. A number of court suits have resulted when patients have suffered burns from the application of heating pads or hot water bottles that were too hot. A solution that is too hot will damage and burn the skin and some patients are much more apt to suffer burns from temperatures that other people might tolerate without discomfort. Nurses are expected to know this and to prevent burns from occurring. When referring to applications of moist heat applied directly to the skin, we frequently use the following temperatures:

Warm	93° to 98°F (34° to 37°C)
Hot	98° to 105°F (37° to 41°C)
Very hot	105° to 115°F (41° to 46°C)

The safe range of water temperature for the hot water bottle when used for most adults and children who have no circulatory impairment is 115° to 125°F (46° to 52°C). In any case, the hot water bottle should be placed in a flannel or cloth cover to protect the skin.

Some patients are less able to tolerate the temperatures listed in the preceding paragraph. When your patient falls into one of these categories, you should reduce the temperature to the low end of the range and avoid the "very hot" range altogether. Those who are much more apt to suffer burns from applications of heat are patients in the following groups: the very young, the aged, unconscious and anesthetized patients, those with edema or swelling of the extremities, and those with circulatory problems. The latter group includes a wide variety of diseases, such as arteriosclerosis, congestive heart failure, diabetes, phlebitis, and shock. This is but a partial list, so you can see that a lot of patients could suffer harm from fluids or electrical pads that are too hot.

To protect your patient from burns due to heat applications, follow these guidelines:

1. Measure the temperature of the liquid if possible. When a thermometer is not available, place the pack against the inner aspect of your arm. If there is any doubt that it is too hot, cool it down.

2. Use a flannel or cloth cover for all hot or cold packs.

3. Observe the condition of the skin frequently for signs of burning or blistering and be attentive to complaints by the patient.

4. Caution the patient and the family not to increase the temperature of appliances or of water in hot water bottles.

Protection from Electrical Shock. Electrical appliances for the application of heat or cold must be used with care to prevent sparks, shock, and even explosions, especially when oxygen is being used. Heating pads that patients bring to the hospital should be inspected for safety by the engineering department before they are used. Any appliance with a frayed or damaged cord should not be used. Avoid using safety pins on heating pads; a metal pin causes a short circuit if it comes in contact with the network of wires within the pad that conducts the electricity and provides the warmth. Pins also can puncture the K-pad; if the fluid leaks out, it is unsuitable for use.

Safety for the Worker

When an electric appliance is used, be aware that it is dangerous to put the plug in the electric outlet in a dark room. Use a light to find the outlet; do not try to locate the outlet using your hand as a guide. Do not handle the plug or put it in the electric outlet when you have wet hands. Do not remove the plug from the outlet by pulling at the cord. Be aware of the cord; it may be stretched across a walking area on the floor. Do *not* trip over it and hurt yourself.

Cost to the Patient

All appliances obtained from Central Service are rented for the patient in most agencies. Some agencies have a daily treatment rate that includes the cost of all treatments and equipment the patient needs. A requisition slip is usually sent to Central Service requesting the item; it is dated and stamped with the patient's name and hospital number. When the appliance is no longer needed, it must be returned to Central Service so that it can be re-processed for the next patient. Do not keep it longer than necessary; the patient may be charged for something that is not being used.

Care of the Equipment

Initial care of the equipment is usually accomplished by the health workers in Central Service. When it is being used by the patient, it is maintained by the health worker who is responsible for the patient's care. It must be kept clean and in good working order. When necessary, report needed repairs to the proper person and replace it immediately (send to Central Service). If equipment is faulty, do not express your concern or annoyance verbally in the presence of the patient or the family. This will only cause unnecessary apprehension or fear.

ITEM 3. USE OF DISPOSABLE HOT AND COLD PACKS

The disposable lightweight pack is a prefilled plastic package containing an exact amount of interreacting ingredients. When these ingredients are mixed by striking, squeezing, or kneading (depending on the manufacturer's instructions), they produce a sustained, controlled temperature. Most of the manufacturers color-code the packs, using blue packages for cold packs and red packages for hot packs.

The packages come in a variety of sizes and shapes. They are made to conform to the body contour (shape) when applied. Sizes range from $4\frac{1}{2} \times 11\frac{1}{2}$ inches for perineal applications to $6\frac{1}{4} \times 7\frac{1}{2}$ inches and $7\frac{1}{2} \times 9\frac{1}{2}$ inches for applications to reduce general swelling and pain.

Hot Packs

The disposable hot pack eliminates the inconvenience of the reusable hot water bottle. Equally important advantages are that its one-time use reduces the probability of cross infection and that its scientifically controlled temperature minimizes the danger of burning the patient. The temperature ranges from $101°$ to $114°F$; the action lasts from 20 to 60 minutes, depending on the size of the pack and the manufacturer's instructions. You must therefore check the specific directions on the product used by your agency.

Cold Packs

The temperature of these packs ranges from $50°$ to $80°F$. Because of the controlled temperature, there is almost no possibility of a freeze burn to the patient. The action lasts from 30 minutes to 4 hours, depending on the size of the pack and the specific product used. Cold packs are used for tonsillectomies, perineal wounds, sprains, nose bleeds, fractures of bones, dental extractions, and reduction of postoperative swelling of some parts of the body.

Most of the packs are intended to be applied directly to the skin surface. The outer covering of the pack is a special material that absorbs perspiration and prevents the cold, damp feel of plastic. Again, there may be a slight variation in this procedure, depending on the manufacturer.

UNIT 34

The fact that the pack is usually intended for one-time use serves to prevent cross infection. If the pack is punctured and the contents leak out, thoroughly and quickly wash the patient's skin with water to remove any of the chemical ingredients. Dispose of the punctured bag and replace it with a new pack. Notify the nurse of the incident.

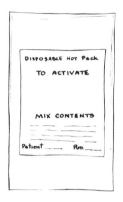

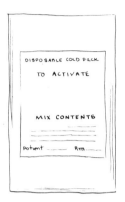

Supplies Needed

Disposable hot or cold pack   Towel
                                     Pins or tape

Important Steps	Key Points
1. Obtain a disposable pack from the storage area.	Universal Steps A, B, C, and D. See Appendix.
2. Wash your hands.	
3. Approach and identify the patient. Explain the procedure.	
4. Provide for privacy as needed.	
5. Mix the contents of the package.	This is done by a striking, squeezing, or kneading motion. The action breaks the internal chambers to permit the contents to mix. Knead until the chemical contents are mixed.

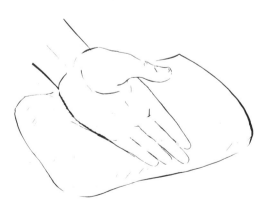

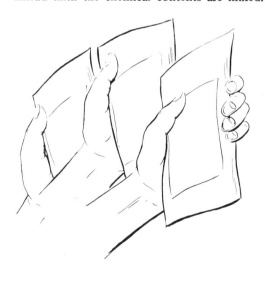

6. Apply the pack to the designated area.

The pack can be applied directly to the area of treatment, e.g., over an abscess on the inner aspect of the right arm.

To keep the pack from shifting, wrap a towel firmly and securely around the area. Fasten the ends with safety pins or tape.

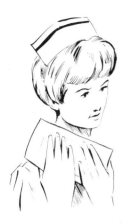

7. Return to the patient at frequent intervals.

See that the pack is producing heat or cold, as required. Observe the patient's skin for an increase or decrease in redness, swelling, pain, and blood circulation. Apply the same general principles and safety precautions that you learned for heat applications in the introduction to this unit.

8. Replace as needed.

The hot pack should be effective for 20 to 60 minutes. Dispose of the packet when it becomes cold. Replace it with a new one p.r.n.

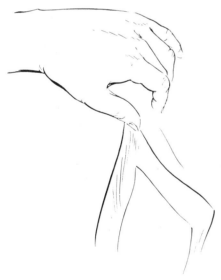

The cold pack should be effective for 30 minutes to 4 hours, depending on the size of the pack and its manufacturer. Dispose of the pack in a waste container when it becomes warm.

U
N
I
T
34

9. Record the treatment on the patient's chart.

Charting example:
1010. Hot pack T 105°F, applied on the inner aspect of the right forearm.

J. Lang, SN

or

0210. Cold pack applied to perineum.

P. Shaw, SN

ITEM 4. THE AQUATHERMIA PAD (K-PAD)

The Aquamatic K control unit is a small, jarlike, plastic unit operated by electricity. There is a temperature gauge on one side and two coupling outlets at the base. The top has a wide mouth with a lid on it so that distilled water can be poured into it. The vinyl Aquamatic K-pad (called K-pad for short) is attached to the coupling outlets at the base of the control unit. The water is heated and circulated through the unit and the pads in a manner similar to that of the hypothermia body unit. The pad is placed directly on the patient's injured area for a continuous heat treatment.

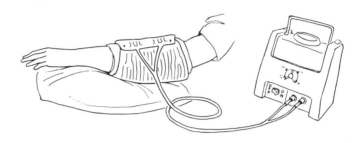

Supplies Needed

Towel   Aquathermia pad
Control unit

Important Steps	Key Points
Carry out Universal Steps, A, B, C, and D. See Appendix.	
1. Check the operation of the unit; set the temperature at 105°F.	The pad should feel warm within 1 to 2 minutes. This is a delicate instrument; be sure it is not dropped or bumped.
2. Place the pad on the patient's injured area.	Secure the pad with a bath towel if necessary. Wrap the towel around the outside of the pad and the injured extremity firmly, evenly, and securely. Fasten it with a safety pin or tape.
3. Check the injured area at frequent intervals.	Note any increased or decreased swelling, redness, circulation, pain, or numbness. Record on the patient's chart as necessary.
4. Remove the equipment.	Remove the electric plug from the electric outlet in the room. *Do not yank or pull the cord; put your hand on the plug and pull the plug.* Unwrap the towel and remove the K-pad.
5. Take the equipment to a sink or utility area, and wash it with soap and water or a disinfectant solution.	*Do not immerse the electric jarlike unit in water. Do not autoclave it.*
Carry out Universal Steps X, Y, and Z. See Appendix.	Charting example: 1930. K-pad applied to rt. shoulder. States pain is relieved by heat.

P. Shaw, SN

To Refill the K-pad and Adjust the Temperature

If you are required by your agency to make adjustments of the temperature setting or to refill the aquathermia unit, refer to the manufacturer's operating manual for instructions or use the following steps as a guideline.

Important Steps	Key Points
1. Unscrew the reservoir cap on the top of the control unit.	All parts are easily visible. Review the equipment operations manual before proceeding. This unit works like the hypothermia machine except that the temperature equipment is applied to a local area for treatment.
2. Fill the unit two-thirds full with distilled water.	
3. Tilt the control unit slowly from the side to let air bubbles escape.	
4. Plug the unit into the electrical outlet.	

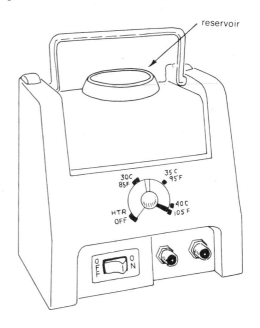

reservoir

5. Fill the K-pad with water by sliding the switch on the right to the "on" position.	Allow it to run at least 2 minutes.
6. Switch the unit off and tilt the control unit again to let air bubbles escape.	
7. Refill the reservoir to the cap level.	
8. Replace the cap, but loosen it 1/4 turn.	
9. Set the desired temperature by inserting a special key into the center of the dial.	Turn the dial until the indicator points to the desired temperature on the dial. Keep the key attached to the machine for p.r.n. changes in temperature.

ITEM 5. ELECTRIC HEATING PAD

||||||||||||||||||||||||||||||||||||||||||||||||||||||||||||||||||||||||||||||||||||||||||||||||||||||||||||||

Supplies Needed

Heating pad   Cover

||||||||||||||||||||||||||||||||||||||||||||||||||||||||||||||||||||||||||||||||||||||||||||||||||||||||||||||

Important Steps	Key Points
Carry out Universal Steps A, B, C, and D. See Appendix.	
1. Check the pad.	Put the plug into an electric outlet. Turn the regulating button to "high" so that the heating mechanism can be checked. The pad should become hot immediately. *Do not use* heating pads if the cords are frayed, worn, or haphazardly repaired.
2. Take the electric pad to the patient's bedside.	Give a detailed explanation to the patient, stressing all the safety measures to observe while the electric pad is being used. Tell the patient that excess heat may lead to burns and that a protective covering prevents blistering of the skin.
3. Place the covered electric pad on the patient's injured area.	Turn the control button to *"low."* *A low degree of heat should always be used when the electric pad is used for the patient.* Put the cloth cover or towel over the pad and apply to the injured area.

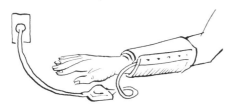

Heating pad.

Important Steps	Key Points
4. Return to the patient at frequent intervals.	Check to see that the appliance is effective. Observe the skin area for increased or decreased redness, pain, or blood circulation. Remove the heating pad and report all unusual changes immediately to the charge nurse.
5. Remove the electric heating pad when the treatment is completed.	Place your hand on the *plug* and pull it from the electric outlet. Remove the protective cover from the heating pad and discard it in the soiled laundry hamper or chute.
Carry out Universal Steps X, Y, and Z. See Appendix.	Charting example: 1610. Electric heating pad applied at low temperature on anterior aspect of lower left leg.
	P. Shaw, SN

ITEM 6. THE HOT WATER BOTTLE

Hot water bottles may be used to provide heat to a localized area of the body. Care must be taken to avoid using hot water that will cause a burn on the patient's skin. Patients with certain conditions such as emaciation, malnutrition, and circulatory problems are less able to tolerate warm water that may be comfortable to your skin. Some agencies may limit the use of hot water bottles for this reason. Given a patient with an inflamed area on the knee, apply a hot water bottle safely.

|||||||||||||||||||||||||||||||||||||||||||||||||||||||||||||||||||||||||||||||||||||||||||||||||||||||||||||||||||||||||||||||||||||

Supplies Needed

Towel   Cover
Hot water bottle   Bath thermometer

|||||||||||||||||||||||||||||||||||||||||||||||||||||||||||||||||||||||||||||||||||||||||||||||||||||||||||||||||||||||||||||||||||||

Important Steps	**Key Points**

Carry out Universal Steps A, B, C, and D. See Appendix.

1. Check the temperature of the water with a bath thermometer.

Burns of the skin occur when the water is too hot. Use the bath thermometer to measure the temperature, and do not use water hotter than $125°F$ ($52°C$), even though some patients may think the water is not hot enough. It will produce the desired effects.

2. Fill the hot water bottle one-half to two-thirds full with hot water.

Do not fill it so full that it is cumbersome and heavy. Lay the bottle on a flat surface.
   a. Expel the excess air until the water level comes to the mouth of the water bottle.
   b. Close the bottle with the screw-top cover or with a special clamp or tab.
   c. Wipe the outside of the bottle dry. Check for leaks and replace it if you find any.
   d. Place in flannel cover, a towel, or a pillowcase.

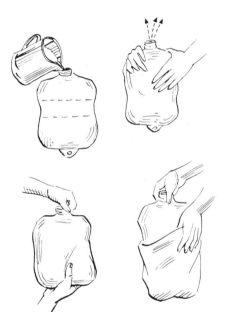

Filling hot water bottle.

3. Put the hot water bottle on the affected area.

Explain the importance of its use in relation to patient's injury or infection. Refer any questions that you are unable to answer to the charge nurse. To ensure effective immobilization, wrap a piece of sheeting or towel firmly and securely around the area. Fasten the ends with safety pins or tape.

U
N
I
T
34

Important Steps	Key Points
4. Return to the patient at frequent intervals.	Observe the skin for an increase or decrease in redness, heat, swelling, pain, and blood circulation. As the treatment continues, empty the cool water from the bottle and refill it with hot water. (Repeat steps 1 through 3.)
5. Remove the hot water bottle.	When the treatment is completed, or if redness, swelling, or pain increases, report immediately to the charge nurse. Put the cover in the soiled laundry bag. Discard the disposable cover in the wastebasket.
Carry out Universal Steps X, Y, and Z. See Appendix.	Charting example: 0900. Hot water bottle applied to right knee. J. Lang, SN

ITEM 7.   THE HEAT CRADLE

The heat cradle is made of metal bands, soldered and shaped in a half-moon form like the cradle used to keep the bedding off the patient's legs. An electric socket with a cord is attached to the center top band at the highest point. A 25-watt electric bulb is used, and the heat from the bulb produces the warmth necessary for the treatment. When in use, the cradle is covered by a sheet or the top bedding so that the heat is kept within the area. The size of the cradle permits air to circulate, and there is no weight on the patient's body to cause discomfort. This method of heat application is generally used on the lower trunk and extremities to promote healing of wounds and to increase the circulation.

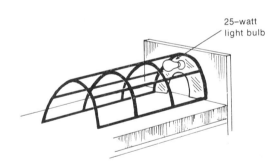

Supplies Needed

Heat cradle with 25-watt bulb   Dressings, as needed

Important Steps	Key Points
Carry out Universal Steps A, B, C, and D. See Appendix.	
1. Place the cradle on the bed and over the body part to be treated.	Replace the top covers. *Make sure that the sheets do not come near or in direct contact with the light bulb.* The heat from the bulb could burn a hole in the sheets and start a fire.

Important Steps	Key Points
2. Plug in the cord and turn on the light.	Plug the cord into an outlet near the bed. Make sure that the cord does not droop or lie on the floor where someone may trip over it and pull the cradle off the bed.
3. Prepare the patient for the treatment.	Position the patient in good alignment, and adjust the position of the bed for the patient's comfort.

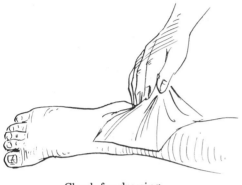

Check for dressing.

The heat cradle treatment may be ordered for a specified period of time or on a continuous basis. Check the physician's order for length of treatment. Also examine the area for necessary dressings. For dry heat and no dressings, the body part is exposed. If dry or moist dressings are required, apply them. Moist dressing should be wrapped with plastic sheeting and covered with a towel.

Important Steps	Key Points
4. Return to the patient at frequent intervals.	Observe the condition of the skin, noting decreased or increased circulation, swelling, temperature, or pain. Note the condition of the dressings. It may be necessary to add saline solution or water to keep the dressing moist. Usually this is done with an irrigating syringe. Leave the heat cradle in place for the *ordered* length of time.
5. Remove the cradle.	If treatment is to be continued at intervals during the day, put the cradle in a safe place in the patient's room. *Do not* set it on the floor. Organisms from the floor could adhere to the cradle and become the source of a secondary infection to the patient.
Carry out Universal Steps X, Y, and Z. See Appendix.	Charting example: 1900. Heat cradle applied to legs for 30 minutes. P. Shaw, SN 1930. Heat cradle removed. Skin looks pink, swelling and pain have decreased. P. Shaw, SN

U
N
I
T
34

ITEM 8.   THE ICE BAG OR ICE COLLAR

Another common method used for the local application of cold is the reusable ice bag or ice collar. Made of rubber or plastic, it can be filled with ice.

Some agencies have ice bags that are pneumatically sealed with a liquid solution inside. They are stored in the freezing unit of a special refrigerator. After the ice melts, the ice bag is returned to the refrigerator for refreezing.

|||||||||||||||||||||||||||||||||||||||||||||||||||||||||||||||||||||||||||||||||||||||||||||||||||||||||||||||||||||||||||||

Supplies Needed

    Ice bag   Flannel cover or towel
    Ice cubes or chips

|||||||||||||||||||||||||||||||||||||||||||||||||||||||||||||||||||||||||||||||||||||||||||||||||||||||||||||||||||||||||||||

Important Steps	**Key Points**

Carry out Universal Steps A, B, C, and D. See Appendix.

1. Fill the open-necked ice bag with ice.

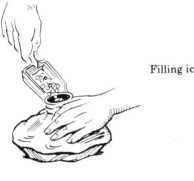

Filling ice bag.

Get a pan of ice cubes or crushed ice from the ice maker. Many hospitals have an ice machine either on the unit or in a centrally located area.
Fill the ice bag three-quarters full.
    a. Expel air from the bag. Lay it on a flat surface and press on the outside to expel the air.
    b. Seal or close the bag.
    c. Wipe outer surface dry and check for leaks.
    d. Put the bag in the cover.

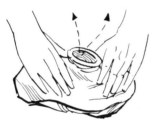

Expressing air from bag.

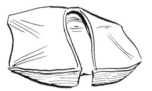

Ice bag with cover.

2. Take the ice bag to the patient and put it on the affected area.

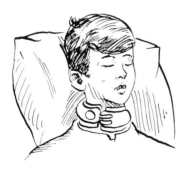

Ice collar.

Explain the importance of its use. Refer questions that you are unable to answer to the charge nurse. To ensure that the bag will remain in place, wrap a towel firmly and securely around the area, and fasten the ends with safety pins or tape.

Important Steps	**Key Points**
3. Return to the patient at frequent intervals.	Check to see if the ice bag is effective. Observe the skin area for increased or decreased redness, swelling, pain, numbness, and blood circulation. Report all unusual changes in the patient's condition immediately to the charge nurse.
4. Remove the ice bag when the treatment is completed or if the skin becomes more red or painful.	Put the linen cover in the soiled laundry hamper (or down the linen chute). Discard the plastic and disposable covers in the wastebasket.
Carry out Universal Steps X, Y, and Z. See Appendix.	Charting example: 1100. Ice collar applied to throat.
	J. Lang, SN

ITEM 9. FULL-BODY HYPOTHERMIA AND HYPERTHERMIA TREATMENT

Hypothermia, or the lowering of body temperature below the normal range, is a useful technique to decrease the rate of metabolic processes in the body. It is used to reduce high fevers, to control gastrointestinal hemorrhages, and to prevent cerebral edema (swelling of the brain) in head injuries or operations; it is also used for certain types of surgery. Usually the body temperature is reduced only a few degrees by cooling the body surface, but for surgical operations it may be reduced to 77°F (25°C) or even lower. Cooling may be achieved by cooling the body surface or by cooling the blood directly.

Hyperthermia may be used to increase the body temperature after it has been lowered by hypothermia. It may also be used to increase the metabolic rate in the body.

The Aquamatic K Thermia Machine, a refrigerated unit with cooling blankets (or pads) attached to it, is used to raise or lower body temperature in a safe, simple, but precise manner. It controls body temperature in neurological, cardiovascular, and surgical procedures. It is also used as a quick means to lower and regulate fevers or high temperatures due to infections and postoperative and traumatic conditions. It is both a labor- and time-saving device in caring for adult and child patients.

U
N
I
T
34

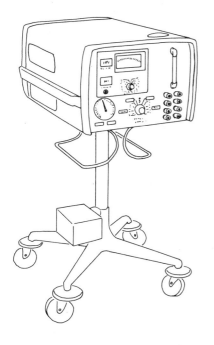

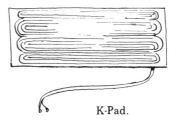

K-Pad.

The machine, an electronically controlled freezing and heating unit, contains a 20 per cent ethyl alcohol and distilled water solution. This solution circulates through the freezing or heating unit to produce the desired temperature (automatic or manually operated). The hollow, cordlike vinyl Aquamatic K-pads, containing the circulating solution, are placed in direct contact with the patient's skin to maintain the body temperature at the desired degree.

Setting Up the Machine. In most hospitals, the hypothermia/hyperthermia control unit and pads are delivered to the nursing unit, ready for use. In these instances, you would proceed directly to the portion of the procedure dealing with its use in patient care. In cases where nursing personnel have to prepare the unit for use, follow the instructions in the manufacturer's manual for the specific unit or use these steps as a guide in preparing the machine for use.

Supplies Needed

Temperature control box
Refrigeration unit and stand
20% ethyl alcohol and distilled
  water (1 gallon)

Thermistor probe
Vinyl K-pads (large or small sizes)
Operations manual

Important Steps	Key Points
1. Plug the electric cord of the machine into the wall outlet.	All Roman numerals in the following instructions refer to the sketches appearing on this and the next two pages.
2. Attach the pads to the unit (I).	Select the number and size of K-pads to be used. There are eight plugs for the pads clearly marked on the machine. Protective couplings remain on any plug not used.

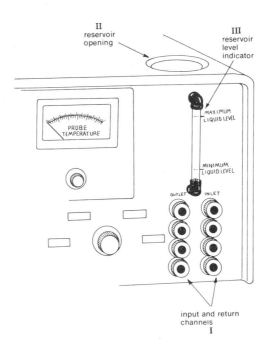

Couplings and plugs of machine.

Important Steps	Key Points
3. Fill the reservoir with the distilled water and alcohol solution.	Observe the reservoir level indicator (III) as a guide to how much fluid is needed, and fill it at least half full.
4. Fill the pads with the alcohol and water solution.	Turn on the pump by setting the heat and cool dials at 80°F (IV). This will pump fluid from the reservoir into the pads. After a few minutes, check the reservoir level indicator (III). Loosen the reservoir cap (II) one quarter turn when the pump is running to prevent a vacuum from developing.
5. Turn off pump and add more fluid to the reservoir, if needed.	More fluid may be added because some was used in filling the pads. It may be necessary to turn the machine off and on several times until the pads are filled.
6. Dial the desired temperature to cool or heat the solution in the pads or blanket.	The blanket temperature will be adjusted from 40° to 50°F, initially, then adjusted to the patient's temperature. This 40° to 50°F is the temperature in the blanket, not the patient's temperature. The patient's body temperature can be raised by setting the "Heat" dial to the desired temperature.

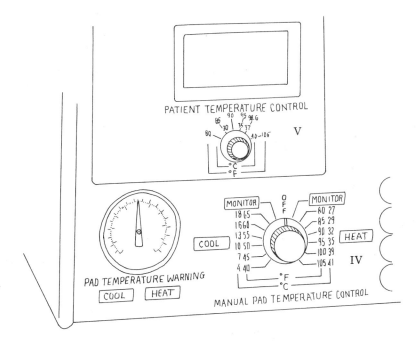

Use in Patient Care

Important Steps	Key Points

1. Place the pads on the patient.

Optimum body temperature control is maintained by having as much of the body covered with the pads as possible.
    a. Put one body-sized pad under the patient so that the pad comes in direct contact with the skin.
    b. Remove the patient's gown and put the second body-sized pad on top of the patient.

Once the patient is on the cooling blankets, his temperature will begin to drop. It may take several hours to reduce the temperature as low as necessary. The doctor prescribes the temperature and the length of time the temperature is to remain at that level. Check the reservoir fluid level frequently. Refill p.r.n.

2. Attach the thermometer unit to the hypothermia unit at the marked connection.

The thermometer unit may be separate from the hypothermia unit. Check your agency equipment. Remove the thermistor probe from its plastic container. Insert the thermistor probe into the appropriate outlet in the control box shown below.

3. Place the thermistor probe into the patient.

Insert the free end of the thermistor probe into the patient's rectum. The continuous, automatic temperature of the patient is recorded on the patient temperature indicator scale shown below (VI). The thermometer indicator will not register unless the probe is inserted in the patient.

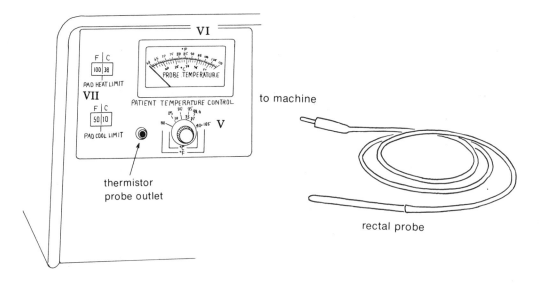

Temperature control unit.   Thermistor probe.

Important Steps	Key Points
4. Set temperature range for pad limits (Dial VII).	This prevents the pads or blankets from getting warmer or cooler than the limits set on the dial.
5. Set the desired temperature for the patient (Dial V).	The patient's actual temperature is indicated on the scale (VI), as the probe automatically provides a continuous measurement of the body heat. When the unit is working, the indicator light will go on. The electronic control device will automatically provide the heating and cooling control within the safety limits set on the temperature dial.
6. Provide for the patient's comfort and care.	Keep the patient from shivering during the cooling process. The shivering action increases the metabolic rate, which produces heat. Shivering can be controlled by various medications.
7. Report and record the indications and use of the procedure.	Charting example: 2030. T. 104.4, p 112, R 24. Placed on hypothermia pad for full-body cooling. 2130. T. 103.1, p. 98, R. 22. No shivering. P. Shaw, SN

To Discontinue the Procedure

Important Steps	Key Points
1. Remove the electric cord plug from the room outlet.	
2. Remove the thermistor probe from the patient.	
3. Disconnect the thermistor probe plug from the unit.	Put it in a safe place, to be returned with the rest of the equipment to the storage area for cleaning. These probes are frequently lost in the linens. They are costly, so be careful.
4. Disconnect the vinyl pads from the coupling outlets in the unit.	
5. Replace the caps to the coupling outlets in the unit.	
6. Remove the pads from the patient.	
Carry out Universal Steps X, Y, and Z. See Appendix.	Charting example: 2330. Hypothermia unit removed. Patient comfortable and quiet. Temperature 98°F. P. Shaw, SN

ITEM 10.   ULTRAVIOLET AND INFRARED HEAT TREATMENTS

Other types of heat appliances that may be used are the ultraviolet and infrared lamps. Usually these treatments are given by the physical therapy staff, but you should know about them. The ultraviolet lamp projects heat rays and produces some chemical reactions that

U
N
I
T
34

inhibit the growth of bacteria; it is also used for the heat it produces. The ultraviolet light seems to be effective in stopping rickets (a vitamin D deficiency disease). Infrared lamps are used for the relief of pain caused by arthritis and rheumatic conditions. Other heat sources are the sun, the electric arc, and the incandescent lamp. Great caution must be observed when these lamps are used, and the patient must be under constant supervision to avoid severe burns.

The lamps act on the skin and tissue like sun rays. If you have experienced a sunburn, you can understand the possible dangers from these lamps. When the ultraviolet lamp is used, specially fitted dark glasses or protective eye coverings are worn by the patient to protect the eyes, particularly the cornea. When the light rays turn to heat rays, the corneal tissue could be destroyed. (The eye tissue would be coagulated like the white of an egg when it is cooked.)

The lamps are used for superficial and deep heat therapy under the supervision of the physical therapist. If the patient is overexposed to the lamp rays, tissue damage can be extreme — a third-degree burn will result. The skin area first becomes red, then blistered, swollen, and burned so badly that the tissue eventually sloughs off. When this happens, there is danger of a systemic infection and an electrolyte imbalance due to the loss of fluid through the open wound. Symptoms to be noted accompanying the burn are nausea, headache, vomiting, and possible kidney malfunctions (anuria). For these reasons, the lamps are used only in the physical therapy department or by specially trained personnel.

Several precautions must be taken when one gives these treatments:

1. Apply to the local area only.

2. Observe the time elements very strictly. The time of the treatment may be limited to as little as 1 to 2 minutes.

3. Know the heat method you are using, its expected results, and the complications that could arise from improper use.

4. Follow directions explicitly for applying the procedure (time, location, distance from light to skin surface).

5. Stay with the patient and observe his or her reactions closely.

CONCLUSION OF THE UNIT

You have now concluded the lesson on Hot and Cold Applications. When you have practiced the procedures so that you know them, arrange with your instructor to take the post-tests. You will be expected to demonstrate your skills in carrying out the required tasks, as well as knowledge of the effects of heat and cold on the body.

PERFORMANCE TEST

In the classroom or your skills laboratory, your instructor will ask you to perform the following activities without reference to any source material. You will need the mannequin or another student to take the part of the patient.

1. Given a patient who has a swollen, stiff, and painful right shoulder, apply a hot water bottle (or disposable hot pack) to the part, being careful not to burn the patient.

2. Given a patient with a circulatory disease of both legs, apply a heat cradle that will be used indefinitely in a manner that will provide comfort and safety.

3. Given a postoperative tonsillectomy patient, apply an ice collar (or disposable cold pack) to the throat in a manner that will provide comfort and safety.

4. Given a patient who is suspected to have cerebral edema (swelling of the brain), set up the hypothermia machine to control body temperature at 95°F (35°C).

If the machine is not available in your agency, describe the steps of the procedure that you would use.

PERFORMANCE CHECKLIST

APPLICATION OF A HOT WATER BOTTLE TO THE RIGHT SHOULDER

1. Wash your hands.
2. Approach and identify the patient.
3. Obtain a hot water bottle and cover from storage.
4. Test the temperature of the bottle with the bath thermometer.
5. Fill the hot water bottle one-half to two-thirds full with hot water.
6. Expel the excess air from the bottle before securing the top.
7. Put a cover on the bottle.
8. Take the hot water bottle to the patient and explain why it is being used.
9. Place the bottle snugly against the patient's right shoulder.
10. Make sure that the patient is comfortable.
11. Record pertinent information on the patient's chart.

USE OF A HEAT CRADLE OVER THE EXTREMITIES

1. Wash your hands.
2. Approach and identify the patient.
3. Obtain a heat cradle and bring it to the bedside.
4. Provide for the patient's privacy by pulling the curtain.
5. Fold back the top covers without undue exposure of the patient.
6. Place the heat cradle over the patient's legs.
7. Plug in the cord and turn on the light.

U
N
I
T
34

8. Check the wattage of the light and the length and position of the cord.

9. Inspect the patient's legs for need of dressings.

10. Replace the top covers over the heat cradle but away from the light itself.

11. Position the patient in good alignment.

12. Adjust the bed for the patient's comfort.

13. Tell the patient that you will check back at frequent intervals.

14. Record all pertinent information on the patient's chart.

APPLICATION OF ICE COLLAR TO THE THROAT

1. Wash your hands.

2. Approach and identify the patient.

3. Obtain an ice collar and cover from storage.

4. If a freeze pack is available, put a cover on it, or fill the ice pack about three-quarters full with ice.

5. Expel air from the pack and wipe the outside dry after closing the top.

6. Wrap the ice collar in a cover or towel.

7. Apply the ice collar securely to the patient's throat.

8. Inform the patient that the pack will be checked frequently.

9. Make sure that the patient is comfortable.

10. Record all pertinent information on the patient's chart.

SET UP HYPOTHERMIA MACHINE AND CONTROL TEMPERATURE OF 95° F

A. *Prepare the Hypothermia Unit*

1. Wash your hands.

2. Obtain a hypothermia machine with all its parts and take it to the bedside.

3. Plug in the cord.

4. Select two large K-pads and attach them to the unit.

5. Fill the reservoir with fluid.

6. Fill the pads with fluid by turning on the machine.

7. Turn the machine off before adding more fluids.

B. *Prepare the Patient*

1. Approach and identify the patient, and explain the procedure.

2. Place one large K-pad under the patient.

3. Remove gown and place a second large K-pad over the patient.

4. Attach a thermometer unit to the hypothermia unit.

5. Insert the thermistor probe into the patient's rectum.

6. Set the dial for limits of pad temperature: $40°$ to $50°F$ ($4.4°$ to $10°C$) for cooling and $100°F$ ($37.8°C$) for heating.

7. Set the desired temperature of $95°F$ ($35°C$) on the patient temperature control.

8. Provide for the patient's comfort and report any shivering.

9. Inform the patient that his or her temperature and the blanket temperature will be checked frequently.

10. Record all pertinent information on the patient's chart.

POST-TEST

Multiple Choice: Select the best answer for each of the questions.

1. A local application of heat to the upper back would cause

    a. a numbness or loss of sensation.

    b. a bluish, mottled color of the skin.

    c. dilation of blood vessels elsewhere in the body.

    d. increased circulation of blood in the area.

2. Metabolism and growth of new cells are stimulated by

    a. oxygen.

    b. cold.

    c. heat.

    d. light.

3. A hot water bottle is filled only one-half to two-thirds full in order to

    a. make the bottle lighter and less cumbersome to use.

    b. keep it from getting too hot and burning the patient.

    c. assure that it is refilled frequently as it cools.

    d. make it easier to expel the air from the bottle.

4. Heat makes the blood vessels

    a. dilate.

    b. contract.

    c. increase.

    d. decrease.

5. Hypothermia can be defined as

    a. decreased blood supply to a part of the body.

    b. a decrease in the temperature of the blood.

    c. an increase in the temperature of the body.

    d. freezing of a part or all of the body.

6. Infrared and ultraviolet lamps are used under the supervision of the physical therapist because

    a. heat produced from the light rays can cause serious burns.

    b. someone must observe the patient frequently.

    c. the rays can coagulate albumin, or the white of an egg.

    d. the lamps must be a certain distance from the patient's skin.

7. A patient can tolerate the dry cold of an ice bag for a longer period of time than a local bath of ice-cold water because

   a. the nerve endings are numbed by the ice bag.

   b. the intensity of dry cold is greater than that of wet cold.

   c. dry cold reduces the contraction of muscles.

   d. water is a better conductor of cold than air.

8. The temperature indicated by the "Cool" dial or button (IV) on the hypothermia machine is used to regulate the temperature of

   a. the fluid in the reservoir.

   b. the patient's body.

   c. the fluid in the K-pads.

   d. the air in the room.

9. When you are working with electrical equipment, such as the electric heating pad or the hypothermia machines, you should always avoid

   a. using the equipment when oxygen is being used in the same room.

   b. touching the controls without an order from the doctor.

   c. using a cover between the electrical pad or machine and the patient's skin.

   d. plugging the cord into an outlet with wet hands.

10. A cold application causes which of the following effects:

    a. an increase in the metabolic rate of the body

    b. a decrease in the blood supply to the area

    c. a reduction in excess tissue fluid, or swelling

    d. more rapid removal of toxins and waste products

POST-TEST ANSWERS

1. d	6. a
2. c	7. d
3. a	8. c
4. a	9. d
5. b	10. b

UNIT 34

Unit 35

GENERAL PERFORMANCE OBJECTIVE

Following this lesson, you will be able to apply bandages and binders to achieve the purpose for which they are being used.

SPECIFIC PERFORMANCE OBJECTIVES

When you are through with this lesson you will be able to

1. Discuss with the instructor the reasons for which bandages and binders are applied.

2. Examine an area that is wrapped with a binder or a bandage for impaired circulation and take immediate steps to remove the impairment.

3. Apply circular, figure-8, spiral, spiral reverse, and recurrent bandages.

4. Apply a scultetus, T-binder, and double-T-binder.

VOCABULARY

bandage—a piece of soft material, like gauze, used to wrap, bind, support, provide warmth, protect, or immobilize a part.

circular bandage—a bandage that is wrapped around and around a part; each turn covers the preceding turn and holds it securely in place.

elastic bandage—a bandage that is stretchable; when pulled tightly, it causes compression. A commonly used elastic bandage is the Ace bandage.

figure-8 bandage—a bandage in which the turns cross each other like a figure-8; generally used over joints to retain dressings or to exert pressure in the case of sprains or hemorrhage.

recurrent bandage—used over the end of a stump of an amputated extremity, such as a leg or a finger.

reverse spiral bandage—special technique in which a part of the bandage is folded back on itself to make it fit more evenly over an area of varying width, such as the lower leg.

roller bandage—a continuous strip of soft gauze or elastic material used to bind up injured parts. It comes in various widths and lengths.

scultetus binder (many-tailed)—a succession of overlapping bands used to provide girdle-like abdominal support following an operation.

spiral bandage—a bandage that consists of a series of circular turns ascending (going up) a part, such as from the fingers to the wrist; each turn is higher than the preceding one and overlaps the previous turn about half the width of the bandage.

T-binder (sanitary belt)—shaped like the letter "T," it is used to hold perineal pads (peri-pads) as well as rectal or perineal dressings in place.

T-binder, double—shaped like the letter T except that it has two tails TT; commonly used to hold the dressings in place on male patients who have had rectal or perineal surgery.

triangular bandage—a bandage that is three-cornered; it holds dressings in place; it is most often used as a *sling*, a swinging bandage to support the forearm or elbow.

734

INTRODUCTION

Bandages and binders are made from many kinds of soft materials such as muslin, gauze, flannel, rubber, and elastic fabric. There are a number of commonly used bandages and binders; you should be familiar with their names and know how to apply them correctly. These bandages, and combinations of them as described in this unit, represent the most generally applied types. The specific method used will not only depend on the part to be bandaged, but on the purpose of the bandage, for example, support, immobilization, and so forth.

This unit describes various methods of bandaging, including the circular bandage, the figure-8, the spiral, and the spiral reverse. Patients expect even beginning level nurses to be able to bandage parts of the body neatly and with a minimum of wasted motion. Selecting the appropriate type and length of bandage is also important to the final result. Various types of binders and the procedures for applying them are described.

BANDAGING AND BINDING

ITEM 1. PURPOSES FOR BANDAGES AND BINDERS

Bandages and binders are used

1. to apply pressure in order to stop bleeding or swelling, and to assist in absorbing tissue fluids.

2. to provide for immobilization of an injured part, such as a fractured (broken) arm.

3. to hold dressings in place.

4. to protect open wounds from contaminants.

5. to provide support and aid in venous blood return, such as when bandaging the leg of a patient suffering from varicose veins or impaired circulation.

Bandages and binders should be applied so that pressure is evenly distributed to the affected area. If a joint is involved in bandaging, it should be supported in its normal position with a slight flexion of the joint. Both the bandage and binder should be wrapped securely to avoid friction or rubbing of the underlying tissue, which could cause severe irritation. Great care must be taken, however, not to make it too tight so that circulation is cut off. It must be tight enough to stay in place but not so tight as to cut off circulation! Remember the signs and symptoms of impaired circulation from Unit 18, Special Skin Care.

Signs of impaired circulation are *paleness* or *cyanosis, swelling, coolness,* and *pain.* It is helpful to leave the tips of the fingers and toes visible on a bandaged extremity so that you can determine whether the circulation is impaired.

When possible, elevate the extremity for 15 minutes before applying a bandage. This aids venous blood flow and helps to reduce swelling in the hand or foot. If the limb is wrapped while swollen, the bandage will become loose and slip when the edema subsides. You can elevate the extremity by having the patient lie with the arm or leg resting on pillows and above the level of the heart.

A bandage or binder should be applied over a clean, dry area as a precaution against microorganisms which grow in warm, damp areas. Be sure that skin surfaces are not bandaged in contact with each other — they will sweat and provide a moist environment in which microorganisms can grow. Always put some kind of padding (4 X 4 or ABD bandage) between adjoining skin surfaces before bandaging or binding. It is also wise to pad over a bony prominence before bandaging to avoid pressure, which could lead to excoriation of the skin. If left unattended for several days, such an irritation could become a decubitus ulcer.

If a bandage or binder is applied to the dressing of a draining wound, it must be changed frequently to keep it as clean and dry as possible. This reduces the chance of pathogenic organisms getting into the wound and causing an infection. Discard the soiled dressings and bandages, and return the binders to the laundry for washing and reprocessing, or discard them if your agency uses disposable items.

ITEM 2. TYPES OF BANDAGES

There are several types of bandages available for use today. The type you select will depend upon the purpose of the bandage and the doctor's preference, if this is specified. The gauze roller bandage is used less frequently for bandaging the arm or leg when there is a difference in the size of the limb. Other bandages that have more elastic or clinging ability provide a firmer wrapping that stays in place and provides better support.

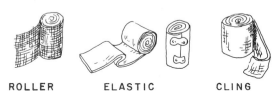

ROLLER   ELASTIC   CLING

Elastic bandages are made of woven material that can be stretched and molded around the part being bandaged. The Ace bandage and stockinette are two types of elastic material. These bandages can be removed, rewound, and used again for the same patient. Do not reuse (1) for a different patient or (2) when a sterile bandage is required to hold a dressing in place over an open wound.

Another popular type of bandage is the cling type. It also stretches but is not elastic. It molds around irregular and hard to bandage areas and is often used for holding dressings in place on the head or on the stump following amputation of a limb. The clinging bandage may then be covered with an elastic bandage that provides firm support.

Approximate lengths and widths needed for bandaging certain body parts:

Type	Length	Width
head bandaging	6 yards	2 inch
body bandaging	10 yards	3 to 6 inch
leg bandaging	9 yards	2 to 4 inch
foot bandaging	4 yards	1½ to 3 inch
arm bandaging	7 to 9 yards	2 to 2½ inch
hand bandaging	3 yards	1 to 2 inch
finger bandaging	1 to 3 yards	½ to 1 inch

You will be expected to apply these bandages and binders safely and correctly. Practice the following procedures with your partner in the skills laboratory.

ITEM 3. THE CIRCULAR BANDAGE

Apply a circular bandage to secure a clean dressing on the posterior aspect of the right forearm.

Supplies Needed

Bandage (elastic, cling, or
  roller), 2 to 2½ inches wide

Dressings, if needed
Soap, water, towels

Important Steps	Key Points
1. Wash your hands.	Universal Steps A, B, C, and D. See Appendix.
2. Obtain your supplies.	
3. Approach the patient and explain what you are going to do.	
4. Provide for privacy and drape as necessary.	
5. Remove the used bandage and wash the area that was bandaged.	Remember that microorganisms grow in dark, moist, dirty places. You may use soap and water or an antiseptic cleansing solution to wash the skin. Apply a dressing if needed. (Check your agency rules.)
6. Place the patient in a comfortable position. Stand directly in front of the patient.	The position should also be convenient for you when you work. The patient may be sitting or prone, depending on where the bandage is required. Standing will make it easier for you to see what you are doing.
7. Unroll the bandage and anchor it in place.	Ask the patient to raise the right arm slightly (about 6 to 12 inches) from the bed, palm upward, so that you can wrap it. If the patient is unable to lift the arm, you may need some assistance.

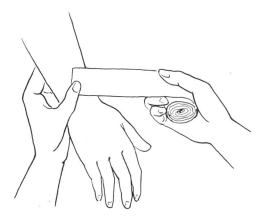

Unwind it toward the right, around the patient's arm. Hold the roll of bandage in your right hand so that it unwinds from the top (reverse hand positions if you are left-handed). Hold the bandage in place with your left thumb with moderate tension. If you hold the bandage too loosely while wrapping, it will come off easily. If the bandage is wrapped too tightly, it will cut off the patient's circulation. You will have to practice wrapping until you judge the proper tension to use.

8. Make two initial circular turns to secure the bandage in place.	Secure the proximal (free) end to the arm directly over the site. For the patient's comfort, the beginning (initial) and terminal end of the bandage are not to be placed directly over the wound, a bony prominence, the inner aspect of a limb, or a part that the patient will lie on.

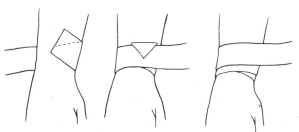

Anchoring bandage in place.

U
N
I
T
35

Important Steps	Key Points
9. Each circular turn goes directly over the preceding turn.	Each successive turn anchors (holds in place) the underlying layer of bandage. Continue unrolling the bandage from right to left around the arm. Use as many circular turns as needed to hold the dressing in place or to immobilize the part.

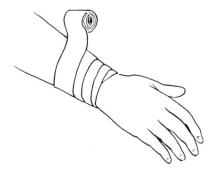

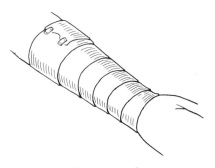

Circular bandage.

10. Secure the terminal end of the bandage.	You can use tape, special metal clips, or a safety pin. Usually the circular bandage is used to keep a dressing in place. Place the patient's arm in a comfortable position.
11. Tidy the work area.	Universal Steps X, Y, and Z. See Appendix.
12. Provide for the patient's comfort.	
13. Record the procedure on the patient's chart.	Charting example: 1010. Dressing changed. Wound of mid forearm is 2½ in. dia., pink, and no drainage. Sterile dry dressing applied with Ace bandage. Fingers warm, slightly swollen, but no pain. M. Victory, PN

ITEM 4. THE FIGURE-8 BANDAGE

The figure-8 bandage may be used by itself or with the circular, spiral, or spiral reverse bandage whenever a joint is included in the wrapping. The figure-8 bandage around the joint protects dressings and keeps them in place, supports and limits the movement of the joint, and promotes the venous blood return, which reduces swelling, or edema. The advantage of the figure-8 bandage is that it can support the joint in a position of flexion, or allow limited movement when this is necessary.

To apply a figure-8 bandage to the ankle, follow these steps.

||||||||||||||||||||||||||||||||||||||||||||||||||||||||||||||||||||||||||||||||||||||||||||||||||||||||||||||||||||||||||||||||||||||||||||||||||||||

Supplies Needed

Bandage (elastic, cling, or roller type),
    1½ to 3 inches wide

||||||||||||||||||||||||||||||||||||||||||||||||||||||||||||||||||||||||||||||||||||||||||||||||||||||||||||||||||||||||||||||||||||||||||||||||||||||

Important Steps	Key Points

Carry out Universal Steps A, B, C, and D. See Appendix.

1. Anchor the bandage over the foot.

To bandage the ankle, place the initial anchoring turns around the foot, beginning near the toes. The anchoring turns generally are placed distal to the joint being wrapped.

2. Make a circular turn over the foot and around the ankle.

For purposes of support, the first turn may be placed at the upper part of the ankle, and each successive turn placed lower over the ankle and heel.

For promoting venous blood return, the first turn is placed lower on the heel and each successive turn overlaps higher onto the ankle. The rest of the leg is also wrapped.

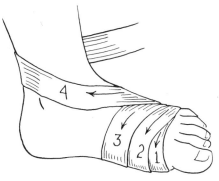

Anchoring turns for figure-8 bandage.

3. Continue to make a spiral turn down over the ankle and around the foot.

4. Alternate the upward and downward spiral turns about the joint.

Overlap each layer all but ½ to 1 inch, and make at least three complete turns. Continue bandaging the lower leg as necessary.

U
N
I
T
35

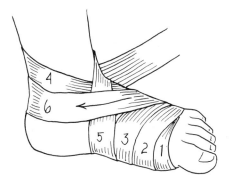

Continue alternate turns around ankle and foot.

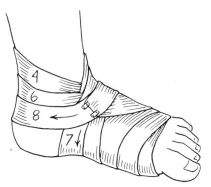

One type of figure-8 bandage.

Important Steps	Key Points
5. Secure the end of the bandage.	Charting example: 1515. Ace bandage applied to right ankle. Slight swelling of foot. Toes pink and warm. <div align="right">P. Walls, RN</div>

Carry out Universal Steps X, Y, and Z. See Appendix.

ITEM 5.   THE SPIRAL BANDAGE

This procedure is used to apply an elastic bandage to an arm or leg. When the leg is involved, an elastic stocking is often ordered instead of the bandage. Read the directions on the package before applying. Frequently observe the circulation in the toes after application. Refer to Unit 16, Dressing and Undressing, for general instructions.

‖‖

Supplies Needed

Bandage (elastic, cling, or roller type), 2 to 4 inches wide

‖‖‖

Important Steps	Key Points
Carry out Universal Steps A, B, C, and D. See Appendix.	
1. Begin by anchoring the bandage with two circular turns.	Most often, you will need to bandage the foot to aid venous blood return when you apply a bandage to the leg. Use the figure-8 bandage and then proceed with the spiral wrapping of the leg.
2. With each succeeding turn of the bandage, angle slightly upward around the leg.	The direction is downward, around, upward, and around, like a spiral staircase, in the same direction as the blood that is returning to the heart. Each turn is parallel to the preceding turn and overlaps about 1/2 to 2/3 the width of the bandage.

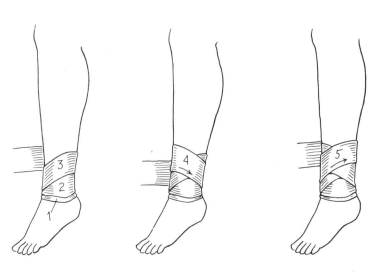

Important Steps	Key Points
3. Wrap the bandage evenly and smoothly.	Hold the limb firmly and wrap it securely. Take care not to wrap it so tightly that you cut off the circulation. As you wrap, ask the patient how it feels. Loosen it immediately if too tight.
4. Continue wrapping in the spiral fashion.	Wrap until the part is thoroughly covered. Do not use excessive bandage. Do not waste motions or material while wrapping.
5. Secure the terminal end of the bandage.	Use tape, clips, or safety pins. As before, do not start or finish the bandage over wounds, bony prominences, and so forth.

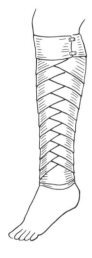

Carry out Universal Steps X, Y, and Z. See Appendix.	Charting example: 0800. Right leg rewrapped with Ace bandage. Toes warm and pink. <div align="right">L. Gomez, SN</div>

ITEM 6. THE SPIRAL REVERSE BANDAGE

This bandage is used to wrap an extremity that has varying thicknesses (such as the thin ankle portion which rises to a thick area like the calf of the leg). This method of bandaging provides a means to make a secure, smooth, even-fitting bandage on an extremity.

Supplies Needed

Bandage (elastic or cling type),
2, 3, or 4 inches wide

Important Steps	Key Points
Carry out Universal Steps A, B, C, and D. See Appendix.	
1. Begin with two circular turns to anchor the bandage.	

U
N
I
T
35

Important Steps	Key Points

2. Make a spiral reverse turn.

This is done at the place on the leg where the bandage will no longer lie smoothly as you continue around the leg.
  a. Place thumb on upper edge of an anterior turn and hold firmly.
  b. Turn the bandage downward over the thumb and toward the lower edge of the previous turn.
  c. Cover about 1/2 to 1/3 of the previous lap and continue the turn.

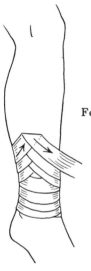

Folding bandage over to make spiral reverse turn.

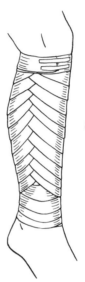

Spiral reverse bandage fits contours of extremity.

3. Continue making spiral reverse turns.

Wind the bandage in the same manner, and place it like the previous layers until the bandage will once again lie smoothly as you unroll it in a spiral direction. The spiral reverse bandage fits the contours of an extremity.

4. Secure the end of the bandage.

Carry out Universal Steps X, Y, and Z. See Appendix.

Charting example:
0925. Right foot and leg rewrapped with Ace bandage. States there is less discomfort today when walking.

L. Gomez, SN

ITEM 7. THE RECURRENT BANDAGE

This type of bandage is applied to hold pressure dressings in place over the tip end of a finger, toe, fist, stump of an amputated extremity or on the head.

This is the type of bandage used on the stump of an *above-the-knee (AK) amputation*. *Below-the-knee amputation is identified as BK amputation.*

||||||||||||||||||||||||||||||||||||||||||||||||||||||||||||||||||||||||||||||||||||||||||||||||||||||||||||||||||||||||||||||||||

Supplies Needed

Bandage (elastic, cling, or roller type);
    width depends on site:
        for finger: 1 inch wide
        for stump or head: 3, 4, or 6 inches wide

||||||||||||||||||||||||||||||||||||||||||||||||||||||||||||||||||||||||||||||||||||||||||||||||||||||||||||||||||||||||||||||||||

Important Steps	Key Points
Carry out Universal Steps A, B, C, and D. See Appendix.	
1. Unroll the bandage and bring over the tip from front to back. Bring bandage over tip.	Hold the top layer of bandage securely on the anterior leg with your left thumb at the highest edge. Unroll the bandage downward over the tip of the stump toward the back. Hold the bandage firmly on the posterior aspect of the leg with the index finger.
2. Make a fold at the back and bring the bandage over the tip to the front.	Move each successive turn alternately to the left, then to the right of the first layer over the tip of the stump in a somewhat spiral manner.
3. Make a fold at the front and hold the folds securely.	
4. Cover the entire surface with overlapping folds.	Continue wrapping until the stump end is well covered, overlapping each layer about 1/2 to 2/3 the width of the previous layer. Continue to hold succeeding layers securely in place with your thumb and index finger.
5. Make several circular turns to hold the folded laps in place. Secure ends with several circular turns.	When the stump is smoothly, evenly, and totally covered, once more reverse the direction of the bandage and make at least two circular turns to cover the gathered ends that you have been holding securely between your thumb and index finger.

Important Steps	Key Points
6. Secure the ends of the bandage.	Secure the final end with tape, a clip, or a safety pin.
Carry out Universal Steps X, Y, and Z. See Appendix.	Charting example: 1100. Right AK stump wound cleansed with antiseptic. No drainage noted. Bandage applied. <div align="right">L. Gomez, SN</div>

ITEM 8. THE SCULTETUS BINDER

The scultetus binder is designed to provide abdominal support after an abdominal operation, post-delivery, or post-paracentesis. The binder is made by sewing heavy flannel strips 3 to 4 inches wide and 4 feet long in overlapping layers of 1/2 inch. The middle third section of the strips is sewed together, leaving about 20 inches free on each end.

Supplies Needed

Scultetus binder   Pins

Important Steps	Key Points
Carry out Universal Steps A, B, C, and D. See Appendix.	
1. Place the binder under the patient's hips.	The solid portion of the binder should be centered under the patient's body, the many-tailed ends lying flat on the bed extending straight out from the patient. All tails on the binder overlap the next one, except for the beginning set of tails on one end. The unlapped beginning tail is placed face up at the lower edge of the hips. As each tail is applied, the next tail is unlapped and can be placed smoothly without wrinkles.

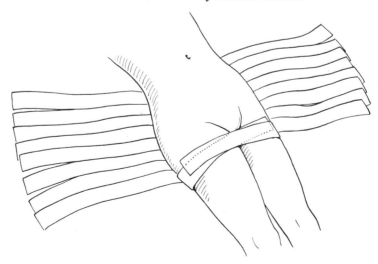

Start applying scultetus binder at the level
of the pubic region, or lower hip.

Important Steps	Key Points
2. Bring the *bottom tail* across the abdomen.	You will begin in the direction in which the tail is going, to provide for smooth, successive spiral-type layers with a 1/2-inch overlap of each layer. Pull tightly. If the end is too long, you may need to fold the free end back on itself, just far enough so it fits smoothly. Incorrect placement of the overlapping tails causes pressure and discomfort for the patient.
3. Alternate tails first from one side of the abdomen, then from the other side.	Proceed toward the waist, slanting each succeeding tail slightly upward.
4. Secure the final tail with a safety pin.	This type of abdominal bandage provides good support for the patient. If you have pulled it securely enough as you criss-crossed each strip and then firmly pinned it, the patient will be able to move freely about without having the bandage come undone.

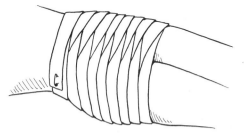

Scultetus binder secured firmly at the waist.

Carry out Universal Steps X, Y, and Z. See Appendix.	Charting example: 0800. Scultetus binder reapplied after bath. Up in chair with no complaints. <div align="right">J. Jones, SN</div>

ITEM 9.   THE SLING

Patients who have an injury to the arm or shoulder often need to support the arm in an elevated position to avoid edema of the hand, pain and discomfort, and fatigue. A commercially made arm support can be placed about the arm and the straps adjusted about the neck. When this type of arm support is not available, you may need to provide a triangular sling bandage to support the injured upper extremity. The triangular sling is made from a piece of cloth 30 to 40 inches square. Fold it diagonally in half to make a double triangle. You can cut it across the diagonal fold if you want a single thickness.

U
N
I
T
35

Supplies Needed

40-inch square, folded in triangle   Pins

Important Steps	Key Points
Carry out Universal Steps A, B, C, and D. See Appendix.	
1. Put one end (1) of the triangle over the shoulder on the uninjured side.	For this lesson, we will say it is the right arm that is injured. Therefore, the end of the triangle will be placed over the patient's left shoulder.

Important Steps	Key Points
2. Place the point (apex) (3) of the triangle toward the elbow.	Ask the patient to bend the injured arm horizontally across the body with the thumb up. Place the bandage under the arm flat against the chest.

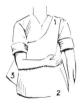 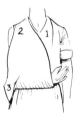

3. Bring the other end (2) over the injured arm and shoulder.	Have the patient keep the elbow bent at right angles across the lower chest. The hand should be slightly higher than the elbow (about 4 inches). This will prevent the fingers from swelling.
4. Tie the two ends with a square knot.	Make the knot to one side of the neck so that it will not be uncomfortable if the patient lies down or will not cause continuing pull on the back of the neck when the arm is in the sling.
5. Fold the apex (or point) of the triangle neatly over the elbow toward the front.	Secure it with a safety pin.

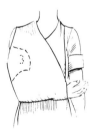

Injured arm supported by sling.

6. Check the circulation in the fingers frequently.	Observe the color of the fingernail beds; they should be pink. Feel the fingers; they should be the same temperature as the fingers on the good hand. If the fingers are cold and pale, report immediately to the charge nurse.
Carry out Universal Steps X, Y, and Z. See Appendix.	Charting example: 1510. Sling applied to right arm. Fingers warm and nailbeds pink. No complaints of pain. J. Jones, SN

ITEM 10. APPLICATION OF A T–BINDER OR DOUBLE T–BINDER

These binders are primarily used to keep peri-pads or rectal and perineal dressings in place. The double T-binder is used for the male patient.

Supplies Needed

Pins
T-binder or sanitary belt

Peri-pad or dressing

Important Steps	Key Points
Carry out Universal Steps A, B, C, and D. See Appendix.	
1. Put on the binder or sanitary belt.	Place the band of the binder around the waist and secure with a pin. Smooth out the tail at the back of the binder.

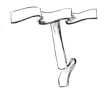
T-binder.

Double T-binder.

Important Steps	Key Points
2. Apply the peri-pad or dressing to the rectal or perineal area.	Avoid touching the side of the pad or dressing that will come in contact with the patient's skin.
3. Secure the pad in place.	Fasten by bringing the free end of the T forward between the legs and securing it snugly at the waist with a safety pin. The double-tailed binder is usually used for the male patient. Bring each tail or strip forward, one on each side of the genital organs, and secure to the waistband with pins.
Carry out Universal Steps X, Y, and Z. See Appendix.	Charting example: 0945. Peri-pad changed. Large amount of foul-smelling sanguineous drainage present. J. Jones, SN

U
N
I
T
35

PERFORMANCE TEST

In the skills laboratory with a partner, you will correctly apply two of the following types of binders or bandages.

1. Scultetus binder.

2. Recurrent bandage.

3. Triangular bandage.

4. Figure-8 bandage.

5. Spiral reverse bandage.

PERFORMANCE CHECKLIST

APPLY THE SCULTETUS BINDER

1. Carry out Universal Steps A, B, C, and D. (See Appendix.)

2. Place the binder under the patient's hips with the unlapped tail at the lower edge.

3. Bring the bottom tail across the abdomen.

4. Alternate tails from one side to the other and pull snugly.

5. Secure the final tail at the waist with pin.

6. Carry out Universal Steps X, Y, and Z.

APPLY A RECURRENT BANDAGE

1. Carry out Universal Steps A, B, C, and D.

2. Unroll bandage and bring over the tip of the stump from front to back.

3. Make a fold at the back and bring over the stump to the front.

4. Make a fold at the front and hold both folds in place.

5. Continue back and forth folds until the entire surface is covered.

6. Make several circular turns to hold the folded laps in place.

7. Secure the ends of the bandage.

8. Carry out Universal Steps X, Y, and Z.

APPLY A TRIANGULAR BANDAGE SLING

1. Carry out Universal Steps A, B, C, and D.

2. Put one end of the triangular bandage on the uninjured shoulder.

3. Place the bandage next to the body with the apex of the triangle toward the elbow on the injured side.

4. Bring the other end over the injured arm and shoulder.

5. Tie both ends at the side of the neck in a square knot.

6. Fold the apex point neatly over the elbow.

7. Check the circulation in the fingers.

8. Carry out Universal Steps X, Y, and Z.

APPLY A FIGURE-8 BANDAGE

1. Carry out Universal Steps A, B, C, and D.

2. Make two turns around the foot to anchor the bandage.

3. Make a circular turn over the foot and around the ankle.

4. Make a spiral turn around the ankle and down over the foot.

5. Alternate upward and downward spiral turns around the joint.

6. Secure the ends of the bandage.

7. Carry out Universal Steps X, Y, and Z.

APPLY A SPIRAL REVERSE BANDAGE

1. Carry out Universal Steps A, B, C, and D.

2. Make two circular turns to anchor the bandage.

3. Make a spiral reverse turn.
    a. Hold thumb on upper edge of an anterior turn.
    b. Turn the bandage down over the thumb and toward the lower edge of the previous turn.
    c. Cover 1/2 to 1/3 of previous lap and continue the turn around the leg.

4. Continue making spiral reverse turns.

5. Secure the end of the bandage.

6. Carry out Universal Steps X, Y, and Z.

POST-TEST

Multiple Choice: Select the one best answer for each of the questions.

1. When you apply a bandage, it is important that the tension of the turns should be

    a. increased at the end of the bandaged part.

    b. sufficient to reduce the venous blood flow.

    c. greater at the beginning of the turn.

    d. evenly distributed over the bandaged area.

2. Bandages are applied over clean, dry skin because

    a. this reduces the odor of the drainage.

    b. dark, moist, warm places promote the growth of bacteria.

    c. washing removes any drainage from the wound.

    d. it is a cooling measure to reduce an elevated temperature.

3. Before applying a bandage to a swollen injured ankle, which one of the following should you carry out?

    a. Carefully do range-of-motion exercise of the part.

    b. Check the circulation in the foot frequently.

    c. Elevate the foot for 15 minutes to reduce some swelling.

    d. Wash the part with antiseptic solution to reduce bacteria.

4. After applying a bandage to an injured extremity, which of the following actions would you carry out?

    a. Check the circulation frequently.

    b. Encourage exercise and motion of the part.

    c. Elevate the extremity to reduce swelling.

    d. Both a and c.

    e. a, b, and c.

5. A tight bandage can cause impaired circulation in an extremity and result in any of the following signs except which one?

    a. Complains of pain in side.

    b. Fingers are cold to touch.

    c. Foot is pale and bluish in color.

    d. Patient is unable to move fingers.

6. The main purpose of the scultetus binder is to

    a. absorb drainage from a wound.

    b. provide firm support of the abdomen.

    c. keep dressings firmly in place.

    d. reduce abdominal swelling.

POST-TEST ANSWERS

1. d
2. b
3. c

4. d
5. a
6. b

Unit 36

MEDICAL ISOLATION TECHNIQUES

GENERAL PERFORMANCE OBJECTIVE

Upon completion of this lesson, you will correctly employ isolation techniques to protect yourself and others when caring for a patient in an isolation unit. You will be able to set up barriers to contain organisms of patients with an infection, and to protect the patient in reverse isolation from possible infection. You will know the principles and practices of terminally disinfecting a unit occupied by a patient who has a communicable disease.

SPECIFIC PERFORMANCE OBJECTIVES

When you have finished this unit you will be able to

1. Describe the difference between medical asepsis used in medical isolation precautions and the surgical asepsis used in reverse isolation and in care of the surgical patient.

2. Prepare a unit for isolation of a patient who has a communicable disease or who needs protection from infection.

3. Use the proper technique to put on and remove a gown worn in an isolation unit.

4. Put on a mask and tell your instructor how to change it in order to retain safe isolation technique practice.

5. Put on and remove gloves using proper technique.

6. Use the double-bagging method to dispose of contaminated dishes, linen, and waste.

7. Collect specimens and transfer them to designated places using proper protection.

8. State methods used to disinfect or kill microorganisms.

VOCABULARY

aerobic—requiring the presence of oxygen to live.
anaerobic—does not need or cannot tolerate oxygen to live.
autoclave—a vessel used to render things sterile by steam under pressure.
bactericidal—a solution that destroys bacteria.
bacteriostatic—arresting (stop or inhibit) bacterial growth.
carrier—one who carries disease germs (usually not currently ill from the disease), such as "Typhoid Mary," a carrier of the typhoid germ who infected others who came in contact with food she handled.
communicable—an illness that may be transferred directly or indirectly from one person to another.
denude—remove a protective layer, as in a third-degree burn.
direct contact—communication of a healthy person with a contagious person (one who has a communicable disease) through *touching* an infected part.

germicide—a solution that kills germs but not resistant spores.

immunity—the state of being resistant to disease; immunity may be brought about by medical practice, such as vaccinations or immunizations.

indirect contact—spread of a contagious disease through some medium other than directly touching the person, such as sputum, dressings, clothing.

isolation—the act of separating, setting apart from others; a method utilized for controlling the spread of communicable or infectious disease.

reverse isolation—a type of isolation technique with barriers to prevent organisms from others from coming in contact with the patient or a part of the body; used when body defenses are impaired or inadequate.

vector—a carrier of microorganisms, such as insects.

venereal disease—a disease usually acquired as a result of sexual intercourse with an individual who is infected with gonorrhea, syphilis, chancroid, Vincent's infection of the genitals, or venereal lymphogranuloma.

viruses—minute (very small) microorganisms, some of which can be filtered and studied; others are nonfilterable; many different kinds and strains exist.

INTRODUCTION

The prevention of the spread of infections and communicable diseases in hospitals and other health agencies presents one of the most common problems health workers must face. The National Communicable Disease Center in Atlanta, Georgia, states the *"handwashing before and after contact with each patient is the single most important means of preventing the spread of infection."*

There are certain additional precautions that must be taken in the case of certain communicable diseases, however. Federal, state, and local public health agencies set forth specific regulations defining which diseases must be reported and isolated, and to what extent, where, and how long. All health agencies are legally required to carry out these regulations.

In this unit, you will learn more about the spread of microorganisms and some of the methods used to control or kill them. Various types of isolation are described, along with some of the diseases that require these precautions. Also included are procedures for donning and removing masks, gown, and gloves; taking vital signs for patients in isolation; and removing contaminated articles from the isolation unit for disposal.

NURSING CARE FOR PATIENTS IN ISOLATION

ITEM 1. SPREAD OF INFECTIOUS DISEASES

The prevention of the spread of infections can be accomplished by controlling one or more of the following elements: the source of the infecting organism, the route of transmission of the organism, and a susceptible host. Susceptibility to the disease is also based on the strength and size of the infecting dose, the organism's ability to survive in the environment in which it finds itself (light versus darkness; with oxygen versus without oxygen) and its ability to resist various disinfection methods.

Microorganisms are transmitted by four general routes:

1. Contact:

   a. *Direct*—actual touching of an infected animal or a person with a communicable disease by a susceptible person. Kissing and sexual intercourse are two means of direct transmission between human beings.

   b. *Indirect*—contact with objects that have been contaminated by an infected person; for example, if you touch the dressings of an infected patient, and neglect to wash your hands, you may transfer microorganisms to yourself by touching your mouth or nose, or by handling food.

c. *Droplet spread*—a spray of mist ejected from the nose or mouth when coughing, sneezing, or talking. These droplets usually travel no more than 3 feet. Most hospital regulations require a distance of at least 6 feet between the beds, as well as the use of proper screening methods.

2. Vehicle: Contaminated food, water, drugs, or blood.

3. Air: Evaporated droplets of an infectious agent. A disease agent that lodges in dust can remain infectious in the air and may be inhaled or digested by a susceptible host.

4. Vector: Organisms that carry disease from one host to another, such as insects or ticks. The mosquito, for example, is a vector for malaria.

Reservoirs (containers) of infection include man, animals, plants, soil, and objects used in daily living. Man is the most common harborer of infection or disease.

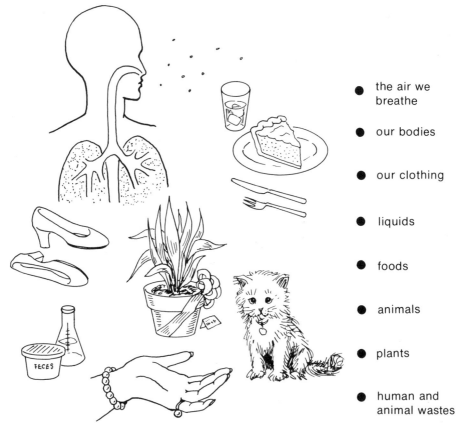

- the air we breathe
- our bodies
- our clothing
- liquids
- foods
- animals
- plants
- human and animal wastes

Disease-causing microorganisms may be found in these places.

ITEM 2. BODY DEFENSES AGAINST INFECTIONS

Human beings are fortunate in having a number of natural body defenses. The unbroken skin serves to protect the body from microorganisms, although microorganisms do enter the body through the respiratory tract and through the oral and genitourinary openings. These sites are also protected, however, by mucus and other secretions and cilia (threadlike projections), which act as barriers to bacteria, as well as by the acid contents of the urine and digestive juices, which kill bacteria.

The skin is called the first line of body defense, and secretions form the second line of defense. If microorganisms break through these two barriers and reach the blood stream, antibodies are formed that fight harmful bacteria.

Fever is another defense. Moderate fever, from $102°$ to $104°F$ ($38.89°$ to $40°C$), is a desirable response to infection, since few bacteria can survive this temperature; however, temperatures higher than this may be destructive to the body tissues.

White blood corpuscles, or phagocytes, are wandering cells in the blood that ingest and destroy bacteria. When the body is injured, they increase in number and surround and engulf invading bacteria. Other phagocytes are fixed in the body, in the liver, spleen, bone marrow, and lymph nodes, which are strategic spots of body function. Destruction of bacteria is also carried out here.

Immunity to Disease

The ability to resist contracting a disease is called immunity. There are two general classifications of immunity—natural and acquired. Natural immunity is the resistance with which one is born. It is inherited and considered permanent. Human beings are subject to many diseases that animals have, but are immune to certain other diseases of animals.

Acquired immunity is developed during life. This is classified further as active aquired immunity and passive acquired immunity. To develop active acquired immunity, the person must have

1. contracted the disease and recovered from it. Example: One who has had measles does not ordinarily have them a second time.

2. had a mild (sometimes unnoticed) infection of the disease.

3. been given a suitable vaccine or antigen (a substance that stimulates antibodies within the person's body). Example: One who is vaccinated with smallpox vaccine will not have the disease.

The process of increasing an individual's resistance to a particular infection by artificial means is called *immunization*.

Passive acquired immunity is made possible by injecting into one person the antibodies from the blood of other persons or animals. This type of immunity is immediate in effect but is of short duration, because the body of the person receiving the antibodies is not stimulated to produce its own antibodies.

Injections of gamma globulin are another method of providing a defense. This substance consists of a fraction of human blood plasma that contains antibodies against certain diseases. Gamma globulin is often used to modify the effects of hepatitis or measles, although we now have a specific vaccine against measles.

Resistance to Disease

The extent of damage from an infection is the result of two factors: the individual's resistance to injury and the microorganism's power to injure.

The person's resistance is influenced by age, state of nutrition, presence of disease (especially of metabolic origin), hormones such as glucocorticoids, adequacy of the blood supply, location of the infection, and natural or acquired antibodies.

The microorganism's power to inflict damage upon the individual is dependent on its ability to produce certain toxins. Toxins may destroy tissues, damage blood vessels and cause hemorrhage, block lymphatic drainage in the body by clot formation, or dissolve blood clots, allowing the infection to spread. In addition, some bacteria are ingested by phagocytes in the body, as mentioned earlier.

To sum up the body's defenses against infection, we are protected by:

1. Healthy unbroken skin and mucous membranes. It is up to you to keep the first line of defense strong.

UNIT 36

2. Removal of bacteria by secretions of mucous membranes and by cilia (hair-like projections) in the nose and bronchial tree. The bacteria are removed by coughing and sneezing.

3. Destruction of bacteria by the gastric juices and the acidic reactions of urine and vaginal discharges.

4. Filtering action of lymph nodes to remove bacteria from the body system.

5. Increased number of white blood cells upon invasion of bacteria.

6. Antibody formation, which keeps microorganisms from multiplying.

7. Inflammatory reaction of the body to an invasion of microorganisms. Inflammation represents warfare between the offending organism and the white cells, as well as the body reaction to the invasion.

ITEM 3. WAYS TO KILL OR CONTROL MICROORGANISMS

Communicable diseases can be controlled by one or more of the following methods:

1. Disinfection: An attempt is made to kill pathogenic microorganisms through either chemical or physical means applied directly. Agents used to destroy microorganisms include:

   a. Steam under pressure (best method), as by autoclave.

   b. Boiling at 212°F or 100°C for 20 minutes, which kills most bacteria.

   c. Dry heat, as in an oven at 320°F or 160°C for one hour.

   d. Open flame or fire.

   e. Direct sunlight for 6 to 8 hours.

   f. Drying, which prevents growth and kills some bacteria because moisture is needed to sustain life.

   g. Cold temperature, which retards growth but is not a reliable method of destroying bacteria.

   h. Chemicals used to inhibit or destroy bacteria (antiseptics, bacteriostatics, germicides, antibiotics, and ethylene oxide gas sterilization).

Concurrent disinfection—the continuous process of disinfection throughout the hospitalization period.

Terminal disinfection—the destruction of infectious material when the disease is over (after recovery, discharge, or death).

2. Isolation. The patient who has the communicable disease is separated from others, either in a private room or in a cubicle in a ward area. Everything inside the isolation unit, except the designated clean areas, is considered contaminated.

3. Handwashing with soap and water.

ITEM 4. COMPARISON OF MEDICAL AND SURGICAL ASEPSIS

In order to control the spread of disease-causing organisms in the hospital, nurses use either medical asepsis or surgical asepsis, or both. Medical and surgical asepsis are different, and different principles are followed for each.

Medical asepsis involves setting up a barrier around the infected person and containing the microorganisms within that boundary in order to prevent the spread of infection to others. The types of isolation precautions described in this unit are primarily for carrying out medical aseptic practices.

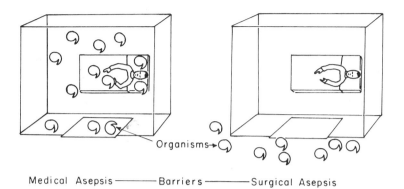

Medical Asepsis————Barriers————Surgical Asepsis

Surgical asepsis sets the barrier around the person who is to be protected from microorganisms carried by other people and present in the normal environment. Principles of surgical asepsis are followed in the operating room, in reverse isolation, in the change of dressings on wounds, and in any procedure that penetrates the skin or cavity of the body. The major differences between medical and surgical asepsis are shown in the following table.

Factor	Medical Asepsis	Surgical Asepsis
Patient	Has infection, lowered resistance to other infections.	Potential host. Lowered resistance makes more susceptible.
Reservoir of infection	The patient.	Other people and the environment.
Objective of barriers	Confine organisms to the room, unit, or locale.	Prevent organism from reaching patient or area.
Equipment and supplies	Disinfect, sterilize, or dispose of *after* contact with patient. Use clean materials.	Disinfect or sterilize *before* contact with patient. Use sterile or clean materials.
Nurse's protective garb: gown, mask, gloves	Clean garb to protect worker from organisms. Discard after contact with patient.	Clean or sterile garb to protect patient. Remedy if contaminated.
Goal of nursing action	*Confine organisms* and prevent spread of infection to others.	*Reduce number of organisms* and prevent spread of infection to patient.

ITEM 5. TYPES OF MEDICAL PRECAUTIONS

There are two main classifications of isolation techniques according to physical set-up. In the *unit type*, a single patient is confined to a location, which may be a room, a cubicle, or a screened area with 6 feet between beds. The *disease type* includes more than one patient in the unit, all with a similar disease; the entire unit is set apart. A tuberculosis unit is an example of the disease type.

When it is known that organisms are discharged from the body through certain routes and not through others, then it is possible to use strict precautions for those exits used.

UNIT
36

Based on this principle, it is possible to employ respiratory precautions, enteric precautions, and wound and skin precautions, as well as strict medical isolation and reverse or protective isolation instituted to guard the patient from infectious organisms.

Respiratory Precautions

Requirements

1. Private room—door must be closed.

2. Gowns—worn by all who have direct patient contact.

3. Masks—must be worn by all persons entering the room.

4. Hands—must be washed on entering and leaving the room.

5. Gloves—not necessary.

6. Articles of use—must be disinfected.

Conditions

1. Chickenpox.

2. Herpes zoster.

3. Measles (rubeola).

4. Meningococcal meningitis.

5. Mumps.

6. Whooping cough (pertussis).

7. German measles (rubella).

8. Tuberculosis.

9. Venezuelan equine encephalomyelitis.

Enteric Precautions

Requirements

1. Private room—needed for children.

2. Gown—worn by all persons having direct contact with the patient.

3. Masks—not needed.

4. Hands—must be washed on entering and leaving the room.

5. Gloves—worn by all having direct patient contact.

6. Articles of use—special precautions necessary for articles contaminated with urine and feces.

Conditions

1. Cholera.

2. Enteropathogenic *Escherichia coli* infection (gastritis from *E. coli*).

3. Hepatitis (infectious or serum).

4. Salmonellosis (typhoid fever).

5. Shigellosis.

Wound and Skin Precautions

Requirements

1. Private room

2. Gowns—must be worn by all who have direct contact with patient.

3. Masks—not needed except during dressing change.

4. Hands—washed on entering and leaving the room.

5. Gloves—worn by all having direct patient contact.

6. Articles of use—special precautions for instruments, dressings, and linen. Special dressing techniques must be used in changing dressings.

Conditions

1. Burns—not infected with *Staphylococcus aureus.*

2. Gas gangrene.

3. Impetigo.

4. Staphylococcal skin and wound infections.

5. Wound infections that are extensive.

Strict Isolation

Requirements	*Conditions*

Requirements

1. Private room—with door closed.

2. Gowns—worn by all persons entering the room.

3. Masks—must be worn by all persons entering the room.

4. Hands—must be washed on entering and leaving the room.

5. Gloves—must be worn by all persons entering the room.

6. Articles of use—must be discarded, or wrapped before being sent to Central Supply for disinfection or sterilization.

Conditions

1. Anthrax inhalation.

2. Burns infected with *Staphylococcus aureus* or Group A *Streptococcus.*

3. Diphtheria.

4. Eczema vaccinatum.

5. Herpes simplex (neonatal vesicular).

6. Rabies.

7. German measles.

8. Smallpox.

9. Staphylococcal enterocolitis or pneumonia.

10. Streptococcal pneumonia.

Reverse, or Protective, Isolation

The requirements for reverse isolation for some patients may involve the use of sterile gowns and gloves, as well as sterile linens and other supplies needed to care for the patient. Other equipment and materials needed must be cleaned or disinfected before being taken into the room. No special care is needed when removing articles from the room.

Requirements

1. Private room—door must be closed.

2. Gowns—must be worn by all who enter the room.

3. Masks—must be worn by all who enter the room.

4. Hands—washed on entering and leaving the room.

5. Gloves—worn by all having direct patient contact.

6. Articles of use—suitable to the condition of isolation.

Conditions

1. Agranulocytosis.

2. Severe, noninfected vesicular or eczematous dermatitis.

3. Immunosuppressive therapy.

4. Lymphomas and leukemia.

5. Burns.

6. Leukopenia from cancer chemotherapy.

UNIT
36

ITEM 6.   GENERAL PRINCIPLES REGARDING ISOLATION

1. Floors are contaminated. Anything dropped on the floor is contaminated and must be discarded or cleaned carefully before reuse.

2. Patients with communicable diseases should be grouped according to the epidemiology of transmission:

   a. Contact through respiratory spread.

   b. Transmission via gastrointestinal tract.

   c. Direct contact with wound or skin infection.

3. Keep dust down. Sweeping compounds or wet-mops with disinfectants must be used for this purpose.

4. Protect the patient from drafts.

5. Establish contaminated and clean zones. The clean areas should include those used by the health worker. Items such as telephones outside the unit should not be used by the patient. There should be a "clean" area in the isolation unit where no contaminated articles are permitted. Items not in the clean area are considered contaminated.

6. Anything that is brought into the isolation area must not be removed except in proper containers, which are then placed in an outside clean container and labeled "isolation."

7. Never rub your eyes or nose, or put your hands near your mouth when you are taking care of a patient in an isolation unit.

8. Never shake linen when you are removing it or placing it on the bed.

9. Wash your hands often. Refer to the Unit 8, Handwashing.

10. Use clean squares of paper or tissue to touch contaminated articles.

11. Paper towels or clean squares of paper provide a clean area on which to place articles within a unit.

12. Keep a water pitcher and a glass in the room. Ice and fresh water are brought to the door and transferred. Use the same technique for food.

13. Faucets should be turned off and on using a paper towel to protect your hands.

14. The same nursing procedures are carried out for these patients as for any patient. However, you have also learned some additional safety precautions (masking, gloving, gowning, and disposal techniques).

15. Inform the charge nurse of skin lesions, sore throat, or other evidence you may have of your own lowered resistance to infection or disease. (You may be reassigned to protect you and the patient.)

ITEM 7. PSYCHOLOGICAL EFFECTS OF ISOLATION

Can you imagine how it would feel to be a patient placed on isolation precautions? Not only do patients feel ill from their disease, but the isolation tends to set them apart and make them feel different. Many patients complain that they are lonely and neglected and that doctors and nurses don't come into the room unless it is absolutely necessary. They feel as if they are contaminated, dirty, and not acceptable. They often feel powerless and not able to control what is happening to them. Being dependent on the nurses and others for care makes some people feel ashamed and depressed. Sensory deprivation is a serious problem for patients in isolation, particularly older patients, who may have impaired vision or not hear well.

It is important that nurses help patients to cope with their feelings about isolation precautions. When providing daily care to patients, take time to listen to their complaints and feelings. If the precautions are causing a problem such as loneliness, frustration because of the feeling of neglect by others, or sensory deprivation, try to plan measures with your nurse or team leader to help solve the problem.

ITEM 8. SETTING UP AN ISOLATION UNIT

Use a cubicle or private room with running water. A sign marked "ISOLATION," or a similar designation used in your agency, should be placed on the outside door or at the entrance to the cubicle. If a cubicle or private room is not available, a selected area of the room can be established as an isolation zone. Screen this area; identify it by hanging an

"ISOLATION" sign on the outside of the screens. Acquaint other workers with the limits of the isolation area. Collect the following items and place them in the patient's unit:

1. The usual patient articles:

    a. Bath basin, soap, and soap dish

    b. Bedpan, urinal, and toilet paper

    c. Water pitcher and plastic drinking cups

    d. Emesis basin, toothbrush and toothpaste

    e. Shaving equipment for males

2. Towels, gown, and linens

3. Paper or plastic bags for collection of articles and refuse

4. Thermometer and holder.

5. Isolation supply unit or special cabinet to hold supplies of masks, gloves, gowns, plastic bags, and so forth

6. Stethoscope and sphygmomanometer

7. Container for contaminated needles and syringes

8. Paper towels and handwashing sink

9. Other equipment as needed for treatment

After you have assembled the supplies and equipment, proceed with the following series of steps.

ITEM 9. PUTTING ON A FACE MASK

When you are to use a mask as part of the isolation garb, follow these principles:

1. Put on the mask before donning gown or gloves or performing a surgical scrub.

2. Use the mask one time and then discard it. Avoid removing the mask from the nose and mouth, and letting it dangle around the neck, as it is grossly contaminated by organisms from the upper respiratory tract.

3. Change the mask when it becomes damp. Masks become moist when you breathe through them, providing a favorable environment for the growth of microorganisms trapped in the material. High-efficiency masks can usually be worn longer than ordinary masks.

U
N
I
T
36

Supplies Needed

Mask

Important Steps	Key Points
1. Take a mask from its container.	Masks may be made of cloth or one of a variety of high-efficiency disposable materials. Handle the mask as little as possible because it will be coming in contact with your face, and you will be breathing through it.

Important Steps	Key Points
2. Put on the mask.	Put it over your *nose* and *mouth*. Tie the mask with the top strings at the back of your head; be sure the strings pass over your ears. Securely tie the lower strings of the mask at the back of your head at the neckline. If you wear glasses, the mask should fit snugly over your nose and under the bottom edge of your glasses. This will prevent your glasses from becoming steamed.

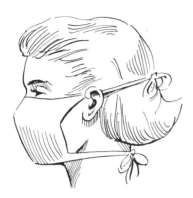

Face mask in place.

Important Steps	Key Points
3. Change your mask as necessary.	Unless it is a high-efficiency mask, your mask will become moist in about 20 minutes as you breathe through it. Change your mask whenever it becomes moist. Germs can grow in a wet environment.

ITEM 10.   USING AN ISOLATION GOWN

Isolation gowns may be made of cloth or of paper, but they should be full length in order to protect the nurse's clothing. The recommended procedure is to use a clean gown each time you enter the room and have direct contact with the patient, then discard the gown upon leaving the room.

The major principle involved in using the gown in medical isolation is that the outer surfaces of the gown are contaminated, especially those areas that come in contact with the patient, the bed, linens, and other articles used or touched by the patient, as well as by organisms carried on air currents within the room.

───

Supplies Needed

Gown (cloth or paper)

───

Important Steps	Key Points
1. Remove your wristwatch and any rings, except a plain wedding band.	Jewelry may harbor microorganisms that could be carried to others outside the isolation unit. If your watch is needed for the TPR, remove it and place it in a small plastic bag or on a clean paper towel at the patient's bedside. (Take the paper towel from the dispenser in the patient's room.)
2. Wash your hands.	Refer to the unit on handwashing. Use a liquid antimicrobial soap.

Important Steps	Key Points
3. Select a clean gown and unfold it.	Hold the gown at the neck opening and let it unfold downward (gowns are usually folded in thirds for neat storage). The open part at the back should face you.
4. Put your arms through the gown sleeves.	Touch only the *inside* of the gown. Holding the inside of the gown, slip one arm at a time into the appropriate sleeve. Pull the gown on as far as possible. Grab the opposite sleeve with your gown-covered hand (see the adjacent diagram); gently pull the sleeve up on your arm and shoulder. When this procedure is completed, go on with the other sleeve in the same manner, always working from the inside of the gown.

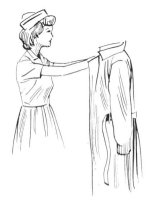

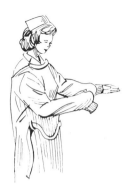

5. Adjust the gown on your shoulders.	Place your fingers *inside* the neckband (at the back) and adjust the gown so that it fits comfortably on your shoulders. Remember to work with the *inside* of the gown: keep your hands clean.
6. Tie the neck tapes (ties).	Handle the ties carefully. Keep your hands clean. Do not touch your hair.
7. Tie the waist belt.	The open part of your gown is at your back. Bring the one side of the gown over the other side of the gown. Adjust the gown so that it fits snugly. Grasp the waist belt at the far (distal) ends, draw them together at your back, and tie them snugly.

U
N
I
T
36

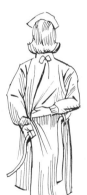

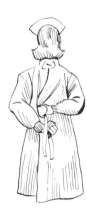

Removing an Isolation Gown

Important Steps	Key Points
1. Untie the waist belt.	The outer surfaces of the gown below the neckline are considered contaminated, so these ties are loosened before you wash your hands.
2. Wash your hands.	
3. Untie the neck ties.	Take care not to contaminate your hands by touching your hair or the *outside* of the gown. Remember, it is contaminated. If you do, you must *rewash* your hands.
4. Remove the first sleeve of the gown.	Place your forefinger *under the cuff* of the sleeve and pull the sleeve down over your hand without touching the outside of the gown.
5. Remove the other sleeve.	With your hand inside the first sleeve, working with your gown-covered hand, draw the second sleeve down over your hand.
6. Slip out of the gown.	Discard it carefully in the soiled linen hamper in the patient's room.
7. Wash your hands.	Wash them according to procedure; dry them thoroughly. Turn off the faucets with a towel and discard the towel in the designated place. *Avoid touching* anything in the room as you leave.

ITEM 11. PUTTING ON GLOVES

When following medical aseptic principles and caring for patients on isolation precautions, it is not necessary to use sterile gloves. Nonsterile, disposable gloves are used for enteric precautions, for skin and wound precautions, and in strict isolation cases. There is no special procedure for putting on nonsterile gloves. Remove the gloves by grasping the cuff and pulling the contaminated outer side in on itself. Discard. Untie the contaminated waist ties of the gown, if used, then wash your hands before untying the neck ties and removing the gown.

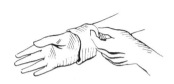

Sterile gloves must be used for all procedures based on surgical aseptic principles. The nurse puts on sterile gloves before performing procedures such as catheterization or change of sterile dressings, the same as is done for any patient not on isolation. Sterile gloves and gown are sometimes required in reverse isolation. Special procedures must be followed to ensure that the outer surfaces remain sterile and are not contaminated. These are described in Volume 3. As a rule, sterile procedures and reverse isolation are assigned to experienced licensed nurses.

ITEM 12. SERVING DIET TRAYS

Many hospitals now prepare a disposable tray with disposable food containers and eating utensils that can be taken to the patient in isolation. After the patient has eaten, the entire tray is disposed of in a bag for the collection of garbage; this bag is then double-bagged at the end of the shift and removed from the room.

In those agencies where disposables are not used, avoid taking the tray into the room each time a meal is served. This practice leads to the accumulation of trays, dishes, and silverware that later must be double-bagged for removal from the room and disinfected before being returned to the kitchens for reuse. The recommended procedure is to keep one tray in the room, use paper plates, and transfer the food from the tray delivered to the unit to the tray in the room. This can be done by two people—one person outside the room and one person gowned and in the room to receive the food if the patient needs assistance in eating—or by one person, who transfers the food to the tray placed near the door of the room.

|||||||||||||||||||||||||||||||||||||||||||||||||||||||||||||||||||||||||||||||||||||||||||||||||||||||||||||||||||||||||

Supplies Needed

Tray   Eating utensils (metal or plastic)
Dishes (paper or plastic)

|||||||||||||||||||||||||||||||||||||||||||||||||||||||||||||||||||||||||||||||||||||||||||||||||||||||||||||||||||||||||

Important Steps	Key Points
1. Take the tray to the isolation door.	Transfer the dishes sent on the cafeteria tray to the tray kept inside the patient's room. Take care not to touch the patient's tray with your hands—it is contaminated. You may do this unassisted or you may have help. Hold the cafeteria tray in your arm as you transfer dishes to the patient's tray.
2. Return the cafeteria tray.	Take it back to the diet cart or to the unit diet kitchen.
3. Serve the patient's tray.	Unless your agency regulations state otherwise, you do not need to put on a gown if you are careful to touch nothing in the patient's room with your uniform. Place the tray on the patient's overbed table. If you are helping the patient eat, however, you will need to gown.
4. After the meal, clear the tray.	If disposable dishes are used, empty liquid contents and soft foods in the patient's toilet. Flush the toilet. Solid foods such as gristle or bones should be disposed of in waterproof bags provided for that purpose. *Do not* throw them into the toilet. This stops up the sewer lines. *Disposable dishes* are then placed in the designated containers in the patient's room. If the dishes and utensils are *reusable*, the liquids and solids are disposed of in the above manner. The dishes are then placed in designated bags.

U
N
I
T
36

ITEM 13. TAKING TPR AND BP

‖‖‖

Supplies Needed

Thermometer and holder   Sphygmomanometer
Stethoscope   Watch with second hand

‖‖

Important Steps	Key Points
1. Wear a gown and mask, if required.	Leave the thermometer, stethoscope, and sphygmomanometer in the isolation room until the patient is discharged or removed from isolation.
2. Place watch in plastic bag or on a clean surface, if needed.	Many hospital rooms are equipped with clocks. If one is not available, however, protect your watch from becoming contaminated by placing it in a clear plastic bag or on a clean paper towel.
3. Follow regular procedure for taking the vital signs.	
4. Wash your hands.	
5. Record the vital signs.	Note your observations promptly on clean paper in the clean area of the unit. Transfer the notes to the patient's chart at the earliest opportunity.

ITEM 14. REMOVAL OF LINENS

Important Steps	Key Points
1. Place the linens in a hamper or plastic bag.	Plastic bags or a laundry hamper with a heavy cloth bag will usually be provided in the patient's room for collection of soiled linens.
2. Remove the linens from the isolation room.	Use the double-bagging technique to remove from the room. The filled laundry bag in the patient's room is placed in a prelabeled clean bag handled by the clean person *outside* the room. Send soiled linens to the laundry room.

ITEM 15. DOUBLE-BAGGING TECHNIQUE

The method of double-bagging is used to remove contaminated material and supplies from the isolation room. The soiled linens, dishes, utensils and trash are placed in plastic or paper collection bags inside the room. These are contaminated, since they have been exposed to infectious organisms in the room.

At the end of the shift, a gowned worker in the room transfers the contaminated bags into a clean bag held by a "clean" nurse outside the room. The clean bag is closed, labeled as contaminated, and handled according to hospital policies for resterilization, disinfecting, and disposal. Clean collection bags are put in the room for the next shift.

Supplies Needed

| Collection bags (plastic, paper, or cloth) | Labels ("Contaminated" or "Isolation") |

Important Steps	Key Points
1. Gather all bags of materials to be removed from the room.	Empty the wastebasket. Collect all used dressings, dishes, utensils, and so forth in the designated disposable bags (waxed brown paper or plastic).
2. Seal the bags securely.	Close with string, tape, or whatever fastener is used in your agency.
3. Clean bag with wide cuff is held open to receive contaminated bag.	The nurse outside the room puts her hands under the wide cuff of the clean bag to hold it open and to prevent being touched by the contaminated bag.

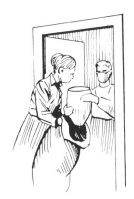

"Clean" nurse holds bag at door of contaminated unit.

4. Place contaminated bag in clean bag and fasten securely.	Secure the bag. The "clean person" then carefully secures the bag with tape, safety pin, or tie, and labels it "Isolation."
5. Dispose of the labeled bags.	Handle the bags according to the hospital policy. Some materials are sent in the double-bags to the Central Supply area to be autoclaved, others are sent to the laundry, and still others are sent to the incinerator.

ITEM 16. COLLECTION OF SPECIMENS

Important Steps	Key Points
1. Secure the appropriate container (urine, sputum, and so forth).	Obtain it from the storage room. Follow the procedures described in the units on bowel and urine elimination and sputum collection.
2. Label the container.	See your agency specifications regarding the name and other information needed on the label.

U
N
I
T
36

Important Steps	Key Points
3. Collect the specimen.	Obtain it in the usual manner. See the previous units on specimen collection.
4. Place the specimen in the container.	Transfer the specimen from the utensil (e.g., bedpan or urinal) to the specimen container.
5. Place the specimen container in a clean, waterproof bag.	The bag should be held by someone "clean" on the outside of the room. Take care not to touch the exterior of the bag. If you touch the bag, you will contaminate it and will need to discard the bag and start over. The "clean person" on the outside of the room will carefully close and secure the opening with masking tape and attach the requisition to the bag.
6. Take it to the designated department.	*Transport* it promptly to the designated department.
7. Record the procedure on the nurses' notes.	Enter the time the specimen was collected, the kind of specimen, and so forth.

ITEM 17. ASSISTING A PATIENT TO SIGN A DOCUMENT

Important Steps	Key Points
1. Place a clean paper towel on the overbed table.	
2. Place the document on the paper towel.	
3. Place another paper towel with its edge close to the line provided for the patient's signature.	The patient's hand will be resting on the paper towel.

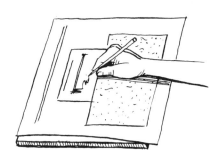

Place paper towel for hand to rest on.

4. When the signature is completed, remove the document from the room.	
5. Wash the pen with soap and water or a specified germicidal solution if it is to be removed from the room; otherwise, place it in the patient's bedside stand.	
6. Wash your hands.	Wash them before leaving the patient's room.
7. Record the action on the nurses' notes.	Designate the time and type of document that was signed.

ITEM 18. TRANSPORTING A PATIENT OUT OF THE UNIT

Occasionally, it is necessary to transport the patient in isolation to another department for special examinations, therapy, or other procedures. In such cases, care is taken to reduce the spread of contamination by wrapping the patient in a clean sheet or bath blanket and instructing the patient not to touch the outer surface.

Supplies Needed

Clean sheet or bath blanket   Stretcher or wheel chair
Mask

Important Steps	Key Points
1. Notify the unit to which the patient is being sent.	
2. Place a clean sheet over the wheelchair or stretcher.	If the patient goes in a wheelchair, place a clean sheet over the chair and wrap it around the seated patient for warmth and privacy. If a stretcher is used, place a clean sheet or cotton blanket on the stretcher, then place the patient on it.
3. Put a blanket on or around the patient.	This provides warmth and privacy.
4. Put a mask on the patient.	*Masks* are *always* worn by patients with respiratory diseases or those who are on strict isolation precautions when being transported in the hallways. (Check your agency procedure.)
5. Transport the patient to the designated area.	Remember to use proper body alignment, balance, and movement for both you and your patient.
6. Return the patient to the room.	Strip the linen from the stretcher or wheelchair. Dispose of it in the patient's linen hamper.
7. Return the used wheelchair or stretcher for cleansing.	

U
N
I
T
36

ITEM 19. TERMINAL DISINFECTION

This procedure is done to clean the room as well as the supplies and utensils when a patient is discharged, expires, or is removed from isolation. Because the room has been exposed to more germs than are usual in a hospital room, *special precautions* must be taken during the final cleaning process before admitting a new patient.

When patients are taken off isolation precautions, many hospitals transfer them to another, "clean," room or unit. The isolation room is stripped of linen and equipment, and contaminated materials are removed. The room is then "fogged" with a disinfectant chemical and allowed to air out. It can then be cleaned in the usual manner by the housekeeping department and prepared for the next patient.

If you are assigned to strip the room and to disinfect the items that were used, you will need assistance. Your coworker should remain "clean" outside the room, ready to receive your supplies and equipment in the appropriate receptacles as you follow these guidelines.

Supplies Needed

Gown, mask, and gloves as required
Labels ("Contaminated" or "Isolation")
Basin with disinfectant and rag or cloth

Collection bags (plastic, paper, or cloth)
Linen pack

Important Steps	Key Points
1. Put on a gown, mask, and gloves if required.	Usually at least a gown is required to protect your clothing while you are working in the contaminated room.
2. Collect all materials, separate them, and place them in bags for removal.	Place all equipment and articles in separate bags according to the method of disposal; examples of the way in which items might be grouped follow: 1. Soiled and clean linens 2. Glasses, dishes, and metal utensils. 3. Opened solutions, packets of dressings, disposable instruments 4. Papers, disposable paper and plastic goods, refuse, and so forth. Remember that great care must be taken in the disposal of needles and syringes. Follow your agency procedure.
3. Prepare a basin with germicidal solution.	
4. Gather instruments and equipment to be disinfected by washing.	*Delicate instruments* such as sphygmomanometers, otoscopes, scissors, thermometers, and *plastic articles* must be wiped off with a cold germicidal solution. They would be melted or destroyed by the high temperature used for autoclave sterilization.
5. Wipe the instruments with germicidal solution.	Articles that cannot be autoclaved should be scrubbed thoroughly with disinfectant solution, taken out of the room, and sent back to the central processing room for further decontamination and storage.
6. Double-bag all bags of materials and remove from the room.	Seal the tops carefully by folding them down several times. Place them in a clean bag held by your clean assistant outside the room. They are then sent to the proper destination for disposal.
7. Remove your isolation garb.	Remove your gown and place it in a clean bag held by the clean assistant, who will close and label the bag securely for transportation to the laundry room.
8. Wash your hands.	

Important Steps	Key Points
9. Notify the housekeeping department that terminal cleaning is required.	Be sure to notify them that it has been an isolation room. They also must take special precautions.
10. Make a closed bed and set up the unit ready for a new admission.	As soon as the housekeeping personnel have finished cleaning the unit, you can prepare the room for the next patient.

ITEM 20. REVERSE ISOLATION TECHNIQUE

Reverse isolation technique is synonymous with surgical asepsis, wherein all things are kept sterile or as clean as possible. In other words, reverse isolation involves the extra precaution that must be taken for patients who have low resistance to infection. We set up as near sterile (free from pathogenic organisms) an environment as possible. Benefiting from reverse isolation technique are patients with extensive burns in which the skin is denuded, patients with open lesions, and patients with low resistance to infection because of a low white blood count or poor kidney function.

Set up the unit in the same way as you would for regular isolation. In reverse isolation, the people entering the room always wear a mask and gown; gloves may also be needed, if direct care is to be given to the patient.

Terminal disinfection is not needed upon discharge in reverse isolation cases, because the room has not been contaminated with infectious organisms. The regular hospital facility terminal cleaning of a unit may be followed.

ITEM 21. KEEPING YOURSELF HEALTHY

It is important that nurses protect themselves against infections. This can be done by keeping your resistance high through good health habits and reducing contamination of your body by observing good aseptic technique. These guidelines will help you avoid infections.

1. Taking a shower daily and shampooing hair as needed (at least once a week).

2. Establishing regular sleeping patterns and sleeping at least 8 hours each night. (Sleep cannot be stored like money in the bank; sleep is required daily for good body resistance to infection and for high performance.)

3. Eating a sensible, well-balanced diet. Avoid crash diets. Use fresh fruits and vegetables for necessary minerals and vitamins. Eat protein foods.

4. Drinking plenty of fluids. Two-thirds of the body consists of water, and because fluid is lost daily by perspiration and elimination, it must be replaced. Drink six to eight glasses of water daily.

5. Developing good habits of elimination. (Do not deny the body urge to eliminate; this upsets the natural function of the body.)

6. Practicing regular habits of oral hygiene. Never neglect your teeth. See your dentist at least yearly.

7. Balancing hours of activity with recreation. Spend some time out of doors in fresh air. Give your body proper exercise.

8. Taking care of your hands. Apply lotion to keep them soft. Cut off hangnails that may tear and produce a gateway for infection. Protect breaks in the skin that may allow microorganisms to enter.

UNIT 36

9. Protecting your eyes when you are in an isolation unit. Do not touch the eyes with your fingers while caring for a patient. (Remember—the most common causes of eye infections are the fingers.) If irrigation fluid happens to get into the eye, rinse the eye immediately with normal saline.

10. Keeping your hands away from your mouth when caring for a patient who is in an isolation unit. Always wash your hands before handling food or eating.

11. Protecting your hair from contamination. Wear a cap when you are in a highly contagious situation.

12. Removing jewelry when you are caring for a patient in an isolation unit. Rings can harbor microorganisms that may not be removed with regular handwashing. Your watch may also harbor microorganisms and interfere with proper handwashing.

PERFORMANCE TEST

1. Discuss with your instructor the differences between isolation technique and reverse isolation technique, as well as the procedure for terminal cleaning following an isolation case.

2. In the skills laboratory with a student partner, correctly demonstrate the isolation technique used in caring for a patient having a staphylococcal wound infection. Demonstrate the procedure for gowning, masking, removing soiled items from the patient's room, double-bagging, and serving and removing a meal tray.

PERFORMANCE CHECKLIST

GOWNING

1. Remove your rings and wristwatch.

2. Wash your hands.

3. Select a clean gown and unfold it.

4. Put your arms into the sleeves, work the arms on, and adjust the shoulders.

5. Tie the neck tapes, close the gown at the back, and tie the waist belt.

REMOVING GOWN

1. Untie the waist belt, push up the sleeves, and wash your hands.

2. Untie the neck ties without contaminating your hands.

3. Remove the sleeves of the gown.

   a. Place your forefinger under one cuff of the sleeve.

   b. Pull the sleeve over your hand without touching the outside of the gown.

   c. For the other sleeve, work it off using the gown-covered second hand.

4. Slip out of the gown and dispose of it in a laundry hamper, taking care not to touch your uniform or shake the gown.

5. Wash your hands as you leave the unit, and turn off the faucet with a paper towel.

MASKING

1. Obtain a mask from the container.

2. Unfold the mask, and place it over your nose and mouth.

3. Tie the top strings at the back of your head.

4. Remove the mask by untying the lower strings, then the top strings, and discard it into the designated receptacle.

5. Change your mask when it becomes moist (or be able to explain when and why you change your mask).

U
N
I
T
36

REMOVAL OF MATERIALS BY DOUBLE-BAGGING

1. Empty waste materials into a designated bag (brown paper or plastic) in the patient's room.

2. Seal the bag securely, for example, with string or tape.

3. Place the sealed bag carefully inside a clean bag being held by the clean person outside the room. Take care to touch only the inside of the bag. (The clean person then closes, secures, and labels the double-bagged package for disposal.)

REMOVAL OF MEAL TRAY

1. Remove all dishes from the tray.

2. Dispose of any liquids down the toilet and flush the toilet.

3. Dispose of solid foods in a brown paper bag(s).

4. Place disposable dishes in the designated receptacle.

5. Place reusable dishes (after foods have been removed) in a brown bag and seal the bag.

6. Hand the sealed bag to the clean person for double-bagging.

7. Close and secure the bag, label it, and transport it for sterilization.

POST-TEST

True or False.   Circle the "T" if the statement is true or "F" if the statement is false.

T   F   1. All articles used for or by the patient in an isolation unit are considered contaminated.

T   F   2. It is necessary to wear a gown when giving a bedpan.

T   F   3. Unused articles and linens are not to be removed from an isolation unit and placed with other articles and linens for use by other patients.

T   F   4. Microorganisms inflict damage to the patient through their ability to produce certain toxins.

T   F   5. Linens removed from an isolation unit must be placed in an additional bag as well as the original bag in which they are placed.

T   F   6. A patient in an isolation unit should not be given a backrub with the bare hands.

T   F   7. The faucet in the isolation bathroom is considered clean and suitable to turn on and off without protection.

T   F   8. Isolation technique dictates that a mask is always worn.

T   F   9. Food trays may be served to the patient in isolation in regular fashion since all dishes are sterilized in the dishwasher.

T   F   10. TPR may be taken without a gown so long as the uniform does not touch anything.

Multiple Choice.   Select the one best answer for each of the following questions.

11. According to the National Communicable Disease Center, the single, most effective way to prevent the spread of disease is by

   a. using antibiotic drugs.

   b. autoclaving contaminated materials.

   c. using the reverse isolation technique.

   d. frequent handwashing.

12. Infectious diseases are spread by which of the following methods?

   a. Contact with someone with the disease.

   b. Breathing smoggy air.

   c. A hot, humid climate.

   d. Close contact with animals.

   e. All of these.

13. The skin and other natural defenses of the body protect it from invasion by microorganisms. Which of the following are natural defenses?

   a. Acidity of the urine and digestive juices.

   b. Moderate fever ($102°$ to $104°$F).

   c. Phagocytic action of white blood cells.

   d. b and c

   e. a, b, and c

U
N
I
T
36

14. A person's resistance to disease can be increased through the process of

    a. inflammation.

    b. allergy.

    c. immunization.

    d. phagocytosis.

15. Which of the following methods of killing bacteria is the least effective?

    a. Boiling materials.

    b. Refrigeration.

    c. Exposure to direct sunlight.

    d. Administration of antibiotics.

16. Medical asepsis is characterized by all of the following factors *except*

    a. disinfection of items taken into the room.

    b. double-bagging of articles removed from the room.

    c. confinement of organisms to a specific space.

    d. confinement of the infection to the patient.

17. The goal of nursing actions is the same for surgical asepsis and for reverse isolation, that is, to

    a. confine the organisms to the infected patient.

    b. protect the nurse from infection.

    c. protect other people from the bacteria.

    d. reduce the organisms in the vicinity of the patient.

18. According to this text, one of the serious problems for patients in isolation, often seen in the elderly, is that of

    a. frustration and anger.

    b. constipation.

    c. sensory deprivation.

    d. loss of appetite.

POST-TEST ANSWERS

1.	T	10.	T
2.	F	11.	d
3.	T	12.	a
4.	T	13.	e
5.	T	14.	c
6.	F	15.	b
7.	F	16.	a
8.	F	17.	d
9.	F	18.	c

THE DYING PATIENT
AND POSTMORTEM CARE

GENERAL PERFORMANCE OBJECTIVE

Following this lesson, you will be able to prepare a body after death. This procedure will involve caring for the skin, body orifices, and tubing, and accounting for valuables left by the patient.

SPECIFIC PERFORMANCE OBJECTIVES

When you have completed this lesson you will be able to

1. Describe the five psychological stages of grieving that dying patients and grieving persons go through.

2. Describe physiological death and its changes in the body in terms of rigor mortis, cooling, and decomposition.

3. Perform postmortem care by cleaning the body, placing it in a restful-appearing position, and readying it for the mortuary.

4. Take care of the deceased's valuables and possessions according to the agency's policies and release them to an authorized person.

VOCABULARY

autopsy—the postmortem examination of the organs of a dead body to determine the cause of death or pathological conditions.
coroner—pathologist (may or may not be a physician) employed by the city, county, or state to examine the bodies of people who have died under unusual circumstances, such as in cases of drownings, shootings, suicides, murders, and auto accidents.
deceased—dead or expired.
morgue—a place where dead bodies are kept before they are released to the mortuary.
next of kin—a person related to the deceased who has legal authority to sign documents; see your agency consent manual for more details.
pathologist—a specialist in diagnosing the morbid (death-related) changes in tissues removed during operations and postmortem examinations.
pathology—the study of the nature and cause of disease.
postmortem—after death.
rigor mortis—temporary rigidity of muscles occurring after death.
shroud—a large sheet, usually muslin or plastic, used to wrap dead bodies.

INTRODUCTION

In our society, death and dying are not regarded as part of the life span by most people. Other people may die, but we don't really believe it will happen to us. We avoid thinking or talking about death because it is a depressing subject and makes us feel uncomfortable. From early childhood we have been sheltered from death and any contact with dying people. Death has been cloaked in a conspiracy of silence and of denial. Only in recent years has there been a move to tear away this curtain of silence and denial in order to examine the universal event — the ending of mortal life.

Much of the information and ideas we have about death can be traced to sources such as books, newspapers, and television. Death as shown on most TV news or dramatic programs is sudden, violent, and mutilative. This view has contributed to the feelings of shock and fear that we associate with death. The truth is, however, that the great majority of deaths are not violent deaths; most people die in their beds.

The major causes of death in the United States are (1) heart diseases, especially the "heart attack"; (2) all forms of cancer; (3) strokes, which are also called cerebrovascular accidents (CVA); (4) accidents of all kinds; and (5) influenza and pneumonia. As you can see, diseases cause most of the deaths, and most occur in sick people who are being treated in hospitals and related health facilities.

Since more than 80 per cent of all deaths in this country occur in hospitals, health workers who care for patients see more of death and dying than do other people. You will be giving care to patients who are in the process of dying. You may also be expected to prepare the body of a patient who has died for the morgue. You will have feelings about the dying patient and death that need to be examined and better understood so that you can cope effectively and help the patient during this trying time.

NURSING AND THE DYING PATIENT

ITEM 1.   COPING WITH APPROACHING DEATH

When patients suspect or learn that they are dying, they are faced with trying to cope with the ultimate loss — that of life itself. Death doesn't come immediately in most cases, but days, weeks, or months later. In the meantime, the dying patient must live each day as it comes. Not only the patient, but the family and those who provide care are involved in coping with the loss.

People go through certain stages as they cope with their feelings about death and dying. Five different stages are described as being characteristic of the grieving process for the last crisis of life. These stages are

Stage 1 — DENIAL	"No, not me." The person cannot believe the fact of death, rejects the information, and discounts the seriousness of the illness.
Stage 2 — ANGER	"Why me?" The person looks for cause or fixes blame and wants to change or reverse the disease but is powerless to control it.
Stage 3 — BARGAINING	"Yes, me, but — " He or she has unfinished business or is unable to let go. Pleas are made to "Make it better" and promises given in return for longer life.
Stage 4 — DEPRESSION	"It's hopeless." The individual has feelings that nothing can be done and mourns impending death. The feeling is that one is no longer in control of one's own life.
Stage 5 — ACCEPTANCE	"I am ready." "Yes, me." The person has the feeling that this task is finished and that it is right to die.

The stages described here overlap one another. Some patients move back and forth and may skip some stages, while others never move beyond the denial stage. In each case, your understanding of the patient's struggle to cope and your concern can help the patient and the family.

When a patient dies, nursing personnel often have a variety of emotions. Some may feel a sense of betrayal because the patient died instead of recovering, especially if they worked very hard to help. Feelings of relief and guilt may result from the death of a patient who was difficult to care for, had complex procedures to carry out, or had unpleasant odors or drainage. Still others may have feelings of dread and fear caused by the death. If you should have these feelings, talk about them with your instructor, the team leader, or another professional, such as a clergyman.

ITEM 2. CARING FOR THE DYING PATIENT

Nurses who care for terminally ill patients must remember that they are living each day of their lives, just as we are. The main difference is that these patients know their future is very limited. Their plans and goals are concerned with the "here and now" or the immediate future. Even though the patient may not live to celebrate another birthday or join in a family vacation trip, he or she can plan on visiting with loved ones, look forward to a sunny day tomorrow, or appreciate the fragrance of flowers.

One of the prime concerns of dying patients is the assurance from family and the nurses that they will not be deserted or left alone. Patients need to know that others "will stick it out" with them. As a nurse, you will continue to provide care, attention, and support during this time of impending loss. Even though the patient may be very weak, just staying at the bedside a few minutes longer and touching or holding hands can provide much comfort and reassurance.

Another concern of the dying person is to be spared unnecessary pain and suffering. You should notify the team leader promptly when the patient becomes restless or complains of pain. In addition, there are other nursing measures you can carry out to help make the patient more comfortable. Giving a backrub, changing the patient's position, or providing a refreshing drink of water or juice may relieve some discomfort.

ITEM 3. RELIGIOUS BELIEFS AND PRACTICES

As people approach the ends of their lives, many receive great comfort from their religious beliefs. Because ideas about death and what is beyond death vary greatly, it is important that you be familiar with some of these beliefs. Members of some religious faiths, such as Catholics, Episcopalians, and Lutherans, believe that baptism is essential for the soul to go to heaven. They will want dying babies and young children to receive this sacrament. Catholics who are dying may wish to receive the sacraments and the anointing of the sick as described in Unit 27, Assisting with Spiritual Care. When a patient of the Orthodox Jewish faith expires, do not prepare the body until the rabbi has performed the final rites.

You should not press your religious beliefs on the dying patient or the family, but stand by to assist in whatever way you can. This might include such things as getting them coffee, calling the clergyman, or assisting with other telephone calls.

UNIT
37

ITEM 4. SIGNS OF DEATH

During the terminal stage of life, the patient's body functions slow down. Death occurs when these stop completely. Generally, the patient is considered to have died when breathing stops or when the heart stops beating. When this happens to the hospitalized patient, the cardiopulmonary resuscitation (CPR) team is called to revive the patient, except in cases where there is a doctor's order for no CPR. In spite of the efforts of the CPR team, some patients die.

Signs of approaching death are as follows:

1. The eyes stare, become fixed, and do not respond to light.

2. Circulation slows, and the hands and feet become cold and mottled in color. The pulse becomes weak and thready; the blood pressure falls.

3. The reflexes gradually disappear and the sphincter muscles relax, causing incontinence of the bowel and bladder.

4. Respirations are of the Cheyne-Stokes type, with slow, shallow breaths, gradually increasing in depth and rapidity, followed by a short period of apnea (no respiration), then a repetition of the cycle with the periods of apnea becoming longer, until all breathing stops.

Hearing is thought to be the last sense to fail. Even though the patient is unconscious, he may still be able to hear, so avoid saying anything in the room of a comatose patient that could have an adverse effect. When breathing or the pulse stops, notify the nurse in charge and call the CPR tream in accordance with your agency's policy.

ITEM 5. AFTER DEATH OCCURS

After the patient dies, the family may need a quiet room in which to discuss matters, including the choice of the mortuary to handle the funeral services. Because this is a highly emotional ordeal, it is important to provide a quiet, secluded room (often near the chapel) where they can have privacy to release their feelings. Offer them coffee or tea. Stay nearby to help if the need arises.

Who Pronounces Death?

The majority of people in this country die in hospitals, so hospital policies state who is responsible for pronouncing the expiration of the patient. The physician is best qualified to determine whether death has occurred and is usually designated as the one responsible to make this decision. Death occurs in different tissues of the body at different times. Brain centers may be dead, for example, even though the body is kept alive by mechanical means. In these cases, the question of whether death has occurred may be difficult to answer.

When people die in community settings, often the first decision that death has occurred is made by police officers, fire fighters, paramedics, or other emergency personnel. The bodies are then taken to the designated morgue, where the circumstances of death are investigated by the coroner's office and other interested departments.

Body Changes After Death

A number of changes take place in the body after death occurs, and these are the basis for the postmortem care procedure that nurses perform. The changes are rigor mortis, cooling of the body, and decomposition.

Rigor mortis begins about two hours after death, reaches its peak by 48 hours, and lasts about 96 hours, then passes. Rigor is the condition where the muscles of the body become contracted and immobilize the joints. It occurs because of a lack of a substance needed for muscle relaxation. Rigor mortis begins with the involuntary muscles of the heart, arteries, and GI tract, and spreads to the voluntary muscles of the head, the neck, and the rest of the body.

Postmortem cooling occurs when circulation stops and no further heat is produced by metabolism. The cooling continues until room temperature is reached, and then the skin of the body feels cool when touched.

When circulation stops, the blood pools in the dependent parts of the body, and the red blood cells break down to cause the appearance of bruising or mottling of the skin. If the patient died lying on the back, the discoloration is seen on the back, the buttocks, the backs of the thighs, and so on. If death occurred while the patient was lying on his side or in a prone position, the mottling occurs on that side. Further decomposition occurs in the digestive tract, where tissues are softened and then liquefied by bacterial action. These changes occur rapidly in hot weather, so the body of the deceased should be placed in cold storage in the morgue. It is best not to keep the body on the nursing unit more than one hour; rather, transfer it to the morgue as soon as possible. In this country, embalming is used as a method of chemically preserving the body indefinitely. A solution is introduced into the body that kills the bacteria and prevents the rapid decomposition of tissue.

Death Records and Releases

The death certificate, which is sent to the local or state health department, is made out by the physician and the undertaker, and by the pathologist if an autopsy is performed. State laws regulate the disposition of unidentified as well as identified bodies. In obtaining permission for autopsies when an unidentified person dies in a hospital, the police and coroner are notified, and they assume responsibility for trying to determine the identity of the body and for burial arrangements.

When a patient dies in the hospital, the RN in charge is responsible for obtaining a form called Release of the Body to the Mortuary and having it properly filled out and signed. There is another form, an autopsy release, which must also be prepared and signed when circumstances require it.

Most state laws require that permission of the next of kin or the guardian be obtained before an autopsy is performed. If circumstances of death necessitate a coroner's inquest, the state is permitted to conduct an autopsy without the consent of relatives of the deceased.

Coroner's Cases

Deaths that result from unusual or unknown causes are investigated by the coroner, regardless of where the death occurred. The coroner has the legal authority to perform an autopsy to determine the cause of death, and no consent from the family is needed. The types of cases that may be investigated include

1. the death of a person within 24 hours after admission to the hospital.

2. the possibility that death resulted from injury, accident, murder, or suicide.

3. the death of a person who has not seen a physician within 72 hours of death.

ITEM 6. POSTMORTEM CARE

Upon the pronouncement of death, you will be expected to carry out the following procedure.

UNIT 37

Supplies Needed

Death care kit or shroud pack:
  Body tags or labels (2)
  Shroud
  Gown, paper (optional)
  Gauze 4 X 4 dressings, or
    cotton balls
  Safety pins

Bag (paper or plastic) for belongings
Valuables list
Basin, water, and towels
Comb or brush

Important Steps	Key Points
1. Gather the necessary equipment and take it into the room.	
2. Draw the curtains around the bed.	When death occurs in a multi-bed unit, provide others with privacy; close the door to the corridor. Wash your hands.
3. Elevate the bed to working height and set it in a flat position.	Lower the head and foot of the bed so the body is in straight alignment.
4. Place the body in a supine position as in sleeping.	Close the eyes; you may use cotton gently applied over the eyelids and held in place by tape if the eyes will not stay closed. Straighten the body, with the arms laid to each side, palms down. Some agencies may prefer to have the arms gently crossed over the body at the waist or across the abdomen. Replace the dentures if required and close the mouth. If the mouth will not remain closed, place a towel rolled as a cylinder under the chin to keep the mouth closed. Place a pillow under the head. Move the body gently to avoid bruises and breaks in the skin.

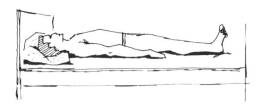

Place body in supine position.

5. Remove any jewelry and list all personal articles.	In general, all rings, earrings, bracelets, beads, hairpins, and so forth, should be removed and placed in a container provided for valuables. Include eyeglasses, cards, letters, keys, religious articles. *Nothing* is too small to be listed on the valuables list, for these articles are valuable to the family.
6. Provide security for the deceased patient's valuables.	Follow your agency's policy for the disposition of valuables. *Never* leave valuables unattended. Place them in the nursing station until they can be stored in a more secure place or released to the family. Whenever possible, the family should be encouraged to take all personal articles home before the patient dies.
7. Clean the body.	Using plain water, wash the areas of the body that may be soiled with blood, feces, or vomitus. If leakage occurs around the rectum, urethra or vagina, place a gauze 4 × 4 over each opening and secure it with tape to prevent further soiling. Following death, sphincter muscles relax, often causing incontinence of feces and urine.
8. Arrange the hair.	Brush and comb the hair neatly. (Review the lesson on hair care if necessary.)
9. Care for drainage and other tubes.	If there *is* to be an *autopsy*, the tubes are generally left in the body; remove the drainage bottles or bags from the tube and fold the tube over twice; secure the end with a rubber band to avoid leakage. If there is no autopsy, tubes usually may be removed. Make sure you deflate the balloon tips so that you do not injure the body tissues upon removal.

Important Steps	Key Points
10. Change the dressings.	Soiled dressings should be replaced with fresh ones. Old adhesive tape marks may be removed with benzene or a similar solution used by your agency.
11. Dress the body in a clean gown for viewing by the family.	If the family wishes to view the body, place it in a sleeping position, supine, eyes closed, arms gently crossed on the lower abdomen. Straighten the bedding (sheet and spread) as though you had completed a bath and prepared the patient for a nap. Remain with the family during the visit.
12. Attach identifying tags to the body.	Label the tag(s) with the patient's name, age, and sex, the date, the hospital number, the room number, and the physician's name. Following hospital policy, tie the tag to the wrist or ankle or tape the label to the patient's anterior chest.
13. Place the body on a shroud if this is your agency's policy.	You may need to tie a bandage lightly under the jaw and up around the head to keep the jaw closed. Also, some agencies lightly bandage the wrists together criss-crossed over the abdomen to prevent the arms from falling off the stretcher when the body is being moved to the morgue.

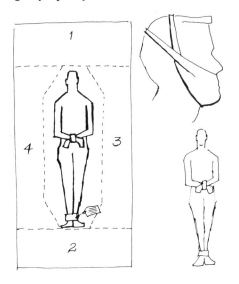

Place body on shroud.

Place the body on the shroud (large square piece of muslin or plastic). As shown in the sketch, wrap side 1 down around the head, followed by side 2 up over the feet. Wrap sides 3 and 4. A large safety-pin or masking tape may be used to keep the shroud in place.

Important Steps	Key Points
14. Apply the outside label.	Tag the outside of the shroud with the patient's name, age, sex, hospital number, room number, physician's name, and the date. Safety-pin this tag to the outside of the shroud.

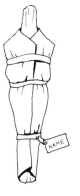

UNIT 37

Important Steps	Key Points

15. Transport the body to the morgue.

Some agencies leave the body in the room until a mortician or coroner's officer removes it. Slide the body gently onto a cart or stretcher. Cover the body with a sheet. In some agencies, the face remains uncovered; in others, it is covered, particularly when the shroud is used. Secure the body with stretcher straps at the chest and knees. Apply the straps tight enough to prevent the body from slipping off but loose enough so as not to cause bruising.

When transporting the body, try to use staff elevators and corridors to avoid encountering visitors and the public. If an elevator is used, secure an elevator key and ask visitors to step off to avoid distress and to make the transfer as fast as possible.

After leaving the body in the morgue, take the stretcher back to the unit, remove the linen and put clean linen on it.

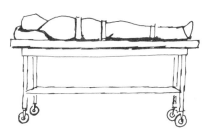

Transport on guerney.

16. Strip the patient's room.

Call the department for room cleaning, or clean the room yourself. Remove the soiled linens, bottles, pitchers, and other articles and put them in the place provided for their processing.

17. Record the procedure.

In your nursing notes, record the time and date the body was taken to the morgue or by the undertaker. If valuables were placed in safe-keeping, indicate this in writing. If valuables were given to the family or friends, record the name of the person(s) to whom they were given, their relationship to the deceased, the time, and the date. Have a coworker who witnessed this action cosign with you in the notes. Charting example:

2010. Transferred to morgue. Valuables (watch, wedding ring, and 2 nightgowns) sent home with son, John.

J. Jones, SN   M. Maye, SN

PERFORMANCE TEST

1. Discuss the five stages of dying with your instructor.

2. In the skills laboratory, prepare the mannequin (Mrs. Chase) as though she were a dead body. You will cleanse her, pack her body orifices, label the body, wrap her in a shroud, label the outside of the shroud, and prepare to transport her to the morgue.

PERFORMANCE CHECKLIST

POSTMORTEM CARE

1. Assemble the necessary equipment in the room.

2. Screen the patient (draw the curtains and close the door).

3. Adjust the bed to working height; flatten the bed.

4. Place the body in the supine position with the eyes closed, dentures in place, arms at the sides or across the chest, and pillow under the head.

5. Remove any jewelry and list personal articles.

6. Clean the body and pack all orifices.

7. Arrange the hair.

8. Remove any tubes (if there will be no autopsy). The tubes remain in if an autopsy is to be performed.

9. Change any dressings.

10. Change the patient's clothing according to your agency's procedure.

11. Identify the body with a labeled tag on the toe, wrist, or chest (follow your agency's procedure).

12. Wrap the body in a shroud and attach a label.

13. Move the body to a stretcher, using correct body movement and alignment.

14. Secure straps above the the knees and chest.

15. Transport the body to the morgue.

16. Return to the room to strip the bed and perform a final cleaning.

17. Dispose of all valuables according to your agency's procedure.

18. Record your activities on the nurses' notes.

POST-TEST

Multiple Choice. Select the one best answer for each of the following questions.

1. The major cause of death in the United States is
   a. automobile accidents.
   b. infectious disease.
   c. heart disease.
   d. cancer.

2. Nurses come in contact with dying more often than other people because what percentage of all deaths occur in hospitals?
   a. 100
   b. 80
   c. 60
   d. 50

3. What stage of grieving is typified by the dying patient's feeling powerless to control what has happened and saying, "Why me? What have I done to deserve this?"
   a. Denial.
   b. Bargaining.
   c. Depression.
   d. Anger.

4. Nurses who care for patients who die have which of the following feelings?
   a. Relief that the patient no longer is suffering.
   b. Feelings of grief, and fear of death itself.
   c. Guilt because of resentment over doing the unpleasant tasks.
   d. Any of these feelings.

5. One of the major fears of the dying patient is that of
   a. being deserted and left alone to die.
   b. being awake and conscious to the end.
   c. becoming addicted to the pain medication.
   d. not being missed by their loved ones.

6. Cheyne-Stokes breathing, often seen in dying patients, is characterized by
   a. difficult breathing with retraction of chest muscles.
   b. cycles of shallow breaths followed by no breathing.
   c. deep, rapid, and gulping type of breathing.
   d. intake of short puffs of air followed by prolonged exhalations.

7. In hospital settings, the patient is pronounced dead by
   a. the first person to discover the condition.
   b. the registered nurse.
   c. the physician.
   d. the CPR team when resuscitation is unsuccessful.

8. The appearance of bruising and mottling of the skin following death is due to

   a. rigor mortis.

   b. injury occurring before death.

   c. decomposition of blood cells.

   d. accidental damage in handling the body.

9. After death, the condition of rigor mortis has what effect on the body?

   a. Relaxation of muscles.

   b. Contraction of muscles.

   c. Discoloration of the skin.

   d. Increased bacterial activity.

   e. Decreased bacterial activity.

10. What types of deaths are legally required to be referred to the coroner for investigation?

   a. Those resulting from unusual or unknown causes.

   b. Those that occurred on the operating table.

   c. Those in which the doctor is not sure of the exact cause.

   d. Those in which CPR was attempted and failed to revive the victim.

POST-TEST ANSWERS

1.	c	6.	b
2.	b	7.	c
3.	d	8.	c
4.	d	9.	b
5.	a	10.	a

APPENDIX:

UNIVERSAL STEPS FOR NURSING PROCEDURES

Important Steps	Key Points and Rationale
A. Collect the equipment needed.	You need to obtain the supplies and equipment needed to carry out the procedure and take them to the bedside for use. If the items are stored in the patient's room or bedside unit, this step could be performed after greeting and identifying the patient.
B. Wash your hands.	Microorganisms abound in hospitals and nursing facilities, as in other places where people congregate, so wash your hands before and after providing care for the patient. Hand-washing reduces the microorganisms on your hands and protects you and others from possible infections.
C. Approach and identify the patient, explain the procedure, and gain patient's cooperation. 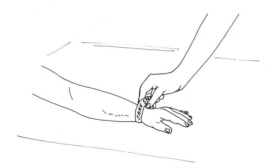	The crucial element is to identify the patient; nothing is accomplished by doing something for the wrong person, and some harm could result from it. Check the identification band; don't just say the patient's name. Be aware that some people respond to any name just to be polite. Explain what you plan to do in simple terms so the patient understands. Gain cooperation by pointing out the benefits or advantages to be gained from the procedure or activity. Patients do have the right to refuse treatment, however, and if this occurs, report to the nurse and discuss the problem.
D. Provide for privacy, and drape the patient as needed. 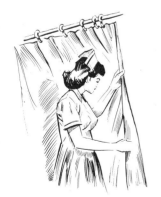	Close the door of the room or pull the curtain around the bed to shield from view of others. Use a gown, sheet, or bathblanket to drape the patient and avoid unnecessary exposure of the patient's body, which might cause embarrassment.

At the completion of the procedure, these steps are routinely carried out.

X. Collect the used items and equipment and dispose of these correctly.

Disposable items such as plastic trays, irrigating sets, catheters, tubes, dressings, and examining gloves are discarded after use. Soiled linens are put in soiled linen hampers.

Equipment and reusable items are cleaned and returned to the storage or processing area (Central Supply). Items belonging to the patient are stored at the bedside or some other designated area.

Y. Provide for the patient's comfort.

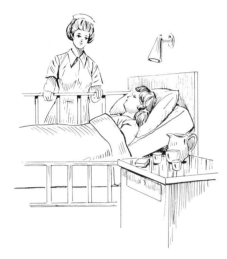

Replace the bedding neatly and raise the side rails, if used. Place the call light within reach, and position the bedside stand or overbed table within reach so patient can get drinking water and personal items.

Leave the bed in a low position.

Z. Record and report the procedure.

Examples of charting are given. The charting should include any complaints of pain, the condition or problem being treated or requiring the procedure; what was done; how the patient responded or reacted; and other nursing observations.

In addition, you should report to team leader or nurse in charge when the procedure is completed, the observations you made concerning the patient's response, and any problems that were encountered.

INDEX

i